Travel Medicine and Migrant Health

EDITED BY

Cameron Lockie MBE BSc(Hons) FRCPEdin FRCGP FRGS

Eric Walker FRCP MRCGP

Lorna Calvert MN RGN

Jonathan Cossar MD ChB

Robin Knill-Jones FRCP FFPHM

Fiona Raeside MN RGN RM

FOREWORD

Professor Sir Kenneth Calman KCB MD FRCS FRSE

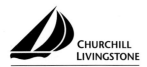
CHURCHILL
LIVINGSTONE

EDINBURGH LONDON NEW YORK PHILADELPHIA ST LOUIS SYDNEY TORONTO 2000

CHURCHILL LIVINGSTONE

An imprint of Harcourt Publishers Limited

© Harcourt Publishers Limited 2000

⟋⟍ is a registered trade mark of Harcourt Publishers
Limited

First published 2000

ISBN 0 443 06242 0

British Library Cataloguing in Publication Data
A catalogue record for this book is available from the
British Library.

Library of Congress Cataloging in Publication Data
A catalog record for this book is available from the Library
of Congress.

Medical knowledge is constantly changing. As new
information becomes available, changes in treatment,
procedures, equipment and the use of drugs become
necessary. The editors, contributors and the publishers
have, as far as it is possible, taken care to ensure that the
information given in this text is accurate and up to date.
However, readers are strongly advised to confirm that the
information, especially with regard to drug usage, complies
with current legislation and standards of practice.

The
publisher's
policy is to use
**paper manufactured
from sustainable forests**

Printed in China

Travel Medicine and Migrant Health

Commissioning Editor: Michael Parkinson
Project Development Manager: Janice Urquhart
Project Manager: Nancy Arnott
Design direction: Erik Bigland
Illustrated by: Ethan Danielson

Foreword

I suspect that most people, professionals and public alike, would be surprise at the scale of international travel at the end of the 20th century. In UK residents there were 45.9 million visits abroad in 1997, 8.9 million of these going to Europe, an 89 fold increase over 1949. As an example of the consequences of this, in the UK there are over 2000 cases of laboratory confirmed cases malaria each year with around 5–10 deaths. New infections are emerging on a regular basis.

The implications of this information for the health of individuals and for the public are readily understood. The numbers of patients with malaria and other tropical diseases, HIV infection and tuberculosis in the world, highlight the problems of real people behind the bare figures. Professionals and the public might also be surprised at the range of conditions which might be encountered, and the public health problems which exist. The whole range of medical practice is covered. Thus most health professionals will at some time have to deal with a clinical referral related to travel, and their own travel experiences will confirm the range, subtlety, seriousness and complexity of the problems.

Those who migrate to this country, or to other parts of the world, suffer special problems. They are a very vulnerable group who not only are dispossessed, homeless, frightened, and perhaps fleeing from danger, but have particular health problems. They need special care and attention, and deserve the highest professional standards of clinical practice.

Much of the work in all of these areas depends on adequate intelligence of prevailing disease conditions and response to treatment with, for example antibiotics. Patterns of drug resistance, local variations in virulence, common concurrent illnesses all need to be known and the information readily available. Thus the importance of information technology and the accessibility of data are essential for good clinical practice. Much time is spent in updating these sources of information, and they are invaluable.

This book is both a reference source and a clinical manual, broad in scope, but practical in detail. However the words of Sir William Osler are salutatory and are particularly apt in the context of this book.

'To study the phenomena of disease without books is to sail an uncharted sea, while to study books without patients is not to go to sea at all.'

Thus this book will not be a substitute for a well taken history which includes questions related to overseas travel, a high index of suspicion, excellent clinical skills, and a wide diagnostic and therapeutic background. Looking after those who have become ill abroad or who are migrants requires a multidisciplinary team approach and an increasingly wide range of skills and expertise.

Travel medicine is a specialty that has almost come of age. It will therefore need to look to the consequences of this. First, there will be the need to maintain and improve standards of clinical practice by those who are part of the speciality. Research and continuing professional development will be essential. Second there will be a tendency for other professionals not to bother to keep up to date, as the 'experts' will do it for them. The range and scope of the problems and their wide range of presentations makes it clear that all doctors and other health professionals need to keep abreast of changes and know when to refer for expert advice. The specialist in Travel Medicine thus has a teaching responsibility to his or her colleagues. Finally there is the importance of public education in this process. Travel medicine, par excellence, needs to be closely involved with the public in giving advice and information. In travel medicine, as in much of clinical work, prevention is better than cure.

This book thus provides a map for the experienced clinician to steer by and a resource for those who need help and guidance.

Kenneth C. Calman. Durham, November 1999.

Sir Kenneth Calman was appointed Vice-Chancellor and Warden of the University of Durham in October 1998. He was born on Christmas Day 1941 and educated at Allen Glen's School in Glasgow. He entered medical school in 1959 and took two years out during this course to gain an Honours Degree in biochemistry. He graduated in medicine (with commendation) in 1967 having obtained a number of distinctions and prizes throughout this course. During the latter part of his undergraduate medical career he developed an interest in dermatology and graduated PhD in 1970. Following his house jobs he moved into the Department of Surgery in Glasgow and proceeded to the Fellowship of the Royal College of Surgeons and an MD Thesis with Honours on Organ Preservation. His clinical interests at this time were in General Surgery, Vascular Surgery and Transplantation. In 1972, he was the MRC Clinical Research Fellow at the Chester Beatty Research Institute in London and returned to Glasgow in 1974 as Professor of Oncology. He remained in that post for 10 years developing particular interests in nutrition, chemotherapy, cancer education, counselling, and patient support groups. In 1984 he became Dean of Postgraduate Medicine and Professor of Postgraduate Medical Education at the University of Glasgow and Consultant Physician with an interest in palliative care at the Victoria Infirmary, Glasgow. During this time he was involved in developing medical education projects and in the supervising of medical education for those in training in the West of Scotland. In 1989 he was appointed Chief Medical Officer at the Scottish Home and Health Department and in September 1991 he became Chief Medical Health Officer in the Department of Health in London. He is a Fellow of numerous Royal Colleges and Faculties and in 1979 was elected a Fellow of the Royal Society of Edinburgh. He has written seven books and over one hundred scientific papers. Sir Kenneth has a number of outside interests including the history of medicine, Scottish literature, cartoons and gardening. He is married with three grown up children and a large dog.

Preface

Travel medicine as an emerging specialty

- What is travel medicine?
- Is it a real specialty?
- Has travel medicine come of age?
- What about the health of emigrants and refugees?

These are the questions frequently asked when the topic of travellers' health is discussed. After reading the opening chapter of this book with its contributions on 'Historical aspects of travel medicine' and 'Emerging infections and their relation to travel', one might wonder why these questions have not already been fully and satisfactorily answered.

Contemporary recognition of the importance of this subject was addressed by the 1st Conference of Travel Medicine held in Zurich in 1988. This was followed by the foundation of the International Society of Travel Medicine (ISTM) in Atlanta, Georgia in 1991. Since then there have been biennial conferences: Paris 1993, Acapulco 1995, Geneva 1997 and Montreal 1999. In addition, the 1st Asia Pacific Travel Health Conference was held in Hong Kong in 1996 and the 2nd in Taiwan in 1998. The development of the ISTM has done much to focus attention on the specialty and integrate the various medical and scientific disciplines involved (Figure 1).[1]

The need for cohesion in this developing specialty is in response to the needs of travellers for expert advice, the increase in travel-related illness and the increasing importance of epidemiology as a basis for the provision of evidence-based prophylactic advice and treatment.

'To travel hopefully is a better thing than to arrive' wrote Robert Louis Stevenson, but to return ill as so many travellers do each year is of

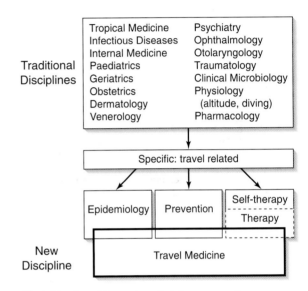

Fig.1 Travel medicine: an interdisciplinary approach.

increasing concern to all those disciplines involved in healthcare provision. Increased awareness of the importance of travel medicine has developed in response to health problems raised by the very rapid increase in international travel over the last 20–30 years. The past decade has been one of the most eventful in a long history of infectious diseases – eventful particularly because of travel.

Travel medicine initially focused upon tourists and business travellers going from richer to poorer countries, and how to help them maintain their health in often very unfamiliar surroundings. However there are other very important groups of travellers with special health needs including migrants – those travelling on a 'one way ticket' (emigration) or involuntarily (e.g. refugees).[2]

This broader and developing concept is considered at various stages in this book including those chapters on emerging infections and their relation to travel; psychological aspects of travel and the long-term expatriate; refugees, disaster relief and migration; ethnic minority and immigrant travellers; the impacts of tourism on host countries.

Also it is increasingly becoming evident that the health, social and economic issues raised by this increase in travel are closely interlinked with other important issues such as the health and economic impact of travel upon the host countries and the concept of emerging and re-emerging infections. The world is seen increasingly to be a 'global village' where health problems in one region rapidly have implications for others.

The UK has been at the forefront of:

- surveillance and the provision of integrated travel health services: Scottish Centre for Infection and Environmental Health (SCIEH) – the Public Health Laboratory Services Communicable Disease Surveillance Centre (CDSC) – the Medical Advisory Service for Travellers' Overseas (MASTA) – the NHS travel health database on the Internet (TRAVAX)
- education – a world first in the development of MSc and Diploma courses in Travel Medicine at the University of Glasgow.

A considerable landmark for the acceptance of travel medicine as a specialty in the UK was the formation of the British Travel Health Association (with over 800 members), launched by Sir Kenneth Calman in May 1998 at the Royal Geographical Society, London.

No specialty can come of age without a sound research and epidemiological basis. The UK now has that basis.

In this new world of rapid, intercontinental transmission of infections, the words of Lopez de Ville Lobus are still appropriate:

Relentless, fierce and strong, the foulest of the age
A curse that ne'er before had reared its head to strike,
Nor had been sung aloud by poet, priest or sage.
Vile was he who gained it, for in his helpless rage
He cast it far and wide to friend and foe alike.

Lopez de Ville Lobus (1498)

Hence the need for national and international recognition for the emerging specialty of travel medicine.

Cameron Lockie   Stratford on Avon

---

1 Steffen R, DuPont HL. Travel Medicine: what's that? Journal of Travel Medicine 1994; 1: 1.

2 Louis Loutan and others: Personal communications and presentations at the 6th Conference of the International Society of Travel medicine (Montreal 1999).

Acknowledgements

Planning and production of any multi-author book is never an easy task. With a subject as broad as Travel Medicine the dilemma of what makes up the content is made ever greater.

The initial stimulus to produce this book was provided by the need to develop a travel medicine textbook, suitable as a reference book for health professionals, studying at the University of Glasgow, distance-learning MSc and Diploma in Travel Medicine. The editors wish to pay particular thanks to past and present students on that course. They have made, via discussion, dissertations and theses, a tremendous contribution to travel medicine. Many are contributors to this book.

The contributors, despite enormous individual work schedules, have done everything possible to ease the editors' work by delivering quality material with enthusiasm and good humour – almost on time!

Our secretarial help has been of the highest calibre and for this we sincerely thank Susan Harvey and Carolyn Ayres.

We are grateful to Harcourt Publishers and in particular Michael Parkinson and Janice Urquhart for their support and patience during production.

The editors would also like to thank Professor Sir Kenneth Calman for writing the Foreword.

Contents

Editors

Lorna Calvert MN RGN*
Travel Health and Immunisation Nurse Specialist at the Scottish Centre for Infection and Environmental Health, core tutor and supervisor for the MSc and Diploma in Travel Medicine courses at the University of Glasgow. Special interest in travel medicine education.

Jonathan Cossar MD ChB*
General Practitioner, Glasgow, part-time Research Associate at the Scottish Centre for Infection and Environmental Health, Deputy Editor of NewsShare, and an Honorary Clinical Senior Lecturer, module author, and core tutor, for the travel medicine courses at the University of Glasgow.

Robin Knill-Jones FRCP FFPHM**
Senior Lecturer in Public Health, core tutor and involved in the course development for the MSc and Diploma in Travel Medicine at the University of Glasgow. Research interests include decision analysis and decision making, epidemiological interests in sports-related injury and occupational influences on reproduction.

Cameron Lockie MBE BSc(Hons) FRCPEdin FRCGP FRGS**
Recently retired General Practitioner, Stratford upon Avon. Previous BA Travel Clinic involvement and professional experience working in Nigeria, the Middle East, the Amazon, and the Black Sea. A Senior Fellow in Travel Medicine, core tutor and course originator for the MSc and Diploma in Travel Medicine at the University of Glasgow. Chairman of British Travel Health Association. Malaria advisory panel for UK travellers.

Fiona Raeside MN RGN RM*
Nurse Epidemiologist at the Scottish Centre for Infection and Environment Health (SCIEH). Honorary Lecturer and member of the core/supervisory group for the Travel Medicine courses at the University of Glasgow. Special interests, travel health and HIV infection.

Eric Walker FRCP MRCGP*
Consultant Physician and Epidemiologist, Scottish Centre for Infection and Environmental Health, Honorary Consultant Physician in Tropical Medicine, West Glasgow Hospitals University Trust, with extensive professional experience working in both Africa and India, Honorary Clinical Senior Lecturer at the University of Glasgow and Editor of NewsShare. Involved in the original development of 'TRAVAX' and the MSc and Diploma Travel Medicine courses at the University of Glasgow. Malaria and Vaccination advisory panels for UK travellers. Author of ABC of Healthy Travel (BMJ).

*Scottish Centre for Infection and Environmental Health (SCIEH), Clifton House, Clifton Place, Glasgow G3 7LN
**Department of Public Health, University of Glasgow, 1 Lilybank Gardens, Glasgow G12 8RZ

Contributors

Abu Saleh Md Abdullah MB BS PhD
Research Associate, Department of Community Medicine, The University of Hong Kong, Hong Kong

James Gordon Avery MD FFPHM DTM&H
Chief Medical Officer, Montserrat, West Indies

Santanu Chatterjee MB BS DTM&H
Medical Advisor and Travel Consultant, Calcutta, India

Peter Chiodini BSc (Hons) PhD FRCP FRCPath
Consultant Parasitologist, Hospital for Tropical Diseases, London, UK

Jane Chiodini MSc (Travel Medicine) RGN RM
Travel Health Adviser in Primary Care, Bidenham, Bedford, UK

Martin Dedicoat BSc MRCP DTM&H
Consultant Physician, Department of Infection, City Hospital, North Staffordshire Hospital, Stoke on Trent, UK

Christopher Ellis MB BS Hons FRCP DTM&H
Consultant Physician, Department of Infection & Tropical Medicine, Birmingham Heartlands Hospital, Birmingham, UK

Michael Farthing MD FRCP
Digestive Diseases Research Centre, St Bartholomew's and The Royal London School of Medicine and Dentistry, University of London, London, UK

Colin Fleming BSc MRCP
Specialist Registrar, Department of Dermatology, Robertson Building, University of Glasgow, Glasgow, UK

Richard Harding BSc MB BS PhD DAvMed MRAeS RAF (retd)
Principal Consultant, Biodynamic Research Corporation, San Antonio, Texas, USA

Anthony J. Hedley MD FRCP FFPHM DsocMed
Head of Department, Department of Community Medicine, University of Hong Kong, Pokfulam, Hong Kong

John Howarth MRCGP (dist) DTM&H
General Practitioner, Cockermouth, Cumbria; Formerly Programme Coordinator for Médecine Sans Frontière. Head of Operations plus Medical Director of MERLIN.

Karen Howell RGN Cert Health Promotion
Director of Travel Health Ltd, Stafford, Staffordshire, UK

Michael Jones FRCP Edin
Associated Specialist at the Regional Infection Unit (RIU), Western General Hospital, Edinburgh and Director and Physician for Care for Mission, Ellen Lodge, Duns, Berwickshire, UK

Dermot Kennedy FRCP Glasg
Lead Consultant Physician, Brownlee Centre, Gartnavel General Hospital, Glasgow, UK

Ted Lankester MA MRCGP
Director, InterHealth, London, UK

Jane Leese FRCP
Senior Medical Officer, Department of Health, London, UK

Iain McIntosh BA(Hons) MB ChB
GP Registrar Training Assessor, Central Scotland and Post-Graduate Medical Educator (Geriatric Medicine), Stirling, UK

Rona MacKie CBE MD DSc FRCP FRCPath FRSE
Head of Department, Department of Dermatology,
Robertson Building, University of Glasgow,
Glasgow, UK.

Bibhat K. Mandall FRCP Edin FRCP Glasg
Consultant Physician, Department of Infectious
Diseases and Tropical Medicine, North
Manchester General Hospital, Manchester, UK.

Jeannett Martin RGN, PN Cert, MA
Senior Nurse, MRC General Practice Research
Framework, MRC Epidemiology and Medical
Care Unit, Wolfson Institute of Preventative
Medicine, Charterhouse Square, London, UK

Brian Mulhall MA MPH FRCP FACSHP DTM&H
Clinical Senior Lecturer, Department of Public
Health & Community Medicine, University of
Sydney, Australia (His contribution was
sponsored by the New South Wales Health
Department and the Commonwealth Deparment
of Health as part of a sexual health program for
travellers).

Andrew Peacock BSc MPhil MD FRCP
Honorary Senior Lecturer, University of Glasgow
and Consultant Respiratory Physician,
Department of Medicine, Gartnavel General
Hospital, Glasgow, UK

Alan Pithie MD BMSc MRCP
Consultant General Physician, Brownlee Centre,
Gartnavel General Hospital, Glasgow, UK

Marlene Simpson RGN, SCM, Cert Travel Med.
Locum Health Adviser, Scottish Centre for
Infection and Environmental Health, Clifton
House, Glasgow, UK

Michael Townend MB ChB(Hons) Diploma in
Travel Medicine
General Practitioner and GP Tutor for West
Cumbria, Cockermouth, Cumbria, UK

Pradhib Venkatesan MA PhD MRCP DTM&H
Clinical Lecturer, Department of Infection and
Tropical Medicine, Birmingham Heartlands
Hospital, Birmingham, UK

Jane Weaver RN RM Dip Trav Med
Occupational Nurse Specialist, Angram House,
Angram, Richmond, North Yorkshire, UK

Philip Welsby FRCP
Consultant Physician, Regional Infectious
Diseases Unit, Western General Hospital,
Edinburgh, UK

Eleanor Wilson RGN SCM FPA Cert. OHNC Rig
Medic Certificate
Nurse Specialist, Travel Section, Scottish Centre
for Infection and Environment Health, Clifton
House, Glasgow, UK

George B Wyatt FRCP FFPHM DTM&H
Senior Lecturer, Consultant Physician and Clinical
Director, Liverpool School of Tropical Medicine,
Liverpool, UK

HISTORY, SURVEILLANCE, RESOURCES, TRAVEL MEDICINE SERVICES

Historical aspects of travel medicine

Jonathan Cossar

Introduction

Although there have been notable medical advances throughout the 20th century, the contemporary traveller is still vulnerable to health hazards. Travel exposes the individual to new, cultural, psychological, physical, physiological, emotional, environmental and microbiological, experiences and challenges.

The traveller's ability to adapt, cope and survive these challenges is affected by many variables that include the individual's pre-existing physical, mental, immunological and medical status. The risk is further affected by personality, experience and behaviour which differs with age, gender, culture, race, social status and education. Travellers at higher risk of infection are:

- the young (less mature/exposed immune system)
- the elderly (immunosenesence)
- the pregnant (altered immunity and also medication restrictions)
- the less experienced (less adept at minimising risks)
- those with pre-existing disease (immune system under stress)
- the immunocompromised (less disease resistance)
- the adventurer or backpacker (increased microbiological spectrum and dose)
- the sex-traveller (high-risk behaviour with a high-risk population).

The final aspect of this challenge relates to the unfamiliar, environmental exposure which includes differences in climate, altitude, sunlight, hygiene, insects, pollution, safety, pathogen presence and disease prevalence.

It is not surprising that health problems have affected travellers throughout history.

The development of travel

Travel continues to be the world's biggest growth industry.

In 1949, 26 million international tourists were recorded (Table 1.1) whereas by 1990 the figure had risen to 429 million[1] (a 17-fold increase), 30% going to the Mediterranean area. If domestic tourists are added, it has been estimated by the World Tourism Organisation that the world total of arrivals at all destinations is now approximately 4150 million.

Since 1949, there has also been a 37-fold increase in scheduled air travellers,[2] and in 1997, 45.9 million visits abroad were recorded by UK residents, a 27-fold rise, with the proportion of those travelling beyond Europe increasing 89-fold to 8.9 million[3] (Fig. 1.1). Those exposed to extremes of climate and culture are showing the most accelerated growth rate.

Groups contributing to this growth in travel include tourists, political representatives, businessmen, technical experts, pilgrims, migrant workers,

TABLE 1.1 Growth in international travel

	1949	1960	1970	1980	1990
			(millions)		
Total numbers of international tourists	26	69	160	285	429
Total numbers of world air travellers	31	106	386	748	1160
Total visits abroad by UK residents	1.7	6.0	11.8	17.5	31.2

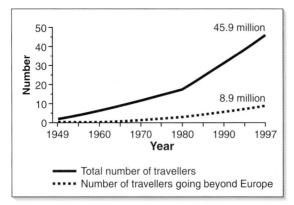

Fig. 1.1 Visits abroad by UK residents.

students, refugees, immigrants, military personnel, sporting participants and followers, and the hotel and travel support services.

Owing to the speed, capacity and frequency of modern travel moreover, travellers are now more likely to return within the incubation period of many infections. For example, since 1948 the fastest, passenger-aircraft, cruising speed has risen from 340 to 1356 miles per hour with Concorde, and the maximum passenger capacity has increased from 40 to over 400 in wide-bodied jets. The long, return, sea journey enabling illnesses acquired abroad to be recognised before return is now rare.

This scale of modern travel means there are no countries in the world where human demographics and behaviour, technological and industrial practices, environmental change, international commerce, microbial adaptation, and changing priorities in public health can occur in isolation, without implications for the potential transmission of infection by travellers.   -

Historical and demographic aspects

Man has travelled from time immemorial, initially from necessity as a hunter-gatherer, then in later times to band together for protection, efficiency of organisation, and for the benefits of extended family or tribal relationships. Further development led to early settlements, thereafter to less nomadic existence but still perhaps seasonal movement of the settlement, and finally to more permanent locations, with travel from there for the purposes of obtaining food, agriculture, trade, employment, conquest and finally leisure. As people came together in greater numbers, the potential for the epidemic spread of infection increased, particularly in the absence of the understanding of disease and an effective public health infrastructure.

In current times, there are continuing population changes in growth, density and distribution. Changed farming practices, with less labour-intensive work, and the lure of potentially richer rewards in cities, act as irresistible forces for changes in population distribution. This is most marked in developing countries where city growth can lead to overcrowding, poor hygiene, inadequate sanitation and unclean drinking water. Not only does this result in high rates of infection in the shantytowns and favellas surrounding these cities, but also in spread to those visiting and mixing with the local population. These visitors may be more immunologically vulnerable if travelling from a country with a more developed sanitation system. Paradoxically, in the 20th century, this is the converse of the history of the conquests of the Americas, when Amerindians of both the north and south with perhaps a lesser genetic diversity,[4] who had been relatively isolated over many centuries, were exposed to diseases that had affected land-linked Europe, Asia and Africa courtesy of the invaders.

COLONISATION

From the early 16th century onwards, smallpox and measles ensured Spanish military success against the Amerindians, Aztecs and Incas. Columbus and his retinue introduced smallpox into Hispaniola with the first native case occurring around 1517. This, along with the depredations of war against the Spanish, led to the population decline of an estimated 2 million Amerindians by 1530.[5] A similar pattern occurred with the expedition of Cortez to Mexico when from 1520 onwards, authoritative estimates attribute 3.5 million deaths to smallpox, more than half the population. A few years later, Pizzaro's conquest in Peru met with equal success when the same disease, aided by civil war, overwhelmed the Incas.

However, the Spanish conquerors were soon affected by the decline in the native population as it created an acute labour shortage. They copied the experience of the Portuguese who had introduced negro slaves to assist with their colonisation of Brazil. The long sea voyages endured by the negroes, in appalling conditions, took a heavy toll in human life. The transit time enabled the infectious processes to exhaust themselves 'en route', and thus survival of the fittest ensured a disease-resistant, imported workforce. For example, many were immune to yellow fever following childhood exposure.

The yellow fever virus, originating from Africa, is dependent upon the mosquito for survival. This water-breeding arthropod provides a reservoir of infection with transovarial transmission of the virus. The presence of suitable water containers on board the ships thus predisposed to the introduction of the virus to the 'New World'.[6] The dwellings and living conditions of the colonists in the West Indies and South America provided ideal conditions for the propagation of the *Aedes aegypti* vector and its transmission of yellow fever, which rapidly took hold. There is concern at the present time for the similar potential for the spread of infectious agents, for example, when organisms taken up in ballast water in one part of the world are subsequently discharged at another.[7]

History was to repeat itself in the colonisation of North America a few centuries later when imported infections took a huge toll of life. This was succinctly summarised by Caitlin who wrote in 1876: 'Thirty millions of white men are now struggling and scuffling for the goods and luxuries of life over the bones and ashes of twelve millions of red men, six millions of whom have fallen victim to the smallpox, the remainder to the sword, the bayonet or whisky.'[8] The further colonisation by emigrants from an overcrowded Europe also helped spread tuberculosis and syphilis but the ambient climatic conditions did not provide the same opportunity for the establishment of an exotic endemic infection like yellow fever.

There are other notable examples of health hazards affecting travellers and indeed influencing history. In the 12th and 13th centuries, the authorities in Venice noted that there was a problem with regular outbreaks of plague affecting the city's inhabitants which occurred shortly after the arrival of ships from the East. As a result, Venice and Rhodes introduced the first regulations governing the arrival of ships in 1377 whereby they were detained at a distance, complete with passengers, cargo and crew for 40 days (quaranto giorni), before being allowed to proceed to their final destination.[9] This measure is generally accepted as the origin of the concept of quarantine and other cities and countries followed this example until some form of sanitary regulation became common place in many countries during the next five centuries.

In an effort to establish international trade independent of England, there was a disastrous attempt to found a Scottish colony on the isthmus of Panama – the ill-fated Darien Expedition of the 1690s. Some 2000 Scots died as a result of appalling local conditions where malaria and yellow fever were rife.[10] This set the seal on the dependency of Scotland on England for trading abroad following the Union of the Crowns (1603) and preceded the Union of the Parliaments in 1707.

Again, a full circle is being completed with the modern-day tourist 'invader' from the developed countries being vulnerable to tuberculosis, hepatitis A and other infections because of lack of exposure in childhood, immunocompromise (transplant recipient, human immunodeficiency virus (HIV) infection, drug abuse), or behavioural risk (e.g. sexual). As well as this vulnerability and indifference to personal hygiene and food safety, there are now risks for both the tourist and the indigenous population from the emergence of a new behavioural sub-culture. For example, there is a growing recognition of an association between prostitution and substance abuse with a sub-culture of sex tourism, sex for drugs, and migration of sex workers from less affluent countries to those where the financial rewards are higher. This has potential for the geographic spread of all the venereal diseases and of hepatitis and HIV in particular.

Economic development and environmental change

The changes in farming practices mentioned earlier are just a small part of the changes in economic development and the environment taking place around the world. The economic demands of a burgeoning population may necessitate major environmental changes: reservoirs and dams for water storage and/or generation of electricity; new roads to be driven into virgin territory; deforestation and re-forestation. Such changes afford the opportunity for the emergence of 'aggressor' strains of flora, fauna, insects and microorganisms, previously contained by a natural balance built up over thousands of years, thereby altering the ecological infrastructure with unforeseen disease consequences. This often means that the pioneer traveller or tourist, anxious to explore the most newly accessible areas in otherwise remote parts of the world, is the first to be exposed to these new hazards.

MISSIONARIES

In the late 19th and early 20th centuries, when European missionaries set out to introduce Christianity to newly opened up Africa, India, China and the Pacific, the Scots supplied more recruits to this cause than any other European country. Study of the health experiences of this group affords a unique insight.[11] Africa presented notable health risks; for example, the missionaries Mungo Park, David Livingstone and Mary Slessor all died in Africa, succumbing respectively to trauma (drowned while under attack by hostile natives), dysentery with internal haemorrhage, and 'exhaustion'. Out of 1427 missionaries studied, 20% retired early because of ill health and a further 11% died in service, these figures being mainly due to infectious illnesses. Those serving in the more climatically rigorous areas like tropical Africa fared less well than those in sub-tropical countries. However, with passage of time there was re-cognition of the association between disease and location, for example, 'blackwater fever' (now known as malignant malaria) and settlement sites on low-lying, swampy ground.

With improvements in the understanding of disease and environmental factors, for example relocating mission stations to higher ground, those serving in later decades experienced fewer problems owing to infection and fewer deaths abroad (Fig. 1.2). Interestingly, missionaries with a medical background experienced fewer problems,

probably because of their knowledge of illness and its prevention. The effect of local climate and environment, and a background knowledge about disease continue to be very relevant to the health experience of the contemporary traveller.

MODERN DAY EXAMPLES

Examples can be found which show the same pattern for today's traveller. New England was rendered virtually treeless in the early 1800s owing to the demands of agriculture. In the mid-1800s, as the westward population migration gathered pace, the forest of the eastern United States was allowed to regenerate naturally. The particular nature of this regeneration provided an ideal habitat for proliferation of deer and a relative dearth of natural predators. Increasing numbers of people visiting for recreational purposes from the USA and abroad offered an ideal opportunity for the Lyme disease spirochete, which is transmitted by tick bite. Lyme disease is now the commonest vector-borne disease in the USA causing problems for both the locals and foreign tourist.[12]

Engineering changes that alter the infrastructure may damage the water table with the potential for contamination of water supplies. Irrigation schemes, environmental degradation and hydro-logical projects in tropical and sub-tropical countries provide the ideal habitat for the spread of the intermediate snail host for schistosomiasis which is now the fourth most prevalent infection worldwide.[13] Again the adventurous (perhaps low budget) traveller, fording streams and rivers, swimming, washing and wading in collections of endemic fresh water while visiting popular river and lake areas in the Nile and Great Lakes Region of East Africa, with high levels of infected snail populations, is at particular risk.[14]

Carbon dioxide emissions and chlorofluoro-carbons (CFCs) are implicated in global warming which directly and indirectly impacts on the exposure of the tourist to unexpected emerging/re-emerging infections. Directly, global warming means an increased opportunity for mosquito-borne viruses and other disease pathogens to gain a foothold in new territories with the attendant risks of malaria and dengue. Indirectly, changed weather systems causing unexpected drought or

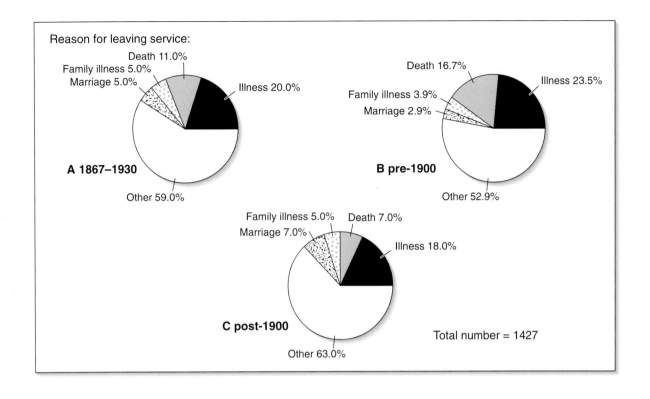

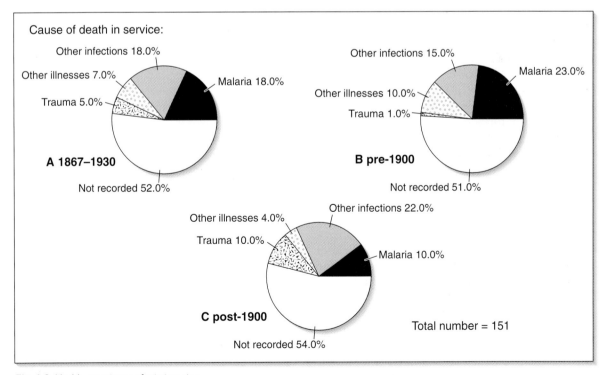

Fig. 1.2 Health experience of missionaries.

flooding can result in contamination of previously safe water and food sources with infectious agents mentioned before. The first indications of these problems may be when a tourist returns with an unexpected illness from an area previously thought to be free from that infection.

Thus changes in economic development and the environment, which are inextricably interlinked, have gone on since the dawning of civilisation. These carry implications for the dissemination of disease which continue today at a faster rate and on a bigger scale than ever before, with an increasing health problem potential for the traveller abroad.

International travel and commerce

EARLIER TIMES

Between 430 and 426 BC, there were two outbreaks of an overwhelming epidemic which decimated the civilian and military population of Athens.[5] Vivid, symptomatic description by the Athenian general, Thucydides, includes intense fever, tormenting thirst, restlessness, violent cough, and suffusion of the tongue and throat with blood. One of the more recent suggestions for this disease is an influenza epidemic complicated by staphylococcal superinfection causing fulminating pneumonia.

Thucydides further described how the port inhabitants of Piraeus were the first to be affected, the disease having spread from Ethiopia, Egypt and throughout the greater part of the Persian empire. From this account, it is clear that the epidemic gained access to Athens via the port trading route. At this time the Athenians were under seige from the Spartans. The decimation caused by the plague is considered by many historians to have made a major contribution to the ultimate defeat of the Athenians in 404 BC owing to the large civilian mortality and also the large proportion of the army and navy who succumbed to the disease.

Episodes of the plague have ravaged mankind over many centuries. During AD 542–750, the Justinian plague, named after the ruling Roman emperor of the time, swept through the Mediterranean nations and is generally accepted to have been bubonic plague. Evidence points to the spread of the disease from the trade routes extending out from the Middle East and beyond. It had a profound effect on the centres of population, and in its wake left greatly weakened Roman and Persian armies which succumbed not long afterwards to the advancing Muslim armies in the 7th century.

Thus the spread of disease travelling along the trade routes was a major contribution to a change in the course of history with the decline of great empires and the emerging dominance of a new culture and religion.

By far the most dramatic example of the epidemic spread of infection was the Black Death which began around 1320 in the Gobi, Mongolia and adjacent region. Over the next 30 years, it spread inexorably along the long-established trading routes of the Mongol empire, ranging across China, India, Asia, Arabia, the Middle East, northern Africa, the Mediterranean, throughout the whole of Europe and north into Russia (Fig. 1.3). It has been estimated that at least one-third of the population of these areas was wiped out by the plague.

RECENT TIMES

It is clear from these historical examples that as traders exchange goods an interface is provided for the exchange of disease organisms. The same remains true today, but the potential scale and diversity for exchange has never been greater. Infected animals may be carried in cargo holds and pathogenic microbes in bilge water tanks. While the Black Death took about 30 years to spread from rural Mongolia in 1320 before reaching northern Europe, there is now no insulating 'time window' as an infected airline passenger can circumnavigate the globe in 68 hours on scheduled services.[15]

There are regular reports of 'airport malaria' caused by the carriage of malaria-bearing mosquitoes aboard aeroplanes or in luggage that somehow defy the control measures specifically designed to eliminate this possibility. A curious example occurred in Switzerland when a 54-year-old man died from malaria. He lived 2.5 km from Geneva Coitrin airport and had no history of recent exposure abroad.[16]

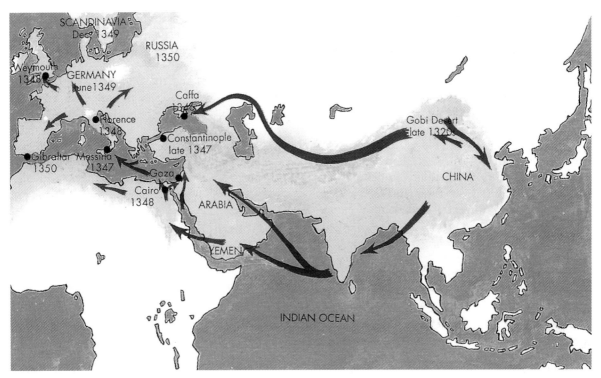

Fig. 1.3 The Black Death.

Travel itself can have direct infectious consequences. In April 1994, a passenger with undiagnosed, resistant tuberculosis, flew from Honolulu to Chicago to Baltimore and returned 1 month later. She died 2 weeks after the flight when the diagnosis became apparent. Following an impressive, contact-tracing exercise co-ordinated by the Centers for Disease Control, Atlanta, Georgia, it was established that transmission of *Mycobacterium tuberculosis* had occurred to five other passengers aboard the inter-continental flight and was associated with the long flight duration and seating proximity to the index case.[17]

Another contemporary travel scenario is the large, often enforced, movement of whole populations or ethnic groups owing to war, pestilence and economic necessity, from their countries of birth to new countries for resettlement. This can introduce disease threats to native populations such as tuberculosis and hepatitis A and B in Vietnamese and other South-East Asians settling in the USA and Canada, diphtheria in East Europeans migrating to Western Europe or in Russian Jews arriving in Israel.

International travel and commerce are here to stay and continue their global expansion. Awareness of the opportunity that this presents for the worldwide dissemination of infections, both new and old, will minimise this threat.

Microbial adaptation and change

Travel gives larger numbers of people the opportunity of exposure to a wider range of unfamiliar pathogens. Not only does this have direct disease consequences for this expanding host population but it also greatly enhances the potential for pathogen diversity and spread.

CHOLERA

The pandemics of cholera that spread across the continents of Asia, Africa, Europe and America in 1817–22 and 1826–32 provide convincing examples of the effective dissemination of one such pathogen around the world, courtesy of travelling man.

Cholera has been endemic in India for the past two millennia, but it was only in the 19th century that it extended beyond the borders of the sub-continent assisted by the presence of a new susceptible host population, the British Army.[18] The disease then travelled with the soldiers and traders to reach the Far East, Middle East and Russia within 5 years.

A further outbreak, in 1826, followed a similar pattern but this time crossed the Atlantic probably with the boatloads of Irish immigrants sailing to the USA, and spread to Central and South America. Millions died in this outbreak, which was made worse by the overcrowded, post-industrial revolution, city conditions, where poverty, poor sanitation and inadequate food were commonplace.

The 7th cholera pandemic started in 1961 and reached a zenith in 1992 when the World Health Organization (WHO) reported a total of 461 783 cases, with 8072 deaths (5291 from Africa alone).[19] This infection, which is potentially preventable by simple basic hygiene and effective sanitation, continues to be a scourge on a global scale with confirmed reports during 1996 from 27 African, 15 Central and South American, 13 Asian and 6 European countries[20] (Fig. 1.4). Despite the knowledge from over 150 years ago on the waterborne spread of this infection, the ability of the pathogen to undergo a change of strain, coupled with the overwhelming ubiquity of tourism/travel in the 1990s, are ensuring a continuing plague.

INFLUENZA

The early part of this century, 1918–19, saw the emergence of a huge influenza pandemic during which the US epidemiologist Edwin Oakes Jordan calculated that 21 million died, more than from the effects of military action in the First World War.[21] Such widespread infection, reckoned to have affected over 1 billion people in one way or another, was only possible because of the improved transport capabilities which had been developed and the consequent, more speedy movements of larger numbers of people.

Sir Patrick Laidlaw, of the UK National Institute for Medical Research, attributed this outbreak to the swine fever influenza virus, and although the source of the virus has not been identified, both major influenza epidemics since 1957 have emanated from the Chinese mainland. Indeed, the same disease as recently as 1969 cost the UK economy in the order of £150 million.

The potential for the emergence of a 'new', antigenic subtype of Type A influenza remains, and with China but a jet flight away via the staging stop of Hong Kong, a fresh epidemic strain can be imported to New York in 16 hours or to London in 14 hours. Thus the forgotten history of 70 years ago may come to life at any time, with even greater vigour thanks to 'jet age' travel.

ANTIMICROBIAL RESISTANCE

The uncontrolled use of antibiotics in some countries also encourages the emergence of more virulent strains of microorganisms; for example, there have been recent concerns about the appearance of a resistant strain of pneumococcus, first isolated in Spain, being transmitted to other countries by tourists.[22–24] The ready availability of antibiotics 'across the counter' in such countries plus the lack of consumer insight regarding the advisability of buying the 'newest' or 'strongest' antibiotic for minor infections are thought to be major contributors to this problem.

There is therefore an obvious potential for the emergence and efficient dissemination of new, more virulent strains of epidemic infections such as influenza and cholera which have occurred throughout the world over many centuries but never with such opportunity for globally affecting so many millions of people so rapidly.

TRAVEL-ASSOCIATED HEALTH RISKS

The contemporary travel phenomenon not only produces economic, environmental, cultural and social repercussions but also medical, epidemiological and medicolegal consequences. Some illnesses may be induced by the travel itself such as motion sickness and upsets to the circadian rhythms; unaccustomed exercise or the effects of altitude may exacerbate pre-existing cardiovascular or respiratory pathology. The effects of exposure to unfamiliar infectious agents and the stress of altered climate, environment and culture may also cause problems for the unwary traveller, which are compounded by differing medical

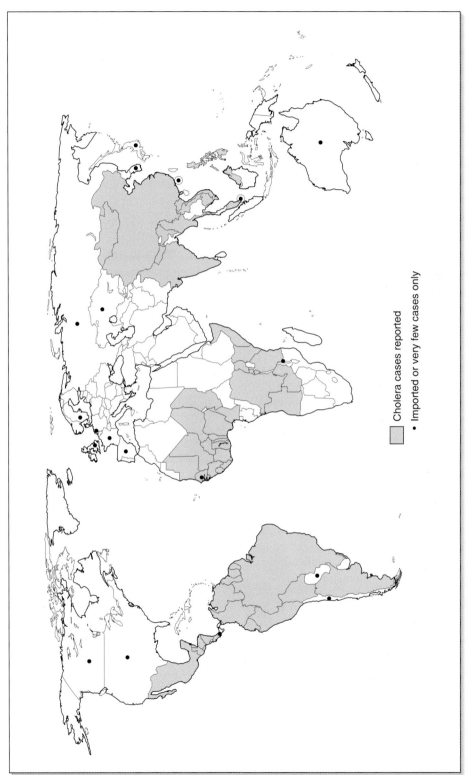

Fig. 1.4 Countries or areas reporting cholera in 1996.

Cholera cases reported

• Imported or very few cases only

practices encountered overseas. This dynamic relationship is illustrated in Figure 1.5.

The higher risk regions include the tropics and sub-tropics of Africa, Asia, and Central and South America. But owing to the wide and changing variations of climate, topography, sanitation, agricultural practices and industrial development found not only within continents but within a single country, the mapping of infections by geography is complex and potentially misleading. Headlines may be made by 'newsworthy', imported infections such as the 2000+ malaria notifications and 7 deaths recorded annually in the UK[25] (> 50% caused by *Plasmodium falciparum*), or the 79% of heterosexually acquired AIDS cases (total number to 31/12/98: 2738)[26] which were contracted abroad (the same pattern as seen for HIV infection) and cumulatively the cause of 1157 deaths (equivalent to 72 per annum since 1982). However, it is only by epidemiological studies that the true perspective of diseases associated with travel can be defined – for example, cases have been recorded of all the infections shown in Table 1.2.[27]

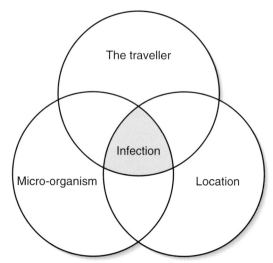

Fig. 1.5 The travel infection 'triad'.

TABLE 1.2 Infections imported to the UK 1978–88	
Acquired immune deficiency syndrome (AIDS)	Legionnaires' disease
	Leishmaniasis
Amoebiasis	Leptospirosis
Brucellosis	Malaria
Campylobacteriosis	Poliomyelitis
Cholera	Rabies
Cytomegalovirus mononucleosis	Salmonellosis
Diphtheria	Schistosomiasis
Dysentery	Sexually transmitted diseases
Giardiasis	Shigellosis
Helminths	Trypanosomiasis
Hepatitis A and B	Tuberculosis
Lassa fever	Typhoid/paratyphoid

Epidemiological studies among travellers

ILLNESS IN TRAVELLERS

In 1973, an outbreak of pneumonia with three fatalities in a group of package holidaymakers returning from Benidorm, Spain to Glasgow, Scotland was subsequently attributed to Legionnaires' disease.[28] This example of travellers returning with a previously unknown disease, which presented diagnostic difficulties and delay in the home country, motivated the development of studies of illnesses associated with travel over the ensuing 12 years.[29–34] These studies showed that the highest attack rates were recorded by the under-40 age groups (Table 1.3), with 41% of the 10–19 age group and 48% of the 20–29 age group reporting illness. Thereafter, attack rates show a progressive diminution with increasing age.

18% of the travellers reported alimentary symptoms, predominantly diarrhoea and vomiting

(Fig. 1.6). Taking all the symptom complexes which include alimentary symptoms, this figure rises to 28% of the total number of travellers and to 76% of all those who reported illness.

Comparing attack rates and the countries visited by the travellers, there is a general trend that the further south and to some extent the further east the travel, the higher the rate for UK residents (Table 1.4). This remains generally true both in summer and in winter. In addition, attack

TABLE 1.3 Age of travellers and reports of illness

Age group (years)	Total (no.)	Unwell (%)
0–9	550	33
10–19	1974	41
20–29	3033	48
30–39	2028	38
40–49	2297	32
50–59	2381	28
60+	1239	20
Not known	725	32
Total	14 227	37

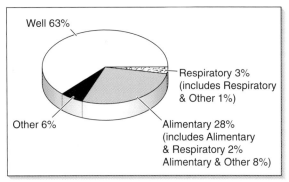

Fig. 1.6 Reports of illness in holidaymakers (n=14 227 1973–85).

TABLE 1.4 Area visited, season, and reports of illness

Area visited	Summer attack rate (%)	Winter attack rate (%)
Europe (north)	19	20
Europe (east)	57	12
Mediterranean (southern Europe)	34	19
Mediterranean (North Africa)	77	32
Average attack rates	37	20

rates were substantially lower in the winter than in the summer, the mean attack rate for winter travellers being 20%[32] compared with 37% for summer travellers.

Undoubtedly, most illnesses encountered by travellers are not recorded, and this is especially the case with less serious (though still troublesome) afflictions such as gastrointestinal problems. Ongoing studies continue in a number of countries to determine the frequency and types of illness encountered by travellers, and to place these in perspective. Although much of the data is incomplete, and depends for its quality on such factors as the enthusiasm of the researcher, meaningful conclusions are still possible, and attack rates can be calculated for different health problems (Fig. 1.7).

MORTALITY IN TRAVELLERS

A review of 952 persons who died while abroad[35] between 1973 and 1988 revealed that, while infection now accounts for only a small proportion (4%) of the mortality, cardiovascular disease was the most frequently recorded cause of death (69%), followed by accidents and injuries (21%). Most deaths occurred in the 50–69 year age range (50%), with the highest cardiovascular mortality (34%) in the 60–69 year age range, and the highest death rate from accidents and injuries (32%) in the 20–29 year age group. The same pattern of mortality was noted in American travellers in 1995[36] and in Australians in 1992–93.[37] This highlights the risks of a strenuous holiday in a warm climate for those with a pre-existing cardiovascular problem and also demonstrates the scope for preventing deaths in younger travellers by improving awareness of hazards such as road accidents and swimming, where alcohol is a frequent, contributing factor.

Several other studies highlight trauma as the commonest cause of death in young travellers abroad and road traffic accidents as the largest single contributor to this group of preventable deaths.[38,39] It is alarming to note that as motor registrations in China, currently 5 vehicles per 1000 population, grow at the rate of 10–20% a year,[40] the current Chinese road death rates are already close to those in the USA which has 770 vehicle registrations per 1000 population,[41,42] quite apart from the future potential for further global warming. As China further opens up to tourism, the hazard to tourists from road traffic accidents will inevitably increase.

Further evidence that lifestyle has a bearing on travellers' problems emerges from the Glasgow

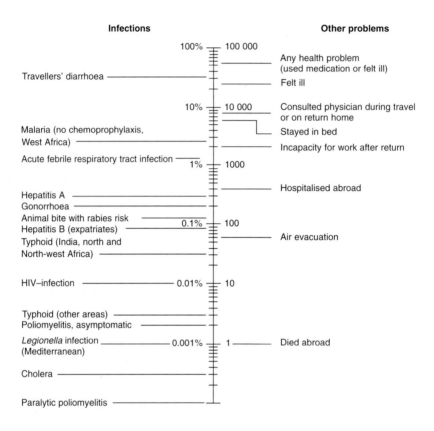

Fig. 1.7 Estimated monthly incidence of health problems per 100 000 travellers to tropical areas. (Source: Steffen R, Lobel H O. Travel medicine. In: Cook G C(ed) Manson's tropical diseases. 20th edn. London, W B Saunders, 1996)

studies: 37% of 2784 smokers reported illness compared with 32% of 7294 non-smokers – a statistically significant difference. No significant correlation was noted between travellers reporting illness and either the reason for travel, the type of accommodation used or the traveller's socio-economic status or the length of stay abroad. However, the highest attack rates were recorded in those who were unskilled or unemployed, and those who set off with pre-existing ill-health.[11]

HOSPITAL ADMISSIONS AFTER RETURN HOME

In attempting to further define the perspective of travel-related illnesses, inpatient data were analysed from the major infectious diseases facility for the Greater Glasgow area (Table 1.5), covering approximately 15% of the Scottish population, 750 000 people.

Out of a total of 1265 admissions, 71 (6 %) were travel-associated, and Asian males accounted for more than one-third of this group; the 20–29 year age group was the most represented (25%). Travel to Southern Asia was associated with 60% of these admissions, correlating with the higher attack rate seen in holidaymakers travelling further south and east; 14% were associated with travel to Spain, probably reflecting the volume of British holiday-makers to that country (5.6 million in 1985).[43]

LABORATORY INFORMATION

Analysis of laboratory isolates of pathogens in travellers collated at the Scottish Centre for Infection and Environmental Health (SCIEH)

TABLE 1.5 Travel-associated admissions 1985

Total admissions	Total travel-associated	Sex	Ethnic origin	Numbers
1265	71 (6%)	M: 44 (62%)	Asian	25 (35%)
			Caucasian	17 (24%)
			African	2 (3%)
		F: 27 (38%)	Asian	14 (20%)
			Caucasian	10 (14%)
			African	3 (4%)

reveals that between 1975 and 1998, there has been an eight-fold increase in the annual total of reports to 1064[44,45] (improved reporting/greater awareness may also be contributory factors to this increase). Cumulative review of the pathogens isolated shows that infections associated with inadequate food handling and poor water supply or sanitation accounted for 88% of these reports in 1998. This figure only represents the small proportion of travellers who were sufficiently unwell to justify further investigation, but the preponderance of isolates associated with gastrointestinal illness mirrors the reports of illness found in the questionnaire surveys. In addition, these figures neither reflect illnesses occurring abroad with a short incubation period, such as influenza, cholera or dengue, nor include illnesses in longer-term travellers, such as expatriates, backpackers and volunteer groups.

COST OF TRAVEL-RELATED ILLNESS

From information supplied by 3049 travellers from the UK who became unwell while abroad, 1% required hospital admission on their return and 14% consulted a doctor.[11] The cost per travel-associated admission in Glasgow in 1997 was given as approximately £630. If the survey figures for Scottish travellers mentioned earlier are used as a basis for calculating the cost of admission to hospital for all ill travellers,[11] it is estimated that over £40 million were spent on this in 1997 in the UK. This amount does not take into account the costs involved with primary care consultations, laboratory investigations, specialist consultations, drug prescriptions, loss of working days and loss of vacation time owing to such illness. Also,

considerable expense is incurred by travellers and their insurance companies from medical treatment obtained abroad.[46]

OTHER STUDIES

While recently published work is sparse, review of comparable studies from other researchers shows that in a study of travellers' diarrhoea in 16 568 randomly selected Swiss travellers, there was a 28% attack rate.[47] Attack rates in other studies ranged from 18% of 2665 Finnish travellers[48] to 41% of 2184 Scottish holidaymakers.[49] All the studies which specified the most affected age group were in agreement[47,49] (i.e. 20–29 years), and similarly where the area was specified, travel to northern Africa[47,48] or Eastern Europe[49] produced the highest attack rates.

The broad correlation of these various findings lends credibility to attempts at detecting patterns of illness derived from the travellers studied, and the use of largely identical methodologies encourages a comparative analysis of relative risk of illness to the travellers, as shown in Table 1.6.

TABLE 1.6 Profile of travellers at risk

Package holidaymakers	> Other travellers
Inexperienced travellers	> Other travellers
Travellers further south, particularly Northern Africa	> Other travellers
Summer travellers	> Winter travellers
Younger age groups (specifically 20–29 years)	> Older travellers
Smokers	> Non-smokers

SEROLOGICAL STUDIES ON TRAVELLERS

Different areas of the world have different health hazards for the traveller. Preventive advice specific to the destination country depends upon the pre-existing health status and the immunity to infection of the individual traveller in addition to the exposure risk, which is affected by lifestyle. Some diseases less common in one country are more prevalent in another and travellers may become complacent about immunisation when travelling to countries where the disease is more common.

For example, a traveller from the UK staying in a slum area in South-East Asia or Africa, who is incompletely immunised and unaware that polio-myelitis is spread by faecal/oral transmission in these areas would be at risk of infection. (1981 cases of paralytic poliomyelitis were reported from these regions to the WHO in 1996.[50])

As a consequence of the recent social catharsis in the former USSR, collapse of public health infra-structure and consumer suspicion of the efficacy of the vaccines and safety of the needles used, herd immunity has now fallen below protective levels for some common pathogens. It is therefore not surprising that in 1992 an outbreak of diphtheria was reported in Russia with 4000 cases[51] rising to 47 802 in 1994 with 1746 deaths.[52] A disease, pre-viously eradicated, has returned to present a threat to the native population and visitors with in-adequate immunity. It also caused difficulties for vaccine manufacturers in meeting the demand.

During the period 1979–82, studies[53] on 470 returning travellers from the West of Scotland indicated that 20% had incomplete immunity to poliomyelitis. 64% of those tested (511 travellers) had antibodies to hepatitis A (ranging from 30%, 10–19 year age group, and rising progressively with increasing age to 89%, age group over 60 years). Only 87% (288 tested) had adequate levels of tetanus antitoxin and 40% of the 225 travellers tested had adequate levels of diphtheria antitoxin.

These results show inadequate protection to poliomyelitis, hepatitis A, tetanus, and diphtheria, putting 1 in 5, 1 in 3, 1 in 8, and 2 in 3 at risk respectively. These data provide a basis for guiding immunisation programmes aimed at the inter-national traveller; for example, the seropositivity profile for hepatitis A supports the cost effective-ness of selective screening in the UK before giving immunoglobulin to older travellers at risk from exposure.[54] The cost of the active hepatitis A vaccine either to the individual traveller, or on the prescriber's budget, also justifies pre-travel screening. Adequate immunisation will provide maximum protection for the traveller exposed to these pathogens, and also protect the community by reducing the risk of local transmission of infection following importation of such pathogens.

Protecting the traveller

While it is important that travellers are advised about the vaccinations appropriate to their des-tination, it should be emphasised that im-munisation and medication can at best only protect against a small proportion (about 5%) of the health hazards to which travellers are exposed. This leaves vast scope for effective, pre-travel health education. The following is a brief résumé of some of the common topics that may need to be covered. All these topics are discussed in greater detail elsewhere in this book.

PREPARATION FOR TRAVEL

Good insurance cover is always strongly recommended. It is a false economy to ignore this issue as the costs of medical care abroad can be financially crippling. Insurance statistics from the USA suggest that three persons in 20 can expect to develop an illness (whether of minor or major significance) every 2 weeks, irrespective of travel. This is of greater significance in those setting out with a pre-existing illness who are more likely to develop a health problem, as indeed are the young, the elderly and the pregnant traveller. It is important that the intending traveller consults for medical advice regarding immunisations in good time to ensure that there is adequate time to complete any complex immunisation schedules.

The journey

The enforced immobility of a long, plane journey predisposes to ankle swelling and deep venous thrombosis. Those on daily medications should carry adequate supplies in their hand luggage, as lost baggage can lead to medical complications in addition to frustration.

The modern passenger jet is pressurised to the equivalent of an altitude of 5000–7000 feet. Reduced oxygen saturation may present difficulties for those with impaired oxygen carrying capacity (e.g. severe bronchitics) or requiring good oxygen saturation (e.g. recent heart attack). As a result of dry air circulation within the aircraft, dehydration can be a problem unless adequate fluids are regularly consumed during a long journey.

Safe water

Water is a prerequisite for life and it can also present particular health hazards for the traveller. Direct ingestion of contaminated water as well as indirect ingestion from food consumption of fish are the most obvious sources of problems. There may also be lack of adequate hygiene and sanitary facilities that predispose to skin and other infections. Water-related disease can be a risk in some countries, for example schistosomiasis in Africa.

Sea

Chemical contamination of recreational water can give rise to gastrointestinal upset, although the risk from ingestion of affected seafood is the likelier source of trouble.

Sun

Awareness of the sun's ability to cause not only short-term discomfort from burning but also long-term risks should be fully appreciated. Sunlight is also synergistic to fungal skin infections. Appreciation of these facts by those with high photosensitivity as well as the amplification of the power of sunlight by the effects of water, snow, sand, altitude, latitude and medication will promote a sensible approach in terms of protective clothing, gradual exposure and the use of appropriate sunscreens.

Sex

The 1991 WHO Report 'AIDS and Mobility' concluded:

> Current studies all indicate that casual sexual contacts are quite common among leisure travellers not being accompanied by the partner. This is most clear in the case of sex tourism.

This report highlighted the importance of safe sexual practices and appropriate health education as the only sure ways to avoid sexually transmitted diseases and AIDS.

Malaria

The important message about malaria is that no current antimalarial measures can guarantee absolute protection, although if mosquito bites can be reduced, then the risk of infection is smaller. Chemoprophylaxis is useful but has limitations as well as advantages.[55] A recent concept is the use of 'stand-by' medication provided by the doctor prior to travel for those at risk from malaria in locations where rapid access to professional care is not possible.

Accidents

Accidents are the second commonest cause of death overall, as well as the main cause of death in younger travellers.

Common causes of accidents include:

- not wearing seat belts/crash helmets
- failure to remember the contra-traffic direction to the home country
- lack of appreciation of differing environmental safety standards (e.g. balcony barrier heights)
- exposure to the risk of assault by straying from usual tourist areas.

Much can be done by travel agents, tour operators and travel couriers to alert the unwary tourist about 'unsafe or no go' areas and to inappropriate conduct. The disinhibiting effect of alcohol, and the natural adventurousness, energy, and disinhibitions of youth clearly highlight the prime, 'at risk' groups.

DISSEMINATION OF INFORMATION ON TRAVELLERS' HEALTH

An inevitable accompaniment to the growth in international travel is that general practitioners and other primary care workers are increasingly contacted by patients seeking advice both prior to travel and following their return, and the intending traveller is faced with a plethora of sources of advice (Fig. 1.8).

Although the travel agent may be the most commonly consulted advice source,[29] there is concern about the availability and quality of that advice.[56] It is clear that no one source can address all the diverse needs of the traveller, but that the general practitioner occupies a pivotal role in this field. There are studies which suggest that general practitioners may encounter problems about giving appropriate advice,[57] that general practice may not be the best location for provision of travel advice,[58] but that general practitioners have a medicolegal responsibility to provide accurate advice.[59]

In recognition of the responsibilities and difficulties which the general practitioner faces in addressing this need, a telephone advice service for the primary care sector was established in Scotland in 1975. Then an online, computerised, health information database (TRAVAX)[60] was established in 1982.

This nationally accessible database, now available via the Internet, includes recommendations on vaccinations for individual countries, malaria prevention advice and information about particular vaccines to help in making a balanced judgement when indications are not clear cut. Details about administration and schedules, interactions between vaccines, advice for those with HIV infection, and current notes detailing known outbreaks and, changes in vaccine availability are included. Many other countries now have similar systems.

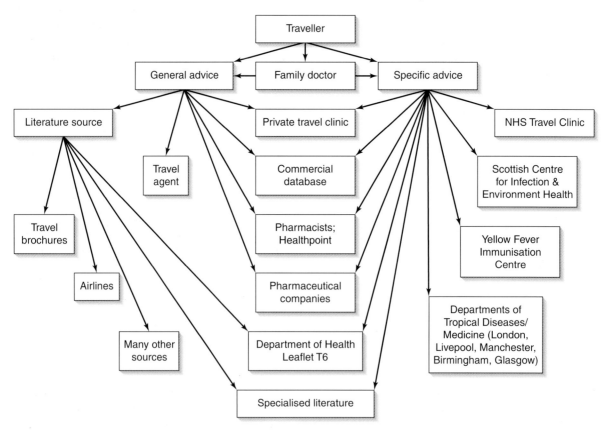

Fig. 1.8 Sources of pre-travel health advice.

A study by Arnold[61] in 1990 involving 899 departing UK travellers at Heathrow airport showed a 65% preference for pre-travel health advice to be provided by the general practitioner. This is logical, as the general practitioner is uniquely placed to advise, having access to the traveller's relevant past medical history, including previous immunisations, allergic reactions, long-term medication and past illnesses, as well as information on the traveller's lifestyle. Such information is essential for the provision of accurate, appropriate advice for the individual traveller.

At the same time, it has to be recognised that it is impractical for all travellers to attend the family doctor prior to departure and indeed there is much information to be disseminated apart from immunisation advice. Such advice may even be better presented by professionals other than the general practitioner. It is therefore important that every opportunity for the dissemination of appropriate pre-travel health advice be taken whenever the consumer interfaces with the travel 'scene', be this the travel agent, airline, currency supplier, visa/government agent, in addition to specifically dedicated medical facilities.

EMERGING AND RE-EMERGING INFECTIONS

Short memories easily 'forget' that only smallpox infection has been eradicated worldwide, and in countries where the public health infrastructure and health education are inadequate, 'old' diseases can readily re-emerge. Similarly, when the impetus of immunisation programmes cannot be sustained, herd immunity falls and epidemic outbreaks return.

Thus the diphtheria epidemic in the former Soviet Union continued for some years with over 47 000 cases reported in 1994 and WHO declaring the epidemic 'an international public health emergency' in 1995.[62] This is a worrying example of the difficulties faced by a country during a period of social upheaval when a competent preventive programme is thrown into disarray from the combined effects of loss of public health direction and control, and consumer resistance because of anxieties about vaccine efficacy and infection transmission from contaminated needles.

Not only does this present an infection risk for the traveller, but it gives cause for review of immunisation programmes in tourist donor countries to ensure that childhood immunisation protection is maintained throughout later life.

The newest 'recruit', in terms of global infection spread by travel, is AIDS (Fig. 1.9). Already the course of history is being charted with the economies of some developing countries under threat of collapse owing to decimation of the workforce and the escalating costs of medical care. Furthermore, the impact on developed countries has raised complex socio-medico-economic issues which have led to fundamental political changes. These have all been brought about as a consequence of the sociosexual interactions of people while travelling, which is as age old as history itself.

Despite these problems, since the 1970s and 1980s, there appears to be a widespread, mistaken belief amongst political decision-makers in the developed world that microbial threats are a thing of the past. Thus university departments of infectious diseases have been disbanded and facilities for dealing with the most dangerous, imported infections such as viral haemorrhagic fever reduced to the absolute minimum. Clearly, this relates to the perception of risk and competition for financial resources in these countries. It is to be hoped that it is never put to the test by, for example, the disaster of the unexpected arrival of a plane-load of returning travellers incubating the Ebola virus.

In 1994, an outbreak of pneumonic plague occurred in Surat, India.[63] Epidemiologists suggested that a cycle of plague, which developed in rats displaced by a severe earthquake in 1993 in a nearby rural area (Beed), spread to cause cases of bubonic plague in the local, rural population. Thereafter, secondary cases of pneumonic plague then passed person-to-person when locals travelled to work in the nearby city of Surat. This highlights the local, public health response, the initial lack of a coordinated, national, public health response, and the widely divergent public health responses from countries around the world, to this perceived 'threat' from infected tourists returning from India. It throws into sharp focus the disarray of public health services around the world in dealing with an international, infectious disease

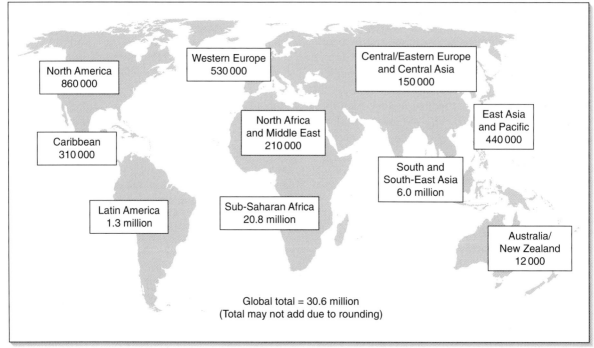

North America
860 000

Western Europe
530 000

Central/Eastern Europe
and Central Asia
150 000

Caribbean
310 000

North Africa
and Middle East
210 000

East Asia
and Pacific
440 000

South and
South-East Asia
6.0 million

Latin America
1.3 million

Sub-Saharan Africa
20.8 million

Australia/
New Zealand
12 000

Global total = 30.6 million
(Total may not add due to rounding)

Fig. 1.9 Estimated number of adults and children living with HIV/AIDS at the end of 1997 by region.

problem and the dangers of further undermining these services. It is obvious from the foregoing examples that the overplay of limited resources coupled with complacency, reduction of facilities, and unexpected population and microbial changes consequent on unforeseen natural and man-made disasters have worrying, worldwide, public health implications.

The response

Effective surveillance means the ability to detect unusual clusters of disease, documentation of the geographic and demographic spread of an outbreak, and estimation of the magnitude of the problem.[12] It can also help the description of the natural history of a disease, identify causal factors, facilitate laboratory and epidemiological research and assess specific intervention efforts. The management of the outbreak of Ebola virus infection in Zaire in 1995[64] exemplifies many of the crucial elements required to respond to the threat of emerging infection. To effect these steps for the welfare of both native and tourist populations, it is necessary to have comprehensive national surveillance to detect outbreaks of

infectious disease, linking with a coordinated global reporting network. This and the development of an internationally accessible database on disease incidence and antibiotic drug resistance with relevant geographic details would be a reassuring move towards improved early detection of future emerging diseases.

Control and education about the indiscriminate use of antibiotics by the general public, medical professionals, veterinary practitioners and food manufacturers will reduce the rate of emerging microbial resistance.

Continued support for vector control programmes still has an important role in reducing the spread of disease. There may need to be greater recognition and financial support for this effort from developed countries in realisation that such programmes may be beyond the financial resources of a developing country and that there are humanitarian benefits which extend beyond the confines of national geographic boundaries.

Ongoing vaccine and drug development is a fundamental part of the continuing fight against disease. The protection of the tourist with appropriate immunisation advice coupled with the continuous review of national immunisation programmes are essential for ensuring the best available pre-emptive protection.

However, for tourists, the biggest single contribution to be made in minimising health problems in general, and infections in particular, is from effective public education and behavioural change. Simple truisms such as 'there is a price to pay for the freedom to travel', 'if travellers do not pick up an infection, they cannot pass it on', and 'immunisations and medications only protect against 5–10% of the problems encountered by travellers, the rest relate to their personal behaviour', have to be appreciated by the consumer and acted upon.

Basic educational messages such as avoid mosquito bites, the rationale of using an impregnated mosquito net, appreciation of behaviour modification in relation to personal hygiene, food handling, sexual behaviour and drug abuse, require continual reinforcement.

EFFECTS OF TRAVEL ON HOST COUNTRIES

Insight for the tourist from a further educational stage beyond the purely selfish is also long overdue. There needs to be appreciation of the social, resource and environmental costs from the apparently insatiable expansion of global tourism. Economically poor countries may realise too late that uncontrolled tourism development not only fails to solve their foreign debt problems but extracts an unacceptable price in loss of native culture, political instability and importation of foreign values and of new disease. Levels of pollution, disease, crime, violence, prostitution, and drug abuse can escalate with direct threats for the very tourists responsible for promoting these changes as well as for the native population. These 'locals' may be left to their own devices when the destination country is given the description 'unsafe' and the tourist moves on to further despoil virgin territory.

The accelerated consumption of resources caused by tourists, for example, for building land, sewage disposal, food and water, can disrupt local agricultural practices with environmental damage and competition for resources with the local population to the detriment of the health and welfare of all concerned. Realisation that the bulk of the profits from tourism, estimated at 80%,[65] return to the affluent, tourist-donor countries with often only temporary low paid, low status jobs for the locals, and the outcomes of depleted resources and social and environmental degradation, may encourage more socially responsible tourism.

Postscript

International travel and tourism are currently the world's fastest growing and, in financial value, largest, industry. Throughout history movement of people from necessity, for commerce, recreation, or military purposes has been associated with transmission of infection. The numbers of contemporary travellers allied to the speed of travel and the repercussions of worldwide changes in demographics, industry, the environment and public health support mean that the opportunities for microbial adaptation and global epidemic spread have never been greater.

Clearly, there are logistic and financial constraints on the individual counselling of every tourist by a healthcare professional. Instead it is more relevant than ever before that individuals are empowered to accept responsibility for their own personal health and welfare when travelling abroad. It is then incumbent on healthcare professionals whether in government service, primary care, public health, travel clinics or health education to ensure that the health information necessary for the traveller is readily available, medically accurate and easily understood. The travel trade must also be involved.

It is also an opportunity to educate about socially responsible tourism, accepting the concept that we all share a 'global village' and that the welfare of our fellow 'villager' is directly related to our own personal behaviour. This insight is far more likely to promote the changes necessary for the individual to reduce the risks from preventable trauma and disease spread, and to halt the other socially and environmentally destructive consequences of global tourism.

Acknowledgements

Figure 1.3 is reproduced with permission from Knight L. Invisible enemies: Epidemics and plagues through history. London: Channel 4 Publications; 1992.

Figures 1.4 and 1.8 are reproduced from the World Health Organization publication, Weekly Epidemiological Record.

Figure 1.7 is reproduced with permission from Cook GC, ed. Manson's tropical diseases. 20th ed. London: WB Saunders; 1996.

REFERENCES

1. World Tourism Organisation (WTO). Tourism compendium, World total. Madrid: WTO; 1990.
2. International Civil Aviation Organization (ICAO). Development of world schedule revenue traffic 1945–1990 statistics. Montreal: ICAO; 1990.
3. Business Statistics Office (BSO). Business monitor annual statistics (MQ 6): Overseas travel and tourism. Table 8A. London: BSO; 1996.
4. Black FL. Why did they die? Science 1992; 258: 1739–1740.
5. Knight L. Invisible enemies: Epidemics and plagues through history. London: Channel 4 Publications; 1992.
6. Velminirovic B. Yellow fever and the HMS Dauntless. Travel Medicine International 1989: 59–63.
7. Carlton JT, Geller JB. Ecological roulette: the global transport of non-indigenous marine organisms. Science 1993; 261: 78–82.
8. Caitlin G. Illustrations of the manners, customs and conditions of the North American Indians. London: Chatto and Windus; 1876.
9. Bruce-Chwatt L. Global problems of imported disease. Advances in Parasitology1973; 11: 75–114.
10. Steel T. Scotland's story. London: Collins; 1984: 133.
11. Cossar JH. Studies on illnesses associated with travel (MD thesis). Glasgow: University of Glasgow; 1987.
12. Lederberg J, Shope RE, Oaks SC. Emerging infections: Microbial threats to health in the United States. Washington DC: National Academic Press; 1992.
13. Scottish Centre for Infection and Environmental Health (SCIEH). Current notes. SCIEH Weekly Report 1995; 29: 95/18.
14. Corachan M. Schistosomiasis in travelers. Journal of Travel Medicine 1995; 2(1): 1–3.
15. British Airways (BA) World timetable. London: BA; 1995.
16. World Health Organization. Airport malaria, a fatal case. Weekly Epidemiological Record 1996; 47: 358.
17. Kenyon TA, et al. Example of transmission of TB aboard a commercial aircraft. Paper presented at the Fourth International Conference on Travel Medicine. Acapulco: 1995.
18. Longmate N. King cholera: The biography of a disease. London: Hamish Hamilton; 1996.
19. World Health Organization. Cholera in 1992. Weekly Epidemiological Record 1993; 68: 149–156.
20. World Health Organization. Cholera in 1996. Weekly Epidemiological Record 1997; 72: 229–234.
21. Collier R. The plague of the Spanish Lady: The influenza pandemic of 1918–1919. London: Macmillan; 1974.
22. Gasc AM, Geslin P, Sicard AM. Relatedness of penicillin-resistant *Streptococcus pneumoniae* serogroup 9 strains from France and Spain. Microbiology 1995; 141 (pt 3): 623–627.
23. Klugman KP, Coffey TJ, Smith A, Wasas A, Meyers S. Cluster of an erythromycin-resistant variant of the Spanish multiply resistant 23F clone of *Streptococcus pneumoniae* in South Africa. European Journal of Clinical Microbiology and Infectious Diseases 1994; 13(2): 171–174.
24. Soares S, Kristinsson KG, Musser JM, Tomasz A. Evidence for the introduction of a multiresistant clone of serotype 6B *Streptococcus pneumoniae* from Spain to Iceland in the late 1980s. Journal of Infectious Diseases 1993; 168(1): 158–163.
25. Public Health Laboratory Service Communicable Disease Surveillance Centre. CDR Review 1997; 7/10: R139.
26. Scottish Centre for Infection and Environmental Health (SCIEH). Surveillance Report: HIV & AIDS. SCIEH Weekly Report 1999; 33: 99/04.
27. Cossar JH, Reid D. Health hazards of international travel. World Health Statistics Quarterly 1989; 42(2): 27–42.
28. Lawson JH, Grist NR, Reid D, Wilson TS. Legionnaires' disease. Lancet 1977; ii: 108.
29. Cossar JH, Reid D, Fallon RJ, et al. A cumulative review of studies on travellers, their experience of illness and the implications of these findings. Journal of Infection 1990; 21: 27–42.
30. Dewar RD, Cossar JH, Reid D, Grist NR. Illness amongst travellers to Scotland: a pilot study. Health Bulletin (Edinburgh) 1983; 41/3:155–162.
31. Cossar JH, Dewar RD, Fallon RJ, et al. Rapid response health surveillance of Scottish tourists. Travel and Traffic Medicine International 1984; 2(1) 23–27.
32. Cossar JH, Dewar RD, Reid D, Grist NR. Travel and health: illness associated with winter package holidays. Journal of the Royal College of General Practitioners 1988; 33: 642–645.
33. Grist NR, Cossar JH, Reid D, et al. Illness associated with a package holiday in Romania. Scottish Medical Journal 1985; 30: 156–160.
34. Cossar JH, Dewar RD, Fallon RJ, Grist NR, Reid D. *Legionella pneumophila* in tourists. Practitioner 1982; 226: 1543–1548.
35. Paixao MTD'A, Dewar RD, Cossar JH, Covell RG, Reid D. What do Scots die of when abroad? Scottish Medical Journal 1991; 36: 114–116.

36. Jong EC, McMullen R. Medicine Manual. Philadelphia: WB Saunders; 1995: 8.

37. Prociv P. Deaths of Australian travellers overseas. Medical Journal of Australia 1995; 163: 27–30.

38. Hardgarten SW, Baker T, Guptil K. Fatalities of American travellers 1975–1984. In: Steffen R, Lobel HO, Haworth J, Bradley DJ, eds. Proceedings of the first conference on international travel medicine. Berlin: Springer; 1989: 55–64.

39. Lustenberger I. Todesfalle von Schweisen in Ausland (thesis). Zurich: University of Zurich; 1988.

40. Roberts I. China takes to the roads. British Medical Journal 1995; 310: 1311–1313.

41. Motor Vehicle Manufacturers Association (MVMA). World motor vehicle data. Detroit: MVMA; 1991.

42. Gouhua L, Baker SP. A comparison of injury death rates in China and the United States, 1986. American Journal of Public Health 1991; 81: 605–609.

43. Central Statistical Office (CSO). Social Trends 15, Table 10.13. London: CSO; 1985.

44. Scottish Centre for Infection and Environmental Health (SCIEH). Surveillance Report: Travel related infections imported into Scotland. SCIEH Weekly Report 1999; 33: 99/03.

45. Sharp JCM. Imported infections into Scotland, 1975. Communicable Diseases Scotland Weekly Report 1976; 76/26: v–vi.

46. Cossar JH. A review of travel-associated illness. In: Steffen R, Lobel HO, Haworth J, Bradley DJ, eds. Proceedings of the first conference on international travel medicine. Berlin: Springer; 1989: 50–54.

47. Steffen R, van der Linde F, Syr K, Schar M. Epidemiology of diarrhoea in travellers. Journal of the American Medical Association 1983; 249: 1176–1180.

48. Peltola H, Kyronseppa H, Holsa P. Trips to the South – a health hazard. Scandinavian Journal of Infectious Diseases 1983; 15: 375–381.

49. McEwan A, Jackson MH. Illness among Scots holidaymakers who had travelled abroad summer 1983. Communicable Diseases Scotland Weekly Report 1987; 87/16: 7

50. World Health Organization. Performance of acute flaccid paralysis (AFP) and incidence of poliomyelitis, 1996–1997 (as of July 1997). Weekly Epidemiological Record 1997; 28: 208.

51. Conradi P. Russia's Diphtheria outbreak worsens. British Medical Journal 1993; 306: 417.

52. World Health Organization. Expanded Programme on Immunisation. Weekly Epidemiological Record 1995; 70: 141.

53. Cossar JH. An immune profile of Scots travellers: a basis for immunization. Proceedings of the second conference on international travel medicine. Atlanta: International Society of Travel Medicine; 1991: 298.

54. Cossar JH, Reid D. Not all travellers need immunoglobulin for hepatitis A. British Medical Journal 1987; 294: 1503.

55. Bradley D. Prophylaxis against malaria for travellers from the United Kingdom. British Medical Journal 1993; 306: 1247–1252.

56. Reid D, Cossar JH, Ako TI, Dewar RD. Do travel brochures give adequate advice on avoiding illness? British Medical Journal 1986; 293: 1472.

57. Usherwood V, Usherwood TP. Survey of general practitioners' advice for travellers to Turkey. Journal of the Royal College of General Practitioners 1989; 39: 148–150.

58. Jeffries M. Booster for GP travel vaccine clinics. Monitor 1989; 2(31): 10–11.

59. Holden JD. General practitioners and vaccination for foreign travel. Journal of the Medical Defence Union 1989; Spring: 6–7.

60. Cossar JH, Walker E, Reid D, Dewar RD. Computerised advice on malaria prevention and immunisation. British Medical Journal 1988; 296: 358.

61. Arnold WSJ. Vaccine information and the practice nurse. Paper presented at the 3rd International Conference on Tourist Health, Venice: 1990.

62. Anon. Diphtheria 'emergency' in former Soviet Union. British Medical Journal 1995; 310: 1222.

63. Chatterjee S. The Indian plague outbreak. Travel Medicine NewsShare 1995.

64. World Health Organization. Ebola haemorrhagic fever. Weekly Epidemiological Record 1995; 70: 149–151.

65. O'Grady A. The challenge of tourism. Bangkok Ecumenical Coalition on Third World Tourism; 1990.

Emerging infections and relation to travel

Dermot Kennedy

Infections have been emerging since the first microbe tried to climb the food chain ladder preying on the protoalgae....Emergence is none other than the dark side of co-evolution, a typical, inexorable biological phenomenon.[1]

'No man is an island' – nor are his diseases. Microbes tend to ignore borders. A new disease that appears in one place may spread rapidly to become a worldwide threat. Influenza A, a supreme example, periodically reminds us that we all live in the global village. We ignore at our peril the problems of the rest of the world. Pathogens furthermore can cross biological – as well as geographical – frontiers, through cross-species transfer. Sometimes that frontier is human, and the consequences serious.

Humans, and the microbes, are the world's most successful life forms engaging intermittently in complex processes of co-evolutionary competition. They share various attributes: adaptability, opportunism and a phenomenal ability to disseminate and to survive adverse environments. However, the bacteria have existed for 30 000 times longer than *Homo sapiens*, a testament to their supreme successfulness. Microbial pathogens have repeatedly proved to be amongst the supreme threats to humanity. They readily find new ways to challenge us. We are, in turn, innovative in the ways that we make ourselves vulnerable to such threats. The result is new diseases.

Medicine creates new names for new problems. 'Emerging infections', for example, is a term first coined in 1989 by Nobel Laureate Lederberg to denote new infections of increasing threat to humans. This is simply a new name for a very old problem. While any particular infection may be 'new' to human experience, the phenomenon of serious epidemics of unknown diseases is as old as recorded time. Many of the epidemic 'new' diseases

of the past became, over time, the familiar endemic infections of our urban civilisation. Their decline in the last 50 years led to predictions of the demise of infectious diseases in the developed world. Indeed, in 1968 the US Surgeon General, W. H. Stewart, announced 'It is time to close the book on infectious diseases.'[2] Such predictions have proved premature. The notoriety of the infectious diseases caused by HIV, hepatitis C, Legionnaires' disease and *Escherichia coli* 0157 and a whole swath of 30 or so, new and emergent diseases has helped to shatter the complacency on this topic. Furthermore, other important, long-standing diseases, once thought to be in irreversible decline, have since re-emerged on a significant scale. Indeed malaria and tuberculosis, once in retreat, together now account for about 10% of all global deaths.[3]

A ground-breaking report 'Emerging Infections: Microbial Threats to Health in the United States' articulated the growing concerns of many US specialists when published in 1992.[4] This also mirrored Europe's anxieties, too, where the WHO Regional Committee noted 'with great concern that all countries of the Region are affected by the emergence and re-emergence of infectious and food borne diseases and by growing antibiotic resistance.'[5] In fact, WHO has labelled the growing threat of infectious diseases as a global crisis[6] and, reflecting its concern, the theme of 'Emerging Infectious Diseases: Global alert, Global response' was chosen for World Health Day 1997, on WHO's historic 50th anniversary.[5]

This section will be divided into five parts. The first will deal with the global scale of infectious diseases as background. The second will focus on the theme of the emergence or re-emergence of diseases. These will be collectively designated as (re-)emergence. To provide a historical context, the third part will chart the rise of the crowd diseases.

Today we understand better the forces which underlay the awesome epidemic outbreaks which once so bewildered its victim communities. Thus the fourth part will analyse the factors, historical and modern, which promote such emergence of disease. While clearly these do vary, there are a number of important underlying themes. These will be reviewed not least because of their value in predicting the future. Given that travel has been such a potent force in the spread of infectious diseases, the last section will examine this phenomenon.

I. The global scale of infectious diseases

Disease activity is a dynamic phenomenon. Over time, the epidemiology of an infection tends to change: in its incidence, its virulence, its geographical distribution or its target population. At best, a snapshot of its epidemiology appears.

While some infections are increasing, others are in decline, perhaps because of immunisation, other public health interventions or to new therapies. An outstanding example has been the impact of glucose/salt solution in dramatically reducing the mortality from infantile gastroenteritis in the developing world. Not so long ago this condition was killing 10 million babies worldwide.

Overall, the global mortality and morbidity from infectious diseases are formidable. Their statistical estimation is however difficult even in developed countries, partly owing to their changing pattern. Nevertheless, an important World Health Report estimated that 52 million deaths occurred globally from all causes in 1995.[3] Collectively, the infectious diseases were the world's principal killer and accounted for an estimated 17.3 million deaths, some 33% of the total (Table 1.7). By comparison, cardiovascular deaths were estimated at 15 million and cancer deaths at 6 million.

By mode of transmission, person-to-person spread was the commonest by far, at 65% of the total. By anatomical groups, lower respiratory tract

TABLE 1.7 Estimated global mortality in millions (M) in 1995 based on a global population of 5800 M (World Health Report 1996)

Aetiology	Deaths	Categories (as % of total infection deaths)		
Infections	17.3 M (33%)	By mode of transmission		%
		•Person-to-person	11.2 M	65
		•Food, H$_2$O, soil borne	3.7 M	22
		•Insect-borne	2.3 M	15
		•Animal-borne	0.006 M	0.3
		By disease group		
		•Lower resp. tract	4.4 M	25
		•Bacterial GI infection	3.1 M	18
		•Tuberculosis	3.1 M	18
		•Malaria	2.1 M	12
		•Hepatitis B	1.1 M	6
		•HIV/AIDS	1.0 M	6
		•Measles	1.0 M	6
Others	34.7 M (67%)			
•Cardiovascular	15 M			
•Cancer	6 M			
Total	52 M			

infections, especially pneumonia, were most frequent followed by gastrointestinal infections. Together these accounted for more than 40% of all infection deaths. By individual disease, tuberculosis and malaria were most important and together accounted for 30% of all infection deaths and 10% of total deaths.

Of outstanding importance for the developing world, infection still remains a significant problem in developed countries. In the USA, infectious diseases are the third most common cause of death.[7] HIV infection leads in those aged between 25 and 44 years[8] though deaths have recently declined with the introduction of antiretroviral therapy. Infection with hepatitis C virus continues to spread, with an estimated 4 million Americans infected and some 8–10 000 deaths in the USA annually.[9] There are about 600 000 cases of pneumonia in the USA annually, resulting in up to 50 000 deaths.[12] Overall, there was a 58% increase in infection-related deaths in the USA between 1980 and 1992.[2]

To estimate global morbidity from infection is much more difficult and in any comprehensive sense it is perhaps impossible. Nevertheless, rough estimates for some important infections are shown in Table 1.8. They provide a sense of the scale of some of the more significant conditions. The data are derived from several sources.[2,10]

Only some of the diseases in Table 1.9 satisfy the definition of emerging infections; others are re-emerging, sometimes on a regional or perhaps on a global basis.

2. Emerging and re-emerging infections

Emerging infections are those that have been recently discovered, have increased in humans in the last 20 years or threaten to increase in the future. Re-emerging infections denote diseases which, once diminishing in incidence, have increased because of ecological changes, public health decline or drug resistance.[11] Both disease concepts, illustrated with notable examples, are defined in Box 1.1.[4,12] These diseases must be defined geographically. Although some diseases,

such as HIV and hepatitis C virus (HCV) infections, are global in occurrence, more typically, (re-)emerging infections are regionally delineated or, at least, at first. Clearly, this can change.

EMERGING INFECTIONS

Emerging infections are new diseases: either newly discovered, exhibiting serious new manifestations, or newly recognised as occurring in a previously unaffected area. Successful emergence depends on a microbe's ability to circumvent the host's innate or acquired resistance, its transmissibility and whether the environment is conducive to its persistence.[4] Microbes, emerging from the evolutionary stream of life, thrive on 'undercurrents of opportunity' provided by behavioural or ecological changes. We cannot determine when a new pathogen or disease has first affected humans. The date of initial recognition is the only 'hard' data available. Retrospective serological studies sometimes identify evidence of even earlier disease occurrence as with HIV or *Legionella* infection. How does recognition of a new pathogen or disease occur? This may be triggered by its degree of severity, especially when there are fatalities, or by its transmissibility. Legionnaires' disease, toxic shock syndrome and *Hantavirus* pulmonary syndrome are acute illnesses with distinctive clinical features, and significant mortalities. An outbreak is quickly recognised as an epidemiological 'event'. By contrast, infection with the chronic blood-borne viruses may take years to manifest clinically. Had HIV-1 and HCV been less transmissible and the extent of infection less widespread, they probably would not have been identified so quickly.

The question also arises: how new is new? Given the extraordinary diversity of the microbial world, how genuinely new formed are 'new' human pathogens? Disease may be recognised only because of increased human contact with a long-standing, though previously unknown, pathogen. *Legionella pneumophila* probably predated the emergence of *Homo sapiens* by many millions of years. Technology, by increasing pathogen-to-human contact, through the circulation of environmental water, was the critical factor. Disease may appear with the transfer of a pathogen across the species barrier, perhaps through increased human–animal contact. This may

TABLE 1.8 Estimates in millions (M) of global scale of some infectious diseases (deaths in brackets)

Diseases	Estimated no.	Disease	Estimated no.
Viral		**Bacterial**	
Hepatitis B	>300 M (1.1 M)	Tetanus	? (0.5 M)
Hepatitis C	170–350 M	Pertussis	40 M (0.4 M)
Rotavirus	> 80 M (0.87 M)	Tuberculosis	12 M (new)
Dengue	50–100 M	Leprosy	12 M
HIV (1998)	30 M (2.5 M)	Meningococcus	1.2 M (0.2 M)
Measles	45 M (1 M)	Trachoma	146 M
Parasite		**Helminthic**	
Schistosomiasis	200 M	Ascaris	1000 M
Leishmaniasis	12 M	Hookworm	900 M
Malaria	300 M (2.1M)	Filariasis	80–200 M
Amoebiasis	500 M (0.1 M)	Ancyclostomiasis	700–900 M

Box 1.1 Definitions and examples of emerging and re-emerging infections

Emerging infections are due to 'new' pathogens or diseases which may be:

- appearing in the human population, possibly for the first time:
  HIV, *Escherichia coli* 0157, new variant Creutzfeldt–Jakob disease, *Vibrio cholerae* 0139, Toxic shock syndrome, influenza A H5N1, *Hantavirus* pulmonary syndrome

- newly identified infections, possibly increasing in incidence:
  Legionella, *Campylobacter*, *Cryptosporidium*, HCV, Lassa, Ebola, Lyme borreliosis, bartonellosis, ehrlichiosis, hepatitis E, *Chlamydia pneumoniae*

- appearing in areas not previously reported:
  dengue, yellow fever, *Hantaviruses*, Ebola, malaria, cholera, viral encephalitis.

Re-emerging infections are known communicable diseases, once declining but now increasing owing to:

- deterioration in public health:
  tuberculosis, diphtheria, cholera (e.g. Russia) gastrointestinal infection (e.g. Central Africa):
  pertussis, leishmaniasis

- change in conditions (e.g. ecological change allowing disease to reassert itself):
  malaria (global), dengue, salmonellosis, yellow fever, cryptosporidiosis

- increase in drug resistance:
  MDR TB, MRSA, vancomycin-resistant enterococci, typhoid, *Shigella*, gonococcus, pneumococcus

HCV, hepatitis C virus; MDR TB, multi-drug resistant tuberculosis MRSA, methicillin-resistant *Staphylococcus aureus*

be influenced by changes in environmental or human ecology as will shortly be described.[4] *Hantavirus* pulmonary syndrome comes to mind. Such species transfer probably occurs more commonly than the evolution of new pathogens and has been called 'microbial traffic' by Morse.[11] However, pathogens may have undergone some evolutionary change by genetic mutation, gene reassortment or acquisition of virulence factors. Examples would include HIV-1 (genetic mutation), new pandemic strains of influenza A (genetic reassortment) and toxin-producing *Staphylococcus aureus* as in toxic shock syndrome or *Escherichia coli* 0157 (acquisition of new toxin). In many instances, however, the pathogen is not new rather than newly recognised either in nature or in humans. By whatever means by which they have emerged, there have been approximately 30 new pathogens or diseases identified in the last 25 years. The major ones are listed in Box 1.2.[12]

Certain of these pathogens are global in distribution. Others such as Ebola, *Hanta* and Sabia viruses are geographically limited in their extent. Certain diseases have come to recognition through technical innovations such as Legionellosis, toxic shock syndrome and hepatitis C. Food-borne diseases have in all parts of the world become a major public health issue through modern methods of animal husbandry and food processing.[13] Yet other infections may emerge owing to intrusion into pristine ecosystems as instanced by many viral haemorrhagic fevers, including those caused by Ebola, various Arenaviridae including Lassa, and various *Hantaviruses*.

RE-EMERGING INFECTIONS

Re-emerging infections consist of old 'enemies' once thought to be in inexorable retreat but increasing once again[11,12] (Box 1.1). A notable European example is diphtheria in the Russian Federation. Amongst various infections re-emerging with the public health chaos resulting from the break-up of the former Soviet regime, this epidemic began in 1990. From 839 cases in 1989, a rapid 57-fold increase occurred producing by 1994 some 47 802 cases, 75% of them in adults.[2] Malaria has shown dramatic increases in many parts of the world with an eight-fold increase in Africa in the late 1980s.[2] A dramatic resurgence of tuberculosis

has occurred globally with a quadrupling of cases since 1985.[2] In Europe, reported cases increased in 1995–96 by 11%.

Diseases have re-emerged in the developed world too, some as the result of antimicrobial drug resistance. As well as bacteria, the latter phenomenon affects parasites, fungi and viruses, too, though antibiotic resistance currently poses the greatest threat. This is hardly surprising. Bacteria are the Earth's first and most successful life form, having evolved 3.6 billion years ago. Since bacteria have, over aeons, survived great extremes of heat, cold and chemical exposure, it is surely no surprise that so many have developed resistance to antibiotics. Speculation about the 'post-antibiotic era'[14] now seems less fanciful. Bacteria have a remarkable ability to transfer resistance factors not just within but also across species. Resistance can thus be disseminated rapidly over wide areas.[15] Indeed, what we are witnessing today is as much a global epidemic of resistance genes as the spread of resistant bacteria themselves.[14] This relates to the gross and inappropriate use of antibiotics today. It is estimated that almost half of the 150 million antibiotic courses prescribed annually in the USA are used inappropriately.[2] Multi-drug resistance is an even greater threat, especially in our hospitals and institutions. Multi-drug resistant *Myco-bacterium tuberculosis*, multi-resistant *Staphylococcus aureus* and vancomycin-resistant enterococci simply represent the notorious tip of a potentially enormous iceberg.[16]

How much of a threat is this new wave of disease? Influenced perhaps by media hysteria, some foresee a veritable epidemic of epidemics in the future[2] with impacts perhaps similar to some

Box 1.2 Major pathogens identified since 1973

1973	Rotavirus	1982	*Escherichia coli* 0157:H7	1989	Hepatitis C virus
1975	Parvovirus B19	1982	HTLV II virus	1989	*Ehrlichia chaffensis*
1976	*Cryptosporidium*	1982	*Borrelia burgdorferi*	1990	Hepatitis E virus
1977	Ebola virus	1983	HIV-1	1991	Guanarito virus
1977	*Legionella* sp.	1983	*Helicobacter pylori*	1992	*Vibrio cholerae* 0139
1977	*Hantavirus*	1985	*Chlamydia*	1992	*Bartonella henselae*
1997	*Campylobacter*		*pneumoniae*	1993	Sin nombre virus
1980	HTLV-I	1986	*Cyclospora*	1994	Sabiavirus
1981	*Staphylococcus aureus*	1988	Human herpes virus	1995	Human herpes virus type 8
	(toxic shock)			1996	Andes virus

HIV, human immunodeficiency virus; HTLV, human T-cell lymphotropic virus plagues of the past. We study history to better interpret the present, to anticipate, and perhaps influence the future. Thus, the emergence of the crowd diseases has important lessons to teach us.

3. The rise of the crowd diseases

While 'infection' per se is as old as time, the communicable diseases of humans – the crowd diseases – are of relatively recent emergence.[17] They appeared with the historically critical transition from hunting and foraging to farming and pastoralism. This created the right circumstances – human-to-animal contact, population growth, increased human-to-human contact – to allow the successful emergence of crowd diseases. Human contact and migration ensured their successful dissemination and, ultimate persistence.[18] Infection was probably less significant for prehistoric man than his urban descendants.[17,19,20] 'Civilisation' and the crowd diseases evolved together[17,21] probably as cause and effect, to become over time inseparably associated. Instead of following herds, man now colonised them, acquiring, through species transfer, many diseases. Diseases such as measles, smallpox, tuberculosis and diphtheria became subsequently of major demographic importance.[17,22] Initially occurring as intense, local epidemics in isolated primitive settlements of, say, Mesopotamia, the crowd diseases would ultimately afflict all mankind as gradually through contact it was to reunite after its interminable phase of dispersal (Fig. 1.11).

Significant contact between large populated regions began during the Classical period, kindling a series of catastrophic epidemics.[18,23] The densely populated, Roman cities provided the fuel for the great fires of epidemic disease which so characterised the ancient world. The Plague of Antoninus, probably smallpox, arrived from the Middle East in AD 166. Over 30 years, it killed perhaps one-third of the Roman Empire, including the legendary Emperor, Marcus Aurelius.[20] A further massive population decline followed the arrival from Ethiopia of the plague of St Cyprian – probably measles – in AD 250. These so weakened

Rome that it could not resist the invasion of various migrating Asian Steppe tribes.[22] In turn, they introduced the first of three great pandemics of plague, a disease endemic to Asian Steppe marmots.[18] The Great Plague of Justinian, probably the worst, killed perhaps half the Mediterranean population.[19,20,24] According to Creighton the great historian of epidemics, 'nothing stands out more clearly as the stroke of fate in bringing the ancient civilisation to an end than the vast depopulation and solitude made by the plague which came with the corn ships from Egypt to Byzantium in AD 543.'[25] Europe, plunged into the Dark Ages, took five centuries to recover. In 1348, the annus terribilis in, for various reasons, an otherwise calamitous century, Mongol invasions brought the second pandemic. Within 4 years, an estimated one-third of the European population died.[18,26,27] With recurrent epidemics between the 14th and 17th centuries, it took almost 250 years for the European population to recover numerically.[18]

European colonial expansion now brought epidemic disaster to the New Worlds. Crosby argues that European domination was ultimately more biological than military.[28] The 16th century Amerindian population, isolated since around 12 000 BC, had no resistance to Old World crowd diseases. About 90% of the MesoAmerican population of 70 million died within 100 years of Columbus's arrival principally from infectious diseases such as smallpox.[29] The Columbian exchange of New World food for Old World diseases had diametrically opposing population effects. The deadly paradox of such exchanges would recur later in Polynesia, Australasia and Siberia when the disease pools of the Old World met the vulnerable gene pools of the New.[28] The ultimate reuniting of the human species had disastrous consequences for one-half of it. Figure 1.9 (p. 20) highlights the geographical relationship of human mobility and lifestyle to the historical spread of disease.

Renaissance Europe itself witnessed new diseases. These included syphilis and typhus.[18] Indeed syphilis affected the military, political and religious balance of 16th century Europe,[30] remaining an important cause of death until the mid-20th century. Typhus, 'a sleeping volcano', could erupt violently with every famine or military campaign stretching from the Thirty Years War to the Napoleonic wars and the First World War. With 20 million Russian victims, Lenin concluded that 'either socialism will defeat the louse or the louse will defeat socialism.'[20] During the Irish famine of 1848–51, 'famine fevers' may have killed up to 20% of the population[20] and these were spread by starving Irish migrants to severely affect mainland cities.

Epidemic disease coincided with the 19th century, mass, internal migration of peasants to increasingly industrialised and squalid cities. Cities amplify disease. For example, in the 19th century, Glasgow experienced 23 separate epidemics involving eight different diseases, four of which killed more than 1% of its population.[31,32] This palled, however, in comparison to the mortality from endemic urban diseases such as tuberculosis, pneumonia and diarrhoeal disease. The panic, induced by the then emerging disease cholera, imported four times into Britain between 1832 and 1866, proved to be a vital sanitary reformer by triggering the great era of public health reform.[33] The paramount 20th century pandemic was influenza in 1918–19 with a global mortality on a unique scale estimated at 23–40 million.[34] Since then, the conquest of many of the crowd diseases, through improved living conditions, immunisation and drug therapy has produced unprecedented levels of health, especially of children in the developed world. The question was posed: had we witnessed the rise and now the fall of the infectious diseases? Had the factors that promote disease so changed that populations, in the developed world anyway, would now be exempt from epidemics of new or resurgent diseases, at least on the scale of the last three millennia? A not unimportant question, but one which can only be answered speculatively and in generalities. While we cannot foretell the future, Lederberg has argued that 'we are intrinsically more vulnerable than before.'[35]

4. Factors underlying the emergence of disease

The processes by which the crowd diseases have emerged provide some limited answers. Many

factors underlay this process, in the past and present. Many of these persist and indeed have intensified. In a 'long look back to the future', Table 1.9 summarises the important themes: diseases by historical era, by increasing population size,[17] by changing human lifestyle or mobility, and by the scale of their impact.

The factors shown in Table 1.9 will now be analysed further, first in their historical then their modern context. Important themes will be emphasised in **bold** print.

LESSONS FROM BIOHISTORY

Disease is rarely random in activity. It relates profoundly to changes in the environment and in human behaviour, acting simultaneously or sequentially. The great underlying forces of demographic history have been biological: foodstuffs and famine, fertility and 'fevers' – in combination with the effects of climate change and human migration. For 95% of history humans were hunter-gatherers and gradually spread, in small nomadic groups, to all habitable continents during glaciations. Initially, humanity was too scattered to sustain crowd diseases. These emerged with the rise of pastoralism and farming. *Pastoralism*, originating in the Middle East, provided a disease bridge between humans and animals through the resultant extensive cross-species contact. Most crowd diseases have probably originated through species transfer from an animal source.[19,22] The biologist Evgeny Pavlovsky estimates that humans have acquired infections from about 300 domestic and 100 wild animals.[20] The difference in scale between them is surely significant. According to biologist Thomas Hull, these domesticated animals include dogs (65 diseases), sheep (46), cattle (45), pigs (42), horses (35), rodents (32), poultry (26) and others (20). *Farming* produced the critical population threshold for crowd disease, and the related development of urban settlements provided the paramount means of their amplification. Measles, for example, requires a host population of 500 000 people in contact, to sustain its circulation; first achieved only after 6000 BC. Measles probably originated either from bovine rinderpest or canine distemper through increased intimacy of animal contact and increasing settled human populations.

TABLE 1.9 Human population, mobility, lifestyle and disease (M, millions; B, billions)

Era	Global population	Mobility and lifestyle	Effect	Diseases	Scale
Pre-history	< 5 M	Nomadic humanity disperses	Limited	Animal/soil/insect based	Limited
Neolithic	5–50 M	Pastoral, isolated settlements	Species transfer	Crowd diseases emerge	Intense local epidemics
Classical	100–200 M	Urban; inter-regional contact	Old World spread	Smallpox, measles, plague	Population decline by $2/3$
Medieval/ Renaissance	300–400 M	Mongols, war, trade	Intense epidemics	Plague, syphilis, typhus	Population decline by $1/2$–$4/5$
Colonial	0.75–2 B	Humanity 're-unites'	New World (NW) spread	Smallpox, measles, etc.	Population decline in NW by $1/2$–$4/5$
Modern	2–6 B	Mass travel migration	Pandemic potential	New and old diseases	$1/3$ global deaths
Future	increase ? 11–30 B	Accelerating change	? Disease increase	Emerging/ re-emerging	Unknown

Cities are vulnerable to disease for internal and external reasons. Internally, they combine a maximum of exposure to disease through **poor hygiene and overcrowding** with a minimum of resistance caused by poor health, poor nutrition, pollution and 'urban stress.'[17] Externally connected, commercially and militarily, with other great population centres, they are subject to diseases which follow the trade routes such as the Silk Road and the Rhine valley. Thus, central to the emergence of the crowd diseases, beginning about 9000 BC and linked to the end of the Ice Age, was the revolutionary change in **human lifestyle**: from nomadic to pastoral, then to an urban type of existence.[19] A gardening metaphor neatly summarises this. Pastoralism brought the 'seeds' of new infection through species transfer of pathogens; farming provided, through population growth, sufficient human 'soil' to sustain these diseases; and cities were the ideal 'climate' for their further growth into perennial and ubiquitous threats. The neolithic revolution allowed large continental populations to develop but in complete biological isolation from each other. Their growing **contact** through trade and conflict had profound disease consequences. As McNeill states: 'Once civilisation has begun, the disease load that it harbours becomes one of the major weapons of its expansion.'[18] This phenomenon is reflected in the step-by-step intensification of disease as shown chronologically in Table 1.9. Here vulnerable populations were serially exposed to unfamiliar infections to produce so-called **virgin soil epidemics**. This phenomenon could be approaching some degree of stabilisation, although it is impossible to predict the future impact of any new infections. As new diseases continue to appear, the background to their emergence is now worthy of analysis.

THE DYNAMICS OF DISEASE EMERGENCE TODAY

In fundamentals similar to the past, the process is now more intricate and has additional new factors. Two elemental themes remain:

- **behaviour** – which means human activity in its widest sense
- **biology** – which concerns all life forms: human, animal, insect and the microbial worlds.

Figure 1.10 attempts to simplify the complexity of the many interacting influences, while still remaining comprehensive. The impact of the diverse consequences of population growth, urbanisation and ecological upset on factors such as human behaviour, lifestyle, susceptibility, and environmental and biological changes are listed in Figure 1.10. All these may influence both microbial adaptation and human vulnerability, so as to tip the balance towards the pathogen's advantage and thus result in emergent disease.

For many reasons microbes have remarkable powers to adapt, and to evolve new or intensified pathogenetic mechanisms, as part of their evolutionary survival strategies.[1]

The overarching human problem now, as in the past, is population growth.[4] This impacts on every aspect of disease dynamics, including human, environmental and biological factors. It is a remarkable fact, to reflect on, that the annual population increase now is as great as the total world population was at the time of Athens. Population growth took until AD 1800 to reach 1 billion. The last billion has taken just 6 years! In the last 25 years, global population has grown from 2.5 billion to 5.8 billion and will likely reach 8.6 billion in the next 25 years.

Growing populations must be fed, which profoundly affects the ecology and biology of rural environments; and housed, which increasingly means in overcrowded urban conurbations. Most of the global population increase is now focused in cities.[36] By AD 2000, 3 billion people, half the world's population, are expected to live in cities including about 25 megacities with populations exceeding 11 million people.[1] Urbanisation and its problems amplify many diseases:

- poor sanitation – gastrointestinal infections
- overcrowding – respiratory infections
- behaviour change – HIV and HCV infections
- ecological change – dengue and filariasis.

The sharing of intravenous devices is a current phenomenon unprecedented in human experience. As a public health threat, it is an incalculable one since we do not know what other diseases it may yet spawn. Our previous complacency about this threat may come back to increasingly haunt us.

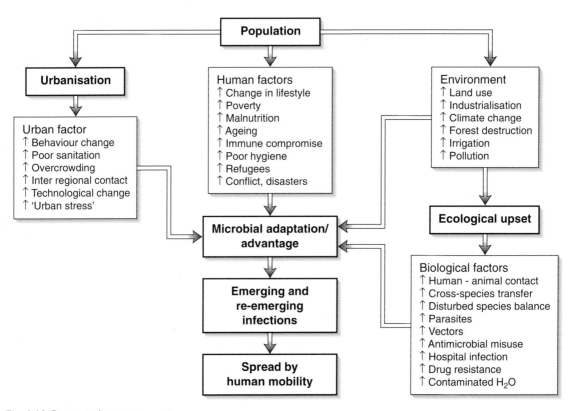

Fig. 1.10 Factors in disease emergence.

Ecological changes are accelerating. The impact of climate change has now, as in the past, profound biological implications. Among these may be an increase in vector and parasite burdens.[1] We may see various epidemics caused by diverse arboviruses, at least 100 of which can affect humans, and the highly fatal *Hantavirus* pulmonary syndrome. Some *Hantaviruses* may be evolving towards human-to-human transmissibility.[37] Disturbance of pristine ecosystems, such as tropical rain forests or savannah regions through deforestation and agriculture, has apparently led to outbreaks of Ebola, Lassa and Machupo virus infections.[38] Damming and/or pollution of environmental water have led to increases in cryptosporidiosis, cholera, schistosomiasis and mosquito-related diseases such as malaria, filariasis and Rift Valley fever.[1,38] Described as 'the destructive generation', humanity's effect on its environment, only since 1970 alone, includes: a doubling of wood and water consumption; an increase by 250% in carbon dioxide emissions; a decline by 50% in fresh water ecosystems; a decline by 30% in marine ecosystems; a decrease by 13% of the world's forest cover.[39] Human behaviour, by individuals, by groups and by nations, is central to all these many changes.

New elements have been added to the dynamics of disease emergence.[1] The vast use of antimicrobial drugs, not just in humans, but also in animal husbandry, has implications still to be grasped. Other technological changes must include those medical interventions that enhance the spread of blood-borne infections such as the hepatitis viruses and retroviruses.[1] Emerging food-borne diseases, a consequence of modern food production, are becoming increasingly a major public health concern.[5,13]

Wilson cogently argues that the world today is in a state of turbulence and rapid change.[40] Emergent diseases represent the instability and stress in the system which results from the unprecedented opportunities for mixing people, animals and microbes – in fact, diverse gene pools – from all geographical areas, in an environment altered by industry, technology, agriculture, chemicals, climate change and population growth. Clearly these new diseases are more readily spread by the increase in human travel and commerce.

5. Human mobility, travel and disease

Disease recognises no borders. It is spread by human – and animal – mobility. As Wilson further states: 'Travel is a potent force in the emergence of infectious disease.'[41] Human migration has been the pathway for disseminating infection throughout history (Fig. 1.11). It will so continue. Disease spread by the trade routes flourished particularly when and wherever war or famine occurred. McNeill has identified three major waves of disease linked to population movement as during: the Roman period, the period of the Mongol Empire and the era of European colonial exploration in the 15th–19th centuries. Their impact has already been described. Geographical seclusion entailed biological isolation, entrenching genetic vulnerability and leading to appalling epidemics when contact subsequently brought new diseases. Of course, the reverse can also hold true: it may be the visitor who is stricken. Some modern examples of disease and travel are shown in Table 1.10.[41]

Table 1.10 contains a broad mix of examples: diseases which are new or re-emerged; spread by trade or pilgrimage, animal export or public health breakdown; travel by air, ship or road; transmission by humans, animals or vectors. Travel today is unprecedented in its scale, impact, frequency, speed and distance travelled. Currently about 500 million people fly across international borders, while, in the early 1990s, about 20 million people were refugees and 30 million were displaced persons.[41] Thus, travel takes many forms: mass migration to escape danger, famine or poverty; economic trade by land, sea and air, which may include animals and other, uninvited, cargoes; warfare, conflict and military manoeuvres; pilgrimage, educational and altruistic visits; and the astonishing modern phenomenon of mass tourism. Travel, certainly in its modern, mass form, can significantly change environments and ecosystems. Travel may have biological consequences for the visitor, the visited and the return community. Humans are only part of the huge biomass that now criss-crosses our shrinking globe.[41]

This biology of travel is highlighted in Box 1.3. The disease consequence of travel may not be immediately apparent if the pathogen is not recognised or if it leads to chronic latent infection. Travel is also one of the signal means of spread of resistant, and multiresistant, pathogens and genes. Furthermore, travellers indulge more readily in permissive behaviours which may enhance the risk of acquiring and/or transmitting infection.

While humans may carry pathogens and their vectors, their transport or trade commodities may also be an unexpected source of disease. The recent, massive cholera epidemic in South America may have originated from a ship's bilge.[41] The huge trade in used Japanese tyres may have introduced, ominously for North America, the hardy tiger mosquito, *Aedes albopictus*, which can readily transmit dengue and yellow fever. Imported monkeys have introduced filoviruses: Marburg virus to Europe in 1967 and the Reston Ebola strain to America in 1990. The trade in animals, living or dead, for food, pets or research is increasing massively. It has caused much concern as reflected in the export ban on British cattle because of new

> **Box 1.3 The biology of travel: what may be imported to and from a destination**
>
> - Infected humans or animals
> - Pathogens
> - Vectors
> - Drug-resistant microbes
> - Virulence and resistance genes
> - Flora and fauna of biological significance
> - Risk behaviour
> - Genetic, medical and cultural vulnerability.

variant Creutzfeldt–Jakob disease. Other life forms accompany human travellers. Historically, rodents and insects alone have caused an unimaginable scale of death from all outbreaks of plague, malaria, typhus and yellow fever. These are old, enduring enemies. A new one is that of drug resistance.

After its appearance about 1945, penicillin resistance in the *Staphylococcus aureus* spread very rapidly around the world; although this has been slower for *Streptococcus pneumoniae* it is still widespread with rates as high as 60% in Spain, a favourite country for vacations. Multi-drug

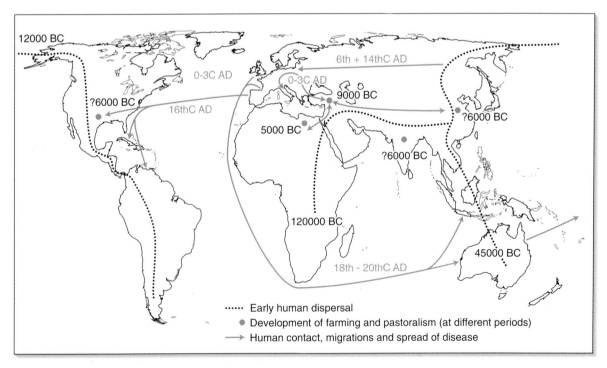

Fig. 1.11 Human mobility and disease: an historical geography.

TABLE 1.10 Recent examples of travel-associated spread of disease

What	Where	When	Comment
Group A meningococcus	Mecca	1987	By pilgrimage
Vibrio cholerae 01	S. America	1990	Probably by ship
Dengue haemorrhagic fever	Cuba	1981	By ship; ? by travellers
Diphtheria	Eastern Europe	1995	Contact with Russia
HIV-1	Global	1980s	Travel in and from Africa
New variant Creutzfeldt–Jakob disease	France	1980s	UK export of cattle

resistance reflects the epidemic of drug-resistant genes criss-crossing the world. Risky behaviour patterns may be introduced to, or acquired from, local populations. These patterns, perhaps sexual or drug-related, may be brought home with their associated diseases. As Luc Montaigne, the discoverer of HIV-1, has stated: 'the globalisation of culture means the globalisation of pathogens.' He described the 'vector' of HIV-1 as being the Boeing 747 aeroplane. Others have implicated the Trans-African Highway in changing the environment, mobility and behaviour patterns of Central Africans.

with greater success than in the past. As in the past, nevertheless, new diseases will continue to emerge. The last words, therefore, go to the Renaissance physician, Hieronymus Frascatorius of Verona.[30] Not only was he the first to give us the concept of microbes ('animalculi') in his book *De Contagionie* (1546), and the term syphilis from his famous poem 'syphilis sive Morbus Gallicus', but he also described the concept of emerging infections with the prediction: 'There will come yet other new and unusual ailments, as time brings them in its course...'

Conclusion

Infection is an inescapable reality of human existence and will continue to ebb and flow over time as new diseases emerge and old ones re-emerge. It is clear that human activity can have a profound impact on this process and may amplify the scale of any newly emergent disease. Travel is critical to the spread of such diseases. We all now live in the global village. The transfer of pathogens from one country to another is frequently quicker than the incubation period of their associated diseases. This is rendering border controls futile. There is thus the need to design an international policy and legal framework for the control of such emerging infections.[42]

The international health regulations, of such value in the past, are currently being revised by WHO. International law will undoubtedly play a role in this global strategy.[43] However, in the end we cannot escape disease. We can only try to limit it and minimise its consequences, and it is 'hoped'

REFERENCES

1. Lederberg J. Foreword. In Scheld WM, Armstrong D, Hughes JM, eds. Emerging infections. Washington DC: ASM Press; 1998.
2. Platt AE. Infecting ourselves: How environmental and social disruptions trigger disease. Worldwatch Paper 129, Washington DC; 1996.
3. World Health Organization. The World Health Report 1996. Fighting disease fostering development. Geneva: WHO; 1996.
4. Lederberg J, Shoape RE, Oaks SC Jr. Emerging infections: Microbial threats to health in the United States. Washington DC: National Academic Press; 1992.
5. Nakajima H. Editorial: Infectious diseases global alert, global response. World Health Organization 1997; 1: 3.
6. Shalala DE (US Secretary of Health). Collaboration in the fight against infectious diseases. Emerging Infectious Diseases 1998; 4: 354–357.
7. Pinner RW, Teutsch SM, Simonsen L et al. Trends in infectious diseases mortality in the United States. Journal of the American Medical Association 1996; 275: 189–193.
8. Centers for Disease Control and Prevention. HIV/AIDS Surveillance Report 1996; 8: 3–4, 30–33. Atlanta, Ga: Public Health Service.

9. Leader: 'Making sense of hepatitis C'. Lancet 1998; 352: 1485.

10. Centre for Disease Control and Prevention. Morbidity and Mortality Weekly Report 1993; 42.

11. Morse SS. 'Examining the origins of emerging viruses'. In Morse SE, ed. Emerging viruses. Oxford: Oxford University Press; 1993: 10–28.

12. Satcher D. Emerging infections: getting ahead of the curve. Emerging Infectious Diseases 1995; 1: 1–6.

13. Special issue on emerging foodborne pathogens. Emerging Infectious Diseases 1997; 3: 415–584.

14. Cohen ML. Epidemiology of drug resistance: implications for a post-antibiotic era. Science 1992; 257: 1050–1055.

15. Tenover FC, Hughes JM. The challenges of emerging infectious diseases: development and spread of multiple-resistant bacterial pathogens. Journal of the American Medical Association 1996; 275: 300–304.

16. Leader: 'Global paradox'. Lancet 1996; 348: 282.

17. McKeown T. The origin of human disease. Oxford; Blackwell; 1988: ch 2.

18. McNeill WH. Confluence of the civilised disease pools of europe: 500 BC to AD 1200. In: Plagues and peoples. London: Penguin; 1976: ch 3.

19. Cohen MN. The history of infectious diseases. In: Health and the rise of civilisation. New Haven: Yale Univesity Press; 1989: ch 4.

20. Karlen A. Revolution. In: Plague's progress: a social history of man and disease. London: Gollancz; 1995: ch 3.

21. Cockburn A. The evolution of human infectious diseases. In: Cockburn A, ed. Infectious diseases, their evolution and eradication. Springfield: Charles C Thomas; 1967.

22. Diamond J. Lethal gift of livestock. In: Guns, germs and steel. London: Cape; 1997.

23. Cartwright FF. Disease in the ancient world. In: Disease and history. London: Granada Publishing; 1972: ch 1.

24. Wills SC. Four tales from the new decameron. In: Plagues: their origin, history and future. London: Flamingo; 1997: ch 4.

25. Creighton C. Epidemics in Britain. London: Frank Cass; 1965 (first edition 1894).

26. Ziegler P. The toll in lives. In: The black death. Stroud: Alan Sutton; 1991: ch 14.

27. Hobson W. The black death. In: World health and history. Bristol: Wright; 1963: ch 3.

28. Crosby AW. Ecological imperialism: The biological expansion of Europe, 900–1900. Cambridge: Cambridge University Press; 1986.

29. McNeill WH. Trans-oceanic exchanges 1500–1700. In: Plagues and peoples. London: Penguin; 1976: ch 5.

30. Dubois R. The evolution of microbial diseases. In: Man adapting. New Haven: Yale University Press; 1965: ch 7.

31. Glaister J. The epidemic history of Glasgow during the century 1783–1883. Glasgow College Library, 1886.

32. Lees REM. Epidemic disease in Glasgow during the 19th century. Scottish Medical Journal 1996; 41: 74–77.

33. Brotherston J. Destitution and disease during the first half of the 19 C and the reform of the Poor Law. In: The early public health movement in Scotland. London: H K Lewis; 1952.

34. Collier R. The plague of the Spanish lady: the influenza pandemic of 1918–19. London: MacMillan; 1974.

35. Lederberg J. Infectious diseases as an evolutionary paradigm. Emerging infectious diseases 1977; 3: 417–423.

36. Krause RM. Emerging infections. San Diego: Academic Press; 1998.

37. Toro J, Vega JD, Khan AS et al. An outbreak of *Hantavirus* pulmonary syndrome, Chile, 1997. Emerging infectious diseases 1998; 4: 687–694.

38. Morse SM. Factors in the emergence of infectious diseases. Emerging infectious diseases 1995; 1: 7–15.

39. Denton P. The destructive generation. World Wildlife News Winter 1998/99; 3.

40. Wilson ME. Infectious diseases: an ecological perspective. British Medical Journal 1995; 311: 1681–1684.

41. Wilson ME. Travel and the emergence of infectious diseases. Emerging infectious diseases 1995; 1(2): 39–46.

42. Plotkin BJ, Kimball AM. Designing an international policy and legal framework for the control of emerging infectious diseases: first steps. Emerging infectious diseases 1997; 3(1): 1–9.

43. Fidler DP. Globalisation, international law and emerging infectious diseases. Emerging infectious diseases 1996; 2(2); 77–84.

Surveillance of travel-related illness

Eric Walker

Introduction

There are some basic principles involved in assessing the appropriate advice, immunisations and other prophylaxis to recommend for travellers. These include continually collecting data from host countries on the potential risks and balancing this against the intended itinerary of the traveller. Electronic communications are opening up new possibilities for both collecting and distributing this information. Changes to the processes involved in reporting outbreaks of international importance are underway within the World Health Organization, and these International Health Regulations are discussed.

Some terms used in travel medicine

SURVEILLANCE

Epidemiological surveillance in this context is the ongoing systematic collection, analysis, interpretation and dissemination of health data concerning travel-related illness. The aim is to allow an accurate assessment of the health risks for any particular traveller, or defined group of travellers, which in turn will allow more effective advice on prevention and management of travel-related illness.

　'Sentinel' surveillance collects data from designated centres or sources, representative of larger populations at risk, simplifying logistics and saving resources.

Surveillance can:
- Estimate the size of a health problem
- Detect outbreaks of disease
- Characterise disease trends
- Allow rational risk assessments in a clinical situation
- Evaluate interventions and preventive programmes
- Assist with health planning
- Identify research needs.

INCIDENCE

- **Incidence** is defined as the number of cases of a particular illness occurring in a defined group of travellers over a specific period of time.
- **Prevalence** is the number of cases present at a particular moment in time.

Do not confuse 'incidence' with 'prevalence'. If a disease is prevalent in a country, there may be a risk to travellers but it is only a crude estimate and does not normally take into account important lifestyle factors such as type of accommodation and duration of stay.

Incidence of travel-related diseases
- The number of cases of a disease occurring in a specified group of travellers over a defined period of time.
- Make sure you are actually talking about 'incidence', which must have a denominator.
- Never forget to define the denominator!

- Numerator: for example, the number of cases of illness that have occurred in the group being studied over a defined period of time.

- Denominator: for example, the number of travellers in the group being studied.

Both the numerators and the denominators can be further refined, for example, to include only those undertaking a particular type of trip such as a package holiday or backpacking; or only those with a pre-existing health problem such as diabetes mellitus.

RISK ASSESSMENT (see also Ch. 4)

This is the attempt, usually in a clinical situation, to evaluate and quantify the health risk(s) for a particular traveller. It depends upon using a combination of numerator and denominator data, mathematics and personal judgement.

- Risk assessment is complicated and inevitably has to be flexible because often travellers vary their plans while abroad.
- Risk analysis is **not** a static process and in most instances needs to be continually revised, as new information becomes available.
- The aim of risk assessment is that it should be 'evidence based'.

Advice based on personal anecdotes, or unrepresentative incidence studies, has often led to travel health advice being far from ideal. Frequently such advice is passed on from book to book, or chart to chart, with a minimum of updating and no obvious reference to the original source of information.

THE HEALTH RISK TO TRAVELLERS IS NOT NECESSARILY THE SAME AS FOR LOCALS WITHIN THE HOST COUNTRY

Data confined to the prevalence or incidence of diseases among local residents in a particular host country are not usually sufficient alone to make a useful risk assessment for travellers, because their intended lifestyle and immune status often differs from that of the local population.

Good accommodation may reduce the incidence of food and water-borne diseases but lack of acquired immunity may make them more vulnerable, for example, to hepatitis A.

It is important to look in detail at the illnesses experienced by different categories of traveller (e.g. package tourists, business travellers, and backpackers), going to specific destinations, carrying out different types of activities and staying for varying periods of time.

Prompt and accurate diagnosis of illness in the returned traveller also depends upon the attending doctor's up-to-date knowledge of travel-related diseases and current risk areas.

Making use of surveillance data

Once a process is established for collecting data, the next stage of surveillance is collating the data, studying trends, looking for causes, identifying 'emerging or re-emerging' infections and using the information to make health risk assessments for the travellers.

DENOMINATORS

Denominators are essential before any useful conclusions or recommendations can be made (i.e. the numbers of travellers potentially at risk of the particular disease being studied). They are often neglected or poorly defined, particularly by the media. Totals of those travelling abroad worldwide (Table 2.1) or those leaving the UK for particular countries (Figs 2.1 and 2.2) can sometimes be used as a broad estimate, as taken from data supplied by the UK Central Statistical Office on a quarterly basis.

TABLE 2.1 International travel (millions) (data from the Central Statistical Office)

	1960	1970	1980	1990	2000
International travellers worldwide	69	160	285	429	670 (estimate)
Trips abroad from the UK	6	12	17	31	50 (estimate)

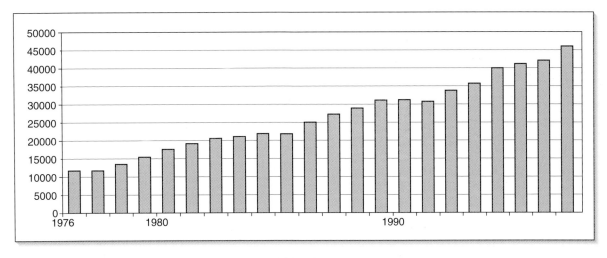

Fig. 2.1 Annual totals of travellers going abroad from the UK (1976–7).

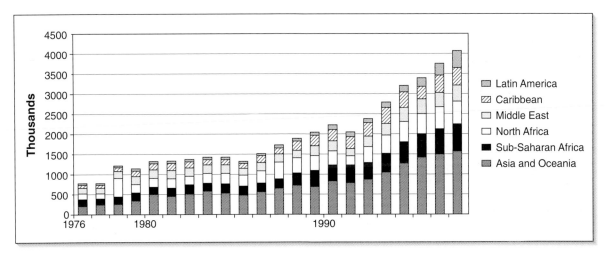

Fig. 2.2 Travellers from the UK going to areas with greater risk of infection.

More specific denominators are often needed. Examples are:

- 'The number of package tourists travelling to Kenya for less than 3 weeks', when looking at the effectiveness of malaria prophylaxis in this particular group of travellers.
- 'The number of children under 1 year of age living for more than 6 months in a rural tropical environment', when looking at the incidence of diarrhoea in this age group under these circumstances.

NUMERATORS

The following are some examples of how 'numerator' data can be collected.

Illness occurring after return in the traveller's home country

Recording 'imported infection' can be a useful way of studying trends and assessing potential risk to the public 'at home' from cross-infection. It must be remembered that imported illness does **not** include illnesses occurring abroad, often because of a short incubation period, such as influenza, cholera or dengue. Neither does 'imported illness' include illnesses such as malaria occurring overseas in longer-term travellers such as expatriates, backpackers and volunteer groups.

Statutory notifications

Statutory (legally required) notifications in the UK do not distinguish those infections contracted at home from those contracted abroad. Malaria, diphtheria or tick typhus are likely to have been acquired overseas but infections common in the UK such as hepatitis A, food poisoning or *shigella* dysentery may well have been contracted abroad.

Laboratory reports

These provide useful information on travel-related illnesses but only for those where laboratory investigations are frequently requested such as diarrhoea illnesses and malaria. Reference Laboratories by the nature of their special interest have a particular role in surveying imported disease. These may include data from reference laboratories for parasitology, *Legionella*, malaria

and potentially dangerous pathogens causing viral haemorrhagic fevers. Annual incidence figures, the month of onset of travel-related illnesses and the age of those affected can, for example, be estimated using laboratory reports.

Table 2.2 shows that there has been a progressive increase in the number of cases of 'imported' *Plasmodium falciparum* malaria over this 6-year period. Extra information provided from the laboratories showed that most 'imported' *Plasmodium falciparum* was contracted in sub-Saharan Africa (Nigeria, Ghana and Kenya) and most *Plasmodium vivax* malaria in Asia (India or Pakistan). These figures do not show the total annual incidence of malaria in UK travellers since many cases occur while the travellers are overseas.

Figure 2.3 shows how the date when laboratory tests are requested can provide a rough estimate of the time of onset of illness. It has to be presumed that the tests are usually performed when symptoms first appear. These figures relate to Scotland and are heavily 'weighted' towards diarrhoeal illnesses since they are so common and often result in a stool sample being sent to the laboratory. The peak incidence coincides with the summer holiday period and most illnesses are contracted in popular holiday destinations such as Spain.

Figure 2.4 shows imported infections occur most commonly in those between 20 and 30 years; the age at which backpacking and perhaps inexperience in taking appropriate preventive precautions is common among young people.

Box 2.1 Statutory notifications of infectious disease in Scotland

(Notification data from the Information Services Division of the Common Services Agency as supplied by Health Boards)

There were no cases reported between 1995 and 1998 of infections in italics that are usually travel-related. Notifications do not record whether an infection is imported.

Anthrax; Bacillary dysentery; Chickenpox; Cholera; *Continued fever*; *Diphtheria*; Erysipelas; Food poisoning; Legionellosis; Leptospirosis; Lyme disease; *Malaria*; Measles; Meningococcal infection; Mumps; Paratyphoid fever; *Plague*; *Poliomyelitis*; Puerperal fever; *Rabies*; Relapsing fever; Rubella; Scarlet fever; *Smallpox*; *Tetanus*; Toxoplasmosis; Tuberculosis; Typhoid fever; Tick typhus; *Viral haemorrhagic fever*; Viral hepatitis; Whooping cough

---

TABLE 2.2 Annual incidence of malaria in the UK (data from the UK Malaria Reference Laboratory surveillance scheme)

	1992	1993	1994	1995	1996	1997
Plasmodium falciparum	900	1048	1178	1112	1283	1401
Plasmodium vivax	532	708	501	742	1014	790
Other species	138	116	208	201	203	173
Totals	1570	1872	1887	2055	2500	2364
Deaths	11	5	11	4	11	13

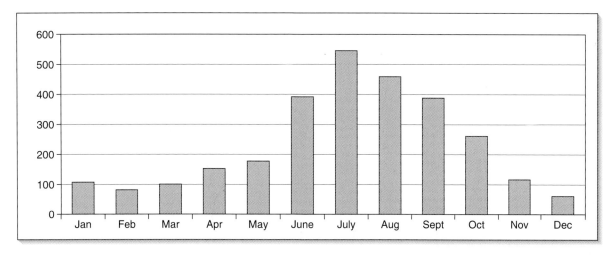

Fig. 2.3 Month of onset of infections contracted abroad (3047 cases between 1992 and 1996 inclusive as reported by Consultants in Public Health Medicine).

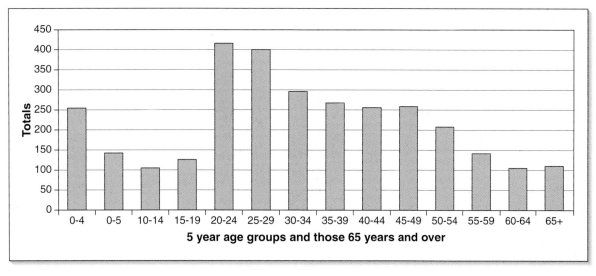

Fig. 2.4 Age of travellers contracting infection abroad (3047 cases between 1992 and 1996 inclusive as reported by Consultants in Public Health Medicine).

The peak in those under 4 years of age probably reflects the greater likelihood that investigations (e.g. stool cultures) were instituted for these children rather than this age group contracting more infections. It is not possible to conclude from this data that infections were more common in these age groups without knowing how many actual travellers there were in each age group (i.e. the denominator).

Identifying changing trends in incidence of travel-related illness

Comparing totals of actual with expected cases can follow trends in the incidence of imported infections. The denominator used here is the estimated number of travellers leaving the home country to go to 'risk' areas taken from data supplied by the UK Central Statistical Office as described above.

Figures 2.5 and 2.6 show that the incidence of hepatitis A and malaria has declined in recent years in relation to the numbers of travellers at risk. This can be due to factors such as better accommodation provided by the tour operators (e.g. with safer food and water), and improved personal precautionary measures including chemoprophylaxis (e.g. against malaria) and vaccination (e.g. for hepatitis A).

Sentinel surveillance of travel-related illness

While laboratory reports may record a recent overseas travel history, it is clear that in many instances the travel association is missed. This may be because the travel history is not mentioned on the investigation request form or not confirmed by the reporting laboratory. Also many travel-related illnesses do not result in a laboratory-

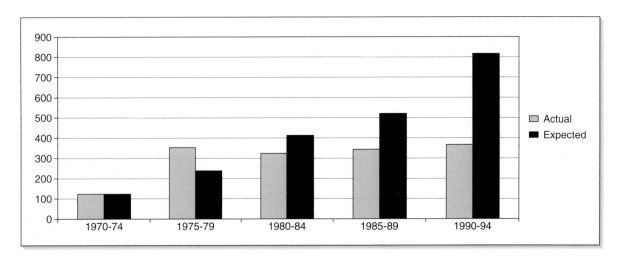

Fig. 2.5 Actual and expected cases of malaria occurring in Scotland from the baseline of the 5-year period 1970–4.

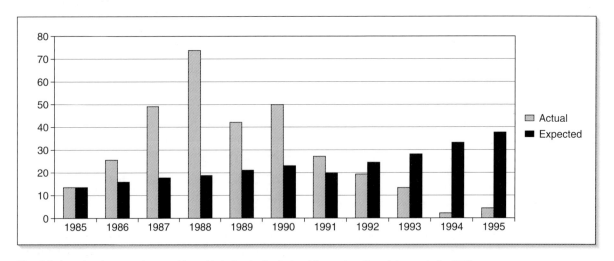

Fig. 2.6 Actual and expected cases of hepatitis in Scotland calculated from a baseline of the totals for 1985.

confirmed diagnosis. This can occur when a firm diagnosis has been possible based solely on the history or examination of the patient or when laboratory confirmation has not been considered necessary (e.g. in influenza, self-limiting diarrhoea or skin infections such as cutaneous larva migrans). Another limitation of laboratory-based surveillance for infections is that treatment may have been administered prior to the laboratory sample being collected, preventing successful culture.

It is therefore becoming increasingly important to document travel-related illnesses, based on symptoms, to complement data from laboratory reports. Initial reporting to the World Health Organization of infections of public health importance, under the International Health Regulations, is soon to be based on major symptoms or syndromes.

This clinical information can be gathered, for example, in collaboration with clinicians in Infectious and Tropical Disease units who see returning travellers. Basic details are recorded of any illness thought to have originated in an overseas country. These details include the country from where the infection is thought to have originated, any confirmed diagnosis and if there is no confirmed diagnosis, the predominant symptom(s). Further details can be obtained later if necessary.

International Health Regulations:

- Currently require notification of a few selected diseases (cholera, plague, yellow fever).
- Will require notification of 'disease syndromes' of international importance (haemorrhagic fevers, diarrhoea, jaundice, respiratory and neurological illnesses).

---

awaiting laboratory verification of the causative agents.

Other sources of information about travel-related illness

FEEDBACK FROM USERS OF PRE-TRAVEL ADVISORY SERVICES

This is an important source of information that can provide advance notice from travellers or their relatives about outbreaks of disease and other health issues abroad causing concern. This information can be reported and confirmed if necessary, through international contacts and the World Health Organization.

RECORDING ILLNESS EXPERIENCED BY DEFINED GROUPS OF TRAVELLERS SUCH AS VOLUNTEERS OR EXPATRIATES

When travellers in these distinct categories can be identified, they may have a medical 'check-up' after return or be asked to return a questionnaire. This is often the only way of determining details about illness occurring while the traveller is actually overseas.

SURVEILLANCE WITHIN GENERAL PRACTICE

This can provide invaluable information about less severe illnesses not requiring hospital referral or laboratory investigations.

International Health Regulations (IHR)

These require World Health Organization member states to notify diseases of international importance: currently (1998) plague, cholera and yellow fever. However, the regulations are being revised to emphasise the importance of notifying all disease outbreaks of immediate international importance. Electronic reporting of specific clinical syndromes should help countries to report more immediately. This, it is hoped, will facilitate a more rapid alert to a potential problem and an appropriate international response while

Emerging and re-emerging infections (see also Ch. 1)

Figure 2.7 shows schematically how the various specialities involved in understanding and in managing travel-related disease interrelate. At different stages in our understanding of a disease and in its control, different disciplines predominate. Note the important arrow to the left of the figure symbolising re-emergence of disease when control mechanisms fail (e.g. owing to economic factors, wars and migration and apathy) and the top, left-hand circle which symbolises the recognition of a newly recognised problem (e.g. HIV infection).

Emerging and re-emerging infection is a relatively new term which describes the continually changing patterns of communicable disease which occur, for example, as the result of the capacity of microorganisms to adapt and change and of human interventions, such as immunisations or the use of antibiotics.

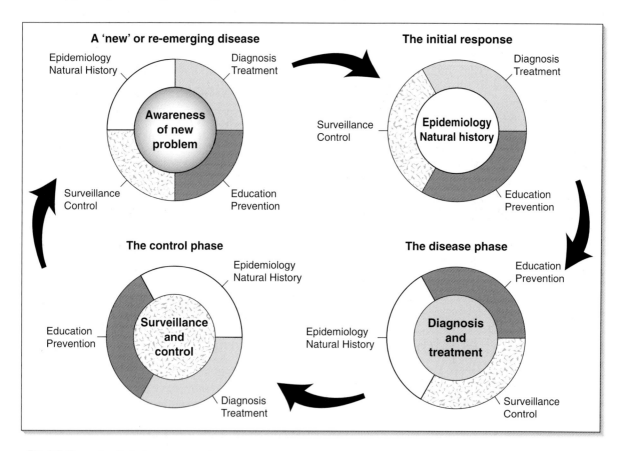

Fig. 2.7 The cycle of infection management.

Examples of 'emerging and re-emerging infections' that have recently caused international concern

Plague in north-west India (February 1995)
This had a serious impact on travel to India although in the event no related cases occurred outside India itself and few outside the affected towns. Precautions were established in many other countries for the containment of any possible imported cases. General practitioners in the UK were advised on the need for vigilance and prompt referral.

Examples of 'emerging and re-emerging infections' that have recently caused international concern *cont'd*

Ebola fever in Zaire (May 1995); Gabon (October 1996); South Africa (November 1996)
Unlike plague, there is no specific treatment for this usually fatal disease. Fortunately, there is less international travel between other countries and Zaire. A less publicised outbreak in Gabon had continued through into 1997. It was concluded that sufferers were unlikely to be able to travel if they had reached an infectious phase of the illness. However, there was the possibility of people arriving during the incubation phases.
In the UK, extracts from the Department of Health's Memorandum on the Control of Viral Haemorrhagic Fevers were distributed to consultants in public health medicine and infectious diseases, general practitioners and port authorities.
Although no possible imported cases were identified, considerable effort was put into contingency planning for future, similar outbreaks. A secondary case occurred in South Africa, which then caused illness in a healthcare worker.

Dengue in India (November 1996)
A large outbreak of dengue in Delhi during 1996 focused attention on the recent spread of this potentially serious disease throughout many parts of Asia and the need for travellers to avoid mosquito bites in the absence of an effective vaccine. A smaller outbreak occurred again in 1997 and a pattern is emerging of annual epidemics in northern India.

Meningococcal infection in the Balearic Islands of Spain (July 1996)
Several cases and small clusters of meningococcal infection occurred in tourists to Spain and there were fears that serious outbreaks might occur in the large numbers of people in close contact with each other in the resorts. The strains involved were not of type A associated with epidemics in Africa. Prophylaxis was offered to those in a hotel complex. Attention was drawn to the potential for spread in large hotels, where people, for example, frequent bars and clubs.

Multi-drug-resistant tuberculosis on a long haul air flight (March 1997)
A traveller on a flight from North America to the UK was found to have been shedding multi-drug resistant *Mycobacterium*. A major, contact tracing exercise was carried out and a number of fellow passengers who had been in seats close to the index case were thought to have been infected. The possible transmission of infections in aircraft is an issue which is gaining increasing attention.

Typhoid in tourists to the Dominican Republic (August 1997)
An outbreak of enteric infections, including typhoid, in tourists resulted in a major British tour company temporarily suspending its package holidays. Tour companies have become increasingly involved in protecting the health of their clients following a directive of the European Community on Travellers' Health.

Influenza H5N1 in Hong Kong (December 1997)
Towards the end of 1997, human cases caused by this strain of influenza, which had been known to be present in poultry for several decades, appeared in Hong Kong. All poultry flocks in Hong Kong were eventually destroyed. However, while there was no convincing evidence of human to human transmission, if this had occurred there would have been concern regarding the possibility of a major pandemic. There was intense international interest and support for the HongKong authorities and regular reports of the current situation were published on the Internet.

Enterovirus type 71 in Taiwan (May 1998)
A major outbreak occurred with an estimated 3–500 000 people affected, mostly children. There were around 50 deaths in infants, mostly from meningo-encephalitis. While few authorities advised avoiding travel to Taiwan, advice was given to travellers about personal hygiene (enteroviruses are spread through the faecal–oral route) and that it may be wise to avoid exposing very young children to crowded situations such as playgroups until the epidemic subsided.

Distribution of information

TRADITIONAL METHODS

There are many ways in which information can be distributed to those advising travellers, caring for those with travel-related illness and involved in health planning. In the UK, for example, there are national committees that meet to determine the best general advice, vaccination advice and recommendations for appropriate malaria prophylaxis. Recommendations traditionally are published in books and information charts.

ONLINE COMPUTERISED DATABASES

These have the potential to allow the results of surveillance to be immediately available, for example, to those involved in providing travel health advice, health care and in planning services. This dissemination increasingly now makes use of continually updated databases on the Internet.

Online computerised databases:
- Speed up data collection
- Allow immediate updating
- New information is rapidly available for:
  the travelling public
  travel health advisers
  clinicians managing travel-related illness
  public health and healthcare planners.

PRACTICE POINTS

- Surveillance is the ongoing collection, analysis and distribution of up-to-date accurate information.
- Epidemiology is the ongoing study of diseases and outbreaks, including emerging and re-emerging infections.

  These are the scientific disciplines that allow sound risk assessments to be made. **Ignore them at your peril!**

FURTHER READING

Benenson AS, ed. Control of communicable disease in man. Washington: American Public Health Association; 1998.

Cook GC, ed. Manson's tropical diseases. 20th ed. London: WB Saunders; 1996.

Walker E, Calvert L, Raeside F, Wilson E. The changing incidence of malaria and hepatitis A in Scotland. In: Proceedings of the 5th Conference of the International Society of Travel Medicine. Geneva; 1997. International Society of Travel Medicine, PO Box 871089, Stone Mountain, GA 30087–0028, USA.

World Health Organization. International travel and health. Geneva: World Health Organization (updated annually).

Sources of information for travel health advisers

Eric Walker

Introduction

Good sources of advice both for the public and healthcare advisers are available but can quickly become out of date and may be inconsistent. This chapter explores some of the available sources of information and tries to help the reader to evaluate their role.

Introduction

There are numerous sources of advice for travellers and their advisers including strictly practical needs such as visa requirements, suitable transport and accommodation arrangements. Essential advice on staying healthy is less easy to define, because the needs of individual travellers can vary greatly according to their itinerary, and previous travel experience. There may be an enormous range of potential health risks depending not only on the travellers' intended destination(s) but also upon intended lifestyle, regional and seasonal differences in incidence of disease, and the possibility of local epidemics of disease. (See also Chapter 4 on Risk assessment.)

One difficulty is a shortage of accurate, up-to-date information as to actual health risks which is hardly surprising when it is considered that travel involves virtually every part of the world. It is difficult enough to quantify risks within a small country such as the UK. The understandable consequence is that much travel advice revolves around personal reminiscences and theoretical risks, sometimes based on studies done many decades previously, and circumstances that may not now be comparable. There is a shortage within travel medicine of reliable and ongoing surveillance and of epidemiological research – one reason for the need for academic courses in travel medicine. (See also Surveillance of travel-related diseases.)

International Society of Travel Medicine (ISTM)

The ISTM is committed to address health problems encountered by travellers, supporting high standards of travel medicine practice, research and publications, education and exchange of information between professionals at an international level. The biennial ISTM conference is the largest, regular, travel medicine conference, with leading experts in attendance.

The society produces a quarterly journal, 'The International Journal of Travel Medicine', and a quarterly 'NewsShare'.

Secretariat: International Society of Travel Medicine, PO Box 871089, Stone Mountain, Georgia 30087-0028, USA. *Tel*: (770) 736-7060; *Fax*: (770) 736-6732. E-mail: bcbistm@aol.com

'Official' and government sources of advice

WORLD HEALTH ORGANIZATION

International Travel and Health, Vaccination Requirements and Health Advice (the 'Yellow Book') is produced yearly with updates included in the WHO Weekly Epidemiological Record (available from HM Stationery Office). This lists compulsory immunisations and the risk of malaria by country and gives the distribution by geographical area of other health risks and appropriate preventive advice. It is aimed particularly at national health administrations and specialised advice centres.

NATIONAL PUBLICATIONS

Many countries produce their own regularly updated booklets on health advice for travellers.

- Costs and charges. The 'Red Book' gives information on remuneration and costings within the UK National Health Service.
- *Immunisation against Infectious Disease* (the 'Green Book' available from HMSO). The Department of Health in England (DOH), the Welsh Office and Scottish Home and Health Department in the UK. It is a very useful source of reference and new editions are produced approximately every 3 years.
- T6 leaflet *Health Advice for Travellers* (available free from Post Offices) is updated annually and contains advice on reducing health risks and a simple list, by country, of compulsory and recommended immunisations. It advises about travel insurance and entitlement to medical treatment at reduced cost, and explains how to obtain an application for certificate E111 (which entitles nationals of the European Community to care in other member states).
- TravelSafe, a leaflet for the public specifically related to avoidance of sexually transmitted disease, including HIV infection, is available from the British Health Education Council.

Travel medicine societies and associations

BRITISH TRAVEL HEALTH ASSOCIATION (BTHA)

Founded in 1998, this association already has 800 members. It organises national scientific conferences and publishes a newsletter. The association's aims include support and education for the health adviser, establishing guidelines and setting standards, and developing education and research initiatives. It relates closely to the ISTM.

Secretariat: BTHA, The Scottish Centre for Infection and Environmental Health (SCIEH), Clifton House, Clifton Place, Glasgow, G3 7LN. *Tel*: 0141 300 1100.

THE ROYAL COLLEGE OF NURSING TRAVEL HEALTH SPECIAL INTEREST GROUP

This is a UK based group of nurses representing a variety of nursing disciplines involved in travel health. The group welcomes applicants from overseas, although its value to overseas members is limited. To join the group contact: The Royal College of Nursing, 20 Cavendish Square, London, W1M 0AB. *Tel*: 0207 409 3333; *Fax*: 0207 335 1379.

IN EUROPE

At the time of writing Denmark, France and the Republic of Ireland also have Travel Medicine Societies.

Travel medicine databases within the UK

There are two online databases and one 'disc-based' system available in the UK. As more health centres make use of electronic-based sources of information, these should increasingly become the 'first port of call' for practitioners looking for up-to-date information.

Online databases have the advantage of updating in 'real time' and information should also be easily printed out in a usable form as information sheets.

- MASTA (Medical Advisory Service for Travellers Abroad) is an online, commercial service mainly used by British Airways Travel Clinics and Occupational Health Departments. *Tel*: 0207 631 4408

- TRAVAX is a National Health Service database available on the Internet and also through the NHS Net from the Scottish Centre for Infection and Environmental Health. *Tel*: 0141 300 1130
- TRAVELLER is also a commercial service distributed on floppy disk which is distributed periodically to general practitioners and provided by Pro Choice Applications Ltd. *Tel*: 0114 285 4443.

SCIEH and MASTA also provide printed materials

- Medical Advisory Service for Travellers Abroad. *Tel*: 01705 553 933.
- Newstel and the Scottish Centre for Infection and Environmental Health. *Tel*: 090655 00059.

AUTOMATED TELEPHONE ADVICE SERVICES

Recorded message answering services in the UK are aimed primarily at the travelling public:

- Hospital for Tropical Diseases in London. *Tel*: 0891 600 350
- Liverpool School of Tropical Medicine. *Tel*: 0898 345081
- Malaria Reference Laboratory. *Tel*: 0207 927 2437.

Specialist travel medicine centres in the UK

The following provide expert advice to healthcare professionals who are having difficulties making decisions about their patients' requirements:

- Department of Communicable and Tropical Disease, Birmingham Heartland Hospital, Bordersley Green Road, Birmingham, B9 5ST. *Tel*: 0121 766 6611
- Department of Infectious Diseases and Tropical Medicine, Monsall Hospital, Manchester, M10 8WR. *Tel*: 0161 205 2393
- Hospital for Tropical Diseases, 180–182 Tottenham Court Road, London, W1P 9LE. *Tel*: 0207 637 9899

- Liverpool School of Tropical Medicine, Pembroke Place, Liverpool, L3 5QA. *Tel*: 0151 708 9393
- Infectious Diseases Unit, Belvoir Park Hospital, Hospital Road, Belfast, BT8 8JR. *Tel*: 01232 491942
- PHLS Communicable Disease Surveillance Unit, 61 Colindale Avenue, London, NW9 5EQ. *Tel*: 0208 200 6868
- Scottish Centre for Infection and Environmental Health, Clifton House, Clifton Place, Glasgow, G3 7LN. *Tel*: 0141 300 1130.

Travel clinics in the UK

CLINICS IN GENERAL PRACTICE

A number of general practitioners within the National Health Service run travel clinics both for their own patients and for referrals from neighbouring practices.

HOSPITAL-BASED CLINICS

There are some specialised travel medicine clinics within the National Health Service based within Infectious and Tropical Diseases Units – these are more common in Scotland. The London Hospital for Tropical Diseases and the Liverpool School of Tropical Medicine hold regular travel clinics.

PRIVATE TRAVEL CLINICS

These include those provided by British Airways and the travel agency, Trailfinders.

Scientific journals

- *The International Journal of Travel Medicine* and a quarterly *NewsShare* are published by the International Society of Travel Medicine (see above).
- *Travel Medicine International* is available quarterly by subscription. Contact: Mark Allen Publishing Ltd, Croxted Mews, 288 Croxted Road, London, SE24 9DA. *Tel*: 0208 671 7521.

Popular 'magazines'

- *Lonely Planet* is a useful, free, quarterly newsletter available from Lonely Planet Publications, The Barley Mow Centre, 10 Barley Mow Passage, Aiswick, London, W4 4PH.
- *Practice Nurse*, *Pulse* and *General Practitioner*, available in the UK, publish charts, listing recommended and compulsory immunisations and give malaria advice.
- *Travelling Healthy – Health Advice for the Global Traveller* is published bi-monthly and is available on subscription from: Travelling Healthy, 108-48 70th Road, Forest Hills, New York 11375.
  E-mail: travelhealth @ aol.com.

Travel agents

Travel agents increasingly have a legal responsibility to make clients aware of potential health risks and any immigration requirements (e.g. The European Directive (90/314/EEC; Art.3, e) on package travel, package holidays and package tours). However, they understandably do not normally highlight health risks as they do other aspects of holidays. Directories, available to the travel trade, giving information on visa requirements, recommended immunisations, currency and customs allowances, and climate, include:

- *The ABC Guide to International Travel*, published quarterly
- *The Travel Information Manual*, published monthly by the International Air Transport Association
- *The World Travel Guide*.

Travel agents will readily pass on information from these sources but it may be out of date and they are not trained to interpret risks for individual travellers, so the advice tends to be dogmatic and frequently focuses only on 'legal' immigration requirements.

Pharmaceutical publications and companies

The *Monthly Index of Medical Specialities* (MIMS) and *British National Formulary* (BNF) contain useful information. These are readily available and are regularly updated, but owing to conciseness, they tend to be inflexible in relation to a traveller's lifestyle.

Pharmaceutical companies also provide customer support lines.

- Medeva Pharma. Vaccine Advice Line, Regent Park, Kingston Road, Leatherhead, KT22 7PQ. *Tel*: 01625 537607
- Pasteur Merieux MSD Information Service, Clivemont House, Clivemont Road, Maidenhead, Berks, SL6 7BU. *Tel*: 01628 773737. This line provides general advice specifically for travel advisers.
- SmithKline Beecham Pharmaceuticals, Medical Information Department, Mundells, Welwyn Garden City, Herts, AL7 1EY (SB Products only). *Tel*(Freephone): 0800 616482.

Literature for healthcare professionals

- *ABC of Healthy Travel*. Walker E, Williams GR, Raeside F, Calvert L (1997, 5th ed). British Medical Journal. ISBN: 0727911384. This book gives a comprehensive overview of travel advice for healthcare professionals.
- *British National Formulary*. British Medical Association and Royal Pharmaceutical Society (6-monthly). ISBN: 0853692563. One of the essential desktop books for those prescribing drugs and vaccines in the UK.
- *Colour Atlas of Tropical Medicine and Parasitology*. Peters W, Gilles HM (1995). Wolfe Medical. ISBN: 0723420696. A colourful and informative book. More comprehensive information than usual from an 'atlas'.

- *Control of Communicable Disease in Man.* Benenson AS (1995) American Public Health Association. ISBN: 087553077X. An invaluable source of reference on common and unusual infections published by the American Public Health Association.
- *Health Information for International Travel.* International Medical Publishing Inc. Center for Disease Control and Prevention (Atlanta, USA) ISBN: 1883205336. The equivalent of the UK Department of Health's 'Green Book'. An essential source of reference for those working in the USA and useful elsewhere.
- *Health, Hazard and the Higher Risk Traveller.* McIntosh I (1993). Quay Books. ISBN: 1856420817. One of the few books on this subject and very readable.
- *Immunisation against Infectious Diseases.* (The 'Green Book'). Published by HMSO for the Joint Committee on Vaccination and Immunisation. ISBN: 011321815X. Detailed information on vaccines, administration and associated problems. New edition roughly every 3 years.
- *Immunisation: Precautions and Contraindications.* Kassianos GC (1998). Blackwell Science. ISBN: 0865428875. A useful basic guide to the different immunisations available. Special section on travel.
- *International Travel and Health – Vaccination requirements and Health advice.* World Health Organization. ISBN: 9241580208. This book is available in the UK from HMSO and published annually. It contains details of international health regulations and regional details on rabies, malaria and drug resistance as well as a lot of other useful information.
- *Lecture Notes on Tropical Diseases.* Bell DR (1990). Blackwell Science. ISBN: 0632024550. An excellent introduction to tropical diseases – clinical aspects and prevention
- *Manson's Tropical Diseases.* Cook GC et al. Saunders. ISBN: 0702017647. An invaluable detailed resource on tropical diseases, providing answers to difficult questions.
- *Medicine for Mountaineering and other Wilderness Activities.* Wilkerson J. (1992,3rd ed). ISBN: 0898863317. A comprehensive reference book for the more adventurous mountaineers and

useful also for healthcare professionals.
- *MIMS (Monthly Index of Medical Specialities).* Haymarket Medical. *Tel*: 0171 938 0705. Regularly updated lists of medical products available in the UK. Special section on travel vaccines and malaria prophylaxis.
- *Textbook of Travel Health.* Dupont H, Steffen R (1997). Decker. ISBN: 1550090372. A multi-author, comprehensive textbook written by an international group of authors, predominantly members of the International Society of Travel Medicine. Also available on CD.
- *The Travel and Tropical Health Manual.* Jong EC, McMullen R (1995). Saunders. ISBN: 0721642144. A multi-author manual from the USA. Crammed with information and a useful source of reference. Focus not confined to the North American reader.
- *Your Child's Health Abroad.* Wilson-Howarth J, Ellis M (1998). Braht Publications. ISBN: 1898323631. A comprehensive account of problems facing child travellers and their parents. Useful for both the traveller and their advisers.

Literature for travellers

- *Bugs, Bites and Bowels.* Howarth J (1995). Globe Pequot. ISBN: 0860110452. An informed chatty book based on personal experience.
- *Flying – No Fear.* Akers-Douglas A, Georgiou G (1996). ISBN: 1840240067. Includes details of courses and tapes and has useful references.
- *Good Health, Good Travel* (previously *Healthy beyond Heathrow*). Lankester T (1993). Interhealth. ISBN: 0952164000. Especially useful health guide for volunteers and long-term expatriates working overseas.
- *Health Advice for Travellers* (currently called the T6 leaflet). It is updated annually by the UK Department of Health. Available free in Post Offices, it contains some general information, legally required and recommended vaccines for different countries, reciprocal health agreements and an E111 application form for travel 'insurance' in other countries in the European Union.

- *Jetlag – How to Beat It*. O'Connell D (1997). Ascendant Publishing. ISBN: 0953134504. One of the very few comprehensive books on this subject.
- Medicine for Mountaineering. Wilkerson J (1992, 3rd ed). ISBN: 0898863317. For the more adventurous mountaineers and useful also for healthcare professionals.
- *Mountaineering First Aid*. Carline JD, et al (1996, 4th ed). ISBN: 089886478X. An excellent practical guide to first-aid, injuries and environmental problems such as hypothermia, dehydration and acute mountain sickness.
- *Nothing Ventured – Disabled People Travel the World*. Walsh A (1991). Harrap Columbus. ISBN: 0747102082. An invaluable series of reminiscences by disabled travellers on problems and pleasures encountered.
- The *Rough Guide* series. Various authors and dates. Harrap Columbus. Travel guides aimed at the adventurous traveller. They contain some health information of varying quality.
- *Travel in Health*. Fry (1994). International Safari Health. ISBN: 0952293900. Aimed at the traveller, an easily read and accurate commonsense guide.
- *Traveller's Health – How to Stay Healthy Abroad*. Dawood R (1992). Oxford University Press. ISBN: 0192618318. Useful for the traveller who wants to be well informed. A lot of detail.

Some specialist associations for travellers

- British Airways Medical Service, Queens Building (N12), Heathrow Airport, Hounslow, Middlesex. *Tel*: 0208 526 7070. Provides a useful booklet *Your Patient and Air Travel* giving advice on fitness to travel and specific contraindications.
- British Diabetic Association, 10 Queen Anne Street, London, W1M 0BD. *Tel*: 0207 323 1531. Leaflets and information including *Travel Guide* to the more popular countries visited abroad, with advice pertinent to the needs of diabetics.
- British Mountaineering Council, 177–179 Burton Road, Manchester, M20 2BB. *Tel*: 0161 445 4747.

- Foundation for Teaching Aids at Low Cost (TALC), Institute of Child Health, 30 Guilford Street, London, WC1N 1EH. A list is available of books and pamphlets for purchase, primarily for medical and paramedical workers concerned with health problems in the Third World.
- Intermedic, 777 Third Avenue, New York, NY 10017, USA. A list of recommended English-speaking doctors in many countries is available to its members.
- International Association for Medical Assistance to Travellers (IAMAT), 57 Voirets, 1212 Grand-Lancy, Geneva, Switzerland or 40 Regal Road, Guelph, Ontario, Canada, NK1 1B5 (see also Websites). Various leaflets and a medical directory of international participating doctors are available.
- National Association for Maternal and Child Welfare, 1 South Audley Street, London, W1Y 6JS. *Tel*: 0207 383 4541. Provides a booklet *The Care of Babies and Young Children in the Tropics* by D. Morley.
- Royal Association for Disability and Rehabilitation (RADAR), 25 Mortimer Street, London, W1N 8AB. *Tel*: 0207 637 5400. A wide range of leaflets and services are available to help the handicapped arrange, insure, and enjoy their travels.
- Transport Users Committee, 1229 Kingsway, London, WC2B 6NN. *Tel*: 0207 240 6061
- Women's Corona Society, 274 Vauxhall Bridge Road, London, SW1V 1BB. *Tel*: 0207 828 1652. Provides advice and contacts for those travelling abroad in any capacity. Booklets and day courses on living overseas are available.

Some useful World Wide Web addresses relating to travellers' health

- TRAVAX, The A–Z of Healthy Travel – travel health advice for healthcare professionals from the Scottish Centre for Infection and Environmental Health: http://ww.axl.co.uk/scieh

- UK Foreign Office safety information for travellers: http://www.fco.gov.uk/reference/travel_advice (also on BBC2 Ceefax p. 470 and following)
- Center for Disease Control (USA) – travel health advice from the USA: http://www.cdc.gov/travel/index.html
- Health advice for travellers from the UK Department of Health: http://www.open.gov.uk/doh/hat/hatcvr.htm
- International Association for Medical Assistance to travellers (IAMAT): http://www.sentex.net/~iamat
- International Society of Travel Medicine: http://www.istm.org/
- Mobility International – comprehensive advice for the disabled: http://www.miusa.org

- Travel Medical Matrix – links to other sites: http://medmatrix.org/index.asp
- Travel Medicine and Vaccination Centres (TMVC) (Australia) – This group runs travel clinics in many parts of Australia, New Zealand and Asia: http://www.tmvc.com.au/about1.html
- The Weekly Epidemiological Record from the World Health Organization: http://www.who.ch/wer/
- Travel Health online: http://www.tripprep.com/country/country.html
- US State Department services – Travel warnings and consular sheets: http://travel.state.gov/travel_warnings.html
- World Health Organization 'outbreaks' – regularly updated notes by World Health Organization: http://www.who.int/emc/outbreak_news/index.html

Linking onto the Internet to access travel health databases

Doctors and nurses who plan to use the Internet often have little experience of accessing websites. While many have equipment, there are those who are confused by the routine of 'linking on'. As experienced users will know, once access has been achieved a few times, the procedure becomes routine – so do not be discouraged!

The following notes may help those who are struggling. The procedure for accessing the British National Health Service database TRAVAX (*The A–Z of Healthy Travel*) is given. Similar procedures apply for other sites.

Step 1
To connect to the Internet it is necessary to subscribe to an **Internet Service Provider** (ISP). If you are linked to the National Health Service NET in the UK, this can act as your ISP without any extra cost. Otherwise, you will have to subscribe to one of the many commercial providers, some of which allow free registration. (You always have to pay for the phone call time although only at local call rates.)

Step 2
The ISP normally gives you software on a floppy disc or CD for you to install on your computer which contains information to allow their system to run. You connect to the ISP through the ordinary telephone line using a special connector called a modem which you have to install separately, although a modem is often already installed in new computers.

Your ISP provides you with your own identification (ID) and unique password to enter their website, which will **not** be the same as your ID and password for the actual travel health database. Most ISPs have telephone helplines if you experience difficulties.

Step 3
Once online, you have to open a **browser** (often a browser is provided by the ISP on their original software on the floppy disc or CD). Common browsers are Internet Explorer or Netscape. Always try to install the most recent version as they are regularly updated.

Step 4
Once the browser is opened, enter the Internet address (URL) for TRAVAX (UK): http://www.axl.co.uk/scieh and press the 'Return' key.

This takes you to the TRAVAX 'Entry and Registration WebPage'. It is possible to set up your computer so that you will automatically (by default) go to this site.

Linking onto the Internet to access travel health databases *cont'd*

Step 5

Now click on 'Request Registration' and fill in your subscriber details. Identification (ID) and your unique password for TRAVAX are sent to you within a few days.

Step 6

When you return to the 'entry and registration page', you now click on *The A–Z of Healthy Travel* and you will be asked to enter your TRAVAX personal ID and unique password, which allow access to the database. Entry is denied if a wrong or incomplete ID and/or password is entered (every letter, number, space, capital, and fullstop. must be correct).

Step 7

Spend some time getting used to the layout and how to access information in advance of using it with a traveller. Remember you can print off advice sheets.

PRACTICE POINTS

The following sources of information should be readily available in the surgery

- Your 'official', national guidelines on vaccinations and malaria prevention, for example in the UK, the 'Green Book' and the latest report of the UK Malaria Advisory Committee.
- A reliable, easy-to-access and continually updated, online database.
- A detailed atlas. This can be installed on your computer.
- Details of specialist support groups such as those for the elderly, disabled travellers or travellers with diseases such as diabetes mellitus.
- Up-to-date vaccine and drug manufacturer's prescribing literature.

Epidemiology and travel medicine

Robin Knill-Jones

Introduction

This chapter aims to introduce some of the terms and techniques needed for a rigorous approach to the investigation of risk and illness in travellers.

Describing the health of travellers

The characteristics of time, place and person are the starting points for understanding diseases which may affect travellers. For example, knowledge about **time** and seasonal patterns of disease is an essential part of most traveller's plans; the **place**(s) to be visited determines the variety of preventive measures which need to be taken; characteristics of **person** such as age, sex, and some personal preferences for smoking, sex and alcohol, which are risk factors for disease, strongly influence advice given to travellers. Careful consideration of the influence of time, place and person on disease is important to everyone who gives advice to travellers about remaining healthy. This triplet is the basic starting block **for understanding disease in populations**, which is a simple definition of epidemiology. Few travellers are epidemiologists but every traveller (an individual) and their advisers (also individuals) make use of epidemiological information (derived from populations of *many* individuals):

- knowledge about the *geography* of disease is essential to inform what preventive measures are appropriate
- knowledge of the *natural history* of a condition, from following up the health of people over time, informs *prognosis*

- knowledge of the causes of disease – *aetiology* – informs *treatment* and *prevention*.

Epidemiological approaches may also be used to measure *health needs* in the travelling population and to evaluate the ability of travel medicine services to meet these needs in an equitable way.

Since much of travel medicine is directed at preventing illness in travellers, it is useful to start with a definition of the three levels of prevention:

- **primary**   preventing harm and avoiding risk in people who are healthy, for example boiling water before drinking, use of condoms – both to prevent infection
- **secondary**   early identification of infection before there are clinical symptoms, for example screening for asymptomatic individuals who have had a possible exposure to *Bilharzia*
- **tertiary**   preventing complications in patients with established disease, for example advice about diabetes and long-distance air travel, with many changes of time zones.

Both travellers and their advisers have to weigh up risks and benefits of each approach to prevention. Not everyone takes advice, and not all advice is well-informed. The epidemiological approach provides the basic data about risk and benefit, providing an answer to the frequently asked question 'What are my chances of becoming ill if...?' Here opinion is no substitute for good scientific evidence about the magnitude of risk, and the effect on that risk by taking certain preventive actions. Combining the data about risk, chance, and outcome can be done by a *formal decision analysis* to assess the relative value of differing ways of preventing disease. This technique provides one approach to *evidence-based medicine*, but is outwith the scope of this chapter – see Sackett et al.[1]

Measuring disease

The basic concepts in epidemiology are summarised in Box 2.2.

Box 2.2 Concepts in epidemiology	
Numerators	Events, illnesses, actions, risk behaviours
Denominators	Populations – geographic, demographic
Measurement	Quantitative – counting; qualitative – exploring
Cause	Are associations between risk and disease real or apparent?
Design	Observational, analytical, experimental

NUMERATORS

If we wish to measure events, illnesses, actions and risk behaviours, then it is essential that we have a definition of what we are trying to measure. The need for this may seem obvious to some, but completely unnecessary to others. Readers falling into the last group may care to write down a definition of traveller's diarrhoea, and of headaches on holiday. Now ask a few colleagues to do the same. There will be little agreement about exactly what is meant by each term. There will be differences about the definition of diarrhoea, and also about the time period covering travel and travel-related symptoms. Smilarly 'headache' will have definitions which vary from those which include some of the characteristics of migraine, to definitions which, when trying to define a significant headache, may include an action such as taking something for pain relief. Similar problems occur when assessing the prevalence of risky behaviours in travelling populations. For example, a change in use of alcohol while on holiday is difficult to measure until one has a good and tested set of questions, which can be shown to be answered consistently by travellers.

Reducing observer variation

Reducing *observer variation* is not easy. Some of the ways in which this can be done are:

1. training, including practice in use of all measurement techniques
2. experience
3. awareness of the existence of variation
4. check on one's own consistency
5. use of validated questions, instruments and laboratory techniques.

It is impossible to overemphasise the importance of considering observer variation in any study which tries to assess health, risk and illness in travellers. If the problem is not addressed, then any results might be suspect, and after many hours of work, found to be useless.

These issues lead on to the design of the questions to be used in a study. Information can be obtained from travellers by an interviewer, by computer or by paper-based questionnaires. First, you need to have a clear *aim* for the study. This serves to focus on the area of interest and should act as a reference point when tempted to try to do too much! The design of the questions to be used must reflect the objectives of the study:

- set out the objectives clearly – relate to *aim* of study
- produce questions related to the objectives
- do a pilot study to see if there are difficulties in understanding the questions/or if there are differences between interviewers
- define your study populations/sample for the main study (see below).

Successful questionnaires have the following characteristics:

1. well-produced
2. the wording is *clear to the person being interviewed*
3. questions are short, unambiguous and free of complex structures
4. simple questions shoud be first; sensitive ones last
5. use established questions from the literature if available
   – this allows comparison of results and also saves time

6. use *closed* questions (fixed alternatives)
7. but include some *open* questions
   – remember you will have to know in advance *how* you are going to use/code the responses to these questions
8. delete questions that are merely interesting and unrelated to the objectives.

DENOMINATORS – THE SAMPLE

Before considering the detailed design of any study, it is necessary to think about the population which is the subject of study. Epidemiology is about health and illness in *populations* and it is essential to define what is the population of interest.

For example, to assess the impact of travel advice on illnesses in travellers (this is an aim), one might wish to use the population of people attending a travel clinic. They would be approached on their return and their travel illnesses assessed by a questionnaire of some kind. Replies come in, and the natural instinct is then to analyse the results. However, there are four problems:

1. Are those who respond a true sample of all those who travelled after attending the clinic? Probably not – the ill might be more inclined to respond and thus *bias* the data.
2. Is there an *adequate response rate*?
3. Since the aim is to assess *impact of travel advice*, where is the comparison population of travellers who do not get advice?
4. Even if travellers who do not attend the clinic are surveyed, *are they a similar population* in terms of age, sex, income, experience, knowledge, and type of travel destinations?

Considerations of sampling are explained in detail in other texts.[2] The main points to be considered are:

- Is the population that is being studied so large that a sample needs to be taken? If so, then a suitable *sampling frame* needs to be designed and a *random* or *systematic sample* of sufficient size approached.
- If the population is small, is it certain that *all the population* is actually approached?

- *Convenience sampling* – for example, one plane load of passengers on a trip to Africa, is unlikely to give a good indication of the travel illnesses in African travellers in general.

Finally, there is a question about the proportion of those sampled who actually reply – the response rate. Most studies which achieve 80% response rates have many fewer biases than studies with response rates below 50%.

A number of procedures can help to improve the response rate to any study:

1. Do a *pilot study* and then use well-designed, clear and short forms, and use simple language.
2. Make the form easy to complete and to return.
3. Use *reminder* mailings or *multiple* approaches.
4. Distinguish *non-delivery* from *non-response*.
5. Provide an incentive for early replies.
6. In the analysis, look to see if there are differences between the early responders and later responders.

DESIGN OF STUDY

There are many classifications of the types of epidemiological study. However, for the purposes of travel medicine the relevant designs are :

Observational studies. These are simple descriptive studies of populations of travellers and their illnesses. They are also called cross-sectional studies as they take a population consisting of travellers to certain *places* at a certain *time*. They often relate findings to characteristics of *person* which may include personal risk factors, and whether preventive action was taken. These studies have limited value as they are not really designed to test *hypotheses* about the cause and prevention of disease. However, they provide an extremely useful *start* to investigating any travel-related health problem. For the more technically-minded, these studies allow the more precise calculation of sample size for the more definitive studies outlined below.

Observational studies can have two different measurement techniques:

1. *objective* (as discussed above under observer variation)
2. *qualitative*.

Box 2.3 Examples of qualitative studies

- **Participant observation** (e.g. watching people on holiday)
  Needs acceptance into the setting
  Amplify by interviews, observational ethnography
- **Focus groups** (group size 2–12)
  Group meeting and largely undirected discussion
  Provides a safe environment, allows interactions; but needs expert facilitation and some record of the content covered by the group
- **Critical incident technique**
  Getting people to talk about a (memorable) event
  Investigate in depth what happened, impressions of risk and behaviour

---

There are several types of qualitative design, which all aim to look at a topic in *depth* (Box 2.3) in contrast to objective studies which aim to look at a topic in *breadth*. It is often useful to consider doing an in-depth qualitative study when investigating a problem for the first time, then using the results to move to more definitive designs. For example, an investigation into reasons for non-compliance with advice about malaria prophylaxis could easily start with a series of in-depth interviews with individuals who have malaria diagnosed in the UK to establish the kinds of thinking and reasons behind their non-compliance. From this beginning, questions can be developed for more widespread use in travellers.

More advanced study designs are described in detail elsewhere.[3] These include *prospective studies* or *cohort studies*. These designs help to show the level of risk for an illness between two populations – a group *with a risk factor* and another group *without that risk factor*. Risk is then the simple ratio of the incidence of illness in the two populations when they are followed up for a period of time (for definition of incidence see p. 37).

As an example, if there were 10 cases of malaria in 100 people *not* taking prophylaxis, and 2 cases in 100 of those *taking* prophylaxis, then the ratio is 10/2 or 5.0. This simple ratio is a direct measure of risk, and in epidemiological studies is termed *relative risk*. Most studies of travellers lend themselves to cohort study design. This is the most powerful of the designs available and is the least likely to be subject to bias.

However, there will be occasions when a retrospective assessment of risk is needed. For this, a *case-control* design is appropriate. For this type of study, the question is posed in reverse. Starting with a group of ill people (cases), and a group of non-ill people (controls), both are interviewed using standard questions about their risk behaviour *before* their illness or their interview (controls). From this study design, incidence of disease cannot be measured because in one sense it has already happened to the cases. So all that can be done is to *estimate* the relative risk; the resulting ratio is called the *odds ratio*. These studies may be the only possible design for rare diseases, or when a result is needed quickly. As always, there is a trade-off – speed and case-control designs bring a serious problem of bias, which usually stems from the accuracy of people's recall about their risk behaviour in the past.

The epidemiology of travel health and illness has one advantage – rigorous cohort designs are relatively easy to perform. The disadvantage is that becoming good at definition of the illnesses and being precise about the populations being covered are both very difficult.

REFERENCES

1. Sackett DL, Haynes RB, Tugwell P. Clinical epidemiology: a basic science for clinical medicine. Boston: Little Brown; 1985
2. Campbell MJ, Machin D. Medical statistics – A common-sense approach. Chichester: Wiley; 1995
3. Rose G, Barker DJP. Epidemiology for the uninitiated. London: British Medical Journal; 1986.

Provision of travel medicine services

Lorna Calvert

Introduction

This chapter will give an overview of the main issues relevant to providing, and successfully running a travel medicine service. It will also outline the main points for consideration when setting up a designated travel clinic, including potential advantages and disadvantages.

Introduction

It has been well established that the numbers of travellers from the UK increases annually and that there is a corresponding need for healthcare advice and pre-travel preparation to enable those travellers to stay well while abroad. Travellers who are well prepared with health advice and vaccines may be less likely to become ill abroad, thus there may be a reduction in the number of post-travel consultations. This would ultimately be cost-effective.

Many general practice surgeries, health centres and occupational health departments already deal with large numbers of travellers seeking advice and immunisation prior to departure but there are still many travellers who do not seek pre-travel advice. The level of service required from each centre or practice will be determined by the needs of the travelling population within it. Regardless of the level of service, there are universal factors that should be considered by all those providing a travel medicine service.

Identifying broad aims and objectives of the service at an early stage can be a useful exercise since these set goals to be achieved. Aims and objectives may change as the service develops, but initially they could include the following examples:

- identify potential overseas travellers
- identify the travellers' key risk factors, that is the risk of health hazards to them while abroad
- identify travellers with special needs, for example the very young, elderly, pregnant and those with underlying medical conditions or disabilities
- provide individually tailored advice to help prevent ill health while abroad and on return
- offer services including immunisation, prescription of prophylactic medications, and provision of travel health equipment.

Providing a travel medicine service – the main issues

PROVIDING AN APPROPRIATE CLINICAL ENVIRONMENT

The area in which the traveller is seen will depend upon who is delivering the service. For example, in some instances the patients are referred to the doctor for planning and prescribing of vaccine schedules and then transferred to the nurse for vaccine administration; in other situations, the nurse decides which vaccines should be given and also administers them. Wherever the consultation takes place, it is important that the environment is suitable such that any emergency situation is not hampered. There should be ample space, particularly in treatment areas. A bed or couch and emergency equipment should be at hand in the event of a faint or anaphylaxis. Ideally, the clinic should be kept cool to minimise the risk of fainting. Space may be required for a vaccine fridge and if travel equipment such as mosquito nets is to be made available, storage space for this will also be needed.

The waiting area can provide an excellent venue for information provision, and it is here that you have a captive audience with time to fill. Vaccine prices can be displayed so that patients know what they can expect to pay; this can save time later on lengthy explanations of costs. Travel health advice leaflets can be placed for easy access and posters promoting healthy travel practices can be colourful as well as educational. Some clinics even show TV or video footage in waiting areas as part of the pre-travel preparation.

ACCESSING RELIABLE AND UP-TO-DATE INFORMATION

This is an essential element for all travel services to be effective and is covered on pages 47–54.

ROLE OF SPECIALIST AND CONTINUING EDUCATION

Travel medicine is a specialised subject and those working in the field are advised to undertake further education to do so effectively. Certain aspects of travel advice are subject to change, so regular updates are also recommended. Specific courses on this subject are now available and these range from short residential courses to lengthy distance learning courses at MSc level. Study days and seminars are also organised through professional groups such as the British Travel Health Association, the International Society of Travel Medicine, the Royal College of Nurses Travel Health Group. Educational activities sponsored by interested pharmaceutical companies are common. In addition, the value of self-learning through textbooks, journals, and professional organisations cannot be overestimated.

The level of education required by different staff members will depend on their involvement with the travel service. 'In-house' initiatives involving all staff members can be invaluable, particularly if problems arise owing to a lack of understanding on the importance of aspects of the service, or why activities are carried out in a certain way.

ALLOCATING RESPONSIBILITIES

Division and allocation of responsibilities must be clearly defined. Allocation of responsibilities will depend on the number of staff who are involved in the clinic and their professional background, experience and capabilities. Sensible allocation of tasks can prevent duplication of work and make best use of time.

- Preparation of case notes or consultative documents, scheduling of appointments and cashier responsibilities are best done by administrative employees.
- Ordering of vaccines, stock control and monitoring of fridge temperatures are activities that require a responsible named person (with a second named person as a stand-by).
- Administering vaccines and providing travel health advice must be carried out by a suitably qualified nurse or doctor.

International laws and guidelines vary greatly, and the role of the nurse and the doctor in different countries is correspondingly diverse. Travel medicine is a good example of this since in many countries doctors carry out the full consultation, including administration of vaccines, from beginning to end, whereas in the UK, many patients attending for pre-travel advice do not see a doctor at all.

It is important that individuals are satisfied with their delegated responsibilities and that the responsibilities are within that person's capabilities. Staff members should be aware of other member's roles as this avoids confusion and ensures that patients are suitably referred to the correct person for a particular reason.

GROUP PROTOCOLS

Once responsibilities have been defined and delegated, practice protocols should be drawn up by all those involved. Although protocols have limited legal value, they do offer certain benefits:

- they offer guidelines and information
- they identify aims and objectives
- they identify roles and responsibilities
- they provide a uniformity of practice.

When drawing up a protocol there are several points to incorporate:

- ensure everyone who will use the protocol is involved in designing it

- current literature on the subject should be read and then adapted for each individual practice
- each protocol should clearly state its aims, objectives, the target group, staff involved, available resources, a date for review and signatures.

Specifically relating to immunisation, the Department of Health 'Green Book', *Immunisation Against Infectious Disease*,[1] states that delegation of the responsibility of administering vaccines to a nurse, can only be considered when:

- the nurse is willing to be professionally accountable for this work
- the nurse has received training and is competent in all aspects of immunisation
- the nurse has received adequate training in the treatment of anaphylaxis.

The UKCC agrees with this and further states that, registered general nurses should only agree to administer vaccines when a written protocol has been drawn up and agreed upon.[2]

More recently, the 'Crown Report'[3] addressed the supply and administration of medicines under group protocols and offered guidance on the drafting and ongoing management of protocols. At the time of writing, the second report, which will address the issues of prescribing, supply and administration of medicines when not using a group protocol, had not been completed.

Protocols do not apply solely to vaccine administration and may be useful in other aspects of the travel service. Figure 3.1 is an example of a protocol on malaria prevention. It does not cover all aspects of malaria prevention and is included only as a guideline to what might be included.

Protocols, policies and the law are discussed in more detail in Chapter 5

PRESCRIBING

It is important to be clear what prescribing actually means. Consider the following definitions:

- prescribe: lay down or impose authoritatively; advise use of (medicines, etc.) to or for patient for complaint; assert prescriptive right or claim direct in writing.

Aims and objectives
1. To deliver advice on the prevention of malaria to travellers visiting malarious areas.
2. To obtain accurate and up-to-date information to determine the appropriate chemoprophylaxis for the traveller.
3. To increase the travellers' awareness that no chemoprophylaxis is completely effective and that other preventive measures are essential.

Target group
Travellers who attend Main Street Health Centre for advice and are going to malarious areas.

Staff involved
Doctors and nurses employed at the Main Street Health Centre, who give advice to travellers.

Available resources
Specified books and references:
(Examples ....
                    ....)

Further advice
e.g. SCIEH advisory helpline, TRAVAX database.

Equipment
Information booklets, insect repellents, mosquito nets, net dipping kits.

Information to be obtained from the traveller
1. Destination(s)
2. Type of accommodation
3. Medical history, including history of depression
4. Current medications etc.

Prescribing an antimalarial chemoprophylaxis
The initial discussion will be with the travel clinic nurse, any problems will be discussed with the doctor and the prescription will be signed by the doctor.

Advice to be given to the traveller
Verbal and written, including TRAVAX printout.

Date protocol commences ....

Date for review ....

Signatures ....

Fig. 3.1 Example of a protocol on malaria prevention (reproduced with permission of Jane Chiodini).

- prescription: physician's direction for composition of and use of medicine; written direction given by the doctor to the chemist for the compounding of medicine suitable to a patient's care.

(The Concise Oxford Dictionary)

Prescribing is an identified task traditionally carried out by doctors, but in the UK, certain nurses in certain settings are increasingly in an ideal position to prescribe. The travel clinic is a perfect example of this and many travel patients are fully dealt with, without ever seeing a doctor.

Prescribers should be suitably qualified and competent individuals who accept responsibility and liability for their actions. When nurses agree to prescribe, it is important that this is clearly defined within a protocol document. The Crown Report[3] deals with the issue of nurse prescribing and further information on this important matter is found in Chapter 5.

The UKCC Code of Professional Conduct[4] requires that nurses decline duties and responsibilities unless able to carry them out in a safe and skilled manner. While nurses should be professionally accountable for their work, it is worth noting that in general practice, the general practitioner, as the practice nurse's employer, remains liable in law for any negligent acts or omissions by the nurse.

ADMINISTERING VACCINES

This is another area that should be covered with a group protocol.

Consent must always be obtained before immunisation. It may be written or verbal. A child under the age of 16 years may give or refuse consent provided he or she fully understands the benefits and risks involved.

Most vaccines are administered by intramuscular (IM), deep subcutaneous (SC) or intradermal injection (with the exception of a few oral vaccines). It is essential that whoever administers the vaccines is aware of the correct mode of administration for each one and has adequate training in administration techniques to ensure that they do not cause harm and that the vaccines are effective. Rabies vaccine given intradermally is only effective when given correctly and BCG given too deep can cause abscess formation. Written information on possible side effects of vaccines, and guidance on what to do if side effects occur, are useful and should be handed out.

Sources of literature such as *Immunisation Against Infectious Disease*[1] and an up-to-date British National Formulary should be consulted for vaccine schedules, cautions and contraindications. Original papers in reliable medical and nursing journals can sometimes offer advice on alternative or quick vaccine schedules that can be invaluable.

When alternative schedules are used and are contrary to the datasheet recommendations, agreement with supervisors and colleagues is imperative.

ANAPHYLAXIS

Anaphylaxis is extremely rare, but it can occur quickly and can be fatal if not dealt with appropriately. It is an acute, allergic reaction to a foreign substance that results in an excessive release of histamine.

It is important that those administering vaccines are aware of the difference between a faint, a fit and a true, anaphylactic reaction.

Signs and symptoms of anaphylaxis:

- Pallor, limpness and apnoea
- Sinus tachycardia with profound hypotension
- Swelling of lips, face, neck or tongue
- Difficulty breathing, speaking or swallowing
- Bronchospasm with dyspnoea and audible expiratory wheeze
- Diffuse erythema
- Development of itchy urticarial lesions
- Peripheral oedema.

As very young children rarely faint, a sudden loss of consciousness should be presumed to be anaphylaxis in the absence of a strong carotid pulse.

Treatment entails discontinuing the causative agent and lying the patient in the left lateral position and maintaining the airway.

The DOH recommends the following drug treatment for anaphylaxis:

Mild anaphylaxis/allergic reactions (slowly progressing peripheral oedema or changes restricted to the skin)

- Oral anthistamines or subcutaneous adrenaline
- Observation and assurance
- Nebulised salbutamol, oral or parenteral steriods, parenteral antihistamine, if necessary.

Severe anaphylaxis (with cardiovascular collapse)

- Administer intramuscular adrenaline immediately. Begin cardiopulmonary resuscitation if required.
- If no improvement after 5–10 minutes, repeat adrenaline (to a maximum of 3 doses).
- Chlorpheniramine maleate (Piriton) may be given intravenously by an appropriately trained person; intravenous hydrocortisone may be given in severe cases.
- Consider volume replacement with fluids.

Treatment of bronchospasm

- Administer nebulised or intramuscular adrenaline.
- Administer steroids.
- Consider other nebulised bronchodilators such as salbutamol and consider parenteral aminophylline.

Treatment of angio/laryngeal oedema

- Administer nebulised or intramuscular adrenaline.
- Administer antihistamines.
- If necessary, intubate.

Recommended emergency equipment for first line treatment of anaphylaxis includes the following:

Adrenaline for IM or SC use 1:1000
Adrenaline for IV use (in extreme emergency) 1:10 000
Chlorpheniramine (antihistamine) for IM or IV use
Hydrocortisone for IM or IV use
Nebulised bronchodilators, for example. salbutamol
Assorted syringes and needles
Selection of venous cannulae with tape, tourniquet and connectors
Crystalline and colloid IV fluids and giving sets
Selection of different size airways
Ambubag with different size face masks
Intubation equipment
Defibrillator.

A designated person, to ensure drugs are within their expiry dates and that all equipment is present and intact, should check emergency equipment daily.

If anaphylaxis occurs, it should be reported with the yellow card system

From June 1992 to June 1995, there were 87 reports of anaphylaxis following vaccination in the UK. In that same period, over 55 million doses of vaccines were supplied to hospitals and general practices.

STORING AND ORDERING VACCINES

All vaccines require to be stored in a refrigerator and failure to do so can result in some vaccines (mainly 'live' vaccines) becoming ineffective. An appropriate storage refrigerator should be large enough to hold vaccines without being over-crowded as air should be able to circulate if a refrigerator is to work effectively. Vaccine storage refrigerators do not normally have freezer compartments, and should ideally have a lock. Food should never be stored in a vaccine refrigerator.

All vaccines have specific storage instructions in their datasheet, and the supplying pharmacist should be contacted in the event of refrigerator power failure or other storage problems. Discrepancies in temperature should also be reported and on no account should vaccines be frozen. Generally, a temperature between 2 and 4°C is suitable. The temperature of the refrigerator should be read and charted daily, by a designated person. The thermometer should either be of an electronic type on the door or a maximum and minimum thermometer placed at the bottom of the refrigerator.

ually better if one designated person is responsible for the ordering of vaccines as that person will become familiar with stock control. Having written guidelines or protocols is helpful, especially as a back-up when the designated person is absent.

It may take some time to settle into a routine whereby the number of vaccines required can easily be predicted. While it is time-saving to have commonly used vaccines available, it is not cost effective to order surplus vaccines that may go out of date. Stock should be rotated so that it is in order of its expiry date. Travel clinics which deal with large numbers of patients may find it cost effective to set up accounts with vaccine manufacturers as often this cuts out a pharmacy handling charge and some manufacturers will offer discounts for bulk-buying. (This is not acceptable in all Health Authorities.) Vaccines despatched by post should not be accepted if it is more than 48 hours since they were posted.

BECOMING A DESIGNATED YELLOW FEVER VACCINATING CENTRE

The International Certificate of Vaccination for Yellow Fever is the sole remaining certificate requirement under International Health Regulations of the WHO. For this reason, yellow fever vaccine can only be administered in a designated yellow fever vaccinating centre. Becoming a designated yellow fever vaccinating centre can attract travellers to a clinic, and can be a source of income generation if desired but the decision to take this on board should not be taken lightly. Travellers to more exotic destinations, who require yellow fever vaccine, are often exposed to a number of other health risks. If it is decided that the travel clinic will cater for these patients by offering yellow fever vaccine, the clinic should also accept responsibility for providing information and advice on the prevention of other illnesses such as malaria or bilharziasis.

To become a designated yellow fever vaccinating centre, the clinic must register with the Department of Health for England and Wales or the Scottish Home and Health Department. These departments broadly monitor centres which administer yellow fever vaccine by advocating that suitably qualified personnel are administering the

vaccine, that the correct vaccine is being used and that it is properly stored. The Department of Health will then supply yellow fever certificates when requested to do so.

DOCUMENTING THE TRAVEL CONSULTATION

Each practice or centre will have its own methods of documentation. Many general practices use the Lloyd George system, although it is debatable how helpful this is with travel consultations. It can be helpful to devise a document for pre-travel consultations, which is useful during the risk assessment (Ch. 4). This can be doubly useful: first, as a helpful tool, and second, as a detailed record.

Some practices find it useful to ask the traveller to fill in a self-complete questionnaire prior to the consultation. It is questionable whether this saves time since any information obtained this way must be checked to ensure that it is correct and that the questions have all been understood. In addition, most travellers will not recognise the significance of certain questions, for example, why exact destinations are needed for precise malaria advice or why a history of depression 10 years ago may affect malaria chemoprophylaxis advice.

A grid system can be useful for planning vaccine schedules when many are required. Once each vaccine has been administered, the person who gives it should sign the document, the date should be noted for future reference, and batch number written (this is useful in the event of an adverse reaction). The pre-travel consultation document should then be filed in the patient's records.

PROVIDING COMMODITIES OTHER THAN VACCINES

Travellers visiting developing countries or tropical destinations should be advised to take preventive measures against food- and water-borne infections, insect bites and sexually and blood-borne infection. Items such as water purification tablets or filters, insect repellents, impregnated mosquito nets and sterile emergency medical equipment are useful to such travellers and they may need to know where they can be purchased.

Some commercial outlets offer a good service with experienced staff available to give advice, but others do not and include a large, mark-up price on commodities. It may be useful to research what facilities are already available within the area, before deciding whether or not to provide this service. Initially, this may seem an unnecessary addition to the service, but it may prove to be a popular one since all the travellers' needs can be catered for in one place.

There are numerous types of water filters and mosquito nets, which can be ordered and delivered from various outlets in the UK and it is best to shop around to find out which outlet provides the best service and products to suit your travellers' needs. If you do not wish to provide this service for your travellers, or see too few to make the effort of ordering and maintaining stock worthwhile, some companies provide a mail order service for travellers themselves, and you could obtain a copy of a catalogue with the relevant information.

Examples of types of travel goods and when they might be used are referred to throughout this book.

PROVIDING LITERATURE

During a pre-travel consultation a great deal of information can be given. Anxiety associated with receiving vaccines and overload of information may cause travellers to forget much of this advice. Because of this, it is often useful to have some sort of written material to give out which the traveller can read at an opportune moment. Written information can reinforce verbal advice, and is a useful back-up.

There are various forms of written information available to travellers ranging from books on general aspects of travel or specific country guides to basic leaflets on travel insurance or prevention of sunburn. The Department of Health produces a general *Health Advice for Travellers* leaflet (T6) which contains form E111 for insurance purposes, and *Travel Safe*, a leaflet on prevention of HIV and AIDS for travellers. T6 leaflet is available from post offices, or alternatively both the T6 and *Travel Safe* are available, free of charge, in bulk by telephoning 0800 555 777. Many local health authorities produce posters and leaflets on aspects of health promotion for the traveller which are often available free of charge.

Travel clinics can produce their own leaflets based on frequently asked questions or an alternative is to use an on-line database and produce print-outs tailored to individual traveller's needs. Combining health advice with a vaccination record in a booklet form may encourage the travellers to take care not to lose the booklet. Occasionally you may be asked to recommend a helpful book for travellers keen to know more, so a handout with short list of literature for travellers (rather than health advisers) is sometimes useful.

GENERATING INCOME

This is an area that always induces much debate and often results in confusion. The level of income that can be generated from a travel clinic service depends upon numerous factors including the following:

- the country in which the clinic is based, as there are national variations
- whether the clinic is NHS, private or fundholding
- whether NHS reimbursement or 'item- of- service' payments can be claimed for administration of certain vaccines
- the types of services provided.

There is no national legislation which outlines the vaccines and other provisions, travel clinics should charge for. This has led to a tremendous variation in practice throughout the UK that is unlikely to change until legislation is made. There are guidelines, however, on claiming for certain immunisations in the general practice setting.

NHS remuneration for immunisations not part of the target (national schedule) system consists of the following:

- Item-of-service payments for immunisations given as part of public policy, as described in Paragraph 27 of the 'Red Book' (England and Wales, Scotland and Northern Ireland)[5]
- Personally administering the immunisations (England and Wales only).

The 'Red Book' lists those immunisations for which a fee – either the higher rate B or the lower rate A – is payable by the FHSA or Health Board (Scotland) as an item-of-service.

Claims for the item-of-service fee are made on form FP73 in England and Wales (form GP73 in Scotland; form VAC in Northern Ireland). Forms should always be filled in completely and travel destinations specified where requested. Errors or omissions can mean delayed or lost payments.

Personal administration fees for vaccines include fees for practice nurses acting on the doctor's behalf. Oral immunisations, such as polio or oral typhoid, are not covered by this scheme; neither are the routine childhood immunisations. However, low-dose adult diphtheria given for travel reasons is reimbursable, as is the Diptet vaccine given to school leavers, as long as it is purchased in a pre-filled syringe.

This scheme works as follows:

1. The vaccine is purchased directly from the supplier or via the local chemist.
2. The vaccine is administered to the patient.
3. A prescription is written on form FP10 for the immunisations given.
4. At the end of the month, all the FP10s are sent to the Prescription Pricing Authority in England (Welsh Health Common Services Authority in Wales) together with a Form FP34D.
5. Between 6 weeks and 3 months later, reimbursement is received.

This scheme can be used for immunisations for which no item-of-service fee may be payable, so hepatitis B, meningitis and Japanese B encephalitis vaccines can all be processed in this way. Yellow fever is specifically excluded.

Another benefit of personally administering immunisations is that the patient does not have to pay a prescription charge. However, it also means that where a fee might have been charged for providing immunisations this will not be possible.

Non-item-of-service vaccines

The patient may be charged where a fee cannot be claimed on FP73 or GP73. The BMA-suggested fee is £18.50 per course, to which should be added the cost of the vaccine. Obviously, it is not then possible to claim any reimbursement under the personally administered drugs regulations. It is fraudulent to claim an item-of-service fee and then charge the patient.

AUDITING YOUR TRAVEL SERVICE

Audit is necessary to ensure that the services provided by the clinic are meeting the demands of the patients who use them. Audit also helps to improve organisation and efficiency and ultimately improves patient care. The audit cycle includes:

- deciding which area needs to be assessed
- agreeing on standards to be met for that area
- collecting data and comparing them with previously set standards
- agreeing on changes
- implementing changes
- measuring performance.

Areas which might require regular audit include vaccine ordering, ensuring relevant aspects of travel health advice are given, patient waiting time, provision of written materials and documentation of the travel consultation.

SETTING UP A TRAVEL CLINIC

It is well known that the increase in international travel has been dramatic over the past 20 years, and it is generally accepted that this trend will continue. As travellers become more adventurous, and high-risk groups travel more, it is reasonable to assume that the need for pre-travel advice and immunisation will also continue to increase.

Most travellers will contact their own general practice or health centre in the first instance, and a large proportion will need go no further. Business travellers may use their occupational health department as first port of call. As travellers' needs become more complex, some practices or centres may need to consider expansion of their travel medicine services, particularly if they need to refer a large proportion of travellers elsewhere. This will be even more important if access to a specialist travel clinic is not available.

In these instances, it might be useful to consider setting up a designated travel clinic as opposed to seeing patients on an 'ad hoc' basis.

All of the previous issues regarding providing a travel medicine service will need to be thought through, but there are a few other points to consider.

Assessing the need for a travel clinic

The purpose of running a travel clinic is to provide a travel service suited to meet the needs of each individual practice or centre. Within the occupational health setting, this will depend upon the business contacts abroad, and new or forthcoming proposals. In general practice, there are numerous variables which contribute to whether a clinic is worthwhile and if so, the level of service required.

The size of the practice population is one of the key factors. Generally, the larger the population the more travellers, although this does not always follow. The age and type of practice population can have an influence and those situated close to universities with a high proportion of students often have a huge demand for travel services. Those practices with an elderly population, despite the increase in this group's travel activities, usually have less demand.

The location and ease of access of the practice are important. Pre-travel health is not always seen as a priority; if a practice is difficult to access from a person's place of work, the individual might be more likely to attend a more central site. Urban practices tend to be busier with travel patients than rural practices. It is possible, though not proven, that more affluent areas have higher numbers of travellers.

It may be wise to conduct research into the need for a travel clinic service prior to setting one up. This may entail conducting a small retrospective study by looking at the notes of all the patients who attended for travel advice over the previous 3 months, for example. It may also be worth noting how many had to be referred elsewhere for vaccines or advice; if more than 25%, then this may indicate that the service requires expansion. Alternatively, a prospective study could be commenced taking note of all patients who attend for travel advice over a 3 month period, noting what they come for and roughly how much time is spent on each patient. A prediction can then be made on how much time will be required for future travel patients over the next 3 months.

Giving out a brief questionnaire to a sample of patients, asking whether they would use a travel clinic service and if so, the type of service they would like (e.g. would they want to be able to obtain yellow fever vaccine or purchase mosquito nets) can also be useful, although this is time-consuming.

Availability of other travel clinics and the types of services they provide will clearly have a strong influence on the need for a new clinic and it is important to investigate what other travel services are available within the area before planning your own.

Allocating the clinic time

One of the most difficult hurdles to get over is identifying the best time to dedicate to the clinic and this may, initially, seem impossible. The time has to be suitable for staff depending on their other work commitments, but it also has to be suitable for the patients. Finding a time that suits both will be crucial for the success of the clinic; many clinics fail simply because patients do not attend at the appropriate time but make appointments outwith travel clinic hours with the practice or centre.

A popular time for travellers is often in the evenings or on a Saturday, as it can be difficult to take time off work, particularly when travel advice is seen to be associated with 'holidays' and therefore not a priority for employers. Evenings and weekends are often less popular with clinic staff for obvious reasons.

Allocating appointment times

A frequently cited problem of advising and immunising travellers in general practice is that of insufficient appointment time. It is difficult to determine in advance how much time will be required for individual travellers and this will vary substantially depending on such factors as destination, purpose and mode of travel and standards of accommodation.

Generally, first time visits take longer than return visits. During the initial consultation, the patient's travel itinerary and medical and immunisation histories are taken, the vaccine schedule is planned, and often the bulk of precautionary health advice is given. Subsequent visits usually involve ensuring that no adverse reactions to vaccines have occurred, administration of booster injections and the opportunity for questions to be asked.

There is never enough time for consultations. To properly provide a travel medicine service, 5- or 10-minute appointments will not be sufficient, particularly for those seeing travellers with complex itineraries or problems. Giving pre-travel advice may be the most time-consuming part of a consultation but it is also the most important. The ideal length of time needed for appointments would be a suitable area for audit, particularly for those setting up a new travel clinic service.

Advertising the service

Putting up a poster in the waiting room will alert patients that the travel clinic is available and the receptionists should arrange appropriate appointments for intending travellers. Some practices welcome referrals from outwith their own population. Local pharmacies and travel agents might help with advertising and agree to display a poster and flyers.

Vaccine stocks

There are several different options for stocking vaccines. Some clinics prefer to keep only UK childhood schedule vaccines such as polio and tetanus in the clinic refrigerator and will write prescriptions for other vaccines. This means there is a considerable gap between the patient being seen initially and receiving the immunisations, particularly if the nearest pharmacy is outwith the practice. In some instances, the patient will need a further appointment in order to have the vaccines administered.

Other clinics keep commonly used travel vaccines such as hepatitis A and typhoid in the clinic and write prescriptions for more unusual vaccines. For busy travel clinics, having stocks of all

the vaccines that could potentially be used, is least time consuming. This requires a degree of skill in stock control and an ability to predict what might be used over a given period of time. This becomes easier as the clinic becomes more established although there might be slight seasonal variations.

Having a designated travel clinic makes ordering easier as it is obvious what has been used and therefore needs to be replaced. It also allows use of multidose vials of vaccines such as yellow fever. This can be cost effective, but only if the whole vial is used during the clinic as it cannot be stored and re-used after reconstitution. Similarly, the intradermal route can be used for rabies vaccine (see Ch. 2), allowing several doses to be used from one vial, therefore reducing costs. Again, this is only cost effective when more than one person can be immunised as rabies vaccine should not be stored and re-used after reconstitution.

Initial costs: time and money

A considerable amount of time and effort is required in setting up the service. Drawing up protocols, devising suitable documents, identifying or producing written materials all takes time. There also needs to be a financial commitment up front. Finances may be required to purchase necessary reading materials and reference sources, equipment may be needed for access to a database and there may be a registration fee. It might be necessary to send some staff members on a travel medicine course. Funds will be needed to purchase vaccines and perhaps travel goods. It may be some time before the money and effort put in at the beginning are seen to reap any benefits.

Decisions must be made about charging patients – how much for what? Those clinics accepting referrals from other practices will also need to decide whether charges will be different for outside referrals to charges for their own practice population. When vaccines are kept on-site, staff must be allocated to deal with finances. This will include someone who will take payments during the clinic and named persons to pay invoices for orders.

If the prime motive for setting up a travel clinic is to generate income, it is worth noting that not all travel clinics make profits and some make losses. The initial research into the need for a clinic is therefore crucial.

Support from colleagues

As with all new proposals, some staff members will be more enthusiastic than others. For a travel clinic to be successful, it is important to have the backing of all those who will be involved, and in a general practice setting, the agreement of all the partners is essential.

Advantages and disadvantages of running a travel clinic

Advantages
- Better organisation
- The database can be set up in advance; posters, price lists, and health advice leaflets can be laid out; anaphylaxis drugs and equipment can be at hand; first-aid kits and mosquito nets can be displayed; vaccine ordering is easier; multidose vials of vaccine can be used
- Better organisation will save time, therefore more patients can be seen
- Better service
- Patients like an on-site service which caters for all their needs
- Staff will be psychologically prepared
- Clear focus – those involved will be in "travel clinic mode"
- Income generation
- An efficient and effective clinic has the potential to achieve these advantages.

Disadvantages
- Initial costs: time and money are required
- 'De-skilling' of other staff members
  Those involved will become more knowledgeable but those who are not involved may become less knowledgeable: this can cause problems when staff are absent, unless suitable precautions are put in place (good communication, regular updates and meetings and useful protocols, can all help to reduce potential problems)
- Implications of patient perceptions of 'specialist' clinics: some patients may perceive that the service they receive should be of a more specialist nature or of a higher quality. This may not cause problems when the service is of a high standard, but it may make matters worse if anything goes wrong.

PRACTICE POINTS

- A travel medicine service should suit its population.
- The need for travel medicine services will increase and become more complex.
- Access to reliable, accurate and up-to-date information is essential.
- Staff roles and responsibilities should be clearly identified.
- Protocols are useful.
- Setting up a travel clinic needs careful planning.

REFERENCES

1. UK Departments of Health. Immunisation against infectious disease. London: HMSO; 1996.
2. United Kingdom Central Council for Nursing, Midwifery and Health Visiting (UKCC). Standards for the administration of medicines. London: UKCC; 1992.
3. UK Departments of Health. The Crown Report: review of prescribing, supply and administration of medicines. London: HMSO; 1998.
4. United Kingdom Central Council for Nursing, Midwifery and Health Visiting (UKCC). Code of professional conduct. London: UKCC; 1992.
5. Statement of fees and allowances payable to general medical practitioners in England and Wales from April 1990 (the 'Red Book'). London: NHS Publications; 1990: paragraph 27 (available from the Health Publications Unit).

FURTHER READING

Chiodini J. Top tips for setting up a travel clinic. Practice Nurse: 1998; 16: 291–296.
Rodriguez P (Europe), Dardick KR, Baker ME (USA and Canada), Ruff TA (Australia), Kong J, Hedley A (Asia). Travel medicine and the travel clinic. In: Du Pont H, Steffan R, eds. Textbook of travel medicine and health. Hamilton, Ontario: Decker; 1997; ch. 7: 34 –45.

Risk assessment

Fiona Raeside

Introduction

Carrying out a thorough risk assessment prior to travel abroad is the initial step in the travel consultation. It is also one of the most important, since it will provide the information on which future action will be based. This action will certainly include delivering health advice and will frequently involve deciding on necessary immunisations and malaria prophylaxis.

As an appendix to this chapter (p. 75), a scheme for using the available information to assess the need for intervention has been included. This scheme can be useful as a teaching tool and sometimes for taking the traveller through the process of risk assessment to show how different factors need to be considered.

It is important to remember that the purpose of the pre-travel risk assessment is to better prepare travellers to enjoy the experience of travel and make their journey safer by providing information tailored specifically to their needs. It should not act as a deterrent to travel by scaring individuals with lists of potential problems they may encounter.

Various steps are involved in the risk assessment procedure:

- gathering information from the traveller
- evaluating and quantifying potential health risks
- providing tailored advice.

Gathering information from the traveller

WHO SHOULD DO THIS?

Ideally, the pre-travel risk assessment should be conducted by a qualified healthcare professional, generally a nurse or doctor, who has undertaken further training in travel medicine. Commonly, a travel questionnaire or form is devised to collect the necessary information. This ensures all the important areas are addressed and acts as a record of the consultation for future visits. It is the practice in some surgeries and clinics for the traveller to fill out a self-complete questionnaire, or for the receptionist to question the traveller, in advance of attending the nurse or doctor for advice. Information obtained in this way should be treated with caution and used only as a prompt, since patients cannot be relied on to accurately self-report details of vaccination history, allergies, current medication or any past or current health problems. A thorough, pre-travel history should always be taken by a suitably qualified individual.

WHAT QUESTIONS SHOULD BE ASKED?

Certain questions need to be asked during the initial, pre-travel consultation in order to help identify actual and potential health risks and determine appropriate advice and immunisations for any particular traveller.

Box 4.1 Topic for risk assessment questioning	
Traveller details	**Journey details**
Age	Destination(s)
Medical history	Date of departure
Medication	Duration of stay
Allergies	Purpose of trip
Previous vaccinations	Type of accommodation
Previous travel	Mode of transport
Pregnancy (actual or	Urban/rural travel
planned)	Availability of medical
Handicaps or special	facilities
needs	Travel budget

These questions fall broadly into two categories and cover the topics shown in Box 4.1.

The travel health adviser should be able to assess the traveller's actual and potential health risks using information provided in response to questions asked about subjects in Box 4.1.

Evaluating and quantifying potential health risks

TRAVELLER DETAILS

Age. Illness in travellers is reported more commonly in those aged < 40 years.[1,2] Death rates for accidents and injuries are also highest in the younger age group (20–29 years).[3–5] In the very young, common ailments, such as sunburn, diarrhoea and vomiting, may have more serious sequelae than for older travellers. The most common cause of death in travellers is cardiovascular disease, particularly myocardial infarction, and this is more likely to be experienced by elderly individuals.[3–5] In addition, the elderly are more likely to have a pre-existing medical condition which may be exacerbated by travelling or necessitate medical intervention while abroad. Age limits may also apply to certain vaccines and antimalarials. (The needs of elderly travellers and children are discussed in Chapter 7.)

Medical history. When individuals have an existing health problem, it is advisable for them to be assessed prior to travel abroad to ensure their condition will not be aggravated by the trip and to allow any necessary pre-travel arrangements and contingency plans to be made.

Travellers who have recently had major surgery may need to be assessed for their fitness to travel. Individuals who have recently suffered myocardial infarction should avoid flying and travellers with chronic gastrointestinal problems may find that travel to a developing area aggravates their condition. Doses of antimalarials may need to be adjusted in certain conditions, for example, renal or liver disease.

Individuals who are physically unfit, or who have a medical condition which precludes strenuous exercise, should avoid adventure and sporting activities beyond their capabilities. Immuno-suppressed individuals should avoid receiving live vaccines and their response to inactivated ones may be suboptimal, whilst travellers without a spleen are more likely to develop severe malaria if infected. In certain countries, HIV-infected travellers may be refused entry.

Emotional and psychiatric disorders are often overlooked when it comes to determining an individual's suitability to travel. Psychological assessments are difficult to carry out unless specially trained to do so, but they are particularly relevant for individuals intending to be abroad for extended periods. Mefloquine is contraindicated when there is a history of convulsions or psychiatric illness.

Travellers with an underlying medical condition, including pregnancy, should ensure their travel insurance covers their condition.

Travellers with underlying medical conditions are dealt with in greater detail in Chapter 7.

Medication. If planning to live abroad for an extended period, travellers on regular medication should check in advance if they will have access to the drugs they require. If it is envisaged that obtaining medication abroad will be difficult, or for the short-term traveller, an adequate supply of personal medication should be carried, preferably in hand luggage rather than the aircraft hold. Insulin should always be carried in hand luggage since temperatures in the hold may drop to near freezing. Immunosuppressive drugs may contraindicate the use of certain live vaccines. Other medications, for example anticonvulsants and beta-blockers, may be unsuitable when taken in combination with certain antimalarials.

Allergies. A previous allergic reaction to a vaccine or antimalarial may contraindicate further doses. More specifically, an anaphylactic reaction to egg would contraindicate yellow fever vaccine. Individuals who respond vigorously to insect bites may require additional advice regarding bite prevention and use of antihistamines. If the traveller has a life-threatening allergy, it may be advisable for the traveller to carry adrenaline for emergency use.

Previous vaccinations. This will help the travel health adviser to plan a vaccination schedule. Determining risk estimates for vaccine-preventable diseases is extremely complex and there are very few studies which have tackled this issue.[6–9]

Previous travel. Experienced travellers tend to have fewer health problems than individuals who have little travel history. They are more likely to be better organised, more extensively immunised and more aware of the preventive measures which should be taken with respect to food, water, insect bites, sun, accidents and sex. They are also less likely to suffer problems related to culture shock and climate.

Pregnancy. Certain vaccines and antimalarials may be contraindicated during pregnancy. Contracting malaria while pregnant can have very serious consequences for both mother and child since the woman is more likely to develop life-threatening illness and the chances of premature labour and spontaneous abortion are increased. Travel to malarious areas during pregnancy should be avoided where possible. Most airlines will not fly pregnant women past a certain gestation, usually about 35 weeks, but sometimes earlier. (Pregnancy is dealt with in Chapter 7.)

Handicaps or special needs. This will determine, to a certain extent, the destination and type of travel undertaken. Some tour operators organise holidays aimed at specific groups of individuals, for example, wheelchair users. This makes it easier to ensure that travelling arrangements and facilities at the destination are appropriate for the individual's particular needs. Airlines and hotels will often provide services, such as special meals, refrigerators in rooms for storing medication, and wheelchair access, but the traveller needs to be prompted to ask about them. (Travellers with disabilities are further discussed in Chapter 7.)

JOURNEY DETAILS

Destination. Geography plays a large part in determining which diseases an individual may be exposed to, since certain infections will only be transmitted within defined geographic boundaries. For example, Japanese encephalitis is only found in South-East Asia, and yellow fever in Africa and South America. Travel to the tropics and developing countries is generally associated with greater risks to health than travel elsewhere,[2] particularly risks associated with contaminated food and water.

As well as risks from infection, the traveller may face other hazards, including those related to standards of medical care and facilities, crime, public road maintenance and transport services, and these may vary between countries. Travelling to high altitude destinations can also lead to problems, particularly if the traveller has an underlying medical condition which may be aggravated by altitude, for example, cardiopulmonary disease or a seizure disorder. (More detailed descriptions of country-specific health problems can be found in Section 7.)

Date of departure. More reports of illness are recorded during the summer months as opposed to the winter.[10] It is preferable if travellers attend for advice well in advance of their trip (at least 4–6 weeks). This allows vaccination schedules to be fully completed and sufficient advice given and discussed. Last minute attendees are all too frequent and they present problems in terms of the advice and protection which can be offered at short notice.

Duration of stay. Risks for short-stay travellers will differ from those for individuals staying longer term. The length and extent of exposure to health risks are generally increased in the latter. Some risks may be seasonal, for example, malaria after the rains and meningococcal meningitis during the dry season

Purpose of trip. This plays a large part in determining an individual's health risks. Reasons for travel are many and varied, including holiday, business, voluntary work, expedition and visiting family.

Degree of contact with the local population is an important aspect to consider since infections spread person-to-person via the respiratory route, such as diphtheria, tuberculosis and meningitis, are more effectively transmitted in prolonged, close contact situations. As a result, travellers most at risk from these infections would include teachers, healthcare workers and missionaries, rather than package tourists who are more likely to mix with fellow tourists than indigenous people. Travellers returning to their country of origin to stay with family are also more at risk from diseases endemic in the indigenous population. This is particularly so with regard to malaria. Individuals returning home after a long absence may believe they are still immune to the parasite, fail to take prophylaxis, and subsequently contract the infection. (Further detail on ethnic minority travellers is contained in Chapter 20.)

Package tours are an extremely popular type of holiday, particularly with tourists from the UK. The package tour has, to an extent, an element of safety attached which the self-organised or backpacking trip lacks. Flights, accommodation, transfers, meals and excursions may all be organised for the traveller by the holiday company and there will be tour representatives on hand to sort out any problems which may arise. Partly as a result of this, tourists on package holidays, particularly teenagers and young adults, often relax their behaviour and attitudes while abroad. If this is coupled with drug-taking and excessive alcohol, it can be a very volatile combination which is often associated with accidents, sexual risk-taking and illness. Sunburn is also very commonly reported in this group.

Backpackers and expedition travellers visit areas of the world which the average tourist would not consider exploring. At the destination, they will often engage in pursuits other than the usual sunbathing and swimming. Engaging in certain activities may increase their likelihood of exposure to insect and animal bites, for example camping or jungle trekking. Other activities, such as scuba diving, rafting, climbing and watersports may be particularly hazardous if facilities, equipment and supervision at the destination are sub-standard. As a result, backpackers and adventure, expedition travellers may be exposed to very particular health risks and may need additional advice, vaccines, equipment, self-treatment medications and insurance. (Further detail on expedition travel is contained in Chapter 19.)

Those going abroad to work will have very specific needs with regard to health advice, vaccinations and malaria, particularly within certain occupations. Doctors and nurses may be more exposed to blood-borne viruses, veterinarians to rabies and teachers to tuberculosis. Business travellers present their own particular problems, whether going abroad for short-term or longer-term business. Lack of preparation before departure, loneliness and isolation, missing family at home, cultural differences, language barriers, over-indulgence in alcohol and sexual risk-taking are some of the problems which may be experienced by this group.

Type of accommodation. Obviously, staying in five-star hotel accommodation with air-conditioning, access to safe water and a decent restaurant will pose far fewer risks to the traveller's health than sleeping out under canvas and purchasing food from street vendors. However, even the best hotels are not immune to problems of hygiene in their kitchens and bars and a degree of caution should be exercised wherever the traveller is staying.

Mode of transport. This is relevant both for reaching the destination and once there. Certain individuals may not be permitted to travel by air, for example those having undergone recent abdominal surgery or pregnant women into the third trimester. Cruising is an increasingly popular type of holiday and it is likely that motion sickness will be a problem for those travelling by sea. Travelling by train, bus, car, jeep or motorcycle/moped presents hazards surrounding personal safety, not only from road traffic accidents, which are a major cause of death and injury in travellers, but also the risk of assault and robbery.

Urban/rural travel. Risks will vary between urban and rural areas. It is often more difficult to access clean water, medical facilities and screened accommodation in rural areas, whereas accidents are more likely to occur in cities. It is common for travel itineraries to involve stays in both urban and rural areas, for example a beach holiday which includes a week-end safari, and this would need to be identified.

Availability of medical facilities. This is particularly relevant for those travellers with an underlying medical condition, pregnant women and children. Most travellers should be advised to carry a first-aid kit containing items such as adhesive strip bandages, a thermometer and antiseptic lotion. For those visiting areas where medical facilities are poor, additional supplies may be required, including needles, syringes, gauze dressings and antibiotics. Taking out adequate travel insurance to cover medical treatment abroad is essential for every traveller, but for those visiting areas with inadequate medical facilities, it is important that the policy also covers repatriation.

Travel budget. Travellers on a tight budget, as most backpackers are, may be at greater risk from food- and water-borne infections, communicable diseases, insect bites and accidents. They will not be able to afford to eat and sleep in better quality establishments and will use cheaper forms of public transport along with local people. Should they become unwell or injured while abroad, they may find it difficult to pay for medical assistance, another good reason for taking out adequate insurance before departure.

Providing tailored advice

The advice travellers require will depend on the outcome of their risk assessment. However, there are a few key areas (Box 4.2) which usually need to be addressed for all travellers, to a greater or lesser extent.

A proper risk assessment will allow the travel health adviser to give tailored advice which will match the needs of the individual. There is no logic in carrying out a detailed risk assessment for each traveller if the advice delivered does not vary based on the actual or potential health risks the assessment has identified.

For example, not every traveller going to India will require the same advice. Giving the same information regarding food and water hygiene to a businessman visiting Delhi for 1 week as to a low-budget backpacker travelling round the country for 6 months is not only inappropriate but also ineffective. The well-used adage about not purchasing food from street vendors would be highly appropriate and achievable for the business traveller whereas the backpacker would dismiss this piece of information as not being relevant. It would be far better to advise the backpacker that when buying food from street stalls, to choose 'cleaner' looking vendors, who are using fresh ingredients and cooking them on the spot until very hot. The backpacker is much more likely to

follow this tempered advice, and while it is no guarantee of an infection-free meal, it may help reduce the risk!

Pre-travel health advice will be most effective if the risk assessment is reliable and based on credible and **up-to-date** sources of information regarding disease incidence, outbreaks, drug and vaccine profiles and traveller studies. Health recommendations for travellers do not remain static, so the travel health adviser must be aware of where to access current information.

There are many different sources of advice available to the travel health adviser to assist them in risk assessment, such as books and publications, wallcharts, electronic databases, telephone advice lines and Internet websites (see Ch. 2). Many individuals involved in the specialty of travel medicine are themselves prolific travellers, and this also helps when advising others, although it is worth bearing in mind that personal reminiscences may not always reflect current problems.

Conclusion

Unless travellers perceive pre-travel health advice as relevant and achievable in their situation, they are unlikely to follow it. A thorough risk assessment, carried out by a competent individual using accurate and current sources of information, will identify actual and potential health risks and aid the delivery of realistic and appropriate advice. It is inappropriate for travel health advisers to impose rules of behaviour just as it is very difficult for them to successfully affect behaviour, particularly with regard to eating, drinking and sun exposure. However, if the advice offered is tailored on an individual basis and to the traveller's personal circumstances, a successful outcome is more likely.

Most importantly, the risk assessment process needs to be two-way and travellers must be encouraged to take responsibility for their own health. Individuals must not only be made aware of the risks they may encounter when they travel but they must also be alerted to the hazards they may present for the populations and environments they are visiting. Although the travel health

---

> **Box 4.2 Key areas for preventive advice**
>
> - Accident prevention (see Ch. 8)
> - Food and water precautions (see Ch. 11)
> - Insect and animal bite avoidance (see Chs 11 and 13)
> - Sun exposure (see Ch. 9)
> - Sexual behaviour (see Ch. 10)
> - Insurance.

adviser can provide useful information and offer vaccination and chemoprophylaxis, ultimately it is individuals who have to make the decision to act to safeguard, not only their own health, but the well-being of the individuals and environment around them. Communication is the key.

PRACTICE POINTS

Risk assessment

- determines the advice, immunisations and chemoprophylaxis a traveller may require
- should be carried out by a suitably qualified individual
- involves obtaining both traveller and journey details
- should be based on sound, up-to-date sources of reference
- facilitates the delivery of tailored advice.

REFERENCES

1. Cossar JH, Reid D, Fallon RJ et al. A cumulative review of studies on travellers, their experience of illness and the implications of these findings. Journal of Infection 1990; 21: 27–42.
2. Steffen R, Rickenbach M, Willhelm U et al. Health problems after travel to developing countries. Journal of Infectious Diseases 1987; 156: 84–91.
3. Paixao MLT, Dewar RD, Cossar JH et al. What do Scots die of when abroad? Scottish Medical Journal 1991; 36: 114–116.
4. Prociv P. Deaths of Australian travellers overseas. Medical Journal of Australia 1995; 163: 27–30.
5. Hargarten SW, Baker TD, Guptill K. Overseas fatalities of United States citizen travelers: an analysis of deaths related to international travelers. Annals of Emergency Medicine 1991; 20: 622–626.
6. Steffen R, Lobel HO. Epidemiologic basis for the practice of travel medicine. Journal of Wilderness Medicine 1995; 5: 56–66.
7. Steffen R. Risks of hepatitis B for travellers. Vaccine 1990; 8: 31–32.
8. Taylor DN, Pollard RA, Blake PA. Typhoid in the United States and the risk to international travellers. Journal of Infectious Diseases 1983; 148: 615–616.
9. Wittlinger F, Steffen R, Watanabe H, Handszuh H. Risk of cholera among Western and Japanese travellers. Journal of Travel Medicine 1995; 2: 154–158.
10. Peltola H, Kyronseppa H, Holsa P. Trips to the South – a health hazard. Scandiniavian Journal of Infectious Diseases 1983; 15: 375–381.

Appendix

A scheme for using the available information to assess the need for intervention

When using any source of information on possible health risks for a particular traveller, this information has to be translated into whether there is a need to actively provide advice to the traveller or whether to suggest prophylaxis. This requires a 'feel' for the likely health risk both to the individual and the community if no intervention (advice or prophylaxis) was provided, balanced against the effectiveness, potential side effects and cost of the intervention. Using the boxes below, the higher the overall total of scores, the more likely intervention is going to be of benefit.

1. Significance to the individual traveller

How serious could the specific health problem be for the individual?

Score	Grading	Signficance to the individual
0	Minor	Rarely a severe illness
1	Moderate	Serious illness, complete recovery usual, death rare
2	Major	Severe illness, complications and death possible
3	Critical	Severe illness, serious or long-term complications common
4	Grave	Severe illness, complications and death are usual

2. Significance to the community

How serious are the public health implications if the traveller was to be affected?

Score	Grading	Signficance to the community
0	Minor	Minimal or no risk to public health
1	Moderate	Potential for spread to close contacts but usually confinable
2	Major	Potential for spread within the population
3	Critical	High probability of spread within a population
4	Grave	Certainty of spread within the exposed population

3. Likelihood of exposure

How likely is the traveller to become affected – considering destination and intended lifestyle?

Score	Grading	Likelihood of exposure
0	Very unlikely	Disease not normally present at destination
1	Unlikely	Disease present, intended lifestyle makes infection unlikely
2	Possible	Disease widespread but traveller likely to be able to avoid infection
3	Probable	Disease widespread. Traveller's lifestyle makes avoiding infection difficult
4	Almost certain	Disease widespread and highly contagious.

4. Evaluation of active intervention such as prophylaxis

How effective and practical is available prophylaxis, considering possible side effects, cost and time available for completing optimal schedule?

Score	Grading	Value of intervention
0	Passible	Marginal benefits, acceptable side effects, may be difficult to deliver
1	Satisfactory	Significant benefits, possible side effects, may be difficult to delivery
2	Useful	Useful and feasible intervention with some measurable benefits and few adverse side effects
3	Effective	Useful and feasible intervention with significant measurable benefits and few or no adverse side effects
4	Ideal	Highly effective and feasible intervention with side effects very unlikely

Managing risk in travel health – policies, protocols and legal aspects

Karen Howell

Introduction

Promoting the health and welfare of travellers going abroad is fundamentally based upon risk assessment. This is applied at different levels to the individual traveller and the healthcare professional and in the travel healthcare provided by an organisation, where the complexity of risk varies depending on whether the business is a service provider or employer sending personnel overseas. Therefore identifying risks within travel health requires a multifaceted approach taking into account professional competence, the public's expectation of a specialised healthcare service, medicolegal issues, health and safety legislation for clinical practice, premises and the duty of care of organisations sending personnel overseas.

The principal areas requiring risk assessment can be categorised into four domains: the individual traveller, healthcare professionals, travel healthcare provision and the organisations responsible for provision such as general practice, charities or companies (Fig. 5.1). The process of risk assessment which takes into account these domains and meets the diverse, organisational, professional, service-provider and legal requirements. It needs to be effectively managed, to ensure it is responsive to changes within the field of travel health. This can be achieved by making it an integral part of an existing organisational framework that will enable its development, implementation, monitoring and evaluation.

There are two, well-established organisational frameworks in which risk management in travel health can be incorporated: a health and safety

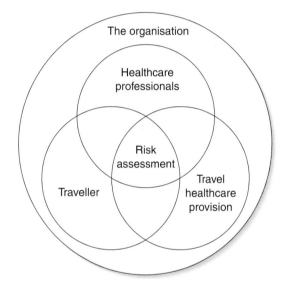

Fig. 5.1 Principal domains for risk management.

policy for an organisation sending personnel overseas and a protocol for travel health service provision. Both these frameworks address a multifactoral approach to the identification of risks in travel health at a individual, professional and organisational level which together will provide effective, competent and quality-driven travel health promotion for travellers going abroad.

Risk assessment in travel health

The principles of risk assessment primarily evolved from health and safety legislation and can be applied to other practice areas where risks can be identified, such as travel health. In risk assessment, it is important to distinguish between the terms 'hazard' and 'risk' and use of 'control measures'.

- *Hazard* is something that can cause harm.
- *Risk* is the degree to which the hazard can cause harm.
- *Control measures* are the interventions in place, either existing or introduced, to reduce the risk.

There are four key areas that underpin risk assessment:

- identification of hazards
- assessing the risk
- implementation of control measures
- monitor and review.

The first three key areas can be applied to the domains for risk assessment in travel health as shown in Box 5.1. Monitor and review are mainly conducted through audit and evaluation.

As shown in Box 5.1, assessment of risk for the traveller easily breaks down into components of hazard and risk. It is slightly more complex for the second example which reflects professional accountability and competence to practice in travel health. The third example for travel healthcare begins to address the infrastructure which underpins this provision of care. Organization takes into account the operational aspects needed to promote the health of travellers.

The process for risk assessment needs to be incorporated as part of a broader framework to ensure all the factors affecting individual, professional, healthcare provision and organisations' risk are identified and effectively managed. Risk management in travel health can be comprehensively directed through travel health and safety policies and protocols, addressing the key elements identified:[1]

- development of a travel health policy and protocol
- organisation and administration
- planning and implementation
- monitoring and audit
- review.

Box 5.1 Domains for risk assessment in travel health

Traveller
Hazard: malaria.
Risk: malaria risk could be high or low depending upon rates of endemicity, resistance to drugs, and prevalent species *Plasmodium falciparum* or *Plasmodium vivax*.
Control measures: malaria chemoprophylaxis and health education for the prevention of malaria.

Healthcare professional
Hazard: no previous education or training in travel health.
Risk: uses an old immunisation chart and gives out-of-date travel vaccine recommendations.
Control measures: appropriate training and education of healthcare professionals is provided.

Travel healthcare
Hazard: failure to establish a current medical condition in a traveller.
Risk: how this condition will be affected by travel, and immunisations and malaria chemoprophylaxis advised.
Control measures: assess the risk to health for a traveller by using a written questionnaire or checklist to ensure all the relevant information is obtained.

Organisation
Hazard: no system in place to identify risks for travel abroad.
Risk: travellers or personnel working overseas acquire travel associated illnesses.
Control measures: develop an organisational framework, a health and safety policy or protocol.

Travel health policies

A policy is a general course of action setting direction for detailed planning that is adopted and followed by a body. It details the organisation and administration, designating levels of responsibility and defining boundaries for making decisions. The policy may embrace the procedures and protocols already in place.

The law and travel health policies

Law is founded on statute or in precedent. There are three principal legal areas to consider that have direct implications for travel health policies in organisations that have a responsibility for personnel sent abroad or are service providers:

- criminal law
- common law
- law of tort.

CRIMINAL LAW

Criminal law is nearly all enacted in statute.[2] There are two sources for this statutory legislation: parliament and European Directives that are implemented as law in the UK. These impose a legal statutory duty of care upon organisations for the health and safety of employees which is enforced usually by penalties under the criminal system.[3] Many Acts of Parliament are developed into codes of practice to facilitate interpretation. Although codes of practice are not in themselves the law, failure to follow their advice will be evidence of a breach in the law.[2]

COMMON LAW

This law is made by the judges and is developed case by case within the reported decisions of courts. Judges are considered competent to make legal rules without reference to Parliament.[2] If the circumstances of a decision do not fit previous decisions, then a judge can make a decision which will further define and develop the common law.

LAW OF TORT

The law of contract and tort (civil liability for unlawful acts) or tort of negligence is part of the common law. The tort of negligence covers the many situations that result in a person suffering injury or ill-health: negligence or lack of care does not automatically give rise to liability; it has to be shown that there was a legal duty to take care, that there has been a negligent breach of that duty and that damage has been suffered by the person to whom the duty was owed because of the breach of that duty.[3]

Employees injured through work usually attempt to prove that their employers are at fault, either through breach of statutory duty or common law negligence. Common law negligence has been evolved by judges in previous cases, where it is considered that an employer must take reasonable care to prevent employees, or any other person within the area of foreseeable risk, from suffering injury to their person.[2] What is reasonable depends on the facts of each case. As with criminal law, the courts may balance the risks against the cost of avoiding it.

Where Parliament has imposed duties on an employer in the criminal law, the judges have in some cases of statutes implied a right in the person for whose benefit the duty was imposed to bring a civil action for damages in addition to the possible criminal prosecution.[2] Not all safety statutes will give rise to civil action.

Geographical implications of the law

Acts of Parliament relating to health and safety, employment law and equal opportunities apply throughout the UK.[2] Laws enacted in the UK apply only to employees who work wholly or mainly in the UK regardless of any term of their contract which claims to exclude UK jurisdiction.[4] The Health and Safety at Work Act (Application outside Great Britain) Order 1989 extends the application of the Health and Safety at Work Act to offshore oil and gas installations, pipeline work, off shore construction and diving operations.[5]

Employees who suffer from ill-health or are injured while working abroad may try to seek compensation from their employing organisation. Their employer may be unwilling to defend the case here or a UK court might decide that the foreign court is more appropriate.[2] When a legal dispute arises between individuals that concerns foreign law, the rules of 'conflict of laws' applies which is that part of the private law of a country which deals with cases having a foreign element: some aspects of the conflict are concerned with a litigant's domicile, the litigant's permanent home, which may govern the law that will be applied to a case.[4]

The following are examples of court decisions that have resulted from legal disputes concerning employees working abroad:

- *Todd v. British Midland Airways (1978).* The extent of employment protection legislation depends upon the country where a person is held ordinarily to work. In this case, an airline pilot who flew from the UK but spent 53% of his time abroad was held ordinarily to work in the UK.[2] It could be argued that he would then be protected by the safety statutes in this country.

- *Square D Ltd and Other v. Cook.* In this case, the employee was sent abroad to work at the main contractor's site in Saudi Arabia where he suffered an injury. It was held that it was throwing too high a responsibility on the home-based employers to hold them responsible for the daily events of a distant site occupied by a third party. As Goldman explains, 'The employer's responsibility to take reasonable care for the safety of the employee cannot be delegated, but the extent of the employer's legal duty depends on what is considered reasonable in the circumstances.'[4]
- *Cawthorn v. Freshfields.* This is a more recent case where a trainee solicitor issued a writ against her firm, claiming personal injury, loss of career as a lawyer and psychological distress, following a business trip to Ghana. She contracted *Shigella* dysentery after eating barracuda while working in Ghana which then developed into irritable bowel syndrome. The claim made against the firm was that she had not been given sufficient advice on eating foods or required inoculations for the country. This case was settled out of court for a sum in the region of £100 000.[6]

It was unfortunate this case did not go through the debate of court where it might have established a primary precedent for the duty of care for employees travelling abroad.

Therefore, for employees working abroad, the process of claiming negligence is convoluted and lengthy. Besides going through the process of proving an employing organisation has a duty of care and that duty was breached resulting in harm, they need to determine the country whose law is most appropriate to the case. In the European Union, health and safety regulations are very similar. The law in many other countries outside Europe is based on the same principles as the UK. Concerns arise in those countries where the process of the legal system has been affected, for example by war or political change.

Legislation affecting travel health policies

There are many areas within legislation that have direct implications for travel health policies. The principal ones to consider are:

- Health and Safety at Work Act 1974.[7]
- Management of Health and Safety at Work Regulations 1992.[1]
- Contracts of employment.

HEALTH AND SAFETY AT WORK ACT 1974

This Act came into force on 1 April 1975. It places on employers statutory duties of care, for organisations with five or more employees. While all the duties described in the Act are relevant, the most pertinent sections that apply to personnel working abroad are:

Section 2: it is the duty of all employers to ensure so far as is reasonably practicable, the health, safety and welfare at work of their employees. The duty is to do that which is reasonably practicable, whether by information, advice or otherwise. It is a difficult for an employer to gauge what level of health and safety is reasonably practicable, especially with travel overseas or personnel living abroad. It may not be possible for an employer to control some risks, such as personal security. Cost–benefit analysis also plays an important role.

Section 2(3): refers to a written policy: 'it is the duty of every employer to prepare and, as often as may be appropriate, revise a written statement of his general policy with respect to the health and safety at work of his employees and, the organisation and arrangements for the time being in force for carrying out that policy and, to bring that statement and any revision to the notice of all his employees.'

Section 3: obliges both employers and self-employed persons to do what is reasonably practicable to protect persons not employed by them who may be affected by their activities. This may apply to consultants or contracted personnel who travel abroad for an organisation or to clients visiting the premises of a travel health clinic.

Section 6: this duty concerns safety require-ments of goods and substances in use (including microorganisms). It includes the course of setting, cleaning, maintenance, dismantling, disposal (goods) and handling, processing, storing and transporting (substances), by a person at work. This relates to clinical practice in travel health.

Section 9: prohibits any employer from charging his employees for any safety equipment provided in respect of any specific statutory requirement. This raises the question of what equipment or supplies an employer should provide for personnel working overseas, such as mosquito nets, sterile injections kits or travel vaccines.

MANAGEMENT OF HEALTH AND SAFETY AT WORK REGULATIONS 1992

The Management of Health and Safety at Work Regulations 1992 and came into force on 1 January 1993. They specify the broad general principles and set minimum standards which apply to virtually all places of work except sea-going ships. No civil action for breach of statutory duty lies in respect of these regulations, but it is likely that they will be regarded by courts as setting new standards of care in common law negligence.[2]

The main focus of these regulations is towards risk assessment and management; they require employers to:

- assess the risks to employees
- implement effective preventive and protective measures
- provide employees with health surveillance
- give information, training and education
- appoint competent persons to supervise a safe system of work.

CONTRACTS OF EMPLOYMENT

A contract is made when one party makes an offer to another and the offer is acceptable. The Employ-ment Protection (Consolidation) Act (EPCA) 1978 protects employees by imposing a statutory obli-gation on employers to put the major terms of the employment contract into writing and to provide employees with a copy.[2] An employee who goes abroad for more than 1 month is entitled to a copy before leaving the UK. It ensures employees are aware of terms and conditions of their contract.

The EPCA was amended by the Trade Union Reform and Employment Rights Act 1993, con-ferring a statutory obligation for an employee starting work to be given a written statement within 8 weeks. Major terms of the agreement should be included such as pay, hours, absence because of sickness or injury, and place of work. It does not cover all the terms of an agreement and does not relate to health and safety at work. The statement should inform the employee of any collective agreements which directly affect the employee's contract. Once a contract is made, neither party can alter its terms without the other's agreement.

As with common law negligence and breach of statutory duty, for those who work abroad it is important to determine the laws of which country are most appropriate to a contract of employment. The Contracts (Applicable Law) Act 1990[4] provides three systems to determine this:

1. Contracting parties may, by an express term, set out the law under which the contract operates and by which any dispute may be resolved.
2. Where there is no express term as the proper law of the contract, a term is to be implied into the contract of employment so that it is governed by the law of the country in which the employee habitually carried out the work which the employee was employed to do.

    Where an employee is required to work in several countries so that there is no 'habitual' place of work, the contract of employment is to be governed by the law of the country that contains the central administration of the employer.
3. If it appears that in considering the contract and its operation, that the laws of another country most closely affect it, the dispute will be settled in accordance with the laws of that country.

Terms and conditions of employment

The written statement of terms and conditions of employment is important evidence when a dispute arises. In English law, regulation of the employment relationship is left to a certain extent to the agreement of the parties. It is sometimes difficult to ascertain the terms of a contract of employment: they may be stated in a contract as express terms which are more clearly defined, or are never put into words but are included by implication, or parties may not express their terms assuming they are obvious.[2]

Express and implied terms

Usually, *express terms* cannot be contraindicated by implied terms. If you want a position to be clear, you should make an express agreement in writing. The country whose law is to apply to an employment contract can be written as an express term: this enables an employee to have a choice of suing in the domicile of the employer, or in the country agreed in the contract of employment.

There is an *implied term* in every contract of employment that the employer will take reasonable care to protect the employee's safety and health while the employee is acting in the course of employment.

Applying the law to travel health policies

Travel health policies provide the opportunity for organisations to state their position, intention and commitment towards the health, safety and welfare of personnel they send abroad. They can be developed in conjunction with the health and safety policy, or as a separate additional policy. Travel health policies play an essential role in the contract of employment where terms and conditions for travelling abroad can be specified.

Using express terms in a contract is the most valid way of defining the position of the employer and employee: they ensure both parties are clear and in agreement with their individual responsibilities for travel health purposes. For instance, there is no implied term in every contract of employment that the employer will provide personal accident insurance for employees who work abroad, or advises employees on the need to take out their own insurance.[2] If employees do not take recommended malaria chemoprophylaxis, they may have breached their contract.[4] As long as the employer has warned employees at the outset of the risk of failing to take malaria chemoprophylaxis, the employer reduces the chance of being found negligent if an employee falls ill and sues for compensation. Employees

who refuse to take malaria chemoprophylaxis, with no medical grounds for this decision, may lead to employers re-assigning them to non-malarious areas or refuse them permission to travel abroad.

The above example can be extended to other travel health policy areas such as accidents: where employees or volunteers are advised to wear crash helmets if riding motorbikes for work purposes while abroad or, by making it compulsory to wear seat belts in the vehicles provided by the organisation.

Benefits of a travel health policy

For travellers, health policies:

- give protection, raising confidence and morale
- create job satisfaction and adaptation
- reduce morbidity and mortality
- provide assurance for the individual and family
- reduce stress and psychological concerns
- offer travel health and safety protection.

For the organisation, a health policy should:

- increase productivity of work
- reduce sickness and absence
- decrease staff turnover
- improve morale in an organisation
- create better teamwork
- ensure appropriate staff are recruited
- improve loyalty and motivation
- protect against litigation
- safeguard public relations or corporate image.

Strategies for developing and implementing travel health policies

The nature, size, complexity and commitment to health and safety of an organisation are important factors to consider for introducing a travel health policy. A difficulty frequently encountered is persuading management of the need to develop and implement a travel health policy. It implies a change for all those who will be affected by that policy in an organisation and may have cost implications. Support is required from management and personnel at various levels in the organisation to make a travel health policy viable.

The introduction, development and implementation of a travel health policy are going to involve change. This process of change needs to be well managed, if it is going to be effective and accepted. To manage this process of change successfully, a strategy needs to be devised. A structured and well considered approach will help to achieve the intended outcomes. Lewin[8] proposed that change is a result of the competition between driving and restraining forces. When a change is introduced, some forces drive while others restrain it. To implement a change, management should analyse the change forces. By selectively removing forces that restrain change, the driving forces will be strong enough to enable implementation.[9]

Other approaches to managing implementation through change are to adopt specific tactics to overcome resistance such as communication, education, participation in the change process, negotiation and coercion by the use of formal powers through top management support. There are various 'management of change' aspects to consider, which will help to plan a suitable strategy for the introduction and implementation of a travel health policy.

Guidelines for developing and implementing a travel health policy

Besides complying with the relevant health and safety legislation and contracts of employment, a travel health policy should reflect the philosophy, values, beliefs, size and functions of an organisation. It is a declaration of intent to protect the health and safety of travellers going abroad, and to enlist the support of all personnel in an organisation towards achieving these ends. The development of a travel health policy should be considered as a living entity, which will continue to evolve and be regularly reviewed.

There is not an ideal travel health policy, it has to be moulded to the individual travel health and safety needs of an organisation. While guidelines to develop a travel health policy cannot cover all situations, they can include the essential components. They need to keep in line with the requirements of the Health and Safety at Work Act 1974,[7] and to include a written policy statement, the organisation and arrangements for carrying it out, such as risk assessment.

The key guidelines for a systematic approach to the development and implementation of a travel health policy are outlined in Figure 5.2 and will be discussed in more detail.

I. IDENTIFY THE NEED FOR A TRAVEL HEALTH POLICY

A travel health policy can be general, or specific covering particular topics in travel health, for example malaria and accidents. Clarify the need for the policy: is it reactive where there is an indication of need, or is it pro-active where you need to decide what opportunities, benefits or advantages will occur as a result?

Within the organisation, identify at an early stage friends or foes to the idea of a travel health

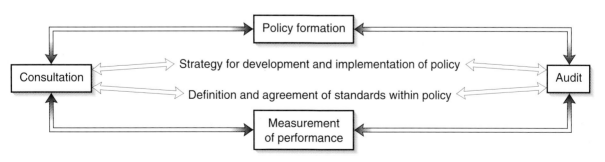

Fig 5.2 Travel health and safety risk management framework.

policy, as advocated by Lewin's management of change theory.[8] Provide information for those who are unsure or against it. Pilot a questionnaire survey to determine the current issues: at the same time this will create awareness of travel health and safety concerns and begin to lay the foundations for the implementation of a travel health policy at an early stage.

2. RESEARCH AND PRESENT THE EVIDENCE

The first aim is to find out what policies are already in place: are any relevant to travel health, such as accident prevention, repatriation, medical insurance and alcohol in the workplace? Existing policies need to be collected and reviewed, as they may need modifying to keep them up to date. You may need to develop an entirely new policy.

Research and analyse the relevant information in travel health and the organisation: include corporate image and data, such as 'absence from work' rates and cost-effectiveness. Collate from this, the evidence to establish the need to develop and implement a travel health policy.

Discuss the research outcomes with management and other key staff. Identify key personnel who need to be involved in the initial discussion. This may include union representatives, other health professionals, safety representatives or a staff member who travels abroad for the organisation. Present your research outcomes to this group. Clearly state the reasons why a travel health policy needs to be developed and implemented, using an evidence-based approach. It may be useful to have an informed advocate at this stage.

3. ORGANISE A WORKING GROUP

Once the need for a travel health policy has been accepted, organise a working group with management's agreement. Create a working team whose members have individual strengths and reflect different aspects of the organisation. Consider the team members' sphere of influence among the managers, employees or volunteers. Representations should be from both sexes, ethnic and disability groups, personnel staff, employees, customers or volunteers who have some experience of travelling abroad with the organisation.

Key individuals in a core group should be selected from:

- managers
- health professionals
- personnel staff members
- safety representatives, to include a safety committee member
- union representatives.

Outline the aims, objectives and agree an action plan for the working group. As the main aim will be to develop and implement a travel health policy, the group will need to be made aware of the rationale supporting a travel health policy. Judge the reactions of the working group members. Some may not agree with the policy. Group work in team-building will be an essential component to enable the group to work together in achieving the aims and objectives. Once the policy has been implemented by the organisation, the team's meetings can develop into review sessions.

4. CONSULTATION WITH PERSONNEL

Discussion should take place with key personnel, particularly those who travel and work abroad. Besides being aware of the issues, they are the ones who will be affected by the implementation of a travel health policy. Consultation can be carried out by:

- *presentation*: to personnel in different sections and at various management levels; the style of presentation should be interactive
- *a questionnaire*: which addresses the key components of a travel health policy, including any ensuing guidelines.

Both these methods would ascertain opinions and problem areas experienced by personnel in travel health relating to their work. This will enable staff to have some ownership and involvement in the development process of the policy, which in turn will enhance its acceptance and compliance.[10,11]

5. DRAFT A TRAVEL HEALTH POLICY

Collate the information from research and consultations with personnel. Then, using a process of brainstorming or presentations, identify and agree upon the key areas of the travel health policy. A policy is not the most appropriate way of covering detailed rules or guidelines, but these should be referred to in the written text. When drafting the policy, consider:

a. The commitment of the organisation

What is the organisation's philosophy and specified commitment to the health, safety and welfare of personnel who travel and work abroad? Does it provide the minimum standards as set out in statutes for health and safety? Does the level of care for personnel take into account the costs of implementing measures that can be considered reasonably practicable. What is the organisation's responsibility to accompanying families of personnel working abroad and to the health, safety and welfare of locally employed staff abroad? What has the consultation process with personnel revealed about the type of advice and support they would like to be given?

b. Travel healthcare provision

How will this be provided? Will guidelines, protocols and procedures be reviewed or developed in line with the travel health policies? What support and advice will be provided to maintain health abroad? What is the organisation's responsibility and position regarding an employee refusing to accept the recommended travel health advice?

c. The organisation and arrangements for carrying out the policy

This section details the systems and procedures an organisation will put in place to:

- carry out a risk assessment to identify travel-related risks and hazards to health
- identify preventive measures
- control travel-related risks and hazards to health
- make staff aware of these risks and their prevention
- define the levels of responsibility.

The policy statement should give the name and where necessary, the business address of the Director, Manager, or Senior Executive who is responsible for fulfilling the policy. Where functional expertise exists to advise line management, then the relationship of these functions, for example occupational health physician, nurse or charity health adviser, should be made clear and the extent of the expert's functions defined in relation to travel health.

While the general responsibility for health and safety rests at the highest management level, all individuals at every level will have to accept degrees of responsibility for carrying out that policy Wherever appropriate key individuals should be named and their responsibilities defined. It should be made clear in the policy that the final level of responsibility rests with each and every individual employee. In addition there should be adequate arrangements to cover the absence of personnel with key safety functions.

The policy may require formulation at more than one level in larger or more complex organisations that are geographically widespread. The highest management level should put in writing the principles of the policy whilst the sub-groups or operational units interpret that policy in a realistic written form to suit the identified needs at the lower levels.

d. Training and education

Identify and specify the training and education needs for those involved in all aspects of the travel health policy. This includes staff who provide travel health advice. In the Health and Safety at Work Act 1974,[7] there is an obligation on every employer to provide such information, instruction, training and supervision as is necessary to ensure, so far as is reasonably practicable, the health and safety at work of all employees.

Therefore, a travel health policy should ensure that personnel are made aware of the:

- risks to health when working abroad
- reasons for health and safety control measures
- roles and responsibilities of management and themselves in maintaining their own and others' health, which includes promoting a safe and healthy working environment.

Reference should be made to further detailed rules and regulations which must be observed. Specify important procedures, such as, dealing with serious situations that may occur abroad, for example war, kidnapping or repatriation for a medical emergency.

e. Setting standards for evaluation

These set criteria against which performance can be measured. The standards should be measurable, achievable and realistic.

f. Revision and review dates

Agree and write in the dates for revision of the draft policy document. Clarify agreed dates for review of the completed policy and specify the criteria for altering the document before this date, for example should new developments arise.

g. Presentation of a travel health policy

A written travel health policy is more effective and likely to be read if it is clear and concise. It should keep to the key areas with detailed reference being made to more specific guidelines, rules, protocols and procedures.

A travel health policy can be presented as:

- a travel health policy statement added to the general written policy statement as required by the Health and Safety at Work Act (1974).[7]
- a single policy document, covering the key areas in travel health, including the organisation and arrangements for carrying it out
- a single policy document for each specific area in travel health.

6. CONSULTATION ON THE DRAFT POLICY

A completed draft policy will need to be sent out for consultation to designated individuals or groups identified and agreed upon by the working group. This may include management, employee representatives, employees or volunteers, safety representatives, safety committee members, union representatives and outside authoritative groups, such as the Health and Safety Executive, or for a specific policy, for example concerning HIV/AIDS, consult with the Terence Higgins Trust or other recognised expert body.

7. IMPLEMENTATION

Achieving successful implementation of a travel health policy requires detailed organisation and arrangements to be operationalised such as:

- The training and supervision required to implement and maintain the aims of the policy.
- Establishing procedures and records. Procedures should be laid down for the recording of accidents occurring abroad or any absence owing to travel-related illness. Any travel health information based on expert analyses should be monitored. The employer should regularly present such records and information to all management levels and the safety committee, so that, if necessary, the policy can be revised. Maintaining records will help to identify travel-related risks and hazards to health: they will define their frequency in an organisation which will affect future policy developments.
- Communicating a travel health policy to all personnel is the most important process of implementation, otherwise the policy is useless. The working group needs to decide on the method that they will use to communicate the policy within the organisation, especially to personnel working abroad. Are there already established methods of communication with personnel in the organisation? Have these been evaluated as being effective in providing information?

Ideally, the written policy document should be distributed to *every* employee for information. This may be difficult and too costly to administer in larger organisations that tend to have a large amount of circulating memos and documents. In the larger or more complex organisations where staff may be based abroad, it may be better to hold the policy documents in a central position in each location for all to see on request, or displayed where all employees could see it. Those who are appointed to a post, which includes travel abroad, should be made aware of any travel health policies.

8. REVIEW, UPDATE AND AUDIT

Any changes or new developments that affect a travel health policy should initiate a revision of the policy. The amended policy is then published and brought to the attention of all the employees. A travel health policy will continually evolve in tandem with the needs of the organisation, its personnel, developments in health and safety legislation and travel medicine.

In order to maintain continuity, the working group will specify a review date and arrange meetings. They can then monitor the content and impact of a travel health policy through audit, which acts as an impetus for making improvements, discussing and incorporating, as agreed, any new developments.

Examples of travel health topics for policy development

A travel health policy can be developed to cover key areas or cover each individual topic area, where the general principles of an organisation need to be stated. All the travel health policies need to identify prime responsibility between the traveller and organisation, bearing in mind cost implications and what is reasonably practicable.

The basic cost issues are who will provide equipment, costs for vaccines, and medical insurance. A fundamental point is who will take prime responsibility: the traveller or the organisation? The following two examples illustrate some of the questions to consider which have implications for more detailed investigation:

EXAMPLE I ACCIDENTS

- Who is responsible for choice and use of vehicles used overseas?
- Will it be specified as compulsory for personnel to wear crash helmets and seat belts?
- Who will be responsible for the maintenance of vehicles abroad, including fitting of seat belts?
- What are the criteria for the recruitment and use of local drivers overseas?
- What is the policy for alcohol?

- Will first-aid training be introduced, by whom, to whom and who will pay?

EXAMPLE 2 MALARIA

- Who provides mosquito nets for personnel?
- Who pays for malaria chemoprophylaxis?
- Should the traveller take stand-by treatment?
- What if a traveller refuses or cannot take malaria chemoprophylaxis?

Travel health protocols

Protocols provide an ideal framework for risk management in travel health and are instrumental in the delivery of clinically effective and quality-driven travel healthcare.

At a practice level, the use of protocols supports the trend in government health policies[12,13] which emphasise quality in healthcare with cost-effectiveness as an underpinning factor: these policies set the direction for putting systems in place to facilitate clinical effectiveness within the healthcare service.

Clinical effectiveness promotes using best available evidence, introducing systems to measure and evaluate healthcare, making efficient use of resources and supporting health professionals to maintain and keep up to date with new developments.[14] It is dependent upon other key areas; information systems, clinical guidelines, research evidence, education and audit. These elements are essential for health professionals to be pro-active in the provision of quality travel healthcare.

The combination of risk management and clinical effectiveness in travel healthcare can be efficiently applied within a protocol to facilitate its operation in practice. A protocol may be defined as written recommendations, rules or standards to be followed for any healthcare service provision or situation where rational procedures can be specified. The process of developing and using a protocol is achieved by using a framework that adopts a systematic approach to travel health service provision. A protocol framework provides the structure, taking into account quality assurance, clinical effectiveness, professional standards, legal requirements and healthcare resources.

Identifying areas of accountability in a protocol

When health professionals take responsibility for providing travel health advice, they then become *accountable* for the service. By taking responsibility as health professionals, they must be satisfied that they have the required knowledge and competence in travel health. Being accountable implies that a situation has been assessed, planned and evaluated.[15] Therefore, through the protocol framework, it is important to identify and assess the key areas of accountability which apply to travel health service provision and their subsequent risk management. Accountability in travel health has several facets which directly or indirectly connect, sometimes causing conflict.

The main areas of accountability are:

- personal
- professional
- medicolegal
- employer/employee
- traveller
- society.

PERSONAL

As individuals, we develop our own personal, ethical principles which may be affected by our professional practice. A health professional may find a personal, moral difficulty in dealing with a traveller's request for the morning-after pill, as an extra measure to prevent pregnancy while on holiday.

PROFESSIONAL

Healthcare professionals must be registered with their relevant, recognised professional body to practise. Doctors register with the General Medical Council (GMC) and nurses with the United Kingdom Central Council for Nursing, Midwifery and Health Visiting (UKCC). These are self-regulatory bodies which are responsible by law for professional standards. Their main purpose is to protect the general public by ensuring doctors and nurses are professionally accountable and work within the standards of their professional codes of practice. Both regulatory bodies take care to point out that health professionals are personally accountable for their own competence in practice.[16,17]

Standards for professional competence to practise post qualification and in specialist areas must be maintained. Nurses are required to show evidence of education and training every 5 years to remain registered with the UKCC.[18] Professional standards to practise for doctors have been questioned following various failures in clinical practice and the ability of medical colleagues to assess clinical competence. This has led to a further development in health service policy with the introduction of clinical governance which will be phased into practice at local levels.[19] The GMC is debating methods for the regular validation of doctors as a measure to ensure professional competence for continued registration.[19]

MEDICOLEGAL

Society has become increasingly aware of health professionals' accountability in providing a standard of healthcare. Failure to meet their expectations of healthcare provision may lead to a formal complaint or litigation. Earlier in this chapter, the background to the principal areas of law was discussed. However, their relevance to accountability for travel healthcare provision to be considered within a protocol framework requires further explanation, particularly regarding:

- criminal law
- common law
- liability.

Criminal law

Health professionals will be affected by criminal law if they commit an offence against a person or become liable through statutory legislation. For example, this applies to laws concerning medicines, infectious diseases and health and safety. An area which has caused professional concern is the legality of nurses administering travel vaccines through the direction of a written *group protocol agreement.*

It is an offence under the Medicines Act 1968 for nurses to administer 'prescription only medicines' unless in accordance with the directions of an appropriate practitioner. The UKCC guidelines on Standards for the Administration of Medicines[20] interpreted this statement within the law as providing the facility for substances to be administered with advanced 'direction' covered by a protocol: this sets out the 'arrangements within which substances can be administered to certain categories of persons who meet the stated criteria'. Such an arrangement under a protocol for the administration of medicines is more accurately termed a 'group protocol agreement'.

The legitimate use of a group protocol agreement has been questioned, with particular, legal uncertainty arising from a protocol being interpreted as 'directions of an appropriate practitioner'. Although the term 'protocol' has not been explicitly stated within the Medicines Act, current nursing practice has evolved beyond the scope of this antiquated part of the law. The Royal College of Nursing, the Medical Defence Union and the UKCC have expressed their support of the use of group protocol agreements for the supply and administration of medicines.[21]

Clarification of the legal position of group protocols became the priority for the Review Team for the Prescribing, Supply and Administration of Medicines. In the resultant Crown Report,[22] the review team defined a group protocol as:

> a specific written instruction for the supply or administration of named medicines in an identified clinical situation. It is drawn up locally by doctors, pharmacists and other appropriate professionals, and approved by the employer, advised by the relevant professional advisory committees. It applies to groups of patients or other service users who may not be individually identified before presentation for treatment.
>
> Crown Report 1998

The Crown Report cautiously supports the use of a group protocol 'for those limited situations where this offers an advantage for patient care, and where it is consistent with appropriate professional relationships and accountability.'[22] Recommendations include the specification of details that clearly state the parameters and criteria for their development and use in healthcare, showing arrangements for professional responsibility and accountability. It confirms the need for legal clarification to ensure health professionals who supply or administer medicines through approved group protocols are acting within the law. The summary of these recommendations are reinforced in the final report for the 'Review of Prescribing, Supply and Administration of Medicines.'[23]

Common law

Legal action taken against health professionals lies in the domain of common law, where they can be sued for negligence. This is when a plaintiff, the person bringing the civil action for harm done, has to prove that the defendant, for example a health professional, was liable. The plaintiff has to prove three outcomes to the satisfaction of a court to win a negligence case:[24]

1. the health professional had a duty of care, which was breached: this breach was considered reasonably foreseeable
2. the health professional did not practise the standard of care required by law and in a way that was acceptable to professional peers
3. as a consequence, harm was done as a result of failure to practise properly.

There are three key areas to consider as part of negligence or duty of care for professional practice which are competence, standards of practice and delegation.

Competence and standards of practice. A health professional's competence to practise is judged according to a standard established in a precedent case in law, known as the 'Bolam test' (1957)[25]: the case held it 'is the standard of the ordinary skilled man exercising and professing to have that special skill. A man need not possess the highest expert skill at the risk of being found negligent . . . it is sufficient if he exercises the skill of an ordinary competent man exercising that particular art.' Therefore, a health professional's practice will be assessed by the standards of professional peers in travel health.

They are not required to be experts, but must have adequate knowledge and skills to practise in travel health. This part of the law is reinforced by professional codes of practice.

Delegation. When delegating travel health advice, it is the duty of the person delegating the task to ensure the health professional carries out that care at a reasonably competent level. The case of *Wilsher* v. *Essex AHA* (1988)[26] set the standard of reasonable care to be expected of students and junior staff: 'The standard is that of *a reasonably competent practitioner*.... You have a duty to ensure that the care which you delegate is carried out at a reasonably competent standard.'

The Department of Health[27] has specified the criteria where a doctor may delegate responsibility for immunisation to a nurse, provided:

1. the nurse is willing to be professionally accountable for this work as defined in the UKCC guidance on the 'Scope of Professional Practice'
2. the nurse has received training and is competent in all aspects of immunisation, including contraindications to specific vaccines
3. adequate training has been given in the recognition and treatment of anaphylaxis.

Equally, a doctor must ensure delegation of travel health service provision is carried out by a nurse who is competent in travel health. It is important to note that practitioners delegating the responsibility of travel health must have a degree of competence themselves in that practice area to ensure appropriate delegation is achieved. New initiatives are being developed encouraging nurses into partnerships with doctors in practice or taking the lead in providing a service where they employ doctors on a sessional basis. For example, a nurse may set up a travel health clinic and employ a doctor for specific clinic times. In this case, nurses must be equally aware of their legal responsibilities as employers and professionals in delegating tasks.

Liability

There are two types of liability to consider 'direct' and 'vicarious'. *Direct liability* is when the employer is responsible for error, such as failing to employ a health professional who is competent in

travel health and it has resulted in harm. *Vicarious liability* means 'indirect' and relates to an employer being held responsible for the actions of employees, even though the employer as an individual has done no direct harm. The Crown Report specifies that an employer is responsible for providing final approval of a protocol in order to ensure full consideration of legal liability and indemnification for staff.[22]

Other legal areas for professional practice

There are several areas in which health professionals must have greater legal awareness to ensure they are providing a good standard of practice. The main areas to consider are:

- consent
- confidentiality
- standards for record-keeping
- health and safety.

EMPLOYER AND EMPLOYEE

There are different aspects of accountability for an employer and employee. Employers have a duty of care to employees and to travellers using the travel health service. They must delegate responsibilities to competent staff and provide the support required for them to deliver the service for which they are contracted. Their responsibility includes health and safety, ensuring travel health advice is given using good standards of practice in a safe working environment.

Employees are directly accountable to their employer for carrying out a service according to their agreed job description in their employment contract. Conflict can arise between professional and employer accountability when a health professional with no prior knowledge or experience in travel health, is delegated the responsibility of providing travel health advice without any provision being made for training and supervision.

TRAVELLER

Healthcare professionals are accountable to travellers for their standards of professional practice and for the travel health service they provide which has been explicitly stated within the

Patients' Charter.[28] The delivery of a travel health service should be developed through consultation with travellers to meet their specific needs.

SOCIETY

There is a legal and professional obligation for healthcare professionals to be accountable for the public health of the community.[29] Protecting the health of a community is an integral function within travel health, particularly in relation to preventing travellers returning with a communicable disease.

The value of protocols to manage accountability in travel health

A protocol enables the use of evidence-based practice and clinical efficiency which improves medicolegal protection. Although background evidence to develop a travel health protocol can be disputed, a protocol does help to distinguish the legal and professional demands required for each travel healthcare team member. A group protocol agreement provides documented evidence of responsible discussion and delegation. When agreeing to implement protocols, nurses should remember that they will still be held responsible for their own actions.[17]

A travel health protocol is a means to providing evidence of the standard of information and advice given to travellers going abroad. In litigation cases, medical or nursing experts would have to testify that a travel health protocol was considered to be at a reasonable standard and relevant to practice.[30,31] This is why it is important to keep protocols up to date; otherwise, they will not be very valid and could, in turn, support the prosecution.

Although protocols have not been put to the test in a court of law as evidence for a health professional's practice, they are considered by legal experts, professional bodies and unions, to supply written documentation to support evidence for the level of care given by a health professional, providing they are based upon current

information. Tingle, a professor in healthcare law points out that the presence of protocols 'shows that healthcare professionals have thought proactively about the care they give and there is written evidence of the standard of care.'[32]

Protocols therefore must be considered essential to the management of the risks associated with the various facets of accountability facing healthcare professionals in the provision of a travel healthcare service.

Benefits of a travel health protocol for health professionals

Developing a protocol enables a multidisciplinary approach to be taken to travel healthcare where roles and responsibilities are clarified to aid teamworking. The Crown Report[22] identified other disciplines, advisory groups and partnerships that need to be involved in the process of development of group protocol. At the same time, a protocol can begin to establish alliances, as advocated in the 1997 health service policy document *The New NHS*,[12] to promote travel health services with travel agents, schools or other commercial organisations.

Collecting information for a protocol supports evidence-based practice and helps health professionals resolve areas where there is conflicting medical opinion or dilemmas in practice: collating data and consultation will support health professionals to reach a consensus for the content of a protocol, from which standards can be set and then measured for audit. Health professionals will be working with uniform information and supportive rationale to provide advice to travellers.

The process of developing a protocol clarifies education and training needs for all the staff involved in providing the travel health service. It facilitates the development of the scope of practice within a professional and legal framework.[33] Having established a protocol, it can then be used as a teaching aid for new members of the travel healthcare team and as a referral point for agency staff. It provides support for litigation as documentary evidence for standards of care and delegated responsibility as well as creating awareness of legal liability between employees and employers.[34]

Advantages for the traveller

The use of a protocol for a travel health service promotes consultation with travellers and the delivery of relevant and uniform information. This will reassure travellers that they are being given quality travel health advice, and will increase their confidence in the service being provided. Consequently, this may lead to a traveller being more compliant with the travel health advice given and result in a more successful outcome to their health.

Advantages for the travel health service

The main benefits of a protocol for the travel health service are to improve standards for clinical effectiveness, make efficient use of resources, establish a safe system of practice for health professionals and travellers and to provide a framework for giving travel health advice which includes auditing and evaluation. In a critical review of 59 published clinical protocols, all but four reported an improvement in the process of patient care.[35]

Disadvantages of a protocol

Although the benefits of a protocol generally outweigh the disadvantages, it is important to identify those areas which may become barriers to developing and implementing a protocol in practice. Health professionals may consider protocols as restricting their individual practice. The process of clarifying roles and responsibilities may be threatening to well-established positions in a practice. It may also be difficult to achieve consensus amongst team members.

A well-recognised difficulty in protocol development is the time factor and commitment of staff. Therefore, a systematic plan of action within a specified timeframe and delegation of tasks must be used to ensure the successful development and implementation of a travel health protocol in practice. Communicating protocol revisions to keep travel healthcare team members informed and up to date may be considered another difficulty to overcome. A reliable system for informing staff of revisions to a protocol needs to be agreed and established, with a staff member designated for this task.

Developing a travel health protocol

This is a comprehensive protocol that will cover all aspects of a travel health service. There are two key elements to developing such a protocol: **the process for developing** and **writing the content using a protocol framework**. These two operations evolve in tandem with each other, with the process setting the direction for writing the content of the protocol. Each of these functions will be addressed separately.

THE PROCESS FOR DEVELOPING A PROTOCOL

The development process comprises the following stages:

- Organise a working group
- Establish an action plan
- Collect evidence and information
- Consultation
- Draft formulation
- Reach consensus and agreement
- Draft approval
- Implementation.

Organise a working group. The working group should be multidisciplinary, representing all staff involved in providing a travel health service, for example, receptionists, nurses, doctors, managers and community pharmacists. Participation by all the key members of the travel healthcare team will give greater ownership of a protocol and, hence, responsibility to adhere to the content. Where there are difficulties in arranging a multidisciplinary group owing to personnel restraints or lack of motivation, then the healthcare professional most active in giving travel health advice may devise a draft protocol for consultation. Working alone on such a document is not easy and is more reliant upon the consultation process to reach both consensus and agreement for the protocol's content and use in practice.

Establish an action plan. In order to successfully achieve the goal of a 'written travel health protocol', an action plan is agreed at the start of the working group. It should be set within a timeframe that is practical and realistic. Points for action should include the delegation of tasks to each member of the group and setting deadlines for completion. Working to an action plan will make more effective use of group members' time and resources, and will manage the progress in developing a protocol more successfully.

Collect evidence and information. Researching the evidence and available information is time-consuming. Once collected, it needs to be analysed and critically evaluated, before it is used as supportive evidence for the content of a protocol.

Consultation. This process should include individuals, outside the working group, who are involved in providing travel healthcare in a practice and those affected by the travel health service, namely the travellers. It is good practice to focus on the needs of the traveller going abroad.[36] A common complaint is that the communication of health professionals with patients is poor, and they feel they are not sufficiently involved in healthcare decision-making.[37] Therefore it is important to identify the needs and views of travellers going abroad: what are their expectations and requirements for a travel health service?

Outside the travel health practice area, identify those individuals with a professional, public health or service interest in travel healthcare, for example local consultants in infectious diseases or genitourinary clinics, public health doctors, community pharmacists and travel agents. All these groups of people will bring expertise to different areas in the development of a protocol. At the same time, it will raise interested groups' awareness of a travel health service, which may be beneficial to working relationships and improve the standards of travel healthcare in a locality.

Draft formulation. Once the draft has been completed send it for comment to the key individuals identified during the consultation. Feedback can be done informally or formally through a questionnaire or interview. Specify a date of return for the feedback information.

Reach consensus and agreement. When comments from the draft protocol have been received, the working group needs to review them and agree their inclusion in the revised protocol. This stage may require further evidence to clarify contentious issues.

Draft approval. The final protocol should be approved by the local professional advisory group and by the employer for use in practice.

Implementation. The completed travel health protocol must be dated, read and signed, by all the healthcare professionals involved in providing travel health advice and their employer to confirm they have agreed and accepted the content. Copies can be circulated to the relevant staff and one must be made available in the setting where travel health advice is given. Travel healthcare professionals must ensure they comply with the competence levels specified in accordance with their relevant professional codes of practice, before signing the protocol.

Part of the implementation process must include arrangements for monitoring, reviewing and communicating any changes made to a protocol as a result of new developments in travel health to make sure the protocol maintains its clinical effectiveness.

USING A FRAMEWORK TO WRITE THE PROTOCOL

Begin writing a protocol by drafting an outline of the main headings under which you can put the written content as it develops. A protocol framework is shown in Box 5.2, which indicates the basic headings required. These headings may alter or be added to as part of the protocol's development. Work towards keeping the written information, clear, concise and easy to read, following a logical sequence. Remember the aim of the written content is to ensure all staff can easily understand the protocol.

Using the protocol framework in Box 5.2, the rationale for the main headings can be explained in more detail as follows:

Aim and objectives. At this first stage, the demand for travel health advice in a practice should be assessed before deciding upon the type of service to be offered: will it be a travel clinic, travel session or service provided through ad hoc appointments? Providing a travel health clinic implies expertise in travel health and might raise travellers' expectations about the standard of service to be provided.

The aim should reflect the general intention of the travel health service to promote the health of travellers, ensuring professional and service accountability is considered to achieve this goal. The objectives break down the aim to specify the main intentions to make this work in practice.

Marketing. How will the service be advertised? Will it be through the practice leaflet, posters or practice newsletter? What about approaching other groups such as personnel managers in companies or organisations to make them aware of the travel health service, such as community pharmacists, travel agents or outdoor shops? An annual article in the local newspaper would also raise the public's awareness both in where travel health is provided, and to seek travel health advice early.

Organisation. This is how the service will be planned, setting the scene for providing travel health advice. Items to consider within this section are:

- appointments
- recall system
- resources
- equipment.

Administration. This section primarily involves the active running of the travel health service and will consider such topics as:

- roles and responsibilities
- immunisation group protocol agreement
- record-keeping
- claim forms
- adverse reaction forms
- yellow fever certificates.

Travel healthcare. This identifies the systematic process of giving travel health advice for a consultation and should include:

- risk assessment for travel
- immunisation
- health education
- returning traveller
- referral criteria
- surveillance and support for staff based overseas.

Obtaining information from a traveller needs to be standardised within a travel healthcare setting to ensure relevant details are not missed. This can be effectively directed using a travel health questionnaire or a checklist.

Monitor and review. Details need to be given about arrangements for updating and evaluating the clinical effectiveness and use of the protocol in practice for the traveller and staff involved. Inclusions for consideration are:

- patient evaluation questionnaires
- audit
- communications for updating.

Box 5.2 Using a protocol framework

AIM AND OBJECTIVES
Achieved through:
- Marketing
- Organisation
  — appointments
  — roles and responsibility
  — recall system
  — resources
  — equipment

- Administration
  — record-keeping
  — claim forms
  — adverse reaction forms
  — yellow fever certificates

- Travel healthcare
  — risk assessment
  — immunisation
  — health education
  — returning traveller
  — referral criteria

- Monitor and review
  — sign and date
  — information systems

Sign and date. The protocol should be signed by all the healthcare professionals actively involved in providing the travel health service and their employer to ensure they have understood and agree with the content. The protocol must be dated to make it a valid document.

Conclusion

Developing a travel health policy and protocol is essential to managing identified travel, organisational and professional risk within travel health. Successful risk management will depend upon ensuring policies and protocols remain reactive and responsive to new developments affecting legal, professional and service provision in travel health.

REFERENCES

1. Health and Safety Executive (HSE). Management of Health and Safety at Work Regulations 1992: Approved code of practice. L21. London: HSE Books; 1992.
2. Kloss D. Occupational health law. 2nd ed. Oxford, Blackwell Scientific; 1994.
3. Hywel T. Insurance and liability. In: Pantry S, ed. Occupatonal health. London: Chapman and Hall; 1995.
4. Goldman L. Caring for expatriates and workers abroad: health issues and ethical dilemmas. In: Behrens RH, Riley W, eds. Proceedings from an International Meeting organised by the Postgraduate Medical Federation, the Hospital for Tropical Diseases, and the London School of Hygiene and Tropical Medicine. London: Postgraduate Medical Federation; 1994.
5. Health and Safety at Work to Offshore gas installations
6. Freshfields reaches £100k settlement with Cawthorn. The Lawyer, 1997; 11(32) 12 August.
7. Health and Safety Executive. A guide to the Health and Safety at Work Act 1974. Guidance on the Act. London: HMSO; 1990.
8. Lewin K. Field theory in social science : Selected theoretical papers. New York: Harper & Brothers; 1951.
9. Daft RL. Management. 2nd ed. Orlando: The Dryden Press; 1991.
10. Chang RY. Mastering change management. Management skills series. London: Kogan Page; 1995.
11. Health and Safety Executive (HSE). Five steps to successful health and safety management. HSE IND(G) 132L C1000 7/93.
12. Secretary of State for Health. The new NHS: Modern–dependable. London: HMSO; 1997.
13. Secretary of State for Health. A first class service: quality in the NHS. London: HMSO; 1998.
14. NHS Executive. Promoting clinical effectiveness. A framework for action in and through the NHS. Leeds: NHSE; 1996.
15. Kendrick K. Accountability in practice. Professional Nurse 1995; 10(April): 7.
16. General Medical Council. Good medical practice. London: General Medical Council; 1998.
17. United Kingdom Central Council for Nursing, Midwifery and Health Visiting (UKCC). Code of professional conduct. London: UKCC; 1992.
18. United Kingdom Central Council for Nursing, Midwifery and Health Visiting (UKCC). Standards for post-registration education and practice (PREP). London: UKCC; 1995.
19. Beecham L. Consultant physicians should be appraised annually. British Medical Journal 1999; 318 (13 February): 419.
20. United Kingdom Central Council for Nursing, Midwifery and Health Visiting (UKCC). Standards for the administration of medicines. London: UKCC; 1992.
21. Unions provide advice to practice nurses on protocols. Practice Nurse 1996; 12(10): 599.
22. Department of Health (DOH). Crown Report: review of prescribing, supply and administration of medicines. London: DOH; 1998.
23. Department of Health (DOH). Crown Report: review of prescribing, supply and administration of medicines: final report. London: DOH; 1999.
24. Dimond B. Legal aspects of healthcare. Edinburgh: Churchill Livingstone; 1995.
25. *Bolam v. Friern Hospital Management Committee*; 1957.
26. *Wilsher v. Essex AHA*; 1988.
27. Department of Health. Immunisation against infectious disease. London: HMSO; 1996.
28. Department of Health. The patients' charter. London: HMSO; 1991.
29. Montgomery J. Health care law. Oxford: Oxford University Press; 1997.
30. Hurwitz B. Clinical guidelines and the law. British Medical Journal 1995; 311: 1517–1518.
31. Dukes J. Patient protocols: A review for those who commission, design and use them. Oxford: Oxford Health Care Management Institute; 1993.
32. Tingle J. Clinical protocols and the law. Nursing Times 1995; 91(29).
33. Parker S. Protocols – protection or penalty? MDU Nurse 1994; 4: 1–3.
34. Dukes J, Stewart R. Be prepared. Health Service Journal 1993; 103: 24–25.
35. Grimshaw J, Russell I. Effect of clinical guidelines on medical practice: a systematic review of rigorous evaluations. Lancet 1993; 342: 1317–1322.
36. Royal College of Nursing (RCN). Protocols and nursing guidelines for good practice. Issues in nursing and health, no 21. London: RCN; 1993.
37. Paley G. A framework for clinical protocols. Nursing Standard 1995; 9(21): 33–35.

SECTION 2

PHYSIOLOGICAL, MEDICAL AND PSYCHOLOGICAL TRAVEL-RELATED PROBLEMS

Health problems associated with air travel (including motion sickness, jet lag, fear of flying and air rage)

Richard Harding

Introduction

This chapter describes some of the physiological hazards which all air travellers, including those who are healthy, may experience. Such hazards involve the problems associated with ascent (hypoxia, hyperventilation and decompression sickness) and with descent from altitude (ear and respiratory sinus barotrauma). Other health problems considered are:

- motion sickness
- jet lag
- fear of flying
- air rage.

Problems associated with ascent to and descent from altitude

Ascent to altitude is associated with a fall in atmospheric pressure (and in temperature and density) so that at 5487 m (18 000 ft), for example, ambient pressure falls to half its value at sea level and the ambient temperature to about –20°C. The fall in total atmospheric pressure and the consequent reduction in the partial pressure of oxygen (PO_2) pose the greatest single danger to anyone who flies: hypoxia. Fortunately, the relationship between oxygen saturation of haemoglobin and oxygen tension, as reflected in the shape of the oxygen dissociation curve, acts to reduce the threat.

The plateau of the curve represents an in-built reserve, which is exploited by aircraft designers, and provides protection against hypoxia up to an altitude of 3048 m (10 000 ft). Ascent to this altitude produces a fall in alveolar PO_2 from the normal 13.7 kPa (103 mmHg) to 8.0 kPa (60 mmHg) but only a slight accompanying fall in percentage saturation of haemoglobin with oxygen. As altitude progressively increases above 3048 m (10 000 ft), the percentage saturation of PCO_2 also falls because of the hyperventilation, and this helps to reduce the difference.

HYPOXIA

The physiological consequences of hypoxia in flight are dominated by the neurological effects both of the hypoxia itself and of the cardio-respiratory responses to it.[1]

The respiratory responses depend upon the manner in which the hypoxic insult is delivered. Thus, the changes which accompany a slow ascent to altitude when breathing air will be different from those seen if the ascent is undertaken when breathing oxygen, and will be different again if hypoxia is the result of a rapid loss of cabin pressure. In general, however, hyperventilation is the ventilatory response to a fall in alveolar PO_2 below about 8.0 kPa (60 mmHg). A fall in alveolar PCO_2 also occurs because of the hyperventilation, and this helps to reduce the difference between inspired PO_2 and alveolar PO_2. Thus, hyperventilation is protective against hypoxia in so far as it reduces the fall in alveolar oxygen tension that would otherwise occur on ascent.

General cardiovascular responses to hypoxia including an elevation in heart rate and cardiac output on ascent to above 1829–2438 m (6000–8000 ft) when breathing air, while stroke volume and mean arterial blood pressure remain unchanged. There is, however, a redistribution of output such that, while most vascular beds respond to hypoxia by vasodilatation, desaturation of the blood by just 20% is sufficient to cause a generalised, rapid and reversible vasoconstriction in the pulmonary circulation. In the cerebral circulation, a conflict exists between the vasodilating effect of hypoxia (at levels of arterial $Po_2 < 6.0$ kPa (< 45 mmHg)) and the vasoconstricting influence of hypocapnia (low Pco_2), itself caused by the ventilatory response to hypoxia.

The early neurological effects of hypoxia are of great practical significance in aviation, particularly for air crew. Thus, when breathing air, performance of novel tasks (which may include responses to emergency situations) may be impaired at altitudes as low as 2438 m (8000 ft), while memory and eye–hand coordination are increasingly affected once above 3048 m (10 000 ft). Choice reaction time (measured as the time to select between two alternatives) is impaired significantly by 3658 m (12 000 ft), although simple reaction time (measured as the time to respond to a single stimulus) is unaffected until an altitude of 5487 m (18 000 ft) is exceeded.

The clinical presentation of hypobaric hypoxia is a combination of the features described, and the symptoms and signs are therefore extremely variable. The speed and order of appearance, and of the severity of symptoms, depend on the rate at which and the level to which the inspired oxygen tension is lowered, and on the duration of exposure.

Even when these factors are kept constant, however, there is considerable variation between individuals, although for the same individual the pattern of effects tends to be the same from one occasion to another: and therein lies the value of regular personal exposure to hypoxia in a decompression chamber as part of air crew education and training. Several other pre-existing circumstances may increase susceptibility to hypoxia, including alcohol (which mimics and enhances its effects) and other drugs (particularly antihistamines), incidental illness, exercise, cold and fatigue.[1]

The overt clinical features of acute hypobaric hypoxia can be summarised:

- Clinical features of hypoxia will begin to develop when ascents to altitudes above 3048 m (10 000 ft) are undertaken. It is for this reason that passenger aircraft are always pressurised to an altitude below this, and usually to an altitude of 1829–2438 m (6000–8000 ft). Pressurisation to sea level is too costly in terms of weight, bulk and finance, although it is occasionally used for aeromedical evacuation flights.

- The cabin pressurisation system provides the means by which thermal comfort is maintained since the temperature and humidity of the pressurising air delivered from the engines can be controlled. Any defect in the pressure hull of the aircraft (such as structural failure or an explosion) will lead to rapid decompression of the cabin and the exposure of its occupants to the 'outside' altitude, with the consequent risk of hypoxia and decompression sickness. Rapid decompression in civil aircraft is extremely rare, however, and the large volume of the cabin combined with a (usually) relatively small defect will tend to prolong the time of decompression and so enable the crew to start a descent. In any case, passengers and crew are provided with oxygen masks that deploy automatically if the cabin 'altitude' exceeds a safe level.

- Those passengers with compromised cardiorespiratory and neurological physiology may, of course, be affected by even the mild hypoxia accompanying ascent to normal cabin altitudes.

HYPERVENTILATION

Hyperventilation is a condition in which pulmonary ventilation is greater than that required to eliminate the carbon dioxide produced by body metabolism. There is a consequent and excessive fall in carbon dioxide levels in the tissues, the blood (hypocapnia) and the alveolar gas. The reduction in arterial P_{CO_2} also leads to a fall in hydrogen ion concentration and so to a respiratory alkalosis.

Although hypocapnia has no effect on arterial blood pressure or cardiac output, the latter is redistributed so that blood flow through skeletal muscle is increased while that through the skin and cerebral circulation is reduced. The intense cerebral vasoconstriction acts to reduce local arterial P_{O_2}, and the neurological features of profound hyperventilation are probably the result of a combination of cerebral hypoxia and respiratory alkalosis.[2]

A reduction in arterial P_{CO_2} to below 2.9–4.0 kPa (22–30 mmHg) produces significant decrements in the performance of both psychomotor and complex mental tasks; and is associated with light-headedness, dizziness, anxiety, and paraesthesiae of the extremities and lips. The ability to perform manual tasks is compromised by the neuromuscular disturbance associated with a fall in arterial P_{CO_2} to 2.0–2.7 kPa (15–20 mmHg), with muscle spasms of the limbs (e.g. main d'accoucheur) and face (risus sardonicus), and augmentation of tendon reflexes. There is also a general deterioration in mental performance. At arterial P_{CO_2} levels at or below 1.3–2.0 kPa (10–15 mmHg), general tonic contractions of skeletal muscle (tetany) accompany gross clouding of consciousness, and then unconsciousness.[3]

Hyperventilation is a normal response to a fall in alveolar P_{O_2} below 7.3–8.0 kPa (55–60 mmHg), so that hypobaric hypoxia may be an important cause of the condition. Furthermore, most of the early symptoms of hypoxia are very similar to those produced by hypocapnia (and the features of the latter may dominate the early stages of hypoxia – hence the need to emphasise for air crew the vital importance of treating any such symptom while airborne as hypoxia).

There are, however, other circumstances which may precipitate hyperventilation in flight, the commonest, as on the ground, being anxiety. While flying is, for most people, an exhilarating experience, many are also anxious at some stage, and mild hyperventilation is probably the norm although seldom clinically overt. Some passengers, however, may be so anxious that they routinely require mild pre-flight sedation. Another, less common, cause of hyperventilation is air turbulence.

BAROTRAUMA

Since the body may be considered to be at a constant temperature, any gas within closed or semi-closed body cavities will obey Boyle's Law on ascent to altitude. Thus, for example, any such gas will have doubled in volume, if it is free to do so, at an altitude of about 5487 m (18 000 ft) where atmospheric pressure is half that at sea level. The lungs, the teeth and the gut may be affected during ascent, while the middle ear cavities and sinuses may be adversely affected during descent.

Although potentially the most serious problem, expansion of gas within the lungs on ascent does not usually present a hazard since the trachea is easily able to vent the expanded volume. The lungs are therefore unlikely to be damaged unless a rapid decompression (loss of cabin pressurisation) of catastrophic magnitude takes place and the glottis is closed at the moment of decompression.

Aerodontalgia – dental pain during ascent – is nowadays uncommon since it does not occur in healthy or correctly restored teeth. The mechanism of pain production remains unclear. It may be a consequence of irritation of a diseased pulp by atmospheric pressure changes, or the result of vascular or neural phenomena responding to the relative increase in pressure within a carious deposit or closed air space left inadvertently beneath a dental filling.

Gas expansion within the small intestine can cause pain of sufficient severity to produce vaso-vagal syncope, but this is unlikely to occur during normal operation of commercial aircraft. Gaseous expansion in the small bowel is, however, aggravated by foods and drinks which produce gas, such as beans, curries, brassicas, carbonated beverages and alcohol; and passengers in commercial aircraft may become aware of waist distension following such dietary intake. Gas expansion in the stomach and large bowel does not usually cause any problems since it is easily released.

Expanding gas in the middle ear cavity vents through the Eustachian tube on ascent, and only rarely causes any discomfort. The symptoms of otic barotrauma develop during descent because air cannot pass back up the tube so readily.[4] Pain, which begins as a feeling of increased pressure on the tympanic membrane, quickly becomes increasingly severe unless the Eustachian tube is able to open and so equalise pressure between the middle ear cavity and the pharynx (that is, the atmosphere); an event known as 'clearing' the ears. Many people can achieve such opening merely by swallowing, by yawning, or by moving the jaw from side to side. Others have to perform a deliberate manoeuvre to open the tube by raising the pressure within the nasopharynx.

Some people find learning these techniques very difficult, and may be unable to do so even after much coaching and practice.

- The *Frenzel manoeuvre* is the most useful of these techniques, and is carried out with the mouth, epiglottis and nostrils closed. Air in the nasopharynx is then compressed by the action of the muscles of the mouth and tongue. This manoeuvre, when performed correctly, generates higher nasopharyngeal pressures than the Valsalva manoeuvre and achieves opening of the Eustachian tube at lower pressures.
- The *Valsalva manoeuvre* consists of a forced expiration through an open glottis while the mouth is shut and the nostrils occluded. The increase in intrathoracic pressure is transmitted to the nasopharynx and then to the Eustachian tubes. The rise in intrathoracic pressure is a disadvantage, however, since it impedes venous return to the heart and may even induce syncope.
- In the *Toynbee manoeuvre,* pharyngeal pressure is elevated by swallowing while the mouth is shut and the nostrils occluded. This is the best technique to use when evaluating normal Eustachian function under physiological conditions: under direct vision, a slight inward movement of the tympanic membrane is followed by a more marked outward movement.

The acute angle of entry of the Eustachian tube into the pharynx predisposes to closure of the tube by increasing pressure during descent. Upper respiratory tract infections, by causing inflammation and oedema of the Eustachian lining, increase the likelihood of developing otic barotrauma and of its ultimate result: rupture of the tympanic membrane. Passengers travelling while suffering from a head cold should be made

aware of the potential problem; and a pragmatic approach is to carry a proprietary nasal decongestant in hand luggage and to use it!

The treatment of otic barotrauma, particularly if blood or fluid is present in the middle ear cavity, should include analgesia, a nasal decongestant and a broad spectrum antibiotic.

The aetiology of sinus barotrauma is similar to that of its otic counterpart. On ascent, expanding air vents easily from the sinuses through their ostia. On descent, however, the ostia are readily occluded, especially if the victim is suffering from a cold. A sudden, severe, knife-like pain characteristically occurs in the affected sinus, and continues if descent is not halted. Epistaxis may result from submucosal haemorrhage.

The development of sinus barotrauma is related to the rate of cabin descent, and its prevention is part of the rationale behind the slow rates of descent employed in commercial aircraft. The possibility of a sinus problem cannot be predicted prior to flight, but flying with a cold will clearly increase the risk. Treatment should again include analgesia, nasal decongestants and a suitable antibiotic.

DECOMPRESSION SICKNESS

Aviators or sub-atmospheric decompression sickness, also known as dysbarism, is caused by the same mechanism and has the same clinical features as the condition that afflicts divers. For more details in relation to diving see Chapter 8.

- Joint and limb pain – 'the bends' – is the commonest clinical manifestation of sub-atmospheric decompression sickness, and is seen in about 74% of cases. The pain is characteristically deep, ill localised, and made worse on movement. Although single large joints are most frequently affected, more than one joint can be involved and at any site. The pain usually resolves during descent.
- Respiratory disturbances – 'the chokes' – are seen in about 5% of cases and have serious implications. Feelings of constriction around the lower chest, with an inspiratory snatch, paroxysmal cough on deep inspiration and sub-sternal soreness are followed by malaise and collapse unless descent is initiated.

- Dermal manifestations – 'the creeps' – in the form of an itchy, blotchy rash (± formication) are seen in about 7% of cases, but are of little significance unless associated with respiratory symptoms, when there may be urticaria and mottling of the skin of the thorax.
- Visual disturbances, with blurring, scotomata and fortification patterns, are seen in about 2% of cases, but there is usually no disturbance of other sensory modalities.
- Neurological disturbances – 'the staggers' – are rare, being seen in about 1% of cases. Regional paralysis, paraesthesiae, anaesthesia and fits may all be features.

Finally, a profound cardiovascular collapse may occasionally occur either without warning (primary collapse) or subsequent to any of the other manifestations (secondary collapse). Rarely, collapse may occur several hours after return to sea level (post-descent collapse).

Fortunately, sub-atmospheric decompression sickness does not occur in healthy individuals at altitudes below about 5487 m (18 000 ft) and is rare below 7621 m (25 000 ft).[5] The condition is therefore infrequently seen in the occupants of commercial aircraft. Above 7621 m (25 000 ft), however, it occurs with increasing severity the higher the exposure. As with divers, the treatment is to re-pressurise the victim, and this is accomplished in aviation by descending the aircraft and landing as soon as possible: this alone is usually sufficient to reverse the syndrome, but occasionally a recompression chamber must be used. Since the underlying cause of decompression sickness is believed to be the evolution of free nitrogen bubbles in the tissues, it is beneficial for the victim to breathe 100% oxygen that will wash out the offending gas.

As with hypoxia, some pre-existing circumstances will increase the likelihood of developing the illness: again, alcohol and drugs are unhelpful, and illnesses, cold, fatigue and hypoxia itself will also have a deleterious effect. And so too will any previous recent exposure to pressure changes, such as repeated parachute descents and, much more commonly, sub-aqua diving.

For military personnel and commercial aircrew, many guidelines and regulations exist concerning the necessary precautions to take before flying after such sporting activities.[6] In the UK, the Ministry of Defence recommendation[7] for flying after diving are summarised in Table 6.1.

For civilians, similar constraints should apply, but a good rule of thumb is to avoid 'with stops' diving for the 24 hours before any flight.

Motion sickness

Motion sickness is a unique problem associated with movement in three dimensions, the principal clinical features of which are familiar to most people: epigastric discomfort is followed by increasing nausea, pallor and sweating. The condition may then rapidly worsen (the 'avalanche phenomenon'), with increased salivation, feelings of warmth and, of course, vomiting. Secondary, less common, features may include hyperventilation, frontal headache, flatulence, depression and drowsiness.

TABLE 6.1 Ministry of Defence recommendations for flying after diving

Type of dive	Time interval between diving and flying	Maximum altitude (or effective altitude in pressurised aircraft)
Without stops	Up to 1 hour	Approx. 1000 ft (300 m)*
	1–2 hours	Approx. 5000 ft (1500 m)
	Over 2 hours	Unlimited flying in commercial aircraft (normally at no more than an effective 8000 ft (2400 m) above sea level)
With stops	Up to 4 hours	Approx. 1000 ft (300 m)*
	4–8 hours	Approx. 5000 ft (1500 m)
	8–24 hours	Approx. 16 500 ft (5000 m)
	Over 24 hours	Unlimited

* e.g. Helicopters

Several theories have been advanced to explain why motion produces what is essentially a poison-response mechanism such as that normally activated within the central nervous system as a protective reaction to the ingestion of toxic substances.

Reason's neural mismatch (conflict) theory, provides a sensible and useful model to explain why certain motion stimuli produce motion sickness but others do not.[8] The theory proposes that, when motion sickness develops, the sensory information provided by the visual, vestibular and proprioceptive apparatus is at variance with that expected by the brain on the basis of past experience. The mismatch not only leads to sickness but also initiates changes within the central nervous system that are responsible for the development of protective adaptation. Such a proposal also accounts for the occurrence of sickness when certain expected motion cues are absent – for example, in flight simulators and large screen (Imax) cinemas – but does not, however, explain why motion sickness takes the form that it does or why it should occur at all.

To explain this aspect, Treisman[9] has extended the conflict theory by postulating that the brainstem mechanisms responsible for orientation and motion are also responsible for the detection of, and response to, poisoning. Motion sickness occurs when sensory inputs to the brainstem are so confusing as to mimic the ingestion of poison. There is convincing evidence that this is so: surgical removal of the vestibular apparatus in experimental animals not only renders them immune to motion sickness but also unresponsive to certain poisons.[10]

So, motion sickness is really a misnomer since it is a normal manifestation of sensory function in response to real or apparent (that is, absent), but unfamiliar, motion stimuli. It is also the activation, by motion, of a primitive response to poison. Its incidence varies with the motion environment so that among those in life rafts in heavy sea states virtually 99% are affected, while in modern commercial aircraft the incidence is usually well below 1% and rises to only about 8% in severe turbulence. It also occurs in significant numbers in environments where expected motion cues are absent – for example, in simulators (10–60%) or in Imax film theatres.

For aircraft (and ship) passengers, pharmacological prophylaxis is a realistic approach.[11] But none of the currently available drugs – including cyclizine (Marazine), dimenhydrinate (Dramamine), hyoscine (= scopolamine) and promethazine (Phenergan) – are fully effective and, as central cholinergic blockers, all have central and/or autonomic side effects.

Comparative studies have generally concluded that hyoscine is the most useful single preparation for both the prophylaxis and the treatment of motion sickness. The effectiveness of transdermal hyoscine is similar to that of the oral preparation but has the additional advantages of ease of use and long duration of action (up to 72 hours). Of course, the latter attribute is really of benefit only for long sea voyages and space flight! Individual variability and visual side effects if use is prolonged are its principal drawbacks.

The effects of motion sickness in passengers may also be minimised by avoiding anxiety before and during a flight and, when affected, by reducing sensory input by keeping the head as still as possible, preferably by lying down with the eyes shut. This will reduce the intensity of the sickness but will not abolish it.

Jet lag – the problem of transmeridional travel

The endogenous circadian system, in which many physiological and psychological rhythms have now been identified, is known to be affected by several environmental factors, including light and dark, clock hour and temperature, although many rhythms continue in the absence of such cues, albeit usually with slightly prolonged periodicity.[12] Such environmental factors assist phasing or entrainment of the rhythms, and are known as synchronisers or zeitgebers (time givers).

Travel across time zones outstrips the ability of synchronisers to entrain rhythms, and desynchronisation occurs so producing the syndrome known as jet lag.

Circadian rhythms need a finite period to become re-entrained to local time (usually estimated at about 1 day per time zone crossed), and westward travel is generally considered better tolerated than eastward. This is possibly because the endogenous system – with a natural periodicity in most subjects of about 25 hours – is more able to adapt to the longer 'day' encountered during westward flight.

The aetiology of the effects of jet lag – sleep disturbances, disruption of other body functions such as feeding and bowel habit, general discomfort and reduced psychomotor efficiency – has been the subject of much investigation which has largely concentrated on underlying hormonal variations.[13] Although a 'jet lag pill' is theoretically possible, and studies involving melatonin have produced encouraging results, even greater knowledge of the neurotransmitter mechanisms involved in entrainment will be needed before such sophisticated pharmacological manipulation is fully a reality. Many methods of reducing or preventing these unpleasant consequences of modern travel have been proposed (implying that none is entirely effective), including careful pre-flight manipulation of sleep and eating patterns, but these are impracticable for most people.

Various simple methods can, however, be employed to minimise the effects, such as sleeping on the aircraft (with or without the benefit of a short acting hypnotic), avoiding heavy meals and excessive alcohol, avoiding important commitments for at least 24 hours after arrival, and generally being aware of an inevitable reduction in physical and mental performance for a few days. Finally, temazepam has been shown to have a beneficial effect on sleep and alertness after transmeridional travel, and to have little deleterious effect on performance; but it did not alter the rate of re-entrainment of physiological rhythms.[14]

Fear of flying

In the UK, an estimated 9 million people suffer anxiety about flying and may miss out on professional and personal opportunities. There is no single personality-type prone to fear of flying and there may be a link with problems at work or home. Fear may develop from a bad experience – such as a rough flight or after a news report of a hijacking or crash. Panic attacks are common (sudden, intense anxiety, sweating and trembling). The sensation is often so frightening that the sufferer will from then on refuse to fly.

Advice for the traveller who is afraid of flying

- Fear of flying is common and the safety record of air travel is good.
- Try distraction by talking with other passengers, watching in-flight films, eating or reading.
- Tell the cabin crew. Seek reassurance about strange sounds.
- A visit to the doctor prior to travel can provide reassurance about general fitness for air travel.
- Consider taking a tranquilliser before departure, but remember that these drugs do not mix well with alcohol.

Cognitive-behaviour therapy can be helpful for more severe cases. Sufferers identify what they actually fear, and then learn different ways of overcoming the anxiety. There are courses and counselling available for those with fear of flying, for example: courses run by Aviatours at Heathrow and Manchester airports (01252 793 250).

Air rage

This term has recently been introduced to describe psychological or physical violence occurring

---

Preventing jet lag

- Try to avoid travelling when you are already tired, and rest before departure. During flight get maximum sleep, aided by a mild hypnotic if necessary.
- Stretch and exercise as much as possible to aid circulation and prevent swollen ankles.
- Drink plenty of water or soft drinks to counteract the dry cabin atmosphere.
- Avoid excessive alcohol and caffeine that increase dehydration.
- Jet lag is made worse by a hangover!
- Breaking very long journeys halfway with a stopover can be helpful.
- Avoid heavy commitments on the first day after arrival.
- Some people find the use of melatonin to be helpful; however, its effect as yet, is scientifically unproven.

within aircraft. It is of particular concern because of the cramped conditions inside an aircraft and the inevitable involvement of not only the cabin crew but other passengers. There have been instances where aircraft have had to land prematurely to offload disruptive passengers.

There is often a developing cycle of events which may include delays, exhaustion owing to lack of sleep, excessive use of alcohol sometimes to combat fear of flying, minor irritations because of behaviour of fellow passengers which elsewhere would largely go unnoticed and sometimes anoxia causing irritability in those with pre-existing hypoxic illnesses.

It has recently been recognised that a common cause is nicotine withdrawal in heavy smokers on long–distance, 'no smoking' flights, which are now being introduced by many airlines. Nicotine gum or a mild tranquilliser may be useful prophylaxis.

PRACTICE POINTS

- Those prone to hypoxia, whether owing to respiratory or cardiac disease, may find their symptoms exaggerated in aircraft. Irritability is an early sign of anoxia.
- Air in aircraft is kept dry to avoid damage to equipment. Alcohol and caffeine aggravate dehydration.
- Prolonged sitting can cause circulation problems in the lower limbs resulting in swelling and occasionally thrombosis.
- Sitting in the front of aircraft can help motion sickness. Those prone to sickness should consider taking an anti-emetic in advance.
- Jet lag can be made worse by tiredness and a hangover!
- Fear of flying to some degree is a very common problem. Treatment is available.

REFERENCES

1. Ernsting J, Sharp GR, revised by Harding RM. Hypoxia and hyperventilation. In: Ernsting J, King PF, eds. Aviation medicine. 2nd ed. London: Butterworths, 1988; 45–58.

2. Lum LC. Hyperventilation and anxiety state. Journal of the Royal Society of Medicine 1981; 74: 1–4.
3. Ernsting J, Sharp GR, revised by Harding RM. Hypoxia and hyperventilation. In: Ernsting J, King PF, eds. Aviation medicine. 2nd ed. London: Butterworths, 1988; 58–59.
4. Harding RM. ENT problems and the air traveller. Travel Medicine International 1992; 10(3): 98–100.
5. Ernsting J. Decompression sickness in aviation. In: Busby DE, ed. Recent advances in aviation medicine. Dordrecht, Holland: D Reidel Publishing, 1970; 177–87.
6. Sheffield PJ. Flying after diving guidelines: a review. Aviation Space Environmental Medicine 1990; 61: 1130–1138.
7. Ministry of Defence (Navy). BR 2806 Diving manual. London: HMSO; 1972 (as amended to change 6) Articles 5121 and 5122.
8. Reason JT. Man in motion – the psychology of travel. London: Weidenfeld and Nicolson; 1974; 26–37.
9. Treisman M. Motion sickness: an evolutionary hypothesis. Science 1977; 197: 493–495.
10. Money KE, Cheung BS. Another function of the inner ear: facilitation of the emetic response to poisons. Aviation Space Environmental Medicine 1983; 54: 208–211.
11. Stott JRR. Management of acute and chronic motion sickness. In: Motion sickness: significance in aerospace operations and prophylaxis. Neuilly-sur-Seine, France: NATO Advisory Group for Aerospace Research and Development, 1991; AGARD LS-175: 11.1–11.7.
12. Mills JN, Minors D S, Waterhouse JM. The circadian rhythms of human subjects without timepieces or indications of the alteration of day and night. Journal of Physiology (Lond) 1974; 240: 567–594.
13. Arendt J, Marks V. Physiological changes underlying jet lag. British Medical Journal 1982; 284: 144–146.
14. Donaldson E, Kennaway DJ. Effects of temazepam on sleep, performance, and rhythmic 6-sulphatoxymelatonin and cortisol after transmeridian travel. Aviation Space Environmental Medicine 1991; 62: 654–660.

RECOMMENDED READING

Dawood RM, ed. Travellers' health. 3rd ed. Oxford: Oxford University Press; 1992.
DeHart RL, ed. Fundamentals of aerospace medicine. 2nd ed. Baltimore: Williams and Wilkins; 1996.
Ernsting J, King PF, eds. Aviation medicine. 2nd ed. London: Butterworths; 1988.
Harding RM, Mills FJ. Aviation Medicine. 3rd ed. London: British Medical Association; 1993.
Rayman R. Clinical Aviation Medicine. 2nd ed. Philadelphia: Lea and Febiger; 1989.

Elderly travellers, individuals with disabilities and fitness to travel

Iain McIntosh

SYNOPSIS

There are few absolute contraindications to travel but some individuals and groups are more likely to have travel related illness or accidents than the average tourist or voyager, including

- the elderly
- individuals with disabilities or handicaps.
- those suffering acute and chronic illness who may find exposure to high altitude, climatic extremes and hostile environments aggravate existing problems.
- those taking medications for chronic conditions who may have more difficulties with compliance when away from home.

Pregnancy and child travellers are discussed on pages 148–157.

Introduction

Earlier retirement has encouraged many elderly, and even very old, people to visit relatives overseas or to fulfil long-standing tourist ambitions. There are also many opportunities for those with serious disabilities to travel abroad.

High rates of illness in travellers are recorded in those with preexisting health problems.[1] Elderly tourists on cruises often suffer from a variety of preexisting illness with resulting difficulties.[2] Those with diabetes mellitus, confusional states and urinary incontinence can have difficulties during air travel. Angina and breathlessness can be made worse at high altitude; even some international airports in Asia (e.g. Katmandu) and South America (e.g. Bogota) are high enough to create problems for those coming from a departure point close to sea level.

The following groups of travellers are considered in this section:

- elderly people, including possible problems on cruises and during air travel.
- individuals who are the physically frail, disabled or handicapped.

The need for pre-travel assessment

A pre-travel health consultation may reveal the need for special advice on the mode of travel, choice of destinations and route, which may prevent health problems. A comprehensive history, clinical examination, review of current medications and careful assessment of intended activities are essential.[3]

With sensible advice,[4] most individuals will be able to travel successfully.

Travel insurance

It is absolutely essential that the elderly and those with disabilities have adequate travel health insurance. It must be remembered that existing health problems usually have to be declared in advance, including any arranged hospital admissions. Many aged travellers pay the insurance premium and remain unaware of exclusions relating to pre-existing illness.[5] Cover may not include those, for example, who have within 6 months had a myocardial infarction or coronary bypass surgery. These oversights may invalidate a later claim.

Even if insurance is adequate, its value, in an emergency, depends upon the quality of available medical, nursing and emergency help. Good facilities may be many miles or even days away from some exotic tourist destinations. Cruise ships and aeroplanes may disembark ill passengers in ports of call with very limited facilities, poorly prepared for the highly technical care elderly patients might expect at home.[6]

Elderly travellers

By the year 2000, about 7% of the UK population will be over 75 years. 20% of the population is currently 65 years of age and over. 35% of those on cruises are over 60 years of age and sometimes most passengers are very old. They are fulfilling long-planned ambitions to travel and their right to do so has to be recognised. However, many do so without addressing potential health risks.[7–10]

Health professionals have a responsibility to identify these health risks and explain their significance to the traveller and offer appropriate advice. A study in Scotland showed that one-third of those over 65 years had travelled outside the UK within the past year and one-third of 75–80-year-olds within the preceding 3 years. Many were unaware of difficulties they might encounter in countries without a health service similar to home and had not considered the possible need for emergency aid and repatriation. There is little in the literature regarding attack rates of travel-related disease in older age groups but the same study suggested a higher attack rate in the elderly. Illness may be severe and more life threatening abroad. A lack of medical facilities and limited repatriation possibilities are common features of many developing countries now commonly visited by

tourists. These factors are more important for older travellers, more likely to require access to such assistance.

The main cause of death in travellers overseas is no longer infection but cardiovascular disease, especially in those over 50 years. It is the most common cause of serious illness in passengers during flights. Deterioration in immune response, pre-existing disease, renal dysfunction and metabolic disorders such as diabetes also put older and chronically ill travellers at greater risk. They may contract and be more seriously ill from pneumonia, Legionnaires' disease, intestinal infections and cerebrovascular accidents.

Physiological effects of ageing

Age itself is not a sole determinant of safe and healthy travel. However, a 90-year-old, fit individual will have pulmonary function only half that of a 30-year-old. Most organ systems lose function at roughly 1% per year after the age of 30 years. Several other elements in the ageing process can also have an effect on world travel.[11–27]

- Slower adjustment to changes in temperature, including decreased sweating.
- Poorer renal function. There is 60% deterioration in creatinine clearance by the age of 65.
- Cardiopulmonary function is poorer. There is a decrease in pulmonary response to hypoxia.
- Achlorhydria may predispose older people to gastrointestinal infection.
- A decreased cell-mediated immune response may mean less ability to fight off infection. There are structural and functional alterations in old age, which impair the host's defences against pulmonary infection. These changes increase the risk of the elderly to complications of influenza and pneumococcal infection. Their relative risk of complications and mortality from these diseases increases by a factor of 1.5–2.5. The case fatality rate for Legionnaires' disease, which can occur in hotels and cruise ships, increases with age to 20% in those over 60 years.[20]

- Possible short-term memory loss may mean that the hassles associated with travel may prove more stressful. The elderly may find it more difficult to cope with and adapt to cultural and environmental change.
- Low body mass and osteoporosis make fractures more likely.
- Poorer balance and postural stability make falls more likely.
- By the age of 65, there is a 25% loss of muscle mass and strength. Aerobic capacity for exercise is also progressively lost with ageing.
- Psychological reaction times are slower.
- Impairment in visual and auditory acuity and sensory deprivation or overstimulation can cause confusion with a minimal of provocation.
- Liver disease such as acute hepatitis A in the elderly is more likely to be serious than in the young. There are 400 fatalities per 10 000 cases in the over 65-year-olds compared to 7 in young groups.

The effects of drugs and existing disease in the elderly

Many of the above may be made worse by the side effects of drug medications commonly taken by the elderly. For example, mefloquine used in malaria prophylaxis can aggravate cardiac conduction problems.[28]

Degenerative changes such as arteriosclerosis, chronic obstructive pulmonary disease, diabetes mellitus, arthritis and dementia increase medical risk during long distance travel. Travel fatigue can be particularly upsetting for elderly people. This is especially so in the early stages of Alzheimer's disease which affects up to 50% of people over the age of 75 years.[29] The tendency for older travellers to remain in their seats in airport concourses and on aircraft can result in venous thrombosis and pulmonary embolism.[30] Elderly travellers may have more problems with time zone changes although this can be compensated for to an extent by less need for sleep.

Diarrhoea, the travellers' scourge, may be more serious in the older traveller if there is marked fluid loss. The associated dehydration may increase the likelihood of angina, arrhythmias including atrial fibrillation, myocardial and cerebral infarction. In a study of 952 travellers who died while abroad, 28% were aged 60–69 years. 82% of those dying from cardiovascular causes were over 50 years. If elderly travellers do become ill, medical facilities may not be as found at home.

Environmental factors

STRESS

Transit and flight delays are stressful[31] and perhaps more so for older people. Combined with fatigue, they can be responsible for cardiac and respiratory problems common in international airports. Stress can increase angina, cardiac failure and blood pressure. Angina may become more troublesome with the increased activity and the low arterial oxygen pressure at high altitude. The unavoidable stresses associated with travel, however, can precipitate an acute confusional state in those so predisposed.

HEAT

Hot climates may aggravate postural hypotension in those on anti-hypertensives or anti-parkinsonism drugs. Minimum daily temperatures above 17°C put elderly people at a much higher risk of stroke and myocardial infarction and arterial thrombosis because of haemoconcentration and thrombocytosis. Serum cholesterol levels are raised by up to 15%. Those with a history of transient cerebral ischaemic attacks are at particular risk. During a heatwave in the UK, there was a three-fold increase in deaths from cerebral vascular accident and a two-fold increase in myocardial infarction.

Electrolyte disturbances in chronic renal insufficiency may be made worse and diuretics may make salt depletion more severe. Elderly men with prostatism may find delays in finding toilet accommodation precipitate acute urinary retention. Patients who are severely anaemic have more hypoxaemia if travelling by air or at high altitudes. Hypothyroidism occurs in around 10% of elderly people over 75 years and they can be particularly heat intolerant.

Chronic illnesses in the elderly

ACHLORHYDRIA

About 60% of those over 60 years have some degree of achlorhydria and many take H$_2$ antagonists. This can predispose to more frequent and severe travellers' diarrhoea.

DIABETES MELLITUS

There may be dietary problems en route and at the destination. Travellers' diarrhoea and resultant dehydration may be more serious. *Candida* infection is more likely in hot, humid environments. Wounds and bites may become more easily infected. Those who are on diets and/or oral medication only can normally travel without problems. The diabetic traveller on insulin should be prepared to adjust the timing of insulin administration – this may be complicated, particularly for the elderly – and must be discussed with the doctor or nurse specialist well in advance. Those on insulin may experience hypoglycaemia during flight and should be prepared to adjust food intake accordingly (see also pp 161–2).

FOOTCARE

Many elderly people have foot and lower limb problems including deformities, nail changes, ulcers and poor circulation. Protective footwear should be used on the sand and in the water. Feet and legs can burn in the sun and protective sunscreens or covering up are needed as for other parts of the body. Moisturisers are helpful especially on heels that crack easily. Moist skin can lead to infection.

ARTHRITIS

This can make going to the toilet difficult where crouching toilets are common and replace the flushing toilet found at home. Toilet paper may not be supplied. Even with 'grab handles' (if fitted) it requires considerable agility to use crouch toilets and they may be beyond the capability of an elderly person with arhritis. People with stiff hips or fixed knees are at a particular disadvantage within the restricted and narrow confines of aircraft.

WOUNDS

Travel-related tissue injuries from insect bites and trauma also tend to heal more slowly with older age. Elderly travellers may suffer from swollen ankles as a result of venous stasis when sitting for long periods in a restricted space, as on aircraft or coaches. Oedematous tissues heal poorly following the minor lacerations and bumps so easily acquired from baggage, seating, trolleys and jostling in crowds. Many older people are poorly protected against tetanus.

It can be helpful to think of the elderly in the following categories:

1. The 'young' elderly who travel to low-risk destinations on short-haul journeys and are physically fit.
2. As in (1) but where travel involves climatic extremes, visits to tropical countries and also the frail elderly and those with pre-existing disease – sound pre-travel advice will be necessary.
3. The physically very unfit, terminally ill and those with pre-existing illness travelling to high-health-risk destinations with food, water and hygiene problems, insect-borne diseases and other major environmental differences from home – very careful planning will be needed and sometimes alternative trips, or even cancellation, may be advisable.

Problems for the elderly during air travel

Only one airline passenger in 7 million dies in the air but many are found seriously ill in transit airports according to the Federal Aviation Administration of USA report of 1997. American airlines reported 15 emergencies per day compared with 3 in 1986. This is an increase that they believe is largely due to the increase in elderly travellers. It has been estimated that 5% of airline passengers suffer from chronic illness, many of these being elderly people.

Airline passengers with lung disease may not compensate adequately for the changes in atmospheric pressure in aircraft cabins – arterial Po_2 levels can fall as low as 30–40 mmHg – and light exercise such as arm movements and walking may lead to dyspnoea, fatigue, light-headedness and dizziness.

Immobility in the restricted space of an aircraft cabin can lead to deep vein thrombosis and pulmonary embolism on prolonged journeys, sometimes lasting up to 23 hours in one aircraft. Anti-platelet medication with a low dose of aspirin should be considered for long-haul aeroplane journeys.

A common reason for illness in airports and on cruises is failure to carry and take routinely prescribed medication. There is a tendency for patients to miss diuretic therapy on long journeys by air or coach so as to reduce the need for going to the toilet – this can precipitate cardiac failure. However, older travellers with profuse diarrhoea should temporarily stop diuretics.

Time zone changes involving the crossing of three or more time zones can seriously disturb mental alertness and cause disorientation.

It is essential to stress to elderly travellers the need to carry adequate medication supplies in hand luggage, in case hold luggage gets separated or there are delays in transit.

Problems for the elderly on cruises[32–35]

Many cruise ships are unsuited for frail, elderly and handicapped travellers. A considerable number of these ships are themselves elderly!

Most ship's doctor consultations are with older patients. One study showed 58% of health problems were found in over 65-year-olds. A commonly reported difficulty is lack of regular medications or knowledge of prescriptions. On one ship, 30% of passengers did not know the name of their medication and in many cases the name was not on the bottle. Limited on-board medical supplies mean that this shortfall cannot always be met. Few of the chronically ill carry a note from their doctors to assist the ship's doctor. The risk of cardiovascular illness and accidents may be increased by over-indulgence in food and alcohol, common on cruises, and this may be combined with a lack of exercise. Over-exposure to the sun increases the possibility of stroke.

MEDICAL CARE AVAILABLE

A survey of cruise liners established that the quality of medical care varies considerably from line to line and ship to ship. Some cruise lines do not require medical personnel to have cardiac life-support training although cardiac emergencies are a common presentation to the ship's doctor. Most ships have electrocardiograms and defibrillators but few have more sophisticated monitoring equipment. Shipboard pharmacy supplies of cardiac support drugs may be limited.

There are no international requirements governing cruise ship medicine and no agency checks to ensure that competent doctors are hired, proper equipment and medications are stocked, or correct emergency procedures followed.

Regardless of the quality of medical care, a ship's infirmary is often unable to provide immediate back-up services such as surgery, blood transfusion, detailed laboratory or radiological investigations.

Urgent specialist care will usually be delayed. Secondary medical care resources and quality will be variable and are often poorer than the passengers expect. Medical evacuation in emergency is dependent upon the ship's position at sea, its sailing itinerary and the next port of call. Onward evacuation for specialist attention in Europe or the USA will depend on frequency and availability of local air services. Ambulances regularly meet cruise ships as they dock. Estimates suggest that one passenger in 5000 requires evacuation and these are usually people of advanced years.

SHIP MOVEMENT AND ACCIDENTS

Ships are inherently unstable owing to sea swell and currents, and the most common mishaps to crew and passengers are falls with resultant contusions and fractures. Walking around the ship in rough weather is more likely to lead to injury in old people with poor balance, limited agility and slow reaction times.

The risks of trauma are high when elderly passengers are required to transfer from ship to shore by small boat tender, which is quite a common practice, especially when going ashore to islands. The ship, the lifeboat, the descent ladder and platform move asynchronously leaving a height and distance gap for the passenger to bridge.

Elderly passengers also injure themselves on trips ashore and may not appreciate that jungle or mountainous hinterlands have inherent health risks.

Physically frail, disabled and handicapped individuals

There are 3 million disabled people in the UK, under the age of 75 years, who are often highly motivated to travel despite physical and mental incapacity. Handicap is not normally a barrier to international journeys. The need for careful travel planning and a medical assessment prior to travel are often important pre-requisites if these travellers are to remain in good health while abroad.

Countries in North America, Scandinavia, Western Europe, Australia and New Zealand usually provide extra services for the handicapped. Inadequate or non-existent facilities for frail and physically disadvantaged travellers are common in poorer countries and over much of Eastern Europe and Asia. Guide dogs cannot accompany blind passengers on international air flights. While UK law (since 1996) makes it an offence for providers of goods and services to provide inferior service to disabled persons because of their disability, the Act on Accessibility 1999 affecting transport applies only to new trains from 1999 and coaches from 2000. It does not apply to air and sea travel.

A useful contact address is the Royal Association for Disability and Rehabilitation (RADAR), 12 City Forum, 250 City Road, London, EC1V 8AF. *Tel:* 0207 250 3222.

Travel-related problems

ACCESS

Wheelchair bound travellers can face access problems on aeroplanes, trains and buses. The newer widebodied aeroplanes carry onboard wheelchairs, which can greatly enhance mobility. Many modern trains still only have accommodation for wheelchair passengers in the guard's van and it may be separate from travelling companions and toilet accommodation. Station concourses may be impracticable for wheelchairs because of a lack of passenger lifts. Facilities for the disabled are good in the USA where all public amenities must be wheelchair accessible. Australia, New Zealand, Scandinavia and Canada are broadly comparable whereas in Europe access facilities are less predictable the further east and south one travels.

INVISIBLE DISABILITIES

Travel agents and airline officials may not easily respond to those with 'invisible' disabilities such as deafness, partial blindness and mobility problems.

Deafness

Deafness affects about one-third of those over 75 years, with 20% over 80 years requiring hearing aids. Deaf travellers run the risk of missing announcements in transit. Many modern international airports have special phone-links for deaf and hard-of-hearing travellers where it is possible to type in queries in a special telephone link and receive a typed reply in response.

Blindness

In 1988, a quarter of a million of the UK population were registered as blind or partially sighted.

Three-quarters of these are over 65 years of age. 20% of 80-year-olds are unable to read newsprint even with prescribed spectacles. Blind people are not usually allowed on cruises and guide dogs are only allowed on flights within the UK. Often the airline will insist on provision of a sighted travel companion.

Mobility problems

Arthritis and hip replacement may restrict access to trains, aeroplanes and coaches and the confined space of long-haul flights can result in cramps and spasms in fixed limbs. British Airways provides

---

A checklist for travellers with existing health problems

1. Arrange a full, medical check-up several weeks before departure.
2. Ensure adequate and inclusive medical insurance cover, including repatriation.
3. People over 65 years age should consider vaccination against influenza and pneumococcal infection.
4. Consider whether the special form should be completed to advise transport agents of disability before departure by air.
5. Advise airlines of special medical, dietary and mobility requirements
6. Re-assess medication before departure. Drug review should pay special attention to diuretics, insulin, hypnotics, H_2 antagonists, anticholinergics, anti-epileptics and interactions with anti-malarials.
7. Adequate medication should be carried in the hand luggage.
8. Be aware of special risks of high altitude and climate extremes.
9. Those with respiratory problems should sit well forward in non-smoking areas in aircraft and consideration should be given to supplemental oxygen.
10. Diabetics may require adjustment of food intake and insulin dosage.
11. On long-haul flights, endeavour to exercise the legs as often as possible and avoid staying immobile for long periods. Consider taking a small dose of aspirin.
12. Be aware that medical facilities en route and at destination may be of poor standard.
13. Elderly, disabled cruise passengers should check the adequacy of medical facilities before booking.

---

wheelchair assistance for 200 000 passengers per year in UK airports. Many elderly and frail people still do not take advantage of this service and risk over-fatigue and physical and medical distress during transfer – prior notice is required. These passengers should also be advised to pre-book aircraft seating with additional leg space.

AIRLINES MAY NEED TO BE INFORMED

Travellers with disabilities and serious, pre-existent, chronic illness are required to inform the relevant airline of their condition prior to departure. The Air Transport Travel Association provides questionnaires for completion by disabled and chronically ill passengers. Many handicapped, partially disabled, often elderly people use airlines without having completed these forms and airline agents can refuse onward transportation in their absence. Part 1 is the record of current incapacity, which has to be completed by the passenger, and the passenger's doctor completes Part 2.

REFERENCES

1. Dessary BL, Robin MR, Pasini W. The aged infirm or handicapped traveller. In: Steffen R, Dupont HL, eds. Textbook of travel medicine and health. Canada: Decker; 1997.
2. Goethe WHG, Watson EN, Jones DT. Handbook of nautical medicine. Berlin: Springer-Verlag; 1984: 185–372.
3. McIntosh I. Travel health and the elderly. London: Quay Books, Mark Allan Publications; 1995.
4. Reid D, Cossar J et al. Do travel brochures give adequate advice on avoiding illness? British Medical Journal 1986; 293: 2.
5. McIntosh I. Travel induced illness. Scottish Medicine 1991; 11(4): 14–15.
6. Mitchell M. Have wheelchair will travel. Travel Medicine International 1995; 13(5): 174–177.
7. Finnerty M, Gong H. Advising patients with respiratory disorders about travel. Travel Medicine International 1991; 9: 399–404.
8. Foulkes I. Are you immune to ageing. Health and Ageing 1998; April: 58–59.
9. D'Paixao RJ, Dewar R et al. What do Scots die of when abroad. Scottish Medical Journal 36: 114–116.
10. Mills F, Harding R. Fitness to travel by air. British Medical Journal 1983; 286(12): 69–71.
11. Ward B. Complete guide to cruising and cruise ships. Princeton NJ: Berlitz; 1997.

12. Barry HC, Eathorne SW. Exercise and ageing. Medical Clinics of North America 1994; 78: 357–376

13. Erb B. The elderly in the wilderness. Wilderness Medicine Letter 1995; Winter: 5–6 Wilderness Medical Society, Indianopolis, USA.

14. Villar P, Wiggins J et al. Structure and function of the ageing lung. Care of the Elderly 1991; 3: 129.

15. Cameron J. Renal function in the elderly. Geriatric Medicine 1991; 21: 29–34.

16. Abram S W, Berrow R. Manual of geriatrics. New Jersey: Merck; 1990.

17. Diguesepai. Why everyone over 65 deserves influenza vaccine. British Medical Journal 1996; 313: 1162.

18. Sankilamo U, Isoaho R et al. Effect of age, sex and smoking on pneumococcal antibodies in the elderly. International Journal of Epidemiology 1997; 26: 420–427.

19. Lieberman D, Lieberman D, Schlaeffer F et al. Community-acquired pneumonia in old age: a prospective study of 91 patients admitted from home. Age and Ageing 1997; 26: 69–75.

20. Ellis CJ. Special considerations for new aged travellers. Geriatric Medicine 1995; 25: 19–20.

21. Markides K, Cooper C, eds. Ageing stress and health. New York: Wiley; 1989.

22. Osgood N, Sontz A, eds. The science and practice of gerontology. London: Kingsley; 1989.

23. Elon R. Low body mass and osteoporosis make fractures more likely with falls. British Medical Journal 1996; 312: 561–563.

24. Dargent-Molina P, Favier F et al. Poorer balance and postural stability make falls more likely. Lancet 1996; 348: 145–149.

25. Creditor MC. Hazards of hospitalisation in the elderly. Annals of Internal Medicine 1993; 118: 219–223

26. Hall M, MacLennan W, Lye M. Medical care of the elderly. Chicester: Wiley; 1993.

27. O'Mahoney S, Woodhouse K. The ageing liver. Update 1993; Feb: 288-9621.

28. Conlon C. The immuno-compromised traveller. British Medical Bulletin 1993; 49(2): 412–422.

29. Dementia in the community. England: Alzheimers Disease Society; 1995.

30. Cruikshank J. Air travel and thrombotic episodes. Lancet 1988; 1: 497–498.

31. McIntosh I. The stress of modern travel. Travel Medicine International 1990; 8: 118–121.

32. Velimirovic B. Health hazards of sea tourism. Travel Medicine International 1990; 8: 69–75.

33. Martinovic N. Morbidity of passengers and crew on the cruiser Adriadne. Travel Medicine International 1997; 15: 194–199.

34. Carter JW. Shipboard medicine on package cruises. British Medical Journal 1972; Feb: 553–556.

35. McIntosh I. Health and safety at sea. Travel Medicine International 1997; 15: 234–237.

FURTHER READING

Walsh A. Nothing ventured: Disabled people travel the world. (Rough Guides series) London: Harrap Columbus, 1992.

McIntosh I. Travel and health in the elderly – A medical handbook. London: Quay Books, Mark Allan Publications; 1992.

McIntosh I. Health hazard and the high risk traveller. London: Quay Books, Mark Allan Publications; 1993.

Dawood R, ed. Travellers Health. 3rd ed. Oxford: Oxford University Press; 1992.

Psychological aspects of travel and the long-term expatriate

Michael Jones

Introduction

Travel has been famously described as loosening the bowels and broadening the mind. While both short-term and longer-term travel is often an enriching and broadening experience, there are some for whom the major stresses of travel prove disabling and detrimental to psychological health. On the day the author arrived in Tanzania to work at a teaching hospital, another doctor was flown home. His obsessional personality traits proved incompatible with the realities of working in a developing world hospital even though it was highly regarded as a centre of excellence.

Definitions

A short-term business traveller or tourist is defined here as one whose visit is measured in days or weeks. Short-term visitors rarely adapt to the host culture to any significant extent and are usually cushioned by Western-style accommodation in hotels with only daytime forays into the surrounding culture.

Protracted visitors, or expatriates, are defined as those who take up residence in another country for occupational purposes returning to their original country when their assignment is completed.[1] The term does not include those who migrate permanently to another country although this chapter will also refer to migrants. The length of stay of protracted visitors will be measured in years, and during this time they will adapt to the host culture, evolving from being monocultural to bicultural. Both during and after the main adaptive process, they will be subjected to varying degrees of cultural stress.

Short-term work commitments

People fulfilling short-term work commitments of 3–12 months are often volunteers. These are usually young people doing gap years before or after university, and are viewed by agencies as less committed than those prepared to take on longer-term assignments. They raise a substantial proportion of, if not all, their financial support and because they are less significant contributors to the budget of the agency often bypass the more rigorous screening and preparation procedures reserved for long-term staff. They may be among the most vulnerable of travellers, lacking preparation, short on life experience, and exposed to all the stressors of cultural adaptation but without the time necessary to complete adaptation or acquire the language skills which make adaptation so much easier.

Backpackers

Backpackers tend to be older, having worked for long enough to acquire the resources to travel at length, immersing themselves in the life of local people, yet detached enough to move sequentially from one culture to another at intervals of weeks or months. This group remains an enigma and virtually no research has been done on psychological profiles and outcomes.

Culture and cultural adaptation

Culture

We only really become aware of the characteristics of our own culture when we start to adapt to another culture. Culture has been helpfully described by Hofstede[2] as *the software of the mind,* and is:

- a collective phenomenon
- learned
- distinct from both human nature and personality.[3]

Burnett observes:

...culture may be likened to a game of chess. To a person who has no knowledge of the game the players seem at first to be moving the strangely shaped pieces at random. With time the observer begins to see that there is an order and pattern for every piece, and then finally he begins to see that there is an overall strategy employed by the players. Culture may be likened to the game itself, whilst the world view is the unseen set of rules which determines how the game can be played.[4]

Cultural differences

Understanding the differences between cultures has been enhanced by the work of Hofstede.[5] Using questionnaire responses from several thousand employees of a large multinational company, he identified four pairs of opposite characteristics which could be applied to national cultures, and was able to give varying weight to the strength of any particular characteristic. The fifth dimension emanates from Chinese sources.

a. High-power or low-power distance (more equal than others)

Power distance is defined as the extent to which less powerful members of society expect and accept that power is distributed unequally (high-power distance cultures accept an unequal power distribution). Scandinavian countries, Austria, Eire and UK are generally low-power distance cultures whereas France, Malaysia, the Arab countries, India and some South American countries are high-power distance cultures.

b. Individualist or collectivist (we and they)

Individualist societies are defined as those in which the ties between individuals are loose and in which

everyone is expected to look after him/herself and his/her immediate family. In collectivist cultures people from birth onwards are integrated into strong cohesive groups which, throughout lifetime, continue to protect group members in exchange for unquestioning loyalty. Third world cultures are generally collectivist, and affluent Western cultures are generally individualist.

c. Masculine or feminine (he, she and (s)he)

Masculine cultures are those in which social gender roles are clearly distinct, expecting men to be tough, assertive and achievement-oriented whereas women are normally more modest, tender and concerned with the quality of life. Women who achieve in such masculine cultures often have masculine characteristics. Feminine cultures view roles as interchangeable. The Nordic countries, Costa Rica, Yugoslavia and Portugal are strongly feminine cultures, whereas Japan, Austria, Italy, Switzerland South America and Eire are strongly masculine with UK slightly lower. According to Hofstede's research, Islamic countries are more weakly masculine than one might expect.

d. Low or high uncertainty avoidance (what is different is dangerous)

This is the extent to which members of a culture feel threatened by uncertain or unknown situations. Some cultures seem to have a need for predictability and handle this with written or unwritten rules. The underlying attitude here is *what is different is dangerous*. Greece, Portugal, Belgium, Japan, Germany and Serbia are high on uncertainty avoidance and UK fairly low. The attitude of low uncertainty-avoiding cultures can be summed up in the phrase *what is different is curious*. Other low uncertainty-avoiding cultures are Singapore, Jamaica, Denmark, Sweden, Hong Kong and Eire.

e. Time orientation

The cultures of East Asia favour a long-term orientation whereas Western cultures generally expect quick results.[6] This is a complex concept but one which has political, economic and religious implications. The difficulties which the last British Governor of Hong Kong, Chris Patten, encountered with the Chinese government over the handover of the colony to China constitute a classic example. He was a child of his Western culture, a man in a hurry. The Chinese government was not.

Germany has low-power distance but is strong on uncertainty avoidance and organisations will work like well-oiled machines in which everyone knows their place and role. In the UK with low-power distance and low uncertainty avoidance, important values are negotiation, communication and mutual adjustment, more like a village market place. In countries with high-power distance and low-uncertainty avoidance (Africa, India and the Far East) society acts more like a family where the father or leader has natural authority but there are few formal rules. President Hastings Banda in Malawi, who ran a paternalistic but increasingly repressive regime for 30 years until 1994, was primarily ousted, not by a Malawian revolt but by outside pressure from Western donor countries. Malawians to whom the author spoke were mostly glad to see him go but would not have considered criticising the President because of cultural mores, even though the human rights abuses were widely known about.

Individualism/collectivism has a major effect on motivation. In individualistic cultures, self-fulfilment and self-respect are motivators whereas in a more collectivist culture, people seek 'face' in relation to others and fulfilment of obligations towards their in-group.

The greater the difference between the characteristics of the host and parent culture of the traveller, the more likely it is that a high level of stress will be experienced in cultural transition.

'Culture shock' and adaptation

Both the travel adviser and the traveller need a degree of understanding of the stress reaction to cultural adaptation and the reasons for it. Storti's *The Art of Crossing Cultures* is written with insight and humour and, for those who have not had the privilege of living in another culture, will provide considerable insight.[7] Cultural adaptation is rarely easy. 'Culture shock' is a rather overdramatic term often used to describe the early manifestations of the process of cultural adaptation, and first coined by Oberg in 1960.[8] The advantage of the term is that it rightly implies that cultural change is a serious and severe test of emotional stability. The disadvantage is that it suggests that it is a short, sharp event rather than a process that may take 2 years or more before it is substantially complete.

Oberg described 'culture shock' as 'the anxiety that results from losing all the familiar signs and symbols of social intercourse', giving rise to rejection of the new environment and regression in which the home environment is glorified.

Symptoms include:

- excessive concern about hygiene, food, drinking and bedding
- fear of physical contact with nationals and personal security
- the absent-minded, far away, tropical stare
- a desire for dependence on those of one's own nationality
- anger about the frustrations of the new country
- a terrible longing to go back home.

The stages, which may alternate and recur, include:

- a fascination with the new over the first few weeks
- a stage of hostility and aggression towards the new country
- a third stage of partial acceptance characterised by an emergent humour
- a final fourth stage in which the visitor starts to operate in the new milieu without a feeling of anxiety, accepting the customs of the country as another way of living with enjoyment.

Adler[9] applies different labels to these stages, of **contact**, **disintegration**, **re-integration** and **autonomy**, while Hiebert[10] rather similarly describes the stages as **the tourist stage, disenchantment, resolution** and **adjustment**.

The phase of disintegration or disenchantment is less acute but has similarities to the process of the overwhelming of the internal map described in post-traumatic stress disorder (PTSD).[11] Without adequate support, psychologically vulnerable individuals may be destabilised.

Cross-cultural migration as transition

Hopson & Adams[12] describe transition as discontinuity in a person's life space and define four types:

1. predictable voluntary (e.g. marriage)
2. predictable involuntary (e.g. national service)
3. unpredictable voluntary (e.g. computer dating)
4. unpredictable involuntary (e.g. unexpected earthquake).

Cultural transition largely falls into the third (unpredictable but voluntary) category whereas PTSD is confined to the fourth (unpredictable and involuntary) category. The transition process may start months, and sometimes years, before departure with candidate selection, orientation, training and a final, and usually emotional, farewell to friends and relatives.

Cross-cultural migration as bereavement

The element of migration which applies to any prolonged absence from one's home country can also rightly be seen as involving loss and any experience of significant loss will produce a bereavement reaction. Huntingdon, drawing on her own research,[13] and the work of others [14, 15] has observed that during migration a fundamental part of the self is lost, and for some the experience of separation from the place and culture called 'home' is devastating. Migration calls into question established personal identity, the sense of self in the world and the boundary between inner and outer reality.[16] Migrants tend to articulate their experience by recourse to the body metaphor 'I feel as if half of myself is missing' and studies in Chilean exiles to the UK,[17] Russian Jewish migrants to the USA[18] and re-housed slum dwellers in Boston[19] all suggest that migrants experience feelings which carry a sense of mutilation.

Factors increasing cultural transitional stress

Several authors have observed that individual vulnerability, combined with cultural stress and lack of social support make the risk of developing psychiatric problems greater.[20] Adler[9] concludes that 'for many individuals transitional experiences of any sort may be more negative ... more harmful ... more destructive ... no matter what degree of cultural dissimilarity.'

Factors that increase cultural transition as a stressor include:

- depth of involvement with the host culture
- the extent of value differences between one's own and a host culture
- the frustrations of the new culture
- temperament differences.[21]

Thus a business person working in a capital city and living in a leafy suburb surrounded by other expatriates is not exposed to nearly as much culture stress as the village-based, aid worker. Temperament is a strong determinant of the extent of transitional stress and those personalities' preferences which make them efficient-stabilisers of institutions may find more difficulty than crisis-solvers who will be fired and stimulated by the challenge of the changes in the new environment. Similarly, those with rigid or obsessional personality traits may have much more difficulty than more flexible, laid-back types. Extroverts are likely to engage more easily and learn quickly compared to introverts who, because they need to withdraw to recharge their batteries in the face of the energy drain of adaptation, may limit their contact with the host culture.

ADAPTATION FROM ONE DEVELOPED NATION TO ANOTHER

Protracted visits to *developed* countries may involve just as much cultural adaptation stress as prolonged stays in the developing world. Some aspects of local culture may *seem* familiar and because the visitor expects things to be the same as back home the process of adaptation may be even more difficult. Americans coming to the UK often find living in the UK much more difficult than they imagined, thinking that the differences in life between the USA and the UK will be minimal. Similarly, British nationals working in France often find the transition difficult as they adapt to a much higher power distance culture than their own, and Japanese business people working in the USA often find the combination of poor skills in spoken English, and a culture in which emotion is revealed openly highly stressful.[22]

Cultural adaptation and children

Children re-entering their parents' culture are not bicultural like their parents.[23] but are third culture kids (TCKs), nurtured in a milieu that is a unique blend of two cultures (the third culture). The term TCK, coined by Useem,[24] applies to those children 'who have spent all or part of their formative years in a culture different to that of their parents, and who have been reared in a unique blend of two cultures, a third culture, not having a sense of belonging to either their parents' culture or the host culture'.[25] TCKs are often restless, and in teenage and early adult life may exhibit behaviour which suggests a desire to recover that elusive third culture. The search for this is often a factor in a desire to return overseas as adults. Conversely, they may remain rooted in a home environment seeking the security which may have been absent in childhood.

Personal change and cultural transition

For most travellers, cultural adaptation, once substantially complete, is a deeply enriching experience and may result in substantial redefinition of values and attitudes. At the start of their assignments, Peace Corps volunteers appeared as middle of the road politically, rather conventional personally and family entrenched. At the end of assignments, they had developed more liberal, political views, were more inceptive, were more self-assured and showed an increase in principled moral reasoning.[26]

Aldous Huxley observed:

> So the journey is over and I am back again where I started, richer by much experience and poorer by many exploded convictions, many perished certainties. For convictions and certainties are too often the concomitants of ignorance. Those who like to feel they are always right and who attach a high importance to their own opinions should stay at home. When one is travelling, convictions are mislaid as easily as spectacles; but unlike spectacles they are not easily replaced.[27]

Hiebert suggests we do not need to give up all our basic assumptions. We must have some assumptions, for without them we do not have any tools for organising a culture or our thoughts.[28] However, our acquired ethnocentrism will reduce, many assumptions and convictions will be challenged, and misunderstandings corrected, as we encounter a wider world. Different people become real people and their culture our culture, as we engage with them rather than regarding them as scenery on the journey.

Stress factors in overseas settings

Several studies have highlighted significant stressors beyond the initial phase of cultural adaptation, and the adverse effect that these may have on mental health has been recognised for many decades.[1] Stress reaction is therefore common in expatriates and in Foyle's study[29] affected 17% of those interviewed.

Categories of stress

De Haan[30] classifies stress into three categories: basic stress resulting from work abroad in an alien environment, and including both cultural adaptive stress and exposure on a chronic basis to stressors not present in the home environment; cumulative stress resulting from prolonged exposure to minor traumas; and traumatic stress caused by sudden unpredictable and involuntary psychotraumatic events.

Stressors

Moorhead[31] identified the most stressful areas as being language (57%), separation from children (33%), children's education (25%) and change of work status (20%). Gish[32] found that some geographical sites carried greater stress than others. For instance, physical dangers and climate were particular stressors in the Philippines while co-workers' paternalism towards nationals figured more strongly in Papua New Guinea and Hong Kong. Strong overall stressors included the need for the expatriate to engage with an unfamiliar culture, confrontation, communication across language and cultural barriers, the energy involved in maintaining relationships with supporting donors, and work volume. Some stressors receded with increasing length of service, for instance the sense of living in a 'fish bowl', typified by being followed everywhere by groups of interested children and adults. Political instability, by contrast, was a greater stress for those working overseas for longer periods than for those on short assignments, probably because they were more aware of the implications and more deeply invested in the host culture.

Foyle[29] identified additional stressors:

Problems related to employment

The job may be quite different to that expected owing to inadequate job description at recruitment or the need has changed by the time the new appointee has arrived. Many expatriates are expected to take more senior posts than they would in their home countries, adding pressure in the absence of the range of professional support that would be available at home. They may also be expected to manage and teach others, without

skills or formal training, enhancing feelings of insecurity during cultural transition. Support may be limited, in stark contrast to that experienced in their home country. A sense of isolation is enhanced at a time when other support structures are also missing. Sickness in expatriate colleagues working in small groups may produce sudden and excessive increase in workloads.

Personal observations of returning expatriates presenting for routine review suggest that married women without employment outside the home have a reduced margin for coping and may find life particularly difficult during the fourth decade of life. Single women are the next most at risk group, and they sustain decreased satisfaction in personal life scores in their early 40s.[33]

Language and cultural anxieties

The author has vivid memories of arriving to take up a medical post in Tanzania. Armed with *Teach Yourself Swahili* as he stepped off the plane, he was totally unprepared for stark realities of living in an environment where English was not understood by most people.

Language acquisition has a high priority for those engaged in rural development, educational, medical or missionary work. Learning a new language alone is a significant stressor but is vital for survival in many countries, and may present a major pressure for those who are less linguistically able. However, while the acquisition of good language skills may be stressful, mastery of the language enables successful adaptation and will reduce stress in later years.

Language difficulties may surface both with nationals of the host culture, and other expatriates. The medium of communication between expatriates from the West is often English but this will be a second language for many and subtle idiomatic language may not be understood. The significant differences between European cultures or North America or Australasia in the use of English, and cultural variation that this represents, are often underestimated.

Interpersonal relationships with other expatriates may be affected by different standards or priorities of training and financial disparity between expatriates from different national groups. Whereas expatriates working for multinationals are usually paid on the same scale whatever their nationality, there are often disparities between different nationalities working with similar non-governmental organisations (NGOs), North Americans often being paid at higher levels than their colleagues from Europe. Conversely, the enormous gap in income between expatriates and their national colleagues may cause major feelings of guilt, even when the expatriates' salaries are substantially less than they would be in the home country.

Housing and security

Armed robbery is a constant threat in some countries, and in many large cities the homes of expatriate workers are surrounded by barbed wire fences with security guards patrolling at night. The threat of robbery may be felt particularly by wives and children when husbands are away on field trips.

Single people in some voluntary organisations may be placed under considerable pressure to share accommodation with other singles with whom they may not be in the least compatible. The resulting tension may blight the experience of otherwise satisfying assignments.

Difficulties in intimate and close relationships

Marital tensions may increase as couples change their degree of overlap, usually moving from low to high overlap marriages, without the normal escapes and supports of the home environment. A survey of single female expatriates working with Christian missionary agencies identified isolation and loneliness as specific stressors.[34] Bereavement reactions following the death of a parent may be complicated by inability to visit during terminal illness or to attend a funeral.

STRESSORS FOR CHILDREN

Foyle[29] identifies exclusion from the selection and orientation process, frequent moves and separation from parents during language school, as particular stressors for children. Educational difficulties may include being educated in a boarding school located hundreds of miles away from parents or the school

may even be located in a third country at some distance from parents. If home education is chosen, they have to relate to their mother in the additional role as teacher. During periods of home leave, the child may move from one education system to another for one or two terms, and if educated in a different national school system may have become fluent in another language and speak English with a distinct accent. Expatriate children may even lose fluency in the language of their parents, and find life very difficult when they return to the parental home country. The author observed this on a visit to Asia with Korean children living in Japan. Korean language and culture are deeply complex and expatriates working in Korea find it virtually impossible to fully adapt and become at ease in their host country. The corollary is that Korean children in Japan may lose not only Korean language skills but find themselves as foreigners to their parental culture. Many then seek tertiary education in the USA as the only viable alternative.

Other issues for these 'oddball' children temporarily entering their parents' culture, include the lack of the same 'TV memory' because they have not shared in the evolution of the latest TV soap operas, or knowledge and taste for particular pop groups and national sports. Their interests are different and their new peers are unable to relate to the wider horizons of the expatriate child.

Psychiatric morbidity in travellers

Psychopathology in expatriates has been extensively reviewed by Richardson,[35] and this section draws heavily on his classification and content. Mental health problems have been identified for many years as the most common cause of repatriation.[36,37] Over 80 years ago, Price analysed over 1000 missionaries working with the Church Missionary Society between 1890 and 1908.[38] 40% did not persevere with their assignments, and in two-fifths this was due to mental health issues. Much more recently Peppiatt found an 11% risk of psychiatric disorder in a study of 212 Methodist personnel.[39]

Organic mental disorders

Age-related illness

Dementia is common in the general population and is likely to surface amongst middle-aged expatriates and those nearing retirement. Gradual deterioration in punctuality, attention to details in work, and appropriate decision making should raise concerns.[35] In Foyle's earlier analysis of her cohort[29] about 4% had age related illness.

Psychoactive substances

Caffeine intoxication may occur in those coping with heavy workloads, and use of benzodiazepines is probably as common amongst expatriates as the populations in their home countries.[35] One study disclosed that 20% of a cohort of nearly 400 missionary expatriates used some form of tranquillizer at some point during their period of service.[40] An initial prescription at a time of crisis may be repeated if measures are not taken to reduce stressor exposure and use may then become chronic. Sudden interruption of supply may precipitate severe anxiety, restlessness agitation and insomnia.

Cannabis is also freely available in many countries and, in the author's experience, its use is a behavioural norm for backpackers and students on short-term assignment overseas. It is not however the benign recreational drug of popular myth. Psychotic reactions caused by cannabis have been described,[41, 42] cannabis has been implicated as an independent risk factor for the development of schizophrenia,[43] and there is evidence that it causes short-term memory loss.[44]

Psychological reactions to physical illness and drug therapy

A wide variety of physical conditions may give rise to mental disorder and these have been reviewed by Lishman.[45] In travellers returning with anxiety, depression and confusional states, endocrine and metabolic disorders should be excluded. Thyroid disease is common and Cushing's disease is rare, but have occurred in travellers in the author's experience. Patients with psychological manifestations of malaria, African trypanosomiasis (sleeping sickness) and typhoid usually have clear signs of severe systemic illness, and are admitted to acute medical units. Psychosis has been described in cerebral malaria,[46] and in typhoid psychosis and confusion occur in 5–10%.[47] Catatonic states occur occasionally in typhoid fever, and in African trypanosomiasis, changes in personality and behaviour may precede the objective development of meningo-encephalitis.[48] Psychiatric symptoms may occur as part of the presentation of viral encephalitis.[49] Severe lassitude occurs in some patients with intestinal amoebiasis, and on occasion patients with amoebiasis have been misdiagnosed and admitted to psychiatric units. Metronidazole will produce a more enduring therapeutic response than antidepressants!

Although both considered safe, antimalarial prophylactics, chloroquine and mefloquine, are associated with acute psychotic episodes. The evidence suggests that the risk is higher with mefloquine,[50] but in addition to acute psychotic reactions, variously estimated during prophylaxis to occur in somewhere between 1:6000–10 000,[50–52] mefloquine has clearly been associated with dizziness, a sense of dissociation from the environment, vivid dreams, nightmares and hallucinations. One bizarre occurrence is described in a British Army soldier. A previously healthy, 63 kg private experienced a visual hallucination of the grim reaper standing behind the chaplain, with an auditory hallucination of incoherent voices.[52] The risk of psychotic reactions during the treatment of malaria with mefloquine is higher, and in one study was estimated at 1:215.[53]

Acute psychiatric syndromes including psychotic disorders

5% in Price's[38] study returned because of acute psychiatric problems. Of German technical aid workers, only 0.4% were repatriated per annum, but psychological disorder was the cause in 35% of those evacuated as an emergency,[36] and in 16% of Peace Corps volunteers.[37] While over half merited psychiatric diagnosis in Foyle's recent substantial study,[1] there were few serious psychiatric disorders.

Brief reactive psychosis is probably the most common, non-organic psychotic disorder among expatriates, particularly since candidate screening will identify the vast majority with chronic psychotic disorders, such as schizophrenia.[35] The trigger is usually an overwhelming crisis or stress in a vulnerable individual.

> A 45-year-old secretary working with a voluntary agency in a developing country heard gunshots from a neighbouring flat where her best friend was living. When she arrived on the scene just after the police, she found her friend lying on the floor dead in a pool of blood with a gunshot wound to the head. Over the next 6 months, she developed delusions of persecution and personal opposition and became unable to draw the line between fact and fantasy. She initiated her own referral for 'healing of the memories' at the same time as her agency was arranging referral to the same healthcare agency. At presentation, she had a clear paranoid psychosis, felt an inappropriate degree of responsibility for the death of her friend and was persuaded with great difficulty that consultation with a psychiatrist was the most appropriate next step. At psychiatric review, she rejected admission to hospital but agreed to the prescription of sulpiride following which she gradually improved.

In general, patients respond well with appropriate therapy and a supportive environment.[35]

While schizophrenia usually arises in the second and third decades, it may develop in later adult life, and is defined by the presence of delusions, hallucinations, bizarre beliefs and behaviour interfering with functioning for at least 6 months.[35]

Affective disorders

Price[38] found that one-fifth of those who were permanently invalided home had delusional states and one-fifth were clinically depressed. Later studies have highlighted depression as the most common condition in expatriates referred for psychiatric assessment,[54] with psychosomatic disorders, anxiety states, alcoholism and acute psychosis occurring less frequently. In Dally's small study,[54] anorexia nervosa was common in children referred, but he acknowledges that his known interest in eating disorders may have introduced referral bias. One-third of the expatriates whom he reviewed collapsed in the first 9 months, and one-half between 9 months and 4 years. Foyle[1] analysing nearly 400 psychiatric interviews with expatriates found about 10% had affective disorders. About 5% had neurotic conditions and slightly more displayed personality immaturity. Hypomania also surfaces from time to time.

> A 35-year-old voluntary worker had completed two tours of service in Central Africa and was reviewed 3 months after commencing home leave. Her last period of home leave had been complicated by personal illness and had been emotionally traumatic. At review, she owned feelings of tension and stress, and although not depressed, had felt very angry when she left her post before taking home leave. She spoke loudly, and took much time to explain small points. She was not weepy, yet described events that should have been deeply hurtful. Hyperactivity was evident at interview and during the few days that she was being reviewed she completely reorganised the kitchen of the flat in which she was staying. There was no family history of mental ill health, but her mother had had thyroid problems. Her resting pulse was 90/minute, and hands were warm but not sweaty, with a minimal finger tremor but no eye signs to suggest thyrotoxicosis. Thyroid disease was suspected but thyroid function was normal and after some delay she was referred by her general practitioner to a psychiatrist who made a diagnosis of hypomania, and instituted lithium therapy. She was unable to return to Africa.

STRESS REACTIONS

Various degrees of stress reaction are very common in expatriates for all the reasons outlined above and occur where exposure to chronic stress exceeds the individual's coping mechanisms. The extent of stress reaction may vary from mild fatigue and loss of enthusiasm for work to severe exhaustion, escalation of personal conflict, and major depressive and anxiety symptoms may be accompanied by suicidal ideation.[35] Aid workers, particularly in refugee camps, may experience such overwhelming need that they continue working without taking necessary rest, relaxation and exercise, and soon become ineffective helpers for those they have come to serve. In a survey of 1300 people returning to the International Committee of the Red Cross (ICRC) HQ in 1996, 10% were diagnosed as suffering from stress, cumulative in a half, basic in a quarter and traumatic in 17%. PTSD was uncommon, only occurring in 7%.[30]

Effective pastoral supervision is essential. Those who just need a good holiday must be differentiated from those who are sufficiently unwell to require direction to take extended leave, which may need to last for several months. Counselling in the early stages of severe stress reaction is largely a waste of time since there is usually insufficient energy left to engage with making changes. If clinical depression is an associated feature, then antidepressant medication should not be withheld. Once recovery has occurred, non-directive problem-solving counselling, during which the overseas worker is able to plan necessary and attainable changes to lifestyle may be enormously helpful. Foyle's popular book *Honourably Wounded* for those working with Christian agencies overseas contains much helpful, practical advice about stress-reducing measures which can be applied to other expatriate groups.[55] De Haan observes that if resistance to stress is to be increased, attention must be paid to improving individual autonomy, improving team relationships, reducing interpersonal conflict and providing effective leadership.[30]

In some geographical locations taking local leave may pose major difficulties. Holidays may lie in tension with cultural expectations, or there may simply be no suitable places to go to in the country. Getting away may take several days by 4-wheel drive vehicle on unmade roads or may involve the expensive charter of light aircraft to fly to another country. The 'catch 22' for some voluntary workers is that they simply do not have the financial resources to develop appropriate escapes in high stress environments.

The author saw a family working in an Islamic country. The parents were poorly remunerated, had four children of whom two were teenage girls and beach holidays had become impossible because of the high level of interest shown in the girls by young male nationals. The parents did not have the financial resources to fly to a neighbouring country with excellent holiday facilities, even though this was a normal holiday resort for other expatriate families.

Where finance is a serious problem, agencies must be encouraged by health carers to rethink their financial policies so that those whom they do send overseas have the resources to withstand the pressures and chronic and cumulative stressors of overseas life.

Anxiety disorders

Generalised anxiety disorder, panic disorder, obsessive–compulsive disorder and post-traumatic disorder are all found amongst expatriates. A positive family history is common in those with panic or obsessive–compulsive disorder, disorders which have significant biological components.[35]

Generalised anxiety disorder presents with persistent, unrealistic or excessive anxiety and worries about the future. Physical tension may manifest with trembling fatigue, dyspnoea, palpitations and neurological or gastrointestinal symptoms.[31] Excessive caffeine use and hyperthyroidism should be excluded.[35]

Panic disorder often emerges after the second decade of life and is associated with the sudden onset of severe anxiety, tachycardia, tachypnoea, trembling, nausea, diarrhoea and a sense of impending doom. Drug therapy assists recovery and cognitive and behavioural therapies may also be helpful.[35]

Obsessive–compulsive disorder is characterised by repeated, intrusive, unwelcome thoughts, with retained insight that these thoughts are inappropriate. Rituals may be developed to deal with the intrusive thoughts. Psychotherapy is only of limited value and drug therapies are usually employed.[35]

Post-traumatic stress

Personal violence is more likely in the developing world than in the developed West, both as a result of war and criminal activity[56] and some organisations e.g. ICRC have seen a transition over the last decade from their workers being relatively protected from personal violence to being deliberate targets.[30] Victims rarely seek help themselves and a history of significant trauma quite often emerges during routine medical review if the physician is able to communicate empathy and allows sufficient time.

> A 30-year-old man presented at a tropical clinic for screening for schistosomiasis. The doctor was able to take longer than usual over history-taking and unwittingly provided the patient with an environment in which he felt able to share more deeply. 8 months previously he had been the leader and truck driver of an overland safari. The convoy was held up by bandits, wholesale robbery ensued and young women were raped in front of their companions, while all were threatened with death by machete. The trauma extended beyond the initial incident as he arranged for hospitalisation of the rape victims and anti-HIV drugs to be flown from another country. At medical review he was still disabled by deep anger and accepted counselling therapy.

The developing world is also more prone to the natural disasters of earthquake, flooding and volcanic eruption, which may also cause trauma, and road traffic accidents[57] are much more frequent. Light aircraft accidents also appear to be common.

POST TRAUMATIC STRESS DISORDER

PTSD is as old as mankind, but was not described until the Vietnam War. The American Psychiatric Diagnostic and Statistical Manual of Mental Disorders (DSM IV)[58] recognises acute, chronic and delayed forms.

Turner has likened the processes involved in PTSD to the overwhelming of an internal map.[59] We carry within us an internal map of the external world that we use to make reliable predictions about the future and this enables us to plan ahead and make good decisions. If the predictions are not realised, we experience loss and undergo a bereavement process during which the internal map is redrawn. Thus if a life partner suddenly dies, the internal map that includes that life partner is found to be inadequate and over the period of bereavement, the internal map is altered to take account of the absence of the loved partner.

In PTSD that emotional processing of the internal map is overwhelmed by the severity of the unpredictable event and affected individuals shut off the painful feelings to protect themselves but are then subject to intrusive recollections of the event that alternate with defensive avoidance. Sometimes the obtrusive recollections may appear years after the event, sometimes precipitated by physical illness.

> A 52-year-old, Canadian pilot worked in Central Africa with a British-dominated, expatriate group. He found integration with this group difficult and was particularly irked by the tendency to regard his views, as the most recent arrival, as of little importance, particularly as he had left a responsible, combined managerial and flying post in Canada. About 2 years after arrival, his wife developed cerebral malaria and needed urgent transport to a competent medical centre. As he attempted to take off, a tyre burst on his single-engine Cessna. He skidded off the runway, and narrowly avoided an accident, then changed the tyre and flew her out.
>
> This stress was however compounded a few months later, when he flew a group of passengers to another town. There was a loud explosion from the engine and the oil pressure dropped to zero. Below him was dense, rocky scrub with no roads in sight on which he could have made an emergency landing. He was certain that he and his five passengers were going to die but to his amazement the engine kept going until he reached an airstrip where he landed safely. At the time he appeared unmoved by the incident, and with his passengers was extremely thankful for a safe outcome. 3 months later, he had a febrile illness, developed painful joints that rendered him unfit to fly and started having recurrent disturbing dreams relating to the near tragedy in

the Cessna. Serology later incidentally identified the probable cause of the arthralgia as Chikungunya virus infection.

The described features of PTSD are:

1. exposure to a recognisable trauma or stressor
2. the trauma is persistently re-experienced in at least one of the following ways:
   — recurrent intrusive and distressing recollections or dreams
   — re-experienced in actions or feelings (or traumatic game playing in children)
   — extensive distress reminders
3. persistent avoidance of stimuli associated with the trauma or numbing of general responsiveness
4. persistent symptoms of increased arousal, not present before, as shown by irritability, sleep difficulties, excessive vigilance, startle responses or reaction to trigger stress
5. criteria 2,3,4 have been present during at least 1 month.

Clinically the disorder presents at some point after the event with either nightmares, flashbacks and panic or repressive phenomena, numbing or restricted capacity for feelings and withdrawal predominating. Many experience guilt, irritability, insomnia, impaired concentration and hyper-vigilance. Some individuals exposed to the same event develop problems while others apparently do not. The reasons for this are not well understood, but the security of childhood experience is probably important. The extent of stressor exposure is the major factor for the development of PTSD,[60] particularly its gruesomeness (multiple deaths, mutilated bodies and the deaths of children) and encounters with death, destruction and violence. Rising or persistent anxiety towards the end of the first week suggests serious disorder and the need for early intervention. Normally, reactive symptoms are present in the days after a serious event but fade within a few weeks.

Victims, perpetrators, rescuers and healthcare workers are all at risk. Treatment may be difficult especially when the disorder is well-established. The central element of most therapeutic approaches is the rehearsal of the trauma story[53]

and standardised, critical incident debriefing is now widely practised and accepted,[61] although sound evidence for sustained benefit is lacking.[62] Other approaches have included cognitive, behavioural and drug therapy.

First-aid and therapy

As soon as practical, daily debriefing sessions should start with individuals or groups, aiming at accurate recounting of events and feelings, free emotional expression and appropriate grieving. Basic ground rules concerning toleration of silence and confidentiality are agreed. The trauma story is rehearsed, re-awakening associated feelings in such a way that they can be tolerated and processed without rapid retreat into avoidance. Helpers should thus encourage free emotional expression in a calm, relaxed setting, free from interruptions and with the opportunity to prolong sessions beyond the traditional 50 minutes. Helpers should however avoid probing too deeply, rather allowing the most painful aspects to surface in an atmosphere of accepting, non-judgemental, empathetic listening. Brief contacts, which do no more than raise the emotional temperature cause distress without helping the victim to process the experience, may be harmful. Talking to the relatives of dead colleagues, attending or watching funerals or memorial services and creating collages illustrating the experiences, or writing about them help victims to face up to loss. The use of tape recorders may be helpful. The story is recorded and then played back on a daily basis assisting the emotional processing, but in the absence of tape facilities reflective listening approaches may also be helpful.

Somatoform disorders and chronic fatigue syndrome

Physical symptoms for which there are no demonstrable organic causes occur regularly amongst expatriate workers. It is vital that physical causes are thoroughly excluded with a detailed medical history, physical evaluation and appropriate investigations, and once this process is complete the patient may be more amenable to exploration of other factors in generating symptomatology.[35]

> A 30-year-old physiotherapist working in a developing country manifested a sequence of physical symptoms that took her through the ophthalmological, ENT, medical and gynaecological departments. All investigations were negative for organic causes and she then developed signs of an acute abdomen but without any changes in her white blood count. A laparotomy was performed, but no pathology was disclosed. Consultation with her agency resulted in her repatriation but she remained unwell and later developed severe neurological symptoms. Referral for psychotherapy followed exhaustive and negative, sophisticated imaging techniques.

In Price's study,[38] 20% were repatriated because of neurasthenia (probably the historical equivalent of chronic fatigue syndrome (CFS)) and this was more frequent in those working in Japan than those working in China, India or Africa. Chronic fatigue is quite common in expatriates,[63] although again it is vital that the possibility of organic causes should be considered and investigated. Anaemia, hepatitis, intestinal amoebiasis, giardiasis, brucellosis and schistosomiasis should be excluded before the label of CFS is applied, but most of these may figure as trigger factors. In the author's experience, 90% of expatriates with CFS have identifiable secondary gains from the illness, although their significance is often denied by the sufferer.[64] Lovell found a more open attitude towards causation amongst patients in her study, and noted that expatriates with CFS tend to be hard working, to have an overactive, premorbid lifestyle and to have experienced stressful life events in the period leading up to the onset of CFS.[63]

Adjustment disorders

Adjustment disorders comprise short-duration, maladaptive reactions to psychological, social or physical stressors and may be characterised by

anxiety, depression, disturbance of conduct, physical complaints, social withdrawal, or withdrawal from work, or academic impairment. The stressor can usually be identified and the disorder usually resolves when stressor exposure is ended. Foyle[1] made this diagnosis in a one-third of her patients, and there was a positive association with four stressors: occupational stress, acculturation, home country anxieties and physical health. Clearly, there is a diagnostic grey area between those with marked degrees of stress reaction and adjustment disorders, but the key factor is that adjustment disorders represent maladaptive responses and the intensity of stressor exposure is insufficient to explain the symptoms. Practical, supportive, directive counselling may shorten the duration of the disorder.[35] Foyle noted a negative association between those with adjustment disorders and a personal and family mental health history. By contrast, those with affective disorders were more likely to have had previous consultations with their family doctor or psychiatrists, and were significantly more likely to have a positive mental health family history.[1]

Personality disorder

'Difficult people' are a common source of stress in expatriate working groups, and in many cases the difficult person has an unhelpful personality trait or a personality disorder. Usually the person with the disorder blames everyone else for the difficulties, and the underlying cause of the conflict only emerges after interviewing a number of stressed individuals who interact with the key figure, the 'problem centre'. It is vital that the cause of relationship stress is accurately identified if appropriate management decisions are to be made. All too often one or two stressed individuals are repatriated because it is assumed that they are the ones who cannot cope with the pressures of expatriate life when the real cause of difficulty is another staff member who is allowed to continue in post to cause difficulty with the next raw recruit.

The concept of abnormal personality is well accepted in psychiatric practice although definition is beset with difficulty. WHO defines these conditions as deeply ingrained and enduring behaviour patterns manifesting with inflexible responses to a broad range of personal and social situations.[65] Those with personality disorder tend to be maladaptive, inflexible and impaired in social and occupational functioning, and leave an indelible, negative, and often painful, mark on their relationships with others. Small groups of expatriates working overseas are particularly vulnerable to the negative impact that such persons have on relationships.

The specific disorder descriptions are idealised and few patients fit exactly with the stereotype. There is a continuum of dysfunction between those with well-developed disorder and those who have personality traits which under stress may become so pronounced that disorder is suspected. The prevalence of personality disorder in the general populations ranges from 2 to 13%[66] so it is inevitable that some people with these disorders will surface in those working overseas.

CLASSIFICATION OF PERSONALITY DISORDERS

Schubert[67] has applied a three-cluster classification to the importance of personality disorders in expatriate life.

Cluster A includes paranoid, schizoid and schizotypal disorders. Those with these three personality disorders are perceived as odd or eccentric and are usually excluded during candidate screening.

Cluster C includes avoidant, dependent, obsessive–compulsive, and passive–aggressive disorders. Persons with these disorders may seem anxious and fearful, or may be overly compliant, meticulous, and not expressive of strong feeling. They usually appear overly sensitive for expatriate life and are also usually screened out. However, avoidant-disordered individuals may do well as pioneers in secure solo settings, although their need for physical security is normally a self-excluding characteristic. Their excessive preoccupation with being criticised or rejected may cause real difficulty in small groups.

Those with dependent personality disorder do well in larger groups because they are compliant,

and their fear of abandonment may go unnoticed. However, in a smaller group this becomes problematic. Obsessional (anankastic)-disordered people are dependable, precise and punctual, setting high standards. They are, however, obstinate, become preoccupied with unimportant detail, and appear bigoted and humourless. Passive–aggressive-disordered persons often appear to others as 'fine people', never overtly angry, channelling anger into procrastination and delay, and discreet refusal to follow orders.

Cluster B causes more difficulty. Included in this group are antisocial, emotionally unstable (borderline), histrionic, and narcissistic disorders. These disorders are more subtle and affected persons may slip past the screening process, unless sophisticated screening measures are in place.

The term antisocial personality disorder belies their behavioural characteristics. They are smooth, good talkers, often good at public speaking and excellent advocates for the work with which they are involved overseas. They are sociable, good fundraisers, but are unable to make moral decisions, tend not to honour financial obligations, and have inconsistent work patterns.

A married man with three children working in the developing world with a Christian voluntary agency demonstrated the 'Swiss cheese' aspect of moral decision-making which such people possess. He took a mistress, fathered a child by her, and the first sign that all was not well noticed by his wife was a deterioration in the helpfulness of his preaching. When the relationship became public knowledge, he was repatriated by his agency and he and his wife were referred for counselling. At interview, he was appropriately grieving for the loss of the relationship with his mistress and their son, but seemed unable to comprehend why his wife was so angry. He was an excellent advocate for the work in which he was engaged and his agency were reluctant to lose him, despite the scandal that his action had brought within the national church. He was however unable to engage with counselling therapy and did not return overseas.

Those with emotionally unstable (borderline) disorder can wreak havoc in small working groups. Their underlying pathology involves an inability to tolerate and understand shades of grey in relationships and their tendency to 'split' affects both personal relationships and interactions within groups.[68] At a personal level, they tend to form unstable, intense relationships, and swing between over-idealisation and devaluation. Not infrequently a colleague may fall from grace in the perception of the borderline sufferer and having been a best friend becomes the number one enemy. Borderline persons may find it difficult to integrate into a new culture, but with groups the danger lies in their tendency to divide members into 'good' or 'bad' categories. The 'good' will favour the borderline person, while the 'bad' see the problem that the borderline personality poses, and the group then becomes a fulfilment of the borderline person's perception, although with time most in the team will perceive the destructive impact of the relationship pattern.

Those with a histrionic disorder are highly emotional, attention seeking, need constant reassurance, praise and approval and desire to be the centre of attention. They have shallow, rapidly shifting emotions and loss and rejection can cause deep distress. Their constant need for reassurance and affirmation wears down other members of the team.

Those with a narcissistic personality disorder think of themselves as special but fall apart with the normal disappointments of life. They have fragile self-esteem, and are unable to accept criticism or to empathise.

Appropriate management of those with personality disorders is their removal from the overseas posting. Motivation for change is usually lacking, insight is limited and the response to prolonged psychotherapy is poor.

Coming home

Final re-entry is also highly stressful and adaptation is often much more difficult and may take longer than the original move to the host country. 'Home may not be so sweet'[69] and home may no longer be home. When the author returned to the UK after 6 years in East Africa, the grass looked unnaturally green and UK hospitals, supposedly under-funded, were to my Africanised eyes, institutions characterised by flagrant

wastefulness. It took a couple of years to feel reasonably comfortable again in the UK, but in common with other expatriates I have found that the process of becoming bicultural has left a permanent mark in my experience and attitudes. Nostalgia literally means the pain of looking back. This is deeply understood by those who have worked overseas for protracted periods, and is easily precipitated by television programmes featuring the former host country.

Research on re-entry stress has received heightened attention over the past two decades.[70–72] There are strong elements of bereavement, with various losses impacting at different points in the leaving process.

The range of response

The experience is usually one of low-grade, chronic, gradually easing discomfort. However, the experience may be acutely painful, falling into the unpredictable-involuntary category described by Hopson & Adams.[12]

FACTORS INCREASING RE-ENTRY STRESS REACTION

Distress may be severe, bordering on PTSD if an exit is suddenly enforced by the outbreak of war, precipitated by severe illness, forced by expulsion by a government or accompanied by a sense of failure related to uncompleted or unsatisfactory assignments. Hiebert[10] notes that individuals who have adjusted most successfully to a new culture have the greatest difficulty re-adapting to their old one. Things that once looked natural, now look extravagant and insensitive, and friends have no real point of contact with the expatriate's own past experience.

A 60-year-old missionary returned after a lifetime of service in an African country where she had also grown up as a 'missionary kid'. She was unwisely advised to make a clean break with the past and arrived in the UK with a couple of suitcases and little to remind her of her life's work. She had only a few ageing relatives and found that being in the UK carried no sense of being at home at all. She was disturbed to find herself in tears for no apparent reason, and found it difficult to speak at public meetings. At interview, it was clear that she was experiencing classical bereavement symptoms, having lost a great part of her personal identity in leaving her adopted country. Therapy involved releasing her from public speaking commitments with which she did not feel able to cope, encouraging her to enlarge photographs she had taken in Africa to decorate her new flat and encouraging her to talk about the life that she had left behind in an environment where she felt safe and accepted. The opportunity developed for her to return to work for another year in the same African country, and during this additional tour she was able to adjust to her final departure with much greater ease, this time returning with important physical reminders of her life's work.

Children 'coming home'

The needs of children are similar but with some specifics. The parental culture is not theirs and the desire to come 'home' may be neither shared nor understood by children. They may be repatriated involuntarily and their transition may be more traumatic than for their parents.[12, 73] Their previous life is incomprehensible and of no interest to their new peer group and for expatriate children this is devastating and a denial of their identity.[13] They do not feel that they belong to their parents' culture but neither do they totally belong to the host culture which nurtured them.[25] TCK teenagers often seem mature, with a breadth of experience of life, having developed independence through travel and exposure to different cultures, but they may be naive about life issues in the West from which they have been protected. Younger children may lack basic skills such as dressing themselves or looking after their clothes and toys, having been spoilt or pampered by an ayah. Whatever the age of the child, tremendous adjustments will need to be made, when parents are often overwhelmed by the re-entry transition themselves.

Psychopathology in returnees

Lovell[63] demonstrated that 46% of aid workers experienced psychological difficulties during or after being involved in aid work, and most of these had not experienced problems before they went overseas. One-fifth developed problems while overseas and the remainder after return. While many had found their time overseas a fulfilling experience, two-fifths reported predominantly negative feelings after return. The range and the depth of the losses associated with return from an overseas posting may precipitate clinical depression or other forms of breakdown in predisposed individuals.

Screening candidates for protracted visits

The screening of employees for psychological risk factors requires a good working knowledge of the stressors associated with cross-cultural transition and working overseas, and expertise in psychological health. It is best conducted by those who have personal experience of work abroad, and training in psychiatry, clinical psychology or counselling. The aim is to obtain a total profile of a candidate that covers many facets of life.[74] Life is uncertain and no process of screening can predict with accuracy the impact of major trauma or illness. Peppiatt & Byass, analysing 212 Methodist personnel, noted that psychiatric illness was the commonest serious problem despite careful screening by a general practitioner with overseas experience and a clinical psychologist.[39] Early enforced return from an overseas posting may itself be psychologically damaging, adding a layer of guilt and personal failure to the illness which triggered repatriation, amplified by the need to explain the reasons for return to friends and relatives. The ripples for those working with voluntary agencies may also spread to financial supporters who may understandably feel that their investment has not been worthwhile. A middle path is needed between unrealistic optimism and an over-rigorous exclusion of any who cause concern, but who, with appropriate support and preparation, may make an outstanding contribution. The process is one of risk assessment and the recognition that perfection is unattainable.

Personal and family history

Foyle's extensive research with expatriates working with Christian agencies[1, 29] demonstrated that half had problems which predated their overseas work. The group with pre-selection problems had a history that was lifelong in 60%, and 70% had a family history involving one or more family members. In the great majority, the symptom pattern was the same as previously, with personality disorder, depression, long-standing neurotic symptoms, deprived childhood with or without serious parental violence and abuse found in order of frequency. Others have shown that a number of factors affect the expatriate's ability to cope during cultural change, including physical stamina, emotional maturity,[75] history of behaviour, and past responses to life experience, which Britt suggests are the best predictor of their future ability to cope.[76]

CHILDHOOD EXPERIENCE

In the half of Foyle's patients with pre-selection problems, these related to poor childhood experiences, with or without abuse.[29] Long-standing symptoms in her patients included fears, feelings of inadequacy or insecurity, and previous attacks of depression. Schubert[77] notes that personality disorders often seem to relate to abnormal, early childhood experience. Two surveys in UK colleges preparing candidates for service overseas suggest that the frequency of traumatic events is the same as in the general population.[78,79] In the first, involving 103 respondents, 14% had experienced parental bereavement before the age of 20 years, and 20% had experienced severe parental quarrelling. 17% as children knew a parent was having an extra-marital affair, 16% had experienced parental separation and 9% divorce. Physical abuse had occurred in 11% and sexual abuse in 10%. Three of 38 women had

undergone termination of pregnancy and one had been raped. The findings of the second survey of 113 students were similar, but physical and sexual abuse were reported more frequently at 15.5% and 13.3% respectively, and affected 27% of female respondents.[79] Sexual abuse in childhood has been shown to triple psychiatric morbidity in adult life.[80]

In Chalmers' survey,[79] over half felt that they had dealt adequately with past painful issues but a substantial minority (27%) still felt the effects of these past events in their current functioning. Some of the symptoms noted by Foyle[29] were thought to relate to poor handling of losses in the past. This is particularly important in childhood where an object of attachment, usually a parent, has been lost or threatened in such a way as to cause intense anxiety, insecurity and an inability to form good adult relationships. This may manifest with either a tendency to withdraw from relationships or an inappropriate dependence.[14,81] Both of these reaction patterns are unhealthy, causing extra pressure for the individual and members of their current family during transition. Appropriate handling of separation is important because of the increased likelihood overseas of periods of separation from a spouse, children or other close friends.[73] For many, this includes children leaving for boarding school, husbands doing field trips and the frequent arrival and departure of colleagues.

PAST ADULT LIFE EXPERIENCE

Inadequately resolved, painful or difficult events, for instance recent bereavement, may feed into the adaptation process exacerbating the stress reaction.

Financial implications for agencies

Most commercial and voluntary agencies appreciate that screening candidates makes good people management and sound financial sense. The financial loss for a commercial organisation that repatriates a staff member as an emergency may range between £50 and £100 000, taking account of the costs involved in relocating the family, perhaps having arranged fee-paying education for children, and recruiting and preparing a replacement. The lower salary levels paid by voluntary organisations greatly reduce these costs but the proportionate loss in terms of the ratio of numbers of personnel to the annual turnover of an agency will be much the same.

The screening process

Psychological assessment interviews are only part of the selection process for most agencies, and should be integrated into selection, and not tacked on at the end when a provisional decision has already been made. To do so places undue reliance on the assessment process, which is one of risk assessment, and converts it into a final hurdle.

The whole family should be screened. Spouses prone to mental ill-health may threaten the ability of a family to remain overseas, and children also need some consideration and should be included in the decision-making process. As a general rule, moving adolescents for the first time into a new location overseas is a mistake. They are already coping with one major area of change as they make the transition to adult life, and adding a major cultural transition may overwhelm their coping ability. Boarding school for adolescents in their home country may be preferable to boarding overseas. The main exception would be TCKs, who are likely to re-adapt more easily to a culture to which they have already been exposed. Application forms should be carefully prepared and provide a breadth of data about the applicant prior to formal screening.

I. REFERENCES

Work references are particularly important and any offer in a written reference to comment verbally should always be taken up. The value of references by friends will depend on the degree of contact, and where references are poor the possibility of hidden agendas should be considered. Those working with Christian agencies may place undue reliance on references from church pastors who may in fact have a low level of contact with some members of their congregation. Some church leaders are unrealistically enthusiastic when one of their young people decides to opt for overseas service, an occurrence which Foyle describes as the 'halo effect',[74] and which has its secular equivalent.

> One referee, an acquaintance of the candidate, commented to the agency to which he had applied: 'He is a strong character with a real twinkle of humour although at times he is slightly eccentric. He is good fun and I think will work well in a team situation.' His line manager however commented: 'He is a likeable but completely tactless and domineering individual and is so utterly eccentric that I am sure he would drive his colleagues round the bend ... there are no circumstances therefore under which I would recommend X for the kind of work in which you are involved.'

Work references are far more useful because they usually reflect the day-by-day experience of the candidate by those with whom they are in regular contact, and who are not necessarily seeing them on their best behaviour. References should be read prior to interview and any inconsistencies between data on the reference and candidate application forms explored.

2. PSYCHOLOGICAL SCREENING INTERVIEW

This is the core of the selection process,[74] and any psychometric scales should always be interpreted in the light of information disclosed at interview. One candidate completed a personality scale with a pattern suggesting paranoid personality trait, but at interview was found to have recently emerged from a lengthy and highly stressful employer's enquiry for misconduct, precipitated by an allegation from a jealous colleague. The enquiry had completely cleared her of any misdemeanour, and further interview with repeat application of the scale was recommended after a period of 9–12 months.

A useful analogy is that the interview is the front door to a house whereas psychometric scales are similar to taking a look through the upstairs windows. Such scales provide an additional valuable view of the way a person functions but are secondary in importance to interview.

The interview should include a personal, mental health history, noting any previous referrals for psychiatric help, counselling, or consultations with the family doctor for any form of emotional ill-health. The history should also clarify whether there are current symptoms of mental ill-health, and any past experience of difficulty in coping. Most candidates have such experiences but if this has occurred several times, then warning bells should sound. Self-understanding and insight into the reasons why the candidate had difficulty in coping would comprise a balancing, important, positive indicator. In Lovell's study of returning development workers, feeling validators appeared less at risk of depression than non-validators.[82] Non-validators may correlate with the term 'brittle personality' employed by Fowke,[83] who may not admit to any stress at all despite working in an objectively stressful environment. Those who are able to talk about life's experiences, and their associated feelings with openness and insight are likely to cope better with chronic and cumulative stressors overseas.

Family mental health history

Foyle's data[1,29] strongly suggest that a positive family history of mental ill-health is an adverse indicator, particularly if present in two or more family members. Mental ill-health history should include grandparents, uncles and aunts who are blood relatives and first cousins; candidates may need reminding that depression counts as a mental illness. She advises that:

> those with heavily loaded psychiatric histories should not be accepted for overseas service unless there is clear evidence that they have remained well for several years, have a good work record in their home country, and have shown a capacity for coping in general, and for maintaining good interpersonal relationships. There must be good personal and medical support in the locations to which they will go.[1]

Childhood

Increasing marital breakdown and the increasing proportion of the population reared in dys-

functional families will take an inevitable toll on adult mental health. The vital issue is whether relationships with parents were felt to be good enough in childhood, and, if not, whether an adequate degree of resolution of the pain associated with the relationship has occurred.

> Ruth, aged 35 years, worked in an isolated refugee camp. Her immediate superior, Susan, was a rather critical, brusque lady who reminded Ruth of her mother. Ruth developed frequent angry outbursts towards Susan, and these reached the point where Ruth's contract was terminated, Susan's parting shot to Ruth being criticism of her emotional insecurity. During therapy, it emerged that Ruth had a serious illness when she was 5 years old at the same time as twin brothers were born. Ruth's mother transferred all her attention and affection to the twins on Ruth's return home, a state of affairs which continued into Ruth's teenage years.

Neither this unresolved issue nor its importance for relationships had been identified during her selection.

Discussion with the candidate should clarify how the candidate actually felt during childhood, and feels now, about parents. Were parents distant, non-demonstrative and constantly critical, or warm, available and reassuring? Detailed notes should be made of any traumatic bereavements, physical or sexual abuse, involvement with drugs and alcohol during school life, and any significant experience of bullying in school.

Adult life

The candidate should be encouraged to talk about relationships in work and due note taken of job changes and the reasons. Frequent job changes cause concern unless this was a normal pattern of professional development. The extent, nature and depth of substance abuse (alcohol, drugs) should be noted. Several years clear of drug misuse should have elapsed before service overseas, and serious caution should be exercised with reformed alcoholics. The development of clear insight into the reasons why abuse had occurred would act as a positive pointer.

Sexual history

While this may appear a personal and private matter, the recent death sentence of an expatriate for adultery in an Islamic country reinforces the view that private areas of morality may become the serious, legitimate and expensive concern of the employing agency. Any information disclosed should be treated with appropriate confidentiality. In some countries, homosexual acts may be treated as criminal or become a source of scandal. Vulnerability in the area of sexuality, and the implications of frequent partner changes, whatever the person's orientation should be discussed, and frequent partner change will have implications for STD or HIV risks. Other individuals should only be informed where there are over-riding pastoral implications and then only with the full knowledge and permission of the candidate.

Marriage and other committed relationships

Marital breakdown overseas may cause the repatriation of the whole family. It is unwise to send families overseas where there is serious marital instability since the stresses of cross-cultural adaptation may have a further detrimental impact on the relationship. An alteration in overlap for husband and wife is a frequent consequence of a move overseas and the increase, or decrease in the interactive time may also increase marital stress.

Single candidates applying to some religious voluntary agencies may expect marital prospects to improve when the reality is that they usually contract. It may be helpful in such circumstances to discuss this and clarify whether the candidate is single by choice, and encourage the development of other relationships which will be life-enriching.

Personal beliefs

Exploration of this area may reveal much about the psychological maturity and personality structure of the candidate. Rigidity of religious views may be a manifestation of personality rigidity, and reflect an underlying insecurity and an inability to tolerate shades of grey. Rigidity keeps the world polarised to secure 'black or white', 'in or out'

categories, and this may make it more difficult to adapt to another set of cultural values.

3. INTELLIGENCE LEVEL

Those with low intelligence levels may find it more difficult to adapt cross-culturally. Educational achievements may be one helpful indicator of intelligence but are not wholly reliable. Some may have been denied educational opportunities while others who have gained diplomas or degrees may in fact only have coped with the intensive help of a more intelligent spouse or friend. While the degree of limitation in such candidates is unlikely to cause difficulty in adapting to an overseas environment, their subsequent performance may not match expectations. Of the various intelligence scales marketed, it is preferable to employ a test that assesses both verbal/numerical and non-verbal skills, and to consider further tests of language-acquisition skills where this is essential for adequate performance in the overseas post. The use of the latter may be triggered by poorer performance on verbal/numerical sections. Intelligence tests may still produce unexpectedly poor results in those who have been denied major educational opportunities.

A 38-year-old, married man took up a post in Europe. After 3 years, he lacked fluency in the language which was essential for his work, while his wife and children had successfully settled into their new environment, which included local schooling in the national language for his children. He had left school at 16 years with only one O-Level and although his CV showed successful completion of a college diploma, it emerged that his wife had helped him write most of the assignments. Assessment at an expert centre for learning difficulties in the UK revealed he had a form of dyslexia and further improvement in fluency was unlikely. He and his family returned to the UK, a move which all family members found deeply disappointing and stressful.

4. PERSONALITY ASSESSMENT SCALES

The Myers–Briggs Type Indicator (MBTI) is a widely used, non-judgemental personality typing indicator which uses three categories originally found in the work of Carl Jung: intraversion/extraversion, sensing/intuition, and thinking/feeling. The mother and daughter partnership of Katherine Cook Briggs and Isabel Briggs Myers independently came to similar conclusions and added an additional category of judging/perceiving.[84] MBTI found early favour with Roman Catholic Orders where its value in helping different personality types to live together with understanding was appreciated. It is now widely used both in commerce and by a wide variety of voluntary agencies. Over 3.5 million scales are now administered annually worldwide and the MBTI has been translated into many languages. Although inappropriate as a screening tool for personality pathology, it may be helpful in the placement and preparation of candidates since it helps individuals to understand their personality strengths and weaknesses. Very high scores may be associated with personality pathology which will become clear in other ways.

The Minnesota Multiphasic Personality Inventory (MMPI) is a clinical tool, is widely used in North America and was first formulated in the USA almost 60 years ago.[85] While standardised in the USA the MMPI has not yet been standardised for UK populations. Most British authorities do not favour it, and it has been criticised for lack of internal consistency and temporal stability.[86]

The NEO Five Factor Personality Inventory examines five domains – neuroticism, extraversion, openness, agreeableness and conscientiousness – and each of the five domains is represented by six more specific scales that measure facets of the domain.[87] It is likely that those who score low on the last three domains may have personalities that encounter more difficulty in cross-cultural work, and those who score more highly on the neuroticism domain will be more emotionally vulnerable. Correlations between particular patterns on the NEO and personality disorder have been established.[88]

The Gordon Personal Profile and Gordon Personal Inventory (GPP-I) together measure eight aspects of personality, and are usually employed as companion instruments.[89] The first four – ascendancy, responsibility (stickability), emotional stability and sociability – give an estimate of self-esteem. Very high scores on responsibility may correlate with rigidity. The second set of four domains comprise cautiousness, original thinking, personal relations and vigour. Norms were established in USA college students but the Church Missionary Society in the UK has established norms for their own candidates. UK candidates tend to score lower on ascendancy and higher on responsibility and self-esteem than USA college students (Stuart Buchanan, personal communication).

In addition to these personality assessment scales, there are several other, well-validated scales available.

5. ASSESSMENT OF CURRENT FUNCTIONING

The Heimler Scale of Social Functioning (HSSF)[90,91] assesses the balance of satisfaction and frustration and the margin for coping. Most candidates manifest scales in a 'super-normal' category, with very high satisfaction and low frustration. In the experience of the author and his co-workers, HSSF may help identify an individual's particular coping strategy under pressure and in particular indicate where these might be self-destructive, or produce behaviour which might threaten others. There are also particular patterns that suggest rigidity or inadequate resolution of past painful issues, and the scale appears to correlate well with clinical indicators of depression. On the basis of preliminary data obtained in expatriates returning with problems, the degree to which childhood was a good preparation for adult life appears an important determinant of subsequent difficulties on the field.

Who to exclude?

Foyle has helpfully summarised positive and negative indicators[29] and others have been added in the list below. Because the emotional stresses of cultural adaptation are considerable, there are solid grounds for excluding certain individuals, including those suffering from:

- **Schizophrenia**
  There is good evidence that schizophrenics are

more prone to psychotic breakdown when their environment is altered. Harrison[20] has reviewed the interaction of migration and mental disorder. Numerous studies have shown that the prevalence of schizophrenia is substantially higher amongst migrants than an indigenous population, reinforcing the contention that cultural transition is a serious psychological stressor. No-one with a history of schizophrenia should be recommended for work overseas and those with a strong family history should be screened by a psychiatrist before being accepted.

- **Bipolar or unipolar affective disorder** (manic depression, or unipolar hypomania or depression)
  These disorders often require lithium therapy for control. Few centres in the developing world have the facilities for monitoring lithium or even thyroid function, which may also be affected.
- **Certain personality disorders**
  The detection of these disorders is problematic. Personality may be assessed from reliable accounts of past behaviour, references, and detection may be assisted by psychometric tests.
- **Alcoholism or past drug use**
  Even if apparently reformed, the stress of cultural adaptation usually proves too great and reformed alcoholics are likely to return to their previous means of coping with stress. Those with a history of recent substance misuse are likely to respond similarly.
- **Chronic fatigue syndrome**
  CFS often recurs, and when it does so, it usually precipitates early withdrawal from the assignment. A history of severe CFS should normally be regarded as a contraindication to service overseas.

Who/what to be worried about?

Those with a history of anxiety or minor/ moderate depression. Any past history of disabling anxiety or depression is important, whether or not a healthcare professional was consulted. Single episodes some

years in the past, without any family history, are not a major worry. Repeated episodes and a positive family history will raise concern. Relevant questions are the length of the episode, the triggers, how it resolved, and what has been learned from the episode.[83] Those who have at times been so anxious or depressed that they were overwhelmed and unable to continue to work may not be suitable for work overseas, unless this was an appropriate response to a very severe stress, and insight has been gained into the reasons for the reaction.

Frequent job changes may indicate an inability to maintain a commitment to a particular avenue of employment and those with frequent job changes in the past may wisely be asked to demonstrate that they can hold down a post in their home country before being accepted for service overseas.

Those who manifest unhelpful personality traits. Those who are abnormally rigid frequently refuse to cooperate with psychological aspects of selection. Their underlying insecurity and fear fuels a need to remain in control during selection, and they often cause problems for selectors. Rigidity may also manifest with obsessive attachments, to which they may regress under stress.[83] The over-mystical may absent themselves from work to resource themselves spiritually, without regard for the work in which they are engaged, and this may cause difficulty for their colleagues.[29] Those with impulsive traits and those with frequent paranoid feelings will cause difficulty in relationships and their personality immaturity may render them unsuitable for overseas work.[29]

Those who have had recent losses including bereavement or broken love affairs should wait for 6–12 months before moving overseas.

Those in the process of major life transitions. Adults who have recently become engaged, married or who have moved into a new committed relationship should wait for 6–12 months, Children over the age of 11 are coping with the major personal change of puberty. Most children entering this life change are too stressed to cope well with a major cultural and geographical transition, unless they have previously lived overseas. For the latter, a return overseas may, in a real sense, be a return home.

Those with a past history of eating disorders. Evidence is needed that they have engaged in personal growth, and have tackled some of the problems that led to them adopting this particular form of behaviour.[83] A period of several years should have elapsed and if the disorder was either life-threatening or has recurred, then the candidate should be rejected. Anorexia may be associated with intangible personality deficits that may be hard to identify at selection but cause difficulty for colleagues overseas.[83] Anorexia may be a life threatening illness and in the author's direct experience has been the cause of urgent repatriation.

Those with a past history of self-injury.[83] When did this occur, and what was the nature of the injury? Will high stressor exposure precipitate a further episode of self-injury? A 19-year-old girl had taken an overdose of vitamin tablets at the age of 13 and the whole family was referred for family counselling. When she volunteered for work overseas the information regarding the incident in early teenage was deliberately withheld from the agency. Her mother, with whom she had an ambivalent relationship, died from breast cancer 3 months before she was due to take up her post. 2 months later in Asia she was overwhelmed with loneliness and cut her wrists. The injury was not life-threatening but she was repatriated at considerable extra expense to the agency with whom she was working.

Those with unresolved earlier problems.[83] A significant proportion of candidates for work abroad come from dysfunctional families, or have experienced childhood abuse. The degree of trauma should be explored and an assessment made of the degree of resolution that has taken place. If it is clear that the issue is still sufficiently painful for it to impinge on current functioning, and motivation for change is present, then referral to a therapist with the appropriate skill level may be arranged and a further review made before a final decision is made. Otherwise it is wise to reject the candidate, both for the candidate's sake and that of the agency.

Who to choose?

Suitable candidates are those with:

- a strong degree of self-insight and who know their own strengths and weaknesses

- insight into the way that they interact with others, and awareness of the patterns of reaction which occur in others with whom they are in relationship
- a willingness to learn, vital for cultural adaptation
- a demonstrable, adequate degree of resolution of traumatic, past problems
- a developed, reasonable degree of autonomy
- a sense of humour.

> A married, female candidate at age 27 had parents aged in their mid-50s. They had separated when she was 9 years old and divorced when she was 13. At interview, it was clear that she still coped with considerable pain over the separation, despite some counselling therapy. Of note was her lack of memory of her father before the separation had occurred, but her closeness to her mother who was a good, caring person. She retained a very strong sense of being let down by her father, and prior to her marriage she had always sought to be in very strong control with boyfriends, rejecting anyone who looked as if they were becoming serious or wanted an element of control in the relationship. Within her marriage, she was experiencing anxiety when conflict occurred and was very keen that it was resolved quickly. During the interview, she was encouraged to look for connections between her past experience and current relationship symptom, and was able to do this in a fresh way. The motivation of the candidate to engage with therapy encouraged the assessors to recommend referral for counselling and she was accepted for overseas work.

This candidate had an unsatisfactory childhood and still carried the pain of parental separation. Most people only start to develop insight, and resolve areas of pain from the past in their 30s and 40s. During their 20s they may have problems about which they have little insight, caused by positive and negative transference of relationships with parents onto present relationships.

Concluding an interview

The general positive and negative findings of the interview, and the results of any psychometric tests employed should be discussed with the candidate. All candidates should sign a form giving permission for a report to be sent and the recipient of the report should be clearly indicated. Only a minority of candidates are usually rejected outright but a larger proportion may have indicators for caution, suggesting the need for avoiding certain types of placement or delay while therapies are applied. Handled in an affirming way, an interview may enable a candidate to enhance self-insight and understanding. This new insight itself may improve the ability to cope overseas, and a sensitively handled selection process may become a stimulus to personal development.

Acknowledgements

The task of writing this chapter was not lightly undertaken but proved far more exacting and stimulating than I had anticipated. I gratefully acknowledge the patience and critical comments of my co-worker and wife, Liz Jones. Much of the experience alluded to in this chapter has been jointly gained. I am indebted to Mary Freeman and Dr Marian Ashton who first taught me the Human Social Functioning (Heimler) method and thus stimulated my interest in the psychology of travel. The research of Dr Marjory Foyle is frequently referenced in this chapter, reflecting the enormous importance of her written work and public lectures for those who care for expatriates. The paper by Dr Jarrett Richardson, psychiatrist at the Mayo Clinic is a model of comprehensive clarity and provided a backbone for the section on psychopathology in travellers. The paper by Dr Esther Schubert was a rich resource of insight into personality disorder. I thank my colleague Dr Anne Tait, consultant psychiatrist at the Western General Hospital in Edinburgh, for casting her expert psychiatric eye over the text and making helpful criticisms. Responsibility for errors and omissions remains my own. Lastly, I am grateful to Dr Cameron Lockie, who on behalf of the editors, invited me to contribute to this new British text, and for his encouragement and patience.

PRACTICE POINTS

- Speed and ease of travel means working overseas for long periods does not necessarily mean prolonged isolation from relatives and friends as previously. However, expatriates now often leave at short notice and are less prepared than their predecessors.
- Culture differences can still, even in our 'global village' be very pronounced and criticism is usually best avoided. It only leads to frustration and loss of friends!
- Differences in time concepts and thought patterns does not make people inferior only different.
- Language differences can lead to serious difficulties at times of stress or illness.
- Sometimes people think work overseas will be an escape from difficulties at home – it rarely is, and separation can lead to unresolved relationship problems which will only resurface later.
- Travel often leads to stress, anxiety and depression both for the new expatriate and also, importantly, after return home.
- Special attention must be given to accompanying children – possible illness, the proximity of good medical care and schooling are important issues. Prolonged periods overseas for the first time during teenage years can be especially stressful.

REFERENCES

1. Foyle MF, Beer MD, Watson JP. Expatriate mental health. Acta Psychiatrica Scandinavica 1998; 97: 278–283.
2. Hofstede G. Cultures and organizations, software of the mind. Maidenhead: McGraw-Hill; 1991: 4.
3. Heider K. Expatriate distress and cultural principles. Unpublished paper given at the 4th Annual Symposium on Expatriate Stress and Breakdown. London: Royal College of Physicians; 1986.
4. Burnett D. Clash of worlds. Crowborough: Monarch Publications; 1990: 12–13.
5. Hofstede G. Cultures and organizations, software of the mind. Maidenhead: McGraw-Hill; 1991: 23–138.
6. Hofstede G. Cultures and organizations, software of the mind. Maidenhead: McGraw-Hill; 1991: 164 et seq.

7. Storti C. The art of crossing cultures. Yarmouth: Intercultural Press; 1990.
8. Oberg K. Cultural shock: adjustment to new cultural environments. Practical Anthropology 1960; 7: 177–182.
9. Adler PS. The transitional experience, an alternative view of culture shock. Journal of Humanistic Psychology 1975; 15: 13–23.
10. Hiebert P. Anthropological insights for missionaries. Grand Rapids: Baker Book House; 1985: 74–77.
11. Turner SW. Post traumatic stress disorder. Hospital Update 1991; August: 644–648.
12. Hopson B, Adams J. Towards an understanding of transition, defining some boundaries of transition dynamics. Adams J, Hayes J, Hopson B, eds. In: Transition – Understanding and managing personal change. London: Martin Robertson; 1976: 3–25.
13. Huntingdon J. Migration as bereavement. Unpublished paper at 2nd Annual Symposium on Expatriate Stress and Breakdown. London; Royal College of Physicians; 1984.
14. Bowlby J. Attachment and loss, vol 3. Harmondsworth: Penguin; 1984: 7–22.
15. Parkes CM. Bereavement: Studies of grief in adult life. London: Tavistock; 1972: 208–211.
16. Furnham A, Bochner S. Culture shock – Psychological reaction unfamiliar environments. London: Methuen; 1986: 161–176.
17. Munoz L. Exile as bereavement: socio-psychological manifestations of Chilean exiles in Great Britain. British Journal of Medical Psychology 1980; 53: 227–232.
18. Schellner DP. The immigrant's challenge: mourning the loss of the home and adapting to the New World. Smith College Studies in Social Work; 1981: Spring.
19. Freid M. Grieving for a lost home. In Duhl LJ, ed. The environment of the metropolis. New York: Basic Books; 1962.
20. Harrison G. Migration and mental disorder. Medicine International 1991; 9: 3978–3980.
21. Dye TW. Stress producing factors in cultural adjustment. Missiology: an International Review 1974; 11: 61–77.
22. Berger M. A Japanese psychiatrist's answer to executive stress. International Management 1987; March: 49–50.
23. Hiebert P. Anthropological insights for missionaries. Grand Rapids: Baker Book House; 1985: 65.
24. Useem R, Downie R. Third culture kids. Todays Education 1976; 65: 103–105.
25. Pollock DC. Being a third culture kid: a profile. In: Echerd P, Arathorn A, eds. Understanding and nurturing the missionary family. Pasadena, California: William Carey Library; 1989: 241–252.
26. Haan N. Changes in young adults after Peace Corps experiences: political–social views, moral reasoning, and perceptions of self and parents. Journal of Youth and Adolescence 1974; 3: 177–194.
27. Huxley A, quoted in Storti C. The art of crossing cultures. Yarmouth: Intercultural Press; 1990: 105.
28. Hiebert P. Anthropological insights for missionaries. Grand Rapids: Baker Book House; 1985: 137.
29. Foyle M. Missionary stress. Voluntary Agency Medical Advisors Newsletter, published by Care for Mission, Carberry, Musselburgh, UK, 1991; June: 2–14.
30. De Haan BB. Stress and psychological issues in humanitarian activities: the experience of the International Committee of the Red Cross. Paper presented at Fifth International Conference on Travel Medicine, Geneva. Program and abstracts, No 110. Atlanta: International Society of Travel Medicine; 1997: 126.
31. Moorhead T. The missionary family. The Christian family in Japan. Major papers from the 22nd Hayama Men's Missionary Seminars, Anogi Sanso, Japan; 1981.
32. Gish D. Sources of missionary stress. Journal of Psychology and Theology 1983; 1: 236–242.
33. Jones ES, Jones ME. The Hiemler scale in the routine debrief of expatriate missionaries. Paper presented at Fifth International Conference on Travel Medicine, Geneva. Program and abstracts, No 34. Atlanta: International Society of Travel Medicine; 1997: 89.
34. College G. Single women in mission. Monograph, published by Evangelical Missionary Alliance, Whitefield House, 186 Kennington Park Road, London; 1985.
35. Richardson J. Psychopathology in missionary personnel. In: K O'Donell, ed. Missionary Care, Pasadena, California: William Carey Library; 1992: 89–109.
36. Mikulicz U. Screening for physical and psychological fitness of persons going to the tropics for a prolonged period. In: Lobel HO, Steffen R, Kozarsky PE, eds. Travel medicine 2. Proceedings of the Second Conference on International Travel Medicine, Atlanta, USA, Atlanta: International Society of Travel Medicine; 1992: 22–24.
37. Hynes NA, Gootnick D. Health related events and risks among Peace Corps volunteers. Paper presented at Fifth International Conference on Travel Medicine, Geneva. Program and abstracts, No 109. Atlanta: International Society of Travel Medicine; 1997: 126.
38. Price G. Discussion on the cause of invaliding from the tropics. British Medical Journal 1913; 2: 1290–1297.
39. Peppiatt R, Byass P. A survey of the health of British missionaries. British Journal of General Practice 1991; 41: 159–162.
40. Parshall P. How spiritual are missionaries? Evangelical Missions Quarterly 1987; 23: 8–19.
41. Rottanberg D, Robins AH, Ben Arie O, et al. Cannabis – associated psychosis with hypomanic features. Lancet 1982; ii: 1363–1366.
42. Carney MWP, Bacelle L, Robinson B. Psychosis after cannabis use. British Medical Journal 1984; 288: 1047.
43. Andreasson S, Allebeck P, Engstorm A et al. Cannabis and schizophrenia, a longitudinal study of Swedish conscripts. Lancet 1987; ii: 1483–1485.

44. Editorial. Short term memory impairment in chronic cannabis users. Lancet 1989; ii: 1254–1255.

45. Lishman WA. Specific conditions giving rise to mental disorder. In: Weatherall DJ, Ledingham JGG, Warrell DA, eds. Oxford textbook of medicine. 3rd ed. Oxford: Oxford University Press; 1996: 4236–4243.

46. Warrell DA. Clinical features of malaria. In: Gilles HM, Warrell DA, eds. Bruce-Chwatt's essential malariology. London: Edward Arnold; 1993; 38.

47. Miller SI, Hohmann El, Pegues DA, Salmonella (including *Salmonella typhi*). In: Mandell GL, Bennett JE, Dolin R, eds. Principles and practice of infectious diseases. New York: Churchill Livingstone; 1995: 2013–2033.

48. Smith DH. Human African trypanosomiasis. In : Weatherall DJ, Ledingham JGG, Warrell DA, eds. Oxford: Oxford textbook of medicine 3rd edn. Oxford: Oxford University Press; 1996: 888–894.

49. Warrell DA, Kennedy PGE. Viral infections of the central nervous system. In: Weatherall DJ, Ledingham, JGG, Warrell DA, eds. Oxford textbook of medicine. 3rd ed. Oxford: Oxford University Press; 1996: 4064–4075.

50. Steffen R, Fuchs E, Schildknecht J, et al. Mefloquine compared with other malaria chemoprophylactic regimens in tourists visiting East Africa. Lancet 1993; 341: 1299–1303.

51. Barrett PJ, Emmins PD, Clarke PD, et al. Comparison of adverse events associated with use of mefloquine and combination of chloroquine and proguanil as anti-malarial prophylaxis: postal and telephone survey of travellers. British Medical Journal 1996; 313: 525–528.

52. Croft AMJ, World MJ. Neuropsychiatric reactions with mefloquine chemoprophylaxis. Lancet 1996; 347: 326.

53. Weinke T, Trautmann M, Held T, et al. Neuropsychiatric side effects after the use of mefloquine. American Journal of Tropical Medicine and Hygiene 1991; 45: 86–91.

54. Dally P. Psychiatric illness in expatriates. Journal of the Royal College of Physicians of London 1985; 19: 103–104.

55. Foyle MF. Honourable wounded. Tunbridge Wells: Monarch; 1987.

56. Frame JD, Lange WR, Frankenfield DL. Mortality trends in USA missionaries in Africa 1945–85. American Journal of Tropical Medicine and Hygiene 1992; 46: 686–689.

57. Smith G, Byass P. Unintentional injuries in developing countries: the epidemiology of a neglected problem. Epidemiologic Reviews 1991; 13: 228–266.

58. American Psychiatric Association. Diagnostic and statistical manual. IVth ed., Washington DC: American Psychiatric Association; 1994: 424–429.

59. Turner S. Post traumatic stress disorder. Hospital Update; 1991; August: 644–647.

60. March JS. What constitutes a stressor? The 'criterion A issue'. In: Davidson JRT, Foa ED, eds. Post-traumatic stress disorder: DSM-IV and beyond. Washington DC: American Psychiatric Association, 1993.

61. Dunning C. Intervention strategies for emergency workers. In: Lystad M, ed. Mental health response to mass emergencies. New York: Brunner/Mazel; 1988: 284–307.

62. Raphael B, Meldrum L, McFarlane AC. Does debriefing after psychological trauma work? British Medical Journal 1995; 310: 1479–1480.

63. Lovell DM. Chronic fatigue syndrome amongst overseas development workers. Journal of Travel Medicine 1999; 6: 16–23

64. Jones ME. Understanding and managing chronic fatigue syndrome in missionaries. In: Jones ME, Jones ES, eds. Caring for the missionary into the 21st century. Care for Mission, Carberry, Musselburgh, UK; 1996: 36–43.

65. World Health Organization. The ICD-10 classification of mental and behavioural disorders. Clinical descriptions and diagnostic guidelines. Geneva: WHO; 1992: 198–224.

66. Marlowe M, Sugarman P. Disorders of personality. British Medical Journal 1997; 315: 176–179.

67. Schubert E. Personality disorders and the selection process for overseas missionaries. International Bulletin for Missionary Research 1991; 15: 33–36.

68. Groves JE. Borderline personality disorder. New England Journal of Medicine 1981; 305: 259–262.

69. Stewart C. Home may not be so sweet. Middle East Expatriate; 1986: November: 2–3.

70. Austin C. Cross culture re-entry – An annotated bibliography. Abilene, Texas: Abilene Christian University Press; 1983.

71. Austin C. Re-entry stress: the pain of coming home. Evangelical Missions Quarterly 1983; October: 278–287.

72. Moore L, Jones BV, Austin CN. Predictors of reverse culture shock among North American Church of Christ missionaries. Journal of Psychology and Theology 1987; 15: 336–341.

73. White FJ. Some reflections on the separation phenomenon idiosyncratic to the experience of missionaries and their children. Journal of Psychology and Theology 1983; 11: 181–188.

74. Foyle MF. How to choose the right missionary. In: O'Donnell KJ, O'Donnell ML, eds. Helping missionaries grow – readings in mental health and missions. Pasadena, California: William Carey Library; 1998: 26–34.

75. Cureton CB. Missionary fit: criterion related model. Journal of Psychology and Theology 1983; 11: 196–202.

76. Britt WG. Pretraining variables in the prediction of missionary success overseas. Journal of Psychology and Theology 1983; 11: 203–212.

77. Schubert E. Personality disorders and the selection process for overseas missionaries. International Bulletin for Missionary Research 1991; 15: 33–36.

78. Jones ES, Jones ME. Strangers and exiles II. Carer and Counsellor 1994; 4: 32–37.

79. Chalmers S. Selection procedures for overseas mission. BA (Hons) thesis, Glasgow University; 1994.

80. Mullen PE, Romans-Clarkson SE, Walton VA, et al. Impact of sexual and physical abuse on women's mental health. Lancet 1988; i: 842–845.

81. Worden JW. Grief counselling and grief therapy. London: Tavistock Routledge; 1991.

82. Lovell DM. Psychological adjustment among returned overseas aid workers. Unpublished D. Clin. Psy. Thesis, University of Wales, Bangor; 1997.

83. Fowke R. Difficult personnel – selection, placement and understanding. In: Jones ME, ed. Caring for the missionary into the 21st century. Papers presented at a 1993 seminar. Care for Mission, Carberry, Musselburgh, UK; 1993: 11–25.

84. Briggs Myers I. Introduction to type. Revised by Kirby LK, Myers KD. Oxford: Oxford Psychologists Press; 1998.

85. Hathaway SR, McKinley JC. A multiphasic personality schedule (Minnesota): I. Construction of the schedule. Journal of Psychology 1940; 10: 249–254.

86. Popham SM, Holden RR. Psychometric properties of the MMPI factor scales. Personality and Individual Differences 1991; 12: 513–517.

87. Costa PT, McCrae RR. NEO PI-R professional manual. Florida: psychological Assessment Resources; 1991.

88. Costa PT, McCrae RR. Personality disorders and the five factor model of personality. Journal of Personality Disorders 1990; 4: 362–371.

89. Gordon LV. Gordon personal profile-inventory, GPP-I, manual. 1993 revision. San Antonio: The Psychological Corporation; 1993.

90. Heimler E. Survival in society. London: Weidenfield and Nicolson; 1975: 15–26.

91. Regis S. What is human social functioning (HSF)? Counselling 1993; August: 193–197.

Women and child travellers

Marlene Simpson

Women's issues and travelling when pregnant

Synopsis

Contrary to popular opinion, world travel and exploration have never been the sole prerogative of man. Intrepid women travellers have long since journeyed independently to the far corners of the earth. Admittedly, until the second half of the 20th century, the 'ease' with which they travelled would have dissuaded all but the most committed 'adventurers'. It is difficult to imagine how these women overcame the social, moral and religious objections that modern women do not face.

However, today's women still share the same age-old problems arising from their physiology and gender. When preparing for a foreign trip many women approach their family doctors or travel clinics for advice regarding immunisations, malaria prophylaxis and general health precautions relating to food and water hygiene. Women may travel accompanied on package tours or, for example on organised business trips unconcerned for their personal safety or health. However, for some the allure of a simple or more adventurous holiday brings its own set of health problems and for the female traveller the added worry of menstruation, contraception, pregnancy and personal safety.

Introduction

An informed travel adviser should be able to give advice on the following issues:

- menstruation
- personal hygiene
- fluid retention
- contraception
- personal safety and security.

Women, who plan either a long trip abroad or to reside in a country where good medical facilities may not be easily accessible, are well advised to have a gynaecological check-up preferably 6 weeks before departure. Those with previous gynaecological problems should have a clear understanding of their medical history and should carry a written note of any problems.[1]

Menstruation

Travel can disturb the normal menstrual cycle. Emotional upset, exhaustion and travelling through different time zones can all contribute to an upset in the menstrual pattern. Periods may become irregular or cease altogether. Irregular menstruation is a very common problem affecting women travellers; excessive exercise and the stress of travel may cause infrequent periods. If this is the case, it may lead to confusion over the timing of oral contraception and great anxiety of unplanned pregnancy. Dysmenorrhoea may also be aggravated by travel, so taking supplies of tried and trusted analgesics would have obvious benefits.

ORAL CONTRACEPTION CAN SUPPRESS MENSTRUATION

Women who prefer not to have periods while travelling may suppress ovulation and inhibit menstruation by taking the oral contraceptive pill. This is achieved by taking the pill continuously, without the usual 7-day break in between packets. A reminder to carry extra packets to allow for this should be stressed. However, this method is not advisable for women taking biphasic or triphasic pills because the dose in the first seven pills is too low to prevent possible breakthrough bleeding. Triphasic brands are probably best avoided for long journeys which cross time zones, since the margin of error is less with this type.[2]

SANITARY HYGIENE

Feminine hygiene for the 'normal', 2-week, package holiday tourist should not pose too big a problem. A packet of tampons or sanitary towels thrown in a suitcase at the last minute or a quick visit to the local chemist or supermarket, while on holiday will usually cover all needs. Although women throughout the world menstruate, not all take the same approach to feminine hygiene.

Tampons and sanitary towels are unobtainable in parts of Africa, Asia and South America, and they are scarce luxuries in many of the former eastern block countries. In developing countries, locally made menstrual supplies are usually available although the standard varies. For example, in poor countries such as Bangladesh, local sanitary towels can look and feel more like a mattress than the kind of slim-line product with which most women in the UK are familiar. However, in many of the under-developed countries, the only facilities available locally could be handfuls of leaves or 're-useable' cloths or towels tied on with string! So if the traveller to a remote area is not sufficiently adventurous as to experiment with these methods taking an adequate supply of her own personal choice of feminine hygiene products is advisable. However, this may not always be practicable when space and weight for carrying luxuries are limited.

Within the country they are travelling women should be sensitive to the cultural and religious attitudes towards menstruation. In some countries, it is forbidden to enter places of worship while menstruating and some cultures will not allow women to touch or even walk near food! To avoid such situations discreet use of and disposal of sanitary towels and tampons would be advisable.

Personal hygiene

Personal hygiene and comfort can cause considerable upset and embarrassment to women when travelling. During prolonged journeys on trains, buses and planes, the female bladder can be under considerable stress owing to the lack or infrequency of 'comfort stops'. The absence or inadequacy of toilet facilities, a common

phenomenon in world travel, can add to female difficulties. In some situations, the lack of privacy when attending to body functions may lead to feelings of embarrassment, anxiety and vulnerability.[3] Western women are often physically and mentally unprepared to squat over a hole in the floor or behind a bush. All travellers should follow this sound advice: 'If you must squat, then squat high'[3] to avoid bites when baring the nether regions in an inhospitable environment!

The temptation not to drink 'too much' can cause problems with dehydration. Women should be encouraged to drink small amounts frequently and to avoid alcohol.

For the remote traveller, perhaps on an expedition, where safe water is rationed for drinking and scarce for toilet and washing facilities, the risk of associated infections can be high. Lack of skin cleansing, sweating and inappropriate clothing can encourage chaffing, open sores and monilial infections in women.

Unfortunately, lower urinary tract and vaginal infections are also commonplace, necessitating the need for antibiotic therapy. Many women indulge in sports activities on holiday and can be exposed to hazards which do not affect men, for example water skiing where the risk of foreign body penetration of the vagina and the inrush of contaminated water can result in ascending vaginal infections. It may be prudent for travellers to take a supply of antibiotics and treatment for monilial infections, particularly if they have suffered in the past.

Fluid retention

Unfortunately, enforced inactivity and prolonged sitting during long journeys encourages swelling of the feet and legs (postural oedema). In older women with poor venous circulation peripheral oedema is common.

If fluid retention is a recurrent problem, then the use of a simple diuretic may be appropriate. Exercise where possible; walkabouts help prevent this problem and, more importantly, the risk of deep vein thrombosis from stagnation of blood flow. If walkabouts are infrequent or not practicable, then it is possible to exercise when sitting. Rotating ankles, twiddling toes and flexing the muscles in arms and legs all aid general circulation.

While travelling, women should be advised to dress for comfort rather than as a fashion statement. Loose fitting skirts or trousers allow for 'waist expansion' and comfortable shoes will prevent the sight of women struggling to replace tight footwear at the end of long journeys.

Contraception

Away from everyday stresses and routines, and far from the influence of anyone who might disapprove, holidays and travel bring relaxation of inhibitions and a time of increased sexual activity both for couples and those travelling alone.[1] The woman traveller heading for fun in the sun without due thought to contraceptive protection could bring home an unplanned pregnancy as a souvenir. Whether travelling alone or with a sexual partner, sex on holiday needs to be organised just like travel arrangements. While in some ways it is perhaps best to remain with familiar, well-tried methods, this may not be appropriate.

Women travelling or living for prolonged periods abroad should be advised to find out what contraceptive services are available to them in the areas they are visiting. The International Planned Parenthood Federation[4] (IPPF) and the Family Planning Association of Britain[5] can provide information on this.

If a woman is sexually active and happy with her chosen method of contraception, she should be encouraged to visit her own doctor or family planning clinic for a routine cervical smear test if due and to obtain any contraceptive supplies required. It would also be advisable to take this opportunity to confirm that the method she is using is appropriate for the length and nature of her trip. Travelling may reduce the efficacy of certain contraceptive methods which are normally perfectly adequate at home. If a method of contraception is being changed or used for the first time, it would be sensible to allow at least two or three menstrual cycles to occur, prior to travel, to enable any side effects or problems to be dealt with.

Discussed below are various methods of contraception available to the woman traveller but, as with vaccine recommendations, the advice should be tailored to the individual.

COMBINED ORAL CONTRACEPTIVE PILL

The combined oral contraceptive pill (hereafter referred to as the pill) is a very popular and familiar method of contraception. When used correctly, its reliability is 99–100%.[1] However, for the woman traveller she should be made aware of situations which could alter the efficacy of the pill.

- Stomach upsets and severe diarrhoea reduce absorption of the pill and may leave inadequate protection. If vomiting occurs within 3 hours of taking the pill, a barrier method should be used as well as using the pill to protect during intercourse, throughout the stomach upset and for 7 days after it has ended – 'the 7 day rule'.[2]
- In the case of combined oral contraceptives, some broad-spectrum antibiotics, for example doxycycline, may reduce their efficacy by impairing the bacterial flora responsible for recycling of the ethinyloestradiol from the large bowel. The Family Planning Association advice is that additional contraceptive precautions should be taken while on a short course of broad-spectrum antibiotics and for 7 days after stopping. If this runs beyond the end of a packet, the next packet should be started without a break. In the case of ED (every day) tablets, the inactive ones should be omitted.[6]
- For courses of doxycycline longer than 2 weeks, resistance to the interference develops.[7] This means that additional contraceptive precautions should be taken for 3 weeks only. If this runs beyond the end of a packet, the next packet should be started without a break. In the case of ED tablets, the inactive ones should be omitted.
- The oral contraceptive pill does not interact with chloroquine, proguanil or mefloquine, but they may cause gastrointestinal upset which could reduce efficacy.
- Women on the pill should be advised that if their 7 'pill-free days' coincide with the '7-day rule', then they should *not* take a break of 7 days but carry on with another packet of pills.

As a consequence, they may only experience slight spotting or no withdrawal bleed.

- Another situation when a woman might not have a 7 day break between packets is when she 'tricycles'. This is a means of chemically postponing menstruation by taking the pill continuously. This method might find favour with the remote traveller who wishes not to have a period while travelling. If this method is chosen, then extra packets of pills should be carried to allow for this.
- Travel can interfere with periods – no more so than on long journeys which cross time zones. For women on the oral contraceptive pill this can cause confusion and the possibility of inadequate protection. The following advice should be given:
  — If time zones are crossed, make sure that the pill is taken every 24 hours, continuing to do so every day at the same time.
  — This might mean waking up in the middle of the night to take the pill – and take it *earlier*, before going to sleep rather than later.
  — No more than 24 hours should elapse between doses in order to maintain full protection and prevent breakthrough bleeding.
- The advice given to women if they run out of or lose their pills is to keep an empty packet to enable a doctor or pharmacist to identify a particular pill from its generic and not the brand name. Brand names of the same variety of pill can differ from country to country. The IPPF[4] have branches worldwide and can help if there is a difficulty obtaining supplies.
- Splitting supplies of any medicines between hand luggage and suitcases/backpacks would be a sensible precaution in the event of theft or mislaid luggage.

PROGESTOGEN-ONLY PILL (POP)

For women taking the progestogen-only pill the same rules apply as with the combined pill. It is slightly less effective, 96–98%, and *must* be taken at the *same* time each day, that is, every 24 hours to remain effective – this could pose problems when crossing time zones. However, it does have the advantage of *not* being affected by antibiotics.

BARRIER METHODS

Condoms

As a method of contraception, the male condom is approximately 95% effective when used correctly and is an absolute must to help protect against sexually transmitted diseases (STD), including HIV. It is particularly useful for women travelling alone and is a good method of protection for the chance sexual encounter. It is also a reliable alternative in the event of problems arising with the pill or expulsion of an intrauterine contraceptive device (IUCD).

The female condom, when used correctly, offers women the opportunity of ensuring their own mechanical protection from potential sexually transmitted diseases and as a means of contraception.[3]

Points to remember if using condoms:

- Reliable condoms are often hard to find in the poorer parts of the world. To ask for them can be very embarrassing for the female traveller, particularly if there is a language and cultural barrier. To avoid this, an adequate supply should be carried with them.
- If the condoms carry the British kite mark or the new European CE mark on the packet, it means that they have been tested to a strict safety standard.
- Ensure that the sell-by-date has not expired and the packaging is not damaged. Rubber perishes with age, and heat, and should be discarded if it displays any signs of being brittle, sticky or discoloured.

Diaphragm and cervical cap

The cervical cap, which covers the cervix, and the diaphragm, which covers the cervix and front wall of the vagina, are as useful as the female or male condoms. However, they *must* be used with a spermicide. Both devices require to be prescribed and fitted by a doctor or family planning nurse and the woman taught how to use them correctly. They should also know how to clean their devices and check for tears or perforations. A diaphragm or cap lasts approximately 6 months to 1 year; it may be advisable for those on long trips to take a spare device in case one is lost or becomes unsafe. As each method comes in a range of sizes, women should be advised to keep a note of the manufacturer and size of their own device, which will help if they have to seek a replacement while abroad. IPPF[4] will give addresses of local family planning clinics worldwide.

Points to remember if using diaphragms or caps:

- They should be stored in a cool, dry place in an airtight container as severe heat can perish rubber.
- Spermicides may loose their efficacy if not stored in cool, dry containers. Creams may melt and be difficult to apply and pessaries, which are designed to melt at body temperature, may become impossible to use. Pessaries wrapped individually in silver foil travel best.

Injectable methods of contraception (Depo-Provera and Noristerat)

This method of contraception is very effective and has several advantages over other chemical methods. Depo-Provera is given by deep *intramuscular* injection into the gluteal or deltoid muscle and is effective for *12 weeks*. Noristerat *must* always be injected deep into the gluteal muscle and particular care taken with administration; it is effective for *8 weeks*.[6] Where possible, women using this method for the first time, who are planning to travel, should allow time for two injections as side effects are common with the first injection. The most common side effects are irregular and, occasionally, heavy bleeding. With subsequent injections, periods may stop altogether which is how the injection should work.

Travel advantages of injectable contraception:

- it is not affected by time zones
- it is not affected by gastrointestinal upsets
- it is not affected by antibiotics,
- chemical induced amenorrhoea makes it an attractive method for those wishing to avoid regular periods and the associated personal and feminine hygiene problems.

Intrauterine contraceptive device

For women travellers who already have an IUCD, they should be advised to have it checked before going abroad. The make of the device used will determine when it requires to be replaced; this can range from 3 to 8 years. If the IUCD is being used for the first time, then it should be inserted well in advance, that is, 2–3 cycles before departure to enable any side effects to be dealt with. Most common side effects are heavy, painful periods. Heavy bleeding can cause feelings of lethargy and have obvious drawbacks with personal and feminine hygiene when travelling.

Advantages of IUCD:

- unaffected by gastrointestinal upset
- unaffected by time zones.

Disadvantages of IUCD:

- can be expelled by the uterus, particularly after a period – women should know how and be advised to check that the threads can still be felt
- if IUCD is expelled, contraceptive protection ceases immediately and another method should be used
- problems associated with heavy menstruation.

Emergency or postcoital contraceptive (PCC)

Emergency or postcoital contraception and advice can be obtained from family planning clinics[5] and general practitioners throughout the UK. When travelling abroad, access to the 'World list of family planning addresses' available from IPPF[4] will give advice on what services are available to the female traveller and how to obtain them.

Personal safety and security

As adults we assume that we know the dangers of our environment; when travelling abroad, we move outside our usual environment and are often ignorant of prevailing conditions.[1] Raising awareness, particularly with women travelling alone, to the possibility of personal danger and how to avoid it is advisable.

ADVICE TO BE GIVEN ON SAFETY AND SECURITY

- When travelling, particularly alone, leave an itinerary of your trip with a responsible person and make contact at pre-arranged times and dates.

- Avoid ostentatious displays of money, jewellery, luggage and dress which can encourage the wrong type of attention.
- When travelling, ' be aware' of where your luggage and belongings, particularly hand bags, are at all times. Do not leave them unattended or hanging on the back of chairs in restaurants. Instead, slip a strap from the hand luggage under a chair leg as this will inconspicuously ensure that it cannot be grabbed.[8]
- Choose your accommodation carefully:
  — try to pick accommodation which is in a safe area, that is, not in the middle of the local, 'red light' district[9]
  — request a room near the lift or stair well
  — not on the ground floor
  — inspect the door locks and window fasteners
  — never open the door to your room until you have identified the caller
  — do not identify yourself on the telephone until the caller has done so
  — keep your money and valuables close by you at night.
- Be alert, listen to the advice of locals and fellow travellers, develop a street sense, try not to be in the wrong place at the wrong time.
- In a confrontational situation, a woman traveller is rarely a physical match for a man. However, the following rules can help:
  — Do not turn a scary situation into a dangerous one if you can help it (e.g. it would be unwise to launch into a physical attack if the man confronting you is just after your money – hand it over and avoid finding out what he may do if provoked).
  — Do not panic or show fear. Do not allow the person confronting you to get the upper hand; try to gain psychological advantage by throwing him off his balance (i.e. compliance).
  — If you do find yourself in physical danger try to anticipate the aggressor's next move and plan ahead for it. As the innocent party in the confrontation, you have the advantage of surprise. If you are forced to strike back physically, make sure it is a crippling blow that gives you a chance to escape.[9]

- If you are worried about your ability to gauge dangerous situations and to defend yourself, then consider joining a women's self-defence course before travelling.

PERSONAL SAFETY WHEN TRAVELLING ALONE

- Insist on inspecting your accommodation before agreeing to stay. If unhappy with the room, request a change or where possible move to different accommodation.
- The lone woman traveller will often be flouting convention simply by her presence. Unfortunately women in the developing world do not have the independence that their western counterparts take for granted. For this reason, their presence, especially unaccompanied, will generate interest within local people of both genders. Male-dominated Muslim countries such as the Middle East, North Africa, Pakistan and parts of India and South America are frequently seen as difficult places for women to visit and travel through.
- Before travelling, find out about the cultural do's and don'ts of the country you are visiting. This will enable you to respect local customs and conventions. For lone women travellers in particular, blending into the background is not only a pre-requisite to understanding and observing a different culture, it also keeps you out of trouble. 'The art of travelling is learning to behave like a chameleon.'[9]
- How you dress is an easy method of self-preservation and the most immediate symbol of respect. Dress codes differ greatly from country to country and to get them wrong would put you at an immediate disadvantage. A culture's standard of dress has a lot to do with what parts of the body are considered to be sensuous or provocative.
- As a general rule, tight and skimpy clothes are inappropriate for most countries outside of Europe and North America.
- Clothing should be conservative and presentable, loose fitting and comfortable. Arms and legs should be covered, especially when visiting places of worship and national monuments. Throughout the Arab world and in

other Muslim countries, hair should be covered by a head scarf.

- When travelling, try to be inconspicuous yet confident, avoiding confrontational challenging situations with men by adopting an assertive, dismissive manner.
- Remember eye contact can be seen as a 'come-on' by many men. The use of dark sunglasses will limit this problem.
- Be prepared to answer questions about yourself, particularly if you are single and travelling alone. The often-asked questions of your marital status and family are ones of genuine interest. To avoid the unwanted attentions of some men, the use of a few white lies about 'your husband' and a fake wedding ring are a useful pretence.

Older women travellers

With the overall ageing of European populations, and earlier retirement, more and more elderly people including women are travelling.[10]

The retired can travel when and as far as they choose. They have the time and, with careful budgeting, the money to indulge in foreign travels. There are now a number of travel companies that provide holidays specifically for older travellers. Most offer packages but there is an increasing demand for holidays that combine the advantages of package deals (easy travel arrangements and the support of large organisations) with independence upon reaching their destination.[9] When giving travel advice to this group of people, an adviser should include the following specific points:

- If suffering from a medical condition, choose a destination that easily meets both physical and mental needs.
- Purchase adequate insurance which covers all eventualities, including the cost of repatriation.
- It is a sensible precaution to have a medical check-up before travelling.
- Ensure an adequate supply of prescribed medication is taken and ask your general practitioner for notification of any significant conditions you may suffer from.
- Dress for comfort and exercise legs on long journeys.

- Pay particular attention to food and water hygiene, and high fluid intake should be encouraged.
- Avoidance of insect bites should be stressed – as older skin takes longer to heal, bites and puncture wounds are potentially more serious.
- Ageing skin can suffer seriously from exposure to the sun which can result in possible malignant changes in the skin. The use of sun screens, hats and loose, long-sleeved clothing should be advised.
- A realistic approach to rest and relaxation should be encouraged. If travelling long journeys, which involve crossing time zones, rest for at least 24 hours on arrival at destination.

If older travellers recognise their limitations and are realistic about their expectations, it is possible to make travel in retirement safe and exhilarating.[9]

Summary

20th century women, of all ages, will not be deterred from travelling to the most remote parts of our planet, plunging to the ocean depths or scaling the highest peaks. Travel advisers can play an important role by giving specific pre-travel counselling that will aid preparation.

The pregnant traveller

'To travel or not to travel that is the question....'

No woman can be realistically assured that her pregnancy will be trouble-free and for this traveller the implications of health problems arising from her pregnancy should be considered. Large numbers of women *do* travel in pregnancy and in recent years travel to countries with poor medical care has become increasingly accessible to the adventurous traveller. The pregnant traveller is more at risk from widely varying standards of medical care and its availability in different countries than the direct effects of travel on pregnancy.[1] However, if travel is planned during pregnancy, there are a number of health issues requiring discussion, the outcome of which should help the woman make an informed decision as to whether her travel plans are adequate and/or prudent.

When a pregnant women is trying to decide whether or not she should travel abroad, she should consider the following:

- It is important in early pregnancy to establish antenatal care and arrange routine blood tests and ultrasound scans. It may be necessary to postpone trips so that blood tests to screen for spina bifida can be carried out at 16–18 weeks. For older women, the possibility of screening for Down's syndrome is carried out at about 16 weeks. During the first 24 weeks, it is common to have an ultrasound examination to confirm the age of the fetus and also to detect abnormalities that might have arisen during the development of fetal organs.
- Unfortunately during the early weeks of pregnancy, the tendency to nausea and vomiting is likely to be aggravated by travel. If vomiting is severe during travel, it may be necessary to use antihistamine or phenothiazine preparations under medical supervision,[6] although they do have some unwanted side effects such as drowsiness, dry mouth and blurred vision.
- Early pregnancy is also a time when miscarriage is more common. Travel itself does not increase the risk of miscarriage. However, the consequences of a miscarriage in a country where medical facilities are poor could be serious.[9] Severe haemorrhage following miscarriage might necessitate the need for a blood transfusion. In many of the poorer countries, the risk of AIDS and hepatitis B from unscreened blood transfusions is high. Facilities for surgery with sterile medical instruments may be difficult to obtain and postoperative drug treatment requiring antibiotics and analgesia non-existent.
- Ectopic pregnancies are usually evident during the first trimester and have the potential to be life threatening. They require surgical intervention: at the least, ospherectomy/ salpingectomy and at the worst hysterectomy. The consequences of this occurring in a

country where medical facilities are poor could be fatal.
- Towards the later stages of pregnancy, premature labour becomes a risk. If labour starts early, but at a time when the resulting baby could live, then the future of the baby would depend on the availability of expert care.[1] Survival of a premature baby depends on immediate access to sophisticated, neonatal, intensive care facilities, and the greater the prematurity, the more important this becomes. Without such care, the risk of a mentally or physically handicapped child is high, if indeed the baby survives.

Vaccines and pregnancy

All vaccines should be avoided as far as possible in pregnancy because of the theoretical risk of damage to the developing fetus. Live virus vaccines especially should be *avoided* and these include oral poliomyelitis, oral typhoid, yellow fever, mumps, measles and rubella, and BCG.

The inactivated or killed vaccines should be used *advisedly* and only when the threat of the disease outweighs any risk from the vaccine, for example, typhoid and diphtheria vaccines can cause a fever-like illness as a side effect which, if severe, may lead to miscarriage. However if, for example, the pregnant traveller was planning to travel to the former Soviet Union where the number of cases of diphtheria has increased greatly in recent years, as a result of low immunisation rates in children, immunisation with diphtheria vaccine may be considered a necessary risk.[11]

During pregnancy, protection against tetanus may be given and if polio is required it can be administered subcutaneously in the form of inactivated poliomyelitis vaccine.

For the pregnant traveller, protection against hepatitis A is recommended for areas of moderate or high hepatitis A virus endemicity, particularly if sanitation and food hygiene are likely to be poor.[12] This protection can be given in the form of human normal immunoglobulin (HNIG). If a yellow fever vaccination certificate is necessary as an entry requirement to a country, then a letter of exemption from a medical practitioner should be obtained. However, if a pregnant woman must travel to a high risk area, she should be immunised since the risk of yellow fever outweighs that of immunisation.[12]

Malaria and pregnancy

- Chloroquine and proguanil are the two safest antimalarial drugs to use during pregnancy. However, drug-resistant malaria continues to spread; large areas of Africa and South America are resistant to chloroquine and the antimalarial drug mefloquine is used. This is a relatively new drug and accordingly, there is insufficient clinical experience, in humans, available to assess possible damaging effects during pregnancy. However, mefloquine is teratogenic when administered to rats and mice in early gestation. In this respect, mefloquine should only be used in pregnancy if there are compelling medical reasons and travel to a highly malarious, chloroquine-resistant area unavoidable – preferably after the first trimester.[13] If proguanil is used, a folate supplement should be taken.
- The problem with malaria in pregnancy, particularly in women visiting malarious areas as compared with local inhabitants, is that malaria attacks tend to be considerably more severe.[9] Malaria increases the chance of fetal malformation and some prophylactic regimes may in themselves be a threat to the developing fetus. There is an increased likelihood of a high rate of abortion, danger of intrauterine retardation and a higher incidence of premature birth. The measures to avoid insect bites (see Ch. 14) must be strictly adhered to. Travel to a highly malarious area during pregnancy should, where at all possible, be postponed.

General advice

Advice given to any traveller, on how to avoid tropical and infectious diseases is doubly important for the pregnant traveller. Any disease that causes dehydration, high fever and requires treatment with any drug therapy can put the fetus at considerable risk. How to avoid insect bites and to be aware of food and water hygiene measures should be reinforced (see 5, Ch. 11).

Large numbers of women do indulge in foreign travel during pregnancy. Experts consider that the most suitable time for travel, provided that there have been no complications or other problems during the first trimester, is after the majority of antenatal tests have been completed and the main risks of miscarriage are over, but before the fetus becomes viable and would need neonatal intensive care facilities if born between the 18th and 24th week of pregnancy.[9] However, travel to high risk countries should definitely be avoided, when possible, throughout the pregnancy.

Insurance when pregnant

When organising travel, particular attention must be given to the type of medical travel insurance cover arranged. Some insurance companies completely exclude cover in pregnancy while others do not recognise pregnancy as a medical illness and only include abnormalities of pregnancy within their policies. It may therefore be necessary to have a special policy prepared which will cover the pregnant woman and her unborn child in the event of illness and/or premature delivery requiring specialised neonatal intensive care. Severely premature babies may not be able to travel for several weeks adding further to the cost of care and living expenses of the mother/ parents.

If travel during pregnancy is considered essential, then it would be wise to find out as much as possible about local medical care, doctors, neonatal intensive care facilities. The British Embassy of the country to be visited should be able to help with this information.

If the woman is British and travelling within the European Community, then she should obtain the leaflet T6 which is available free from Post Offices.[14] Contained within the leaflet is an application form E111 and a list of European and other countries which have reciprocal arrangements with the UK for free, or reduced cost, medical care.

Travel in pregnancy

Although the optimal time for foreign travel is between weeks 18 and 24, most pregnant women, if well, may choose to travel beyond these dates. If planning travel late in pregnancy, it should be noted that most airlines will not carry women beyond the 32nd week, although some may allow travel up to the 36th week if a medical certificate of fitness is provided.[9] These rules differ for domestic and international flights and are based on the risk and expense of having to divert the flight if premature labour occurs while on board.[15] It should be noted that shipping lines are also hesitant to allow travel after the 36th week.[7]

Air travel does not pose any particular threat for the pregnant traveller. On a commercial jet aircraft, cabin pressure is maintained at approximately 1829 m (6000 ft) regardless of outside altitude. However, pregnant women and those in the first month after delivery have a small but definitely increased risk of developing a deep vein thrombosis. This can be avoided by not sitting in a cramped position for long periods, having a walkabout and encouraging the circulation in the legs by stretching calf muscles and wriggling toes (see Ch. 6).

This advice should also be followed when travelling by road or rail.

Advice to ensure maximum comfort when pregnant and travelling

- To avoid feeling sick or even faint, if a meal is missed while travelling, it is advisable to carry a light snack such as fruit, biscuits or peanuts.
- Plan to travel at a slower pace. Take frequent rest particularly during the third trimester when increased size makes most women tired and uncomfortable.
- Recognise how often there will be a need to find a toilet. 'You will need to go to the toilet more often than you thought physically possible.'[15] It would be wise to dress for quick and convenient toilet visits.
- Clothes should be loose and comfortable, for example, loose cotton dresses or trousers. Cotton underwear that is not tight fitting is essential as yeast and fungal infections of the vagina are common in pregnant women anywhere; however, travelling in hot climates exacerbates the problem, and it may be a wise precaution to carry antifungal creams or oral medication.

Summary

As travel advisers, we should remember that pregnancy is not an *immediate* contraindication to travel. With careful planning and specific advice, most healthy pregnant women should enjoy travel.

Travelling with children

Travelling with children – a nightmare scenario or the most fantastic adventure a family can experience?

Introduction

With careful planning, travelling with children, of any age, need not be the stressful experience first imagined. As parenthood is an international condition, many parents find that barriers erected by race and language fall away in the presence of children. The world, when seen through a child's innocent reaction to new sights and experiences, can seem less jaded.

When consulting a travel adviser, parents and guardians would expect information about immunisations and specific travel health advice relevant to the areas to be visited. However, highlighting problems uniquely associated with 'small travellers' will help parents when planning their trip. It may be useful to supply written advice in the form of a brochure or leaflet to reinforce oral advice given and to summarise the main points about travelling with children.

Information available from airlines, travel agents and professional organisations should not be ignored. Publications such as *Lonely Planet Travel Guide: Travel with Children*[15] and *Your Child's Health Abroad: A Manual for Travelling Parents*[16] offer excellent sources of anecdotal and detailed information ranging from a 2-week package trip to 'expatriate life'. Organisation and preparation are not optional extras, when travelling with children – they are vital.

Planning for travel

The age of a child is an important factor to consider when preparing for travel. Infants, although small, can require a lot of equipment!

FEEDING IMPLEMENTS

- For infants and younger children, take bottles, feeder cups, spoons, plastic bowls and bibs.
- A supply of sterilising tablets and containers for all the above equipment.
- A lightweight, folding, reclining stroller which can double as a chair in a restaurant when no high chairs are available.
- Unless camping, bedding is usually provided. It may be advisable to bring a waterproof sheet for all small children as occasional accidents do happen even to reliably toilet-trained toddlers.

CLOTHING

- Pack clothing appropriate for the country to be visited and varying climates. Lightweight, loose, cotton clothing is the only material that can be worn comfortably in the tropics but a warm sweater and waterproof jacket may still be required. Correct clothing is essential as a means of protection against the sun and biting insects.
- Hats should be worn by all children when exposed to the sun. Peaked caps leave the tips of ears exposed to the sun; this area is a common site for skin cancer. Bush hats protect this vulnerable area and also help protect the back of the neck which is so easily burned.[16]
- Children should be encouraged to wear some form of protection on their feet at all times in hot climates such as open sandals, thongs, light canvas or plastic shoes. Beaches, pavements, paths and tracks in many developing countries

offer health hazards such as worm infections, parasites and bacteria from animal and human faeces to the barefooted. In many countries, it is also advisable to wear some form of footwear when paddling in the sea or wading in rock pools to protect against sharp coral or shells and any creatures that may be lurking.[15]

NAPPIES

- Cloth nappies, while cheaper, are not as convenient as disposable nappies. They will require to be soaked, washed and dried on a daily basis which may pose difficulties for the more mobile traveller. Supplies of sterilising solution, soap powder and a suitable container for soaking the nappies in will also be required. Another factor to consider is that the climate may not be conducive to the wearing of plastic pants over cloth nappies; in humid conditions, fungal infections are common.[15]
- If disposable nappies are used, then an adequate supply should be taken. They are bulky but light and will make little difference to luggage allowances. Disposing of nappies, in many developing countries, where there is no refuse collection can pose difficulties. Placing soiled nappies in a sealed plastic bag and leaving them with other local rubbish may be the only option.

Logistics of travel

PASSPORTS

In most countries, parents can have children added to their own passport. While the fee for this will be less than separate passports for children, the drawback is that the children can *only* travel with the parent whose passport they appear on. Getting separate passports for children, while an additional expense, will allow freedom of travel with either parent, grandparents or other adults, for example school trips abroad. In this respect, it is worthy of note that, in the UK with effect from 5 October 1998, all children require to have their own passports. The new 'one person, one document' system applies even to babies. The rules have been changed to make child abduction more difficult and to improve identification procedures. (Children who are currently included on their parent's passport will still be permitted to travel on this passport, for the time being. However, when this passport expires, or the child reaches 16 years of age, these children will require to obtain their own passport.)

VISAS

Children with their own passports require visas just like adults. However, if the children are included on the parent's passport, a visa is often only required for the parent, this can result in a considerable saving.[15]

TRAVEL INSURANCE

Those travelling with children should ensure that they have adequate health and travel insurance which covers their dependent children if medical and/or dental assistance is required.

PRE-TRAVEL CHECK-UPS

- Routine dental examination is a sensible precaution, particularly for travellers to more remote areas where dental treatment could be basic or non-existent.
- A pre-travel medical check-up for children, who require regular drug therapy for asthma or diabetes, will ensure that they have an adequate supply of their medication for the length of travel. If further supplies are required during travel, it is advisable to take the original packaging showing the generic rather than the brand name of a drug as this will help with replacements, particularly if the drug requested is not available locally.
- An extra pair of spectacles should be taken and, where possible, a copy of the child's current eye prescription which will make replacement lenses easier to obtain.
- Immunisations and specific travel health advice for children should be sought for the country to be visited. Where possible it would be advisable to wait until a child's primary schedule of

immunisations has been completed, in particular diphtheria, tetanus and polio. The suitability and efficacy of vaccines associated with travel for children are detailed in another chapter.
- Malaria chemoprophylaxis, avoidance of mosquito bites and stand-by treatment are extensively covered in Chapter 13. However, it should be noted that getting some young children to take antimalarial medicine can be very difficult. Chloroquine, for example, is the only antimalarial drug available in syrup form. It is extremely bitter and the bitterness so persistent that it is undisguisable when mixed with jam, rice or fruit juice. Tablets when crushed and mixed with any of the above may be more palatable but some children are notorious for finding and spitting out 'the bits' they do not like.
- Parents should be encouraged to persevere and be very vigilant in protecting their children from mosquito bites.

Medical kit for children

A small, basic medical kit put together with special thought for children's ailments should be recommended[15] and should include:

- Infant/child analgesia with measuring spoon or dropper
- Rehydration solutions (e.g. Dioralyte, Rehidrat available in sachets)
- Antihistamine – useful for allergies, itches from insect bites or stings, as a decongestant or to help prevent motion sickness
- Antiseptic solution/creams (e.g. Savlon and Sudocrem)
- Calamine lotion
- Thermometer
- Steristrips, bandages, cotton wool and gauze
- Creams for nappy rash (e.g. Sudocrem)
- Teething gel
- Sunscreen, suntan lotion, chap stick and insect repellent suitable for children's skin
- Antibiotics – useful if travelling well off the beaten track but should be used with caution.

Preparation

For any would-be traveller to a new country, finding out as much as possible for example about local customs and legends, places of interest, foods available, and dominant language can enhance and benefit the forthcoming trip. Children should be encouraged to look at travel brochures and to get books from the library, especially if they have colour photographs and stories relating to the country to be visited. Even young children can be read stories about places they are going to and what they might see. Similarly, for children going to more rural areas, where the ubiquitous pizza and chips will not be available, introducing them to some 'local foods' before travel, may help to broaden their palate and gain their acceptance of strange foods.

Choice of schooling is very important for intending expatriate families. For older children, boarding school away from the overseas family home may have to be considered if there would be serious, local language difficulties or compatibility of courses with the desired examinations for entry into higher education. Teenage children often find changing schools difficult and if this also involves changing countries serious adaptation problems should be expected. Many would advise against families going abroad as expatriates for the first time if they have teenage children.

The journey

Keeping children occupied, comfortable and as safe as possible may make a journey less stressful.

COMBATING BOREDOM

Babies, when not sleeping or feeding, can be pacified by nursing, playing or even singing to them.

Toddlers can be very difficult to keep entertained. It can require Herculean efforts to amuse and distract them.[15] Having a supply of favourite books, small toys, snacks and an adult's undivided attention can keep them occupied for a few hours.

From age 3–4 years on, children can amuse themselves with drawing and simple games. They can listen to music or story tapes through headphones or the children's channel if available as in-flight entertainment. Allowing them to bring their own small backpacks with favourite toys, and perhaps a few surprise games and books put in for them to find, will add to their enjoyment.

Teenagers are usually content with a window seat on a plane, a few magazines or books, headset, music, in-flight movie and food!

COMFORT WHEN TRAVELLING

Comfort is the main consideration in deciding what to wear. A layer system of clothing works well. Track suits with a T-shirt underneath and a light jacket on top will allow for stripping down, or bundling up if it gets cold. Airports and aircraft can appear very cold because of air conditioning. For babies and toddlers, sleeveless body suits that fasten over nappies can be worn easily under track suits and all-in-one, stretch, sleep suits are good for babies when the temperature drops.

Motion sickness, painful ears during ascent/descent when flying, circadian rhythms, transmeridianal travel and jet lag are covered in Chapter 6.

Journeys to most foreign countries usually involve air travel. When booking with airlines, it is advisable to book 'children's meals' where possible. Many airlines allow infants and young children to travel at approximately 10% of the adult fare. While economically appealing, the reality is that parents or guardians will have children on their laps for the duration and are expected to bring food for them! In this respect, on long-haul flights, it would be beneficial to pay for a child seat (usually 50–67% of the adult fare). Sky cots or bassinets, if required, must be arranged at the time of booking.

Infant carriers/capsules for use in motor vehicles can be used in flight, when a seat has been booked for the child. During take-off, landing or turbulence, very young children should be properly restrained. Standard airline seats are unsuitable for very young children as the child can slip underneath or out of them. Special children's restraining seat belts, which anchor onto the adult's seat belt are available and should be requested. It is important that the child is not placed inside a standard seat belt with an adult, as the weight and the momentum of the adult during any deceleration or turbulence may crush the child. Children are best held securely in the arms of an adult where no other option is available.[17]

Keeping children healthy when abroad

Children and young adults are generally more liable to become ill while travelling than older adults in terms of travel-related illness attack rates.[17] Their behaviour may place them in risky situations and they expose themselves to more pathogens through poor hygiene. In many countries, children and adults can be at risk from serious illness.

Immunisation or chemoprophylaxis is available for many of these diseases as discussed in other chapters. For those diseases where there is no vaccine or prophylactic medication, it is essential that knowledge and awareness of risks and how to avoid them are explained, for example, how to avoid insect bites or how to make water safe for drinking. However, the most common illnesses experienced may include ear and eye infections, common colds, skin rashes, sunburn, diarrhoea, chest infections and trauma. All travellers with children should know how to treat minor ailments and when to seek medical treatment.

Common ailments

FEVER

The fear of exotic tropical infections makes fever a much more worrying complaint in children overseas than at home. Although malaria is an ever-present worry, the vast majority of fevers in children are viral nose and throat infections, such as coughs, colds and tonsillitis. Symptoms may include mild fever of less than 38.5°C, general malaise, loss of appetite, cough and runny nose with perhaps a sore throat.

Treatment should include: stripping the child of most of their clothes and sponging with a cloth dipped in tepid water, gently patting the skin dry and leaving excess moisture to evaporate and cool the skin. Give paracetamol, at the appropriate dose, and cool drinks.

Adults, however, should be aware of the warning signs of more severe fever if a child displays any of the following symptoms:

- a very high fever, temperature >39°C, with headache – possible malaria or typhoid
- severe headache and vomiting with neck stiffness and a temperature >39°C – possible meningitis
- child appears jaundiced and pyrexial – possible hepatitis or malaria
- child is pyrexial and has blood in stools or severe diarrhoea – possible dysentery
- burning sensation on passing urine – possible urinary tract infection.

In short, medical advice should be sought for a fever with or without other symptoms, that does not respond to tepid sponging and antipyrexial medication.

THE CHILD WITH DIARRHOEA

The seriousness of diarrhoea depends on how much fluid is lost from the body. A child's total fluid volume is greater in proportion to body weight than an adult's. Therefore, the effect is greater the younger the child; a baby can become dehydrated within a few hours of the onset of severe diarrhoea.[1] Any kind of diarrhoea can cause dehydration and adults with children must be able to assess whether their child is becoming dehydrated.

The following advice is based on a checklist contained within the publication *Your Child's Health Abroad*:[16]

How to replace fluid loss

- Replacement of fluid loss is the most important part of treatment. Children should be offered plenty of clear fluids such as juice, water and/or oral rehydration solution (available in sachets) (Dioralyte, Rehydrate). Give children below 2 years half a cup (100 ml) after each loose stool and children. 2–10 years one cup (200 ml) after each loose stool.

- Using the dehydration checklist, assess every few hours whether the child is getting dry.
- Although the appetite is often reduced, if the child feels like eating, high calorie, low residue foods (e.g. bananas, biscuits and bread) should be encouraged.

Drug treatment for diarrhoea

This is *only necessary* for some specific types of diarrhoea such as typhoid, cholera and giardiasis. Antidiarrhoeal agents such as kaolin, codeine, diphenoxylate and over-the-counter mixtures should be avoided in children. Medical attention should be sought if diarrhoea persists for more than 3 days and/or there are very frequent bowel movements, blood in the stools, repeated profuse vomiting or fever.

SUNBURN

Bathe the affected area with cool water or cold compresses. Apply calamine lotion and administer an analgesic such as paracetamol. If the area is blistered, keep it dry and covered as a burned area can easily become infected. In children, if sunburn is extensive, they can be at risk of losing a lot of body heat and can become hypothermic. Medical advice should be sought (see Ch. 9).

Prickly heat

Prickly heat is a common complaint in hot, humid climates and can be particularly troublesome for children. It is caused by the sweat glands becoming congested as the skin sweats more in an attempt to get cool. It leads to a distressing prickly sensation under the skin (usually on the neck, back and chest) accompanied by a fine, red rash with tiny blisters. Treatment is to bathe in cool water, pat dry and powder with talc or apply calamine lotion. Keep the child in the shade as much as possible in loose 100% cotton clothing.

Cuts, sores and insect bites

In hot, moist climates, any wound or break in the skin is likely to let in infection. The area should be

---

Dehydration checklist

Does the mouth and tongue appear dry and lacking in saliva?

Does the child seem thirstier than normal?

⇒ Offer more fluids to drink.

If a child displays any of the following signs, they require medical attention **as soon as possible**:

- Children who are becoming significantly dehydrated pass very little urine and it will become dark or tea-coloured. (A child will normally pass urine every 4 hours.)
- Eyes which appear sunken with dark rings.
- Skin which has lost its natural elasticity. You can test for this by pinching a fold of skin; if it continues to stand proud after 2 seconds, then a serious problem exists.
- Children who are unable to drink, become listless and unresponsive.

---

cleaned and then kept dry and clean. This may require the use of a sticking plaster or a non-stick dressing (e.g. Melolin). If the wound becomes infected, it will appear inflamed and painful. An infected wound will probably require a course of oral antibiotics. All children should complete the primary schedule of tetanus injections before travel. A non-immunised child with a deep, dirty wound should have an injection of tetanus immunoglobulin as soon as possible within 4 days of the injury.[16]

Animal bites

Children should be encouraged to avoid and mistrust any dogs or other mammals because of the risk of rabies and other diseases. Any bite, scratch or lick from a warm-blooded, furry animal should immediately be thoroughly cleaned. Clean the wound by scrubbing with soap and running water for at least 5 minutes, then apply an alcohol solution or diluted iodine. The wound should be covered with a clean, dry dressing. If there is any possibility that the animal is infected with rabies, immediate medical assistance should be sought. For those children who have received immunisation against rabies, a reinforcing dose will still be required. For the non-immunised, a course of rabies vaccine and rabies immunoglobulin will be required.

Summary

The key to travelling with children is to remind parents that time spent preparing and planning their journey will lead to more successful and enjoyable travel.

PRACTICE POINTS TO CONSIDER IN ADVANCE

Women travellers
- Menstruation in unfamiliar surroundings
- Fluid retention in the heat
- Availability and choice of contraception
- The possibility of pregnancy
- Personal safety and security.

Child and infant travellers
- Choice of feeds (breast-feeding is usually simpler and more hygienic)
- Breaking long journeys and relieving boredom
- Appropriate clothing and hygiene facilities
- Onset of dehydration, and heat and cold injury tend to be more rapid
- The risk of accidents
- Care to avoid bites – insects and animals
- Available medical care and schooling.

REFERENCES

1. Dawood R, ed. Travellers health: How to stay healthy abroad. 3rd ed. Oxford: Oxford University Press; 1992: 328–352.
2. Cowper A, Young C. Family planning: Fundamentals for health professionals. 2nd ed. London: Chapman and Hall; 1992: 52–74.
3. McIntosh IB. Health hazard and the higher risk traveller. Lancaster: Quay Publishing: 1993: 86–89.
4. International Planned Parenthood Federation. Contraceptive services abroad. Regent's College, Regent's Park, London, NW1 4NW; 1996.
5. Family Planning Association of Britain, 27–35 Mortimer Street, London, W1N 7RJ.
6. British Medical Association and Royal Pharmaceutical Society of Great Britain British National Formulary 33(March) 1998 Chs 4,7.
7. Ganley Y. Handbook of travel medicine. London: Science Press; 1996: 17–22, 27.
8. Wood K. Globe trotter's bible: A guide to budget travel around the world. London: Harper Collins; 1996: 103–105.
9. Brandenburger C, Ogilvie C, eds. The traveller's handbook. 6th ed. London: Wexas; 1994: 277–281, 284–291.
10. McIntosh I. Travel induced illness: a GP based survey. Scotish Medical Journal 1991; 11(4): 14–15.
11. Lea G, Leese J, eds. Health information for overseas travel. London: HMSO; 1995: 10.
12. Salisbury D, Beggs N, eds. Immunisation against infectious disease. London: HMSO; 1996: 87–91.
13. Roche Data Sheet: Lariam (mefloquine) May 1997. Roche Products Ltd, PO Box 8, Welwyn Garden City, Herts AL7 3AY.
14. T6. Health advice for travellers anywhere in the world. Department of Health, PO Box 410, Wetherby, LS23 7LN.
15. Wheeler M. Lonely Planet travel guide: travel with children. Hawthorn, Australia: Lonely Planet Publications; 1995: 9–22, 135–138.
16. Howarth-Wilson J, Ellis M. Your child's health abroad: A manual for travelling parents. Bucks, England: Bradt Publications; 1998.
17. Leggat P, Speare R, Kedjarune U, et al. Travelling with Children 1998; 5(3): 142–145.

Travellers with pre-existing health problems

Eric Walker   Lorna Calvert

Introduction

When advising intending travellers about possible health risks, it is important to be aware of any existing health problems they may have. Existing health problems can, in extreme circumstances, make travel unwise. They can also influence decisions, for example, about the suitability of vaccinations. More often, knowing about existing health problems can allow advice to be given so that complications may be avoided.

Information on the following can be found in other sections of the book:

- difficulties during air flights in those with middle ear disease, hypoxia and following internal surgery (Ch. 6)
- the elderly and those with disabilities (pp. 108–113)
- those who may have psychological difficulties (pp. 119–138)
- Gynaecological problems and travelling with very young children (pp. 142–157)
- interactions between existing medications and vaccinations (Ch. 12)
- Interactions between existing medications and malaria prophylaxis (Ch. 13).

This chapter will consider travel health advice for travellers with the following conditions: gastrointestinal, liver, cardiac or respiratory disease; renal disease and renal failure; epilepsy; skin problems; eye problems; diabetes mellitus; and immunocompromised status.

Insurance and details of medical conditions

Adequate health insurance including cover for repatriation on medical grounds is always important but especially so for those who are more likely to need medical attention when abroad. Travellers may need to be reminded that medical care can be very difficult to obtain in many countries, and it can also be expensive.

It is wise for the traveller with a medical problem to carry a doctor's letter containing a recent medical summary and details of any current prescriptions. Wearing a bracelet or neck chain which gives information on an individual's condition and treatment (such as those available from Medic-Alert or SOS Talisman) can save valuable minutes in an emergency.

Medications

All travellers with underlying medical conditions which require regular and emergency medications and equipment should be sure to take adequate supplies. Availability, names and dosages of medications may vary in the country to be visited. All medications should be clearly labelled. Ensure a supply is available in hand luggage in case of delays. In some instances, carrying stand-by treatments for emergencies should be considered.

Gastrointestinal disease

EXISTING GASTROINTESTINAL DISORDERS

Most people think of diarrhoea as a common travel-related problem but constipation can also result from dietary change in countries where less roughage and cereals are available. Constipation can be aggravated by the dehumidified atmosphere of aircraft cabins and hot climates and by dehydration.

Prevention is often easier than cure and maintaining an adequate fluid intake is essential. For those who know that constipation can be a problem, taking a bulk forming agent regularly can be helpful.

Any abrupt change in bowel habit such as diarrhoea or constipation can exacerbate existing bowel conditions, including irritable bowel syndrome, diverticulitis, ulcerative colitis and Crohn's disease. Giardiasis can be difficult to distinguish from irritable bowel disease and a proportion of those who contract giardiasis will go on to develop irritable bowel disease. Use of an antibiotic as prophylaxis against travellers' diarrhoea may be indicated for those with these pre-existing conditions (see Ch. 11).

PEPTIC ULCERATION

Bleeding from a peptic ulcer or gastro-oesophageal varices can be difficult to manage in remote areas or areas with poor medical facilities. If the bleeding is significant, access to safe, screened blood or blood products may not be possible. Travelling with a peptic ulcer is less of a problem now than previously because of the use of more effective drug treatments. Those with active ulcers may be wise to postpone travelling until symptoms are under control. It should be remembered that those on the highly effective H2 antagonists and proton pump inhibitors, which reduce gastric acidity, are loosing their 'acid barrier' to infection and may be predisposed to infective diarrhoea and complications such as septicaemia.

Liver disease

Patients with liver failure who wish to travel should follow much of the advice given to those who are immunocompromised (see later).

LIVER DISEASE AND ALCOHOL

Travellers often consume more alcohol while abroad than at home. This is common to both holidaymakers and business travellers. Those with alcoholic liver disease may slip into liver failure. It is not uncommon to see delirium tremens occurring in this group of travellers if they become ill and are unable to keep up their alcohol intake.

Cardiovascular disease

CARDIOVASCULAR PROBLEMS

Immobility from any cause including sitting still during a long flight can result in venous thrombosis with the danger of pulmonary emboli. This is particularly risky for those with a previous history of thrombosis, or if there is a degree of cardiac failure, or following recent major surgery. Encouraging as much activity as possible – leg movements and walking – and taking a small dose of aspirin (75 mg daily) are wise precautions in these circumstances.

Those on anticoagulants should ensure that their clotting time is stable prior to departure. Taking a new medication can alter clotting times, for example proguanil can reduce the metabolism of warfarin and lead to an increased prothrombin time.

Some antimalarial drugs can interact with anti-arrythmics and other cardiac drugs. Mefloquine taken together with β-blockers or calcium channel blockers can result in marked bradycardia. Always check cautions, contraindications and drug interactions.

Travellers with pacemakers or metallic implants should alert security staff in airports to avoid unnecessary embarrassment when passing through metal detectors.

Respiratory disease

RESPIRATORY DISEASES

Individuals with chronic obstructive airways disease may find their symptoms exacerbated by the dust in dry, hot countries. Traffic and other pollution which are increasingly common in large cities, particularly in developing countries, can also worsen symptoms.

The availability of cheap cigarettes and stress caused by travel may lead to an increase in smoking and secondary chest infections may occur. Legionnaires' disease is more common in smokers.

The effect of change in climate on asthma is unpredictable and can be positive as well as negative. The traveller with asthma should be sure to carry adequate, routine medications. Ensure a supply is available in hand luggage in case of delays. All medications should be clearly labelled. In some instances, carrying stand-by treatment for emergencies such as aminophylline suppositories, should be considered. This should be discussed with the doctor or nurse who manages the patient prior to travel.

Those with pre-existing lung disease should consider both influenza and pneumococcal vaccination prior to travel. The flu season may occur at a different time of year in the country to be visited than in the UK, and this needs consideration for 'at risk' groups.

An occasional area for concern is the risk of aggravation of symptoms caused by hypoxia in the traveller with chronic respiratory failure who flies straight into an airport which is at high altitude. This is possible, for example, in the Andes and Himalayas. Those with marked respiratory deficiency may wish to seek advice from their general practitioner or respiratory physician prior to departure as well as informing the airline concerned (see also Ch. 8).

Renal disease

RENAL FAILURE

Those with chronic renal failure who need to maintain a high fluid intake while at home may find this very much more difficult in hot climates, especially when clean drinking water is difficult to obtain. The result can be a rise in creatinine and 'acute on chronic' renal failure. This can be further compounded by an episode of travellers' diarrhoea. Dosages of diuretics and use of other drugs such as selective serotonin re-uptake inhibitors which can cause hyponatraemia, may need to be re-assessed.

It is now possible for patients to travel when on renal dialysis and 'networks' of support are available from dialysis units in more developed countries. The traveller's own renal unit or the embassy in the host country may be able to help

with providing contacts. The availability of materials for continuous ambulatory peritoneal dialysis needs prior planning and arranging access to medical contacts at the destination is essential in the event of an emergency.

VACCINATIONS AND MALARIA PROPHYLAXIS IN RENAL FAILURE

There is normally no problem with the administration of vaccines unless the patient is immunocompromised (see later). Antimalarial drug dosages may need adjustment and this should always be discussed with the traveller's own renal physician.

Guidelines in the UK are that in mild failure (creatinine clearance >20 ml/min), chloroquine and/or proguanil can usually be used in the short term (chloroquine at the normal dose and proguanil at half the normal dose). In severe or moderate failure (creatinine clearance <20 ml/min), travel may need to be discouraged, especially to hot or tropical areas where diarrhoea and/or dehydration may add to the traveller's problems.

Side effects from both chloroquine and mefloquine (including convulsions) are more common in renal failure. Doxycycline may be the safest drug for essential travel to areas with substantial chloroquine resistance.

RENAL CALCULI

A high fluid intake is important in the prevention and management of renal calculi, which is a well-known problem in expatriates living in hot climates. Cystitis is also said to be more common for those living in hot climates.

Epilepsy

Travellers with epilepsy should ensure that their travelling companions are aware of their condition and know how to react in the event of a seizure. Travelling when seizure control is poor can clearly lead to difficulties. Those with poor seizure control should consider carrying emergency treatment and companions should know how and when to use it.

Swimming without adequate supervision, especially at sea, may be dangerous. Travellers who would not normally drive should not be tempted to drive in countries where there is no legislation to prevent this.

As with all travellers with existing medical conditions, it may be wise to carry a doctor's letter and it is important that they take adequate medication with them since brands and their dosages may be different abroad. Organising access to medications abroad can be more problematic for short-term or transient visitors than for long-stay expatriates.

Mefloquine and chloroquine are contraindicated for use in patients with epilepsy as they can cause convulsions even in those with no previous history (this is rare, approximately 1:10 000). Chloroquine can also interact with anticonvulsants, rendering them less effective and leading to breakthrough seizures.

Skin problems

Wounds and skin ulcers are more easily infected in the heat and in areas with poor hygiene. Care to thoroughly clean and cover any existing wounds is important. Travellers should carry sufficient supplies of creams, ointments and dressings whenever possible.

Mosquito bites may become infected resulting in streptococcal cellulitis or staphylococcal sepsis. This occurs more often in those with existing venous or lymphatic stasis. Tinea infections of the skin can become worse following exposure to sun.

Those with psoriasis should not take chloroquine as an antimalarial as it can aggravate the condition.

Eye problems

In sunlight, use of sunglasses is important for prevention of damage to the eye, including the long-term prevention of cataracts. Use of sunglasses can be essential if mydriatics are being used and they provide comfort for the wearer.

Dust and dehydration can make the wearing of contact lenses uncomfortable. Carrying plenty of cleaning and wetting solution is advisable and having a pair of conventional spectacles is wise. Contact lens wearers should be careful when handling lenses if DEET-based repellants are used as direct contact with DEET on a lens can damage it.

Diabetes mellitus

The British Diabetic Association, 10 Queen Anne Street, London, W1M 0BD provides leaflets and information, including travel guides to the more popular countries visited abroad, with advice pertinent to the needs of the traveller with diabetes. This includes the availability of different types of insulin in different countries, information on different types of food available and a list of useful translations.

THE JOURNEY

Adequate supplies of medications and equipment should be carried in hand luggage where they can be easily accessed during the journey. This is important in the event of delays or if hold luggage goes missing. Taking a supply of carbohydrate in hand luggage is also recommended in case of delays, and for access during long journeys. Those who suffer from travel sickness should consider taking an anti-emetic as vomiting can predispose to hypoglycaemia. Travellers with diabetes should ensure that their travelling companions are aware of their condition and know how to react in the event of hypo- or hyperglycaemia. Those with unstable diabetes may be wise to wear some form of identification such as Medic-Alert or SOS Talisman.

INSULIN SCHEDULES ON FLIGHTS

All international flights east or west involve crossing time zones. Travellers who take insulin should seek advice in advance, especially those with 'brittle' diabetes. They should remember to monitor sugar levels, especially on long journeys and plan a schedule for taking insulin but be prepared to alter it later if delays occur.

INSULIN STORAGE

Although some manufacturers state that insulin can remain stable for up to 1 month at normal room temperature, extremes of temperature can reduce its activity. Whenever possible, vials should be kept in a cool, dark place. Polystyrene containers, vacuum flasks and face cloths in a sandwich container are all useful. Special 'travel-carry' systems are available from specialist suppliers. Storage is an important issue in cold climates, as insulin should not be allowed to freeze.

CLIMATE

The rate of insulin absorption may be affected in a warm climate and patients should be aware. Maintaining a high fluid intake to compensate for loss is important. Glucose strips should be carefully stored as humidity can affect accurate readings.

ACTIVITIES

Some people are more active on holiday and others are less so, therefore diet, oral glycaemic medication and insulin may need to be adjusted to compensate.

FOOD AND DRINK

Caution is advised to prevent infections. Gastrointestinal upset including vomiting and diarrhoea can lead to hypoglycaemia.

FOOTCARE

Extra attention to footcare in the sun is recommended to prevent burning or blistering. Wearing adequate footwear for protection against injury is also advised, expecially on the beach where hidden hazards may lie.

The HIV-positive and immunocompromised traveller

Immunocompromise can result from the presence of disease or the taking of medication.

AIDS is a classical example of severe immunocompromise caused by disease. Lesser degrees of immunocompromise can result from liver or renal failure, drug addiction, blood dyscrasias and even malnutrition.

Corticosteroids and immunosuppressing drugs used to treat malignancy or to prevent rejection of organ transplants can predispose to infection. This may occur during short, high-dose courses of corticosteroids (e.g. above 60 mg a day) or after more prolonged therapy at lower dosages.

Stress related to travel can lower resistance to infection for reasons that are not always clear. This may be seen, for example, in refugees following enforced displacement. It is known that stress can re-activate tuberculosis – this was well-recognised prior to the advent of anti-tuberculous drug therapy when rest and diet were the mainstays of therapy.

Immunocompromise causes problems for the traveller because infection can be more severe and can be unexpectedly caused by organisms not normally harmful to the healthy individual – the so-called 'opportunistic' infections. At home, in familiar and clean surroundings, exposure to potentially opportunistic infections may be minimal and prevented even further through the ability to control food, water and household hygiene. This is not always the case when abroad in unfamiliar surroundings.

OPPORTUNISTIC INFECTIONS

All immunocompromised travellers, and in particular those with HIV disease, are at greater risk of contracting opportunistic infections. There is the possibility of contracting infections that can 'naturally' persist and cause problems later on when the illness is more advanced (e.g. tuberculosis, strongyloides, cryptosporidiosis, toxoplasmosis, cytomegalovirus). All seriously immunocompromised travellers must be aware of the importance of personal preventive measures such as boiling drinking water, avoiding partially cooked meats and taking care to avoid skin sepsis.

INTERACTIONS WITH MEDICATION AND THE POSSIBLE NEED FOR SPECIALISED MEDICAL CARE

There may be interactions between antimalarial chemoprophylaxis and the complicated drug or antiretroviral regimens that immunocompromised patients often take. Co-trimoxazole, however, used in a high dosage for the prophylaxis of pneumocystis pneumonia, has a useful antimalarial effect (except in areas with a high degree of chloroquine and proguanil resistance).

At the destination there may be a shortage of availability of familiar and emergency care including medications. Language and confidentiality issues can also cause difficulties. As with all travellers who have a medical condition, it is often helpful if a trusted companion knows about the problem.

VACCINATION IN THE IMMUNOCOMPROMISED

Those immunocompromised may have a poor response to active vaccination. Sometimes a higher dose may improve the response.

Live vaccines are usually avoided because of the risk of disseminated or serious infection. It is particularly important to avoid administering BCG because a severe, local or miliary BCG infection may occur.

VACCINATIONS FOR THOSE WITH HIV INFECTION

Table 7.1 gives recommendations on when vaccines can be given 'safely' to those with HIV infection. The advice does not necessarily apply to those with other immunocompromising conditions.

The HIV viral load usually increases temporarily following vaccination. This increase is less evident when the patient is on effective antiretroviral therapy. While the clinical significance of this increase is unclear, it is prudent

TABLE 7.1 Vaccination for those with HIV

HIV	Symptomatic	Asymptomatic
BCG	No	No
Cholera (inactivated)	Yes	Yes
Cholera (live oral)	No	No
Diphtheria	Yes	Yes
Hepatitis A	Yes[1]	Yes
Hepatitis B	Yes[1]	Yes
Influenza	Yes	Yes
Measles	Caution[2]	Yes
Meningococcal A and C	Yes	Yes
Mumps	Caution[2]	Yes
Immunoglobulin	Yes	Yes
Pertussis	Yes	Yes
Pneumococcal	Yes	Yes
Live oral poliomyelitis	Caution[2,4]	Yes
Inactivated poliomyelitis	Yes	Yes
Rabies	Yes	Yes
Rubella	Caution[2]	Yes
Tetanus	Yes	Yes
Typhoid Vi	Yes	Yes
Typhoid oral (live)	No	No
Yellow fever	Caution[2,3]	Caution[2,3]

Notes
[1]Double the dose of hepatitis A and B vaccine in immuno-compromised patients.
[2]Vaccination against measles, mumps and rubella can be given at the discretion of the clinician in charge if the risk of contracting infection is high.
[3]There have been no reports of any adverse reactions after vaccination of the immunocompromised against yellow fever. However, there is little experience in HIV-positive patients.
[4]Oral polio vaccine may be given to children who are known to be infected with HIV provided that their household contacts are not immunocompromised. In these cases, inactivated polio vaccine may be used.

to advise vaccinations only when there is a significant infection risk to the traveller.

ENTRY RESTRICTIONS FOR HIV POSITIVE TRAVELLERS

Some countries operate restrictions for travellers who are known to be HIV-positive. These can vary from complete prohibition of entry to access permitted but working or studying prohibited. It is recommended that those who are HIV-positive find out the current restrictions prior to travelling. Those who are taking antiretroviral and some other medications, who do not declare their HIV status, risk being 'found out' if luggage is searched at customs. Seeking expert advice before travel is advised – with careful planning, most trips can be arranged safely.

BIBLIOGRAPHY

Alder M. ABC of AIDS. London: British Medical Journal Publications; 1993.

Bollinger R, Quinn T. Tropical diseases in the HIV infected traveller. In: Broder S, Merigan TC, Bolognesi D eds. Textbook of AIDS medicine. Baltimore: Williams and Wilkins; 1994: 311–322.

British National Formulary – for drug dosages and interactions in various medical conditions. London: British Medical Journal Publications.

Kumar P, Clark M, eds. Clinical medicine. 4th ed. London: WB Saunders; 1998.

Walker E, Calvert L, Raeside F, Williams GR. The 'ABC' of healthy travel. 5th ed. London: British Medical Journal Publications; 1997.

PRACTICE POINTS

- Always enquire about existing illnesses when advising intending travellers.
- The phone number of the traveller's own doctor may be useful to give to medical attendants abroad.
- Airlines should be told about any serious medical conditions that may cause difficulties in aircraft. They may be able to supply special seating or other facilities.
- Remember to consider possible interactions between antimalarials and other medications.
- Vaccines may be less effective in the immunocompromised and live vaccines should usually be avoided.
- Adequate medications and equipment should be taken since the same preparations may not be available, or easily obtained abroad.
- Travellers with diabetes mellitus can obtain very useful advice from the British Diabetic Association.
- A travelling companion should know about any illness that may require urgent treatment.
- It may be important to check in advance about local available medical facilities at the destination.

TRAVEL-RELATED RISKS: PHYSICAL

Accidents and injuries experienced by travellers

J. Gordon Avery

A man must carry knowledge with him if he is to bring back knowledge.

Samuel Johnson

Introduction and epidemiology

In contrast to the highly privileged, wealthy, well-educated and intrepid travellers of the 19th century, the modern traveller includes those from a much wider range of backgrounds. These range from the rich passenger on a luxury liner to the backpacker on a world tour prior to settling down to relatively humdrum, urban life or academic studies.

In between these extremes there is a wide range of activities ranging from camping and package tours to cycling, and canal holidays, adventure activities and other sporting and leisure activities. Those travelling include regular business travellers, contract workers, volunteers and missionaries.

With such a wide range of activities we can expect a considerable variety of accident and injury experience ranging from road traffic accidents to dog bites. If anticipated, most accidents and injuries can be prevented. However, because the traveller is often in an unfamiliar environment, defences may be relaxed and the potential for accidents is often very much higher than at home.

It is difficult to obtain accurate information on the injuries experienced by travellers abroad. We may assume that many sustain injuries owing to activities similar to those practised at home.

Some of the best information we have is on deaths and on the injuries resulting in repatriation on health grounds. Even here the information is limited and may be difficult to interpret.

Information on travellers from England and Wales is not available but in Scotland,[1] during the 16 years between 1973 and 1988, trauma was the second most common cause of death (Table 8.1). During this period 654 (68.7%) out of 952 recorded deaths were for cardiovascular disease and 197 (20.7%) for trauma. Of these traumatic deaths, 80% were in males, 60% were in those between 20 and 39 years and 25% in those aged between 40 and 59. Two-thirds of the deaths in the 20–39 group were due to trauma.

For travellers from the USA, the risk of death from trauma is around 25 times that from infection. The death rates for trauma in young American adults (aged 15–44) abroad are increased by a factor of two to three times compared with those at

TABLE 8.1 Causes of death in Scottish travellers abroad 1973–88

Cause of death	Age Group					Total	%
	0–19	20–39	40–59	60–79	80+		
Cardiovascular	3	43	240	342	22	654(4)	68.7
Trauma	17	113	51	14	1	197(1)	20.7
Infection	2	3	9	19	1	34	3.6
Other disease	8	9	22	20	1	61(1)	6.4
Not stated	0	2	1	3	0	6	0.6
Totals	**30**	**170**	**323**	**398**	**25**	**952** (Age not known 6)	**100**

home. These deaths are due mostly to road traffic or drowning accidents. A résumé of fatalities experienced abroad by citizens from the USA and Switzerland is shown in Table 8.2.[2–4]

One source of information on the causes of repatriation to the UK on health grounds is the Travellers' Medical Service.[5] This group insures around 1 in 5 of travellers from the UK (total insured journeys outside UK are approximately 22 million per annum). Trauma accounts for nearly 30% of their repatriations (Table 8.3) and diseases of the heart and circulation only 8%. There is a problem with classification of the trauma since 802 (36.3%) are due to undefined 'other causes' (Table 8.4). The major defined causes are falls from standing, 597 cases (27.0%) and winter sports, 359 cases (16.2%). Just over 1 in 10 of the trauma repatriations were due to road traffic accidents.

Overall, trauma is the second most common cause of death in UK citizens travelling abroad (Table 8.1) but is most common between birth and 39 years. It accounts for nearly one-third of repatriations on health grounds (Table 8.3). The most serious injuries to travellers occur from falls during winter sports and accidents on the road.

It is worth reflecting that the major cause of death for males aged 1–44 years and females aged 1–35 years in most developed countries is accidents. When abroad, the traveller has a similar or increased risk of accidents, far greater than for any other

disease, including malaria and other infectious diseases. The risk of death as a result of trauma remains higher even with older travellers while, as expected, cardiovascular disease is more common.

TABLE 8.3 Major causes of repatriation of UK citizens on health grounds by the Travellers' Medical Service in 1993 (7424 cases)[5]

Infection	557
Cancer	29
Hormonal	28
Blood	38
Mental illness	66
Nervous system	190
Heart and circulation (7.8%)	577
Respiratory	922
Gastrointestinal	1101
Genitourinary	352
Skin (includes 144 insect bites)	396
Musculoskeletal	192
Trauma (29.8%)	**2211**
Dental (includes unspecified number of trauma cases)	228
'Curtailment' (e.g. family illness at home)	537
Total	**7424**

TABLE 8.4 Major causes of injury to selected UK citizens repatriated on health grounds in 1993[5]

Road traffic accidents	230	10%
Vehicle occupants	(153)	
Moped riders	(40)	
Pedestrians	(37)	
Water sports	39	2%
Fall	740	33%
Standing	(597)	
From height	(143)	
Assault injury by third party	41	2%
Winter sports	359	16%
Others	802	36%
Total	**2211***	

*Including 242 head injuries, 66 spinal injuries (48 with cord damage.)

TABLE 8.2 Fatalities abroad amongst travellers from Switzerland and the USA

Cause of death	USA: 1975 and 1984 % (n = 2463)	Switzerland: 1987 % (n = 315)
Cardiovascular	49	15
Trauma	25	28
Road traffic accidents	(7)	(13)
Air	(2)	(6)
Drowning	(4)	(5)
Other injuries	(12)	(4)
Infection	1	1
Other illnesses	–	4
Unknown	25	52

AUSTRALIANS ABROAD

An analysis of deaths in 2 400 000 Australians who travelled overseas during a 12-month period in 1992–93 showed the overall risk of dying was probably little different from that while staying home.[6]

The low numbers of deaths from infections suggest it might be more important to remind prospective travellers, especially to developing countries, about the possibility of accidents often related to alcohol and sometimes drugs.

The leading cause of the 421 deaths (35%) was ischaemic heart disease but the second major cause (26%) was trauma. In those under 50, trauma was the leading cause of death, being responsible for over half those in young men and two-thirds in women. The overall ratio of male to female deaths was 4:1. The riskiest destinations were Central and South America, Central and Southern Africa and Mainland Europe.

AMERICANS ABROAD

Although about 5000 Americans die overseas each year, they travel less internationally than Australians. Americans have a lower death rate. Most of them die in the developed countries of Western Europe. The pattern of their causes of death is very similar to those who stay at home,[3] being ischaemic heart disease, injuries, suicides and homicide rather than infectious diseases. Older Americans tend to go to Europe, whereas those younger have much wider horizons, and many more go to less developed countries. Their main cause of death, wherever they go, is from trauma.

Transport accidents

ACCIDENTS ON THE ROAD

In road trauma, the relative risk for tourists in many countries is much higher than for locals. In Bermuda, the risk of a motorcycle accident to a tourist is five times that of the locals.[7] In Crete,[8] visitors who are used to driving on the 'wrong side of the road' are more likely to be involved in road traffic accidents (RTAs) than other visitors. Alcohol abuse and 'drink-driving' are also more common than in locals. The unfamiliar holiday environment, greater freedom, a relaxed attitude towards risk-taking, use of rented vehicles and different road laws all contribute to a higher injury potential. RTAs by visitors are a major cause for concern. In Crete, while the ratio of foreigners to Greeks presenting to hospitals in Heraklion is only 1:18 for all accidents, it is 1:3 for RTAs. Apart from the common causes of death like a coronary and cerebrovascular disease in the older traveller, the commonest cause of death in travellers abroad is RTAs.

Geographical location and safety

- The safest places on the road are Northern Europe and Japan. Still relatively safe are most parts of North America, Australia and New Zealand. This is not due to fewer vehicles on the roads but to better-maintained roads and vehicles and stricter adherence to road safety legislation.
- Less safe are Southern and Eastern Europe, Russia, China and the Indian sub-continent.
- Least safe are most of the African countries, Central and south America, parts of the Middle East. Some parts of Asia like Thailand the Philippines, Cambodia and Vietnam are 'unsafe', whereas some densely populated but developed areas like Singapore and Hong Kong have amongst the lowest death rates in the world for RTAs. Travellers to many of these countries are 'taking their life in their hands' whether crossing the road, going by bus or taking a taxi and even if using a bicycle, or driving a self-hired car. Using a scooter or moped in places like Corsica or some of the Greek Islands is very risky.

ACCIDENTS IN AIRCRAFT

Air crashes are very rare – air travel is the safest of all forms of transport per passenger mile travelled. In spite of the few, well-publicised, jumbo-jet disasters, usually the bigger the planes, the safer they are. You have to be extraordinarily unlucky to be involved in an air disaster.

Precautions when travelling by road

- When crossing the road, remember the traffic may come from the opposite direction to the one in your country; drivers often do not observe pedestrian crossings or light signals.
- When driving, strictly observe speed limits and traffic signs; never drink and drive; watch all sides back and front – and up above as well (vehicles have been known to flip over fly-overs). For security reasons, lock your doors at all stopping points.
- Be very careful on rough, potholed roads.
- Think twice about taking an overloaded, up-country bus.
- Forget about hiring a scooter!
- Take the underpass to the beach!
- Check over any hire vehicle very carefully for mechanical defects.

To reduce the risk of being involved in an air accident

- Travel on scheduled routes on regular airlines such as North American, Western European, Antipodean, South African, Japanese and most Asian airlines.
- Avoid charter flights with recently established companies.
- Avoid cheaper flights and older, fully loaded planes common in some poorer countries.
- Avoid small planes if the weather is bad (it may be exciting but hair-raising and potentially dangerous).

Precautions reducing risk within an aircraft

- Choose a seat in the middle over the wing.
- Study and observe the correct 'safety drill' to be carried out in the event of an accident.
- Keep calm; do not panic (you are in the hands of the airline pilot and crew).

Accidents on railways

Apart from the Orient Express and a few other routes, the days are long gone when the rich travelled in luxury with servants and meals at every stopping place. In most parts of the world, travel by train is hot, cramped, noisy and uncomfortable. Of course, there are exceptions like certain French and Swiss railways.

The accident risk is small. Obstacles on the line, derailments, floods and collapsed bridges are rare. The survival rate is usually high with more chance of survival in the middle of the train and possibly amongst a large number of passengers where you can cushion each other. Baggage falling off racks is perhaps the greatest risk.

ACCIDENTS AT SEA

In spite of the Titanic, Zebrugge and Estonia disasters, the traveller on high standard luxury liners and the majority of modern ferries is usually quite safe. There is always the risk of falling down the gangway in rough seas or being injured during deck games but the resultant injuries are generally minor sprains and bruises. The extremely rare, 'man overboard' incidents are often deliberate suicides.

Cargo ships with 'flags of convenience' registration and crew with dubious qualifications, are of more concern. Ships of this type do regularly get lost at sea through bad weather, poor navigation, fire or mechanical failure. Be prepared for a dramatic rescue by helicopter or several days in an open boat! Coastal, river and sea-ferries in some parts of the world, notably the China Sea, the Caribbean, Africa, India and Bangladesh, are frequently overcrowded, old and haphazardly managed and navigated. For the adventurer this is exciting stuff but if you are wise, you will keep on deck at all times, ready to make a quick getaway – but do not forget the sharks and crocodiles! Make careful note exactly where the (effective) life-jackets, life-rafts and boats are situated. People have survived for several weeks in open boats often with very little food and water.

By definition, the traveller is going to use some form of transport. Even pedestrians still have to watch out for motor vehicles, cyclists, thugs, robbers, muggers, terrorists, passing gunfire, rabid dogs and potholes. So just weigh up the odds. And if you still think it is worth it – as the Australians say, 'Go for your life!'

Domestic accidents

Accidents in and around the home environment are just as likely to occur to the traveller as they are at home. If camping or staying in a rented property, then it could even be higher because of unfamiliarity. In many parts of the world heating, cooling and electrical appliances may be faulty or in poor repair. The standards for product safety may not be as rigorous as many of those in northern Europe, North America or Australasia.

There are special problems in high-rise flats and hotels (e.g. in Mediterranean resorts) from being caught in lifts, falling down stairs or lift shafts or off balconies. These are all relatively rare but the traveller must be aware of the possibilities, especially for their children.

Taking one's own portable adapters and reliable electrical equipment may solve and prevent problems. Otherwise, even greater care is required than that exercised at home.

Fire and burns and scalds are dangers, especially with open fires, paraffin and gas heaters, convectors and hot water taps which have excessively hot water. Because there are no regulations on the temperature of water outlets, most UK residents are aware of this and know how to mix the water in their baths. In countries like Denmark strict regulations apply to the temperature of water coming out of domestic taps and the necessary controls are built into domestic appliances. Leaking gas mains causing explosions or carbon monoxide poisoning have also caused problems on the Algarve in Portugal and in other countries in the past.

Accidents at work

A small but significant proportion of travellers go abroad to work. Typically this may be short-term contract work in the military, technical, academic, educational or health field, or in the engineering construction, transport or oil industries. Travellers may be involved with voluntary and missionary work. In addition, some 'round-the-world' travellers or backpackers take on casual work, for example, as farm hands and bar tenders or work in hotels or in the leisure industry.

Often hazards associated with injury are similar to those experienced in the same jobs at home. However, there may be important differences that should be noted by all overseas workers and not taken lightly.

Possible differences in work conditions abroad

- Variable standards of Health and Safety at Work legislation and regulations.
- Religious and legal culture which, in any dispute or accident, may not favour the foreigner (e.g. in many Muslim countries, the law or sharia directly follows the teachings of the Koran).
- Difficult working conditions owing to remoteness, poor communications and extremes of climate.
- An unskilled or only minimally skilled labour force.
- Psychological problems because of culture shock, distance from home and living in an alien culture.
- Unpredictable use of alcohol and drugs (e.g. officially forbidden, with strict penalties for use or possession) but still widely available.
- Misunderstandings and lack of cooperation by officialdom, local staff and colleagues as a result of language or cultural differences.
- Stress and fatigue caused by any of the above, unregulated working hours, unaccustomed excessive exercise, recreation and increased alcohol consumption.

There are often other problems specific to local situations which make working abroad that much more difficult.

If inadequate or different medical care facilities are expected, a basic course in first aid is important and also a readiness to learn from people who have worked in the area. Media reporters, the military, missionaries and volunteers working in war zones and disaster areas may be familiar with and trained to deal with these special problems. For many, the thrills and excitement of the job far and away offset the considerable risks they are often taking.

Sport/leisure accidents

The traveller abroad may often have the opportunity to engage in sport and leisure activities not normally considered at home. There is a wide range of opportunities varying from surfing in Hawaii, scuba diving on the Great Barrier Reef, bungee jumping in the USA or New Zealand, skiing in Switzerland, white water rafting in Norway, mountaineering or riding in Nepal, paragliding in the South of France or swimming off the Greek Islands.

Each of these activities has its own special risks. Some, like skiing, result in fatalities and casualties every year. Lack of experience and skill, being unaware of the potential hazards and lack of fitness are often compounded by an excess of alcohol or other drugs. Expert instruction and supervision may be expensive or unavailable, so there may be a very strong temptation to 'go it alone'.

Golden rules for safety

- Beware of any unfamiliar activities.
- Find out about all the possible or unexpected local hazards like underwater rocks, strong tides, whirlpools, rapids, avalanches and storms.
- Obtain good instruction.
- Avoid becoming too fatigued.
- Company – have somebody close by to support, observe or supervise.
- Avoid alcohol and drugs which increase bravado but reduce competence.
- Beware of extreme weather conditions:
  — hyperthermia and dehydration follow excessive exertion in hot, dry climates
  — hypothermia can develop quickly in cold or wet climates if caught out, for example, with a broken leg in an isolated area.
- Use all the recommended safety equipment and make sure appropriate rescue or life-saving services are readily available.

If the basic precautions are observed and the necessary skills acquired, there is no reason at all why the younger person – and even older people – should not engage in and thoroughly enjoy a range of new sporting and leisure activities while travelling or on a holiday.

SWIMMING AND DIVING

A common and not fully appreciated hazard abroad is drowning or neck injuries when swimming and diving (see also pp. 184–189).

Drowning is the second most common form of traumatic death in travellers after RTAs, typically in an apparently quiet stretch of river or beach where the current or tide is much stronger than expected or where there are rocks or snags under water. Another potentially tragic scenario is the sudden impulsive plunge into the shallow end of a pool or off a rocky foreshore into shallow water. Every year young people are brought home permanently paralysed from the neck down following such accidents.

When planning to swim – a few simple rules

- Do not do so if you have been drinking alcohol.
- Be aware of the water temperature and the tides and currents, especially the undertow.
- Swim where other people are around.
- If there is a beach patrol or lifeguard service, only swim in the approved places.
- Be very careful when using airbeds or inflatable dinghies if there is an offshore wind – if in doubt, do not proceed. It is very easy to be blown out to sea then panic, jump off the raft, and find yourself too tired to swim. Invariably it is better to stay with anything that floats, try to attract attention and await rescue.

There are a few special circumstances during sporting and leisure activities that need to be considered in more detail.

Sunburn

Sunburn will occur in individuals who are exposed to an excess of sunlight above their normal or tolerable exposure. The degree of sunburn depends on the intensity of the sun, the length of exposure and the pigment in the skin. The lighter and more freckled the skin and the redder or more blonde the hair, the greater the chances of severe sunburn. During acclimatisation, and even afterwards, the use of a sunscreen cream will prevent excessive burning; the higher sun protective factors (SPFs) give the greatest protection. An adequate intake of fluid and salt during the acclimatisation period will help to avoid sunstroke (see also Ch. 9).

Bites and stings

In many parts of the world, travellers may be bitten by animals or stung by insects. Most bites should be treated as at home, but there are increased risks from a wide range of exotic creatures. These range from bites, and rarely suffocation, by snakes in Australia, India, Africa and South America, stings from scorpions in North Africa, attacks from 'game' animals in Africa and India, to unfamiliar insect stings. The bite of the *Anopheles* mosquito can result in malaria.

There are hazards from the sea. Apart from the well-publicised shark attacks, other possibilities range from barracuda bites and starfish and jelly-fish stings, to cone shell poisoning and coral grazes. Local knowledge is most valuable, in order to be aware of the risks and the remedies. It is beyond the scope of this text to list them all here (see also Ch. 11).

Managing dog and other animal bites

- All animals can be affected by rabies, but dogs spread it to humans most frequently because they are domesticated.
- The wound should be carefully cleaned and an injection of tetanus toxoid and prophylactic antibiotics may be required. (Consider a tetanus booster before travelling.)
- Active rabies vaccination (primary courses or boosters) should be considered if the traveller has been to a rabies endemic area. Rabies-specific immunoglobulin can be used for recent bites in high-risk situations when the patient has not previously been vaccinated (see also Ch. 12).
- Monkey bites can result in monkey-pox, a smallpox-like illness with generalised vesicular rash after a 5–17 days' incubation period. The illness is usually mild but deaths have occurred in children. Treatment is supportive.
- Herpes virus (type B) can be contracted from rhesus or Macaque monkey bites from the Old World, usually Africa, and causes a serious, predominantly neurological, infection. Treatment is supportive but aciclovir may help.

Extreme environments

The very adventurous and intrepid traveller may seek out more extreme environments of high mountains, deserts, ice caps and the ocean. In all of these areas, special precautions are required.

One problem that catches out quite a few travellers to more exotic places is mountain sickness. This can affect anyone, including experienced mountaineers, at over 2500 m if the proper acclimatisation has not taken place. The increasing popularity of trekking in the Himalayas has exposed a new group of people not always fully prepared. There are three forms of high altitude sickness – acute mountain sickness, high altitude cerebral oedema and high altitude pulmonary oedema (see pp. 198–199 and Ch. 18).

Winter sports injuries

Downhill and cross-country skiing, snowboarding and tobogganing are becoming increasingly popular.[9–16] Over 1 million people from the UK take skiing holidays each year in the Alps of France, Switzerland and Italy, also in Spain, Austria, Norway and the USA. Other winter sports enthusiasts also travel long distances to the slopes.

In contrast to the regular skiers in the alpine and snow-covered countries, many of the occasional followers of winter sports are inexperienced and unfit. Lack of awareness of the hazards, poor clothing and equipment, excessive alcohol and bravado may contribute to accidents and injuries.

Another contributing factor is the degree of enforced slope management. In the USA, for example, alcohol is positively discouraged on the slopes and antisocial or dangerous antics may result in withdrawal of a ski pass. Professional winter sportsmen and women earn their living from the sport so it is in their interest to remain fit and avoid injuries but they are taking their activities to the limit and so are more exposed to injury than the casual winter sports enthusiast.

Sledding and tobogganing are often done in a more casual way with improvised equipment, sometimes in the dark, and in unfamiliar surroundings. A more recent fashion is snowboarding, sometimes regarded as one of the 'adventure' or 'extreme' sports. Participants not only descend ski slopes at high speed, but they also may engage in gymnastic and acrobatic activities that can easily result in serious injury, both to themselves and others.

SKI INJURIES

The overall rate of ski injuries varies with activity and age and experience but it ranges between 2 and 10 injuries per 1000 ski days. The rates have fallen steadily in most ski centres around the world, but a change in the pattern of injuries has resulted in more upper than lower limb injuries. The injury rates are generally higher in the younger skiers, with the highest rate of all being in those under 10 years. Key risk factors are extreme youth, being male, inexperience, doing a late run, excessive speed and an excess of alcohol. School parties may be more at risk than others because of bravado and inexperience. Showing off, doing complicated aerial manoeuvres and pole planting (sticking ski pole into the snow to execute a rapid turn) are all contributory factors.

The injuries sustained in winter sports vary with the activity and the equipment used. Skiing injuries are typically sprained ankles and knees, fractures of the lower or mid tibia, contusion of the anterior cruciate ligament of the knee and avulsion of the thumb, especially on dry ski slopes where the thumb gets caught in the matting ('skier's thumb'). Alpine or fast downhill skiing is an inherently dangerous sport with a high risk of injury.

Snowboarders typically get fractures or sprains of the wrist, shoulder contusions or dislocations and other upper limb injuries. Both groups, along with tobogganers, can get facial, head, neck and spinal injuries and concussion, usually from colliding, hitting an object or falling headfirst.

Collisions are responsible for only around 10–15% of winter sports injuries, although they can sometimes be very serious. Being overwhelmed by bad weather or an avalanche is a rare but often tragic event and usually happens when skiers are 'off piste' in unsupervised areas.

SKI EQUIPMENT

There is concern that there has recently been an increase in concussion and head injuries, especially in the younger skiers. While the value of helmets is beyond doubt and often compulsory in some sports, for example competitive horse-riding and mountain biking, their use remains controversial in skiing. The benefits of a lightweight, aerodynamic ski helmet need to be weighed against the possible impairment of vision and hearing. The balance is probably in favour of younger skiers wearing helmets. It is particularly important for younger children to be equipped with modern, well-maintained equipment and not with ill-adjusted, 'hand-me-downs' from older siblings. Good quality ski boots and correctly adjusted, quick-release ski binders have reduced ankle injuries. There remains controversy over hard versus soft boots, as the harder and more rigid the boot, the greater the chance of high torsion forces. This should of course be offset by correctly adjusted ski bindings. Correctly fitting boots and binders, using correctly adjusted, release equipment according to age, height, weight and experience, have all contributed to reducing below-knee injuries. Modern ski bindings do not, however, prevent injury to the knee.

NUTRITION, FLUID INTAKE AND FATIGUE WHEN SKIING

Skiers and other sports participants, at home and abroad, often neglect to take account of their carbohydrate and fluid and electrolyte needs. They require a high muscle, glycogen build-up using a high carbohydrate (pasta) diet the day before exercise, and continuing, high carbohydrate intake during and after exercise. They also require copious fluid intake, using sports drinks with glucose polymers and electrolytes as well as water. A golden rule, seldom observed, is to drink until your urine is pale.

The use of stretching and warming-up exercises prior to skiing is very important, but seldom practised, and 'just one more run' when fatigued and with tired muscles is a recipe for increased injury risk. Injuries are more common 'before lunch' and when the slopes are about to close.

Other winter sports activities include mountaineering and trekking, ice-climbing and high altitude canoeing, rafting and hang-gliding. In all of these activities, some of which can also be classed as 'extreme sports', the participants

To reduce winter sports injuries

- Get fit in advance of your holiday.
- Be fully trained for the degree of skill required.
- Avoid excessive fatigue – keep up your carbohydrate and fluid intake.
- Exclude alcohol.
- Be fully familiar with the terrain and the hazard involved, including avalanche potential.
- Keep on a piste suitable to your level of competence.
- Keep a constant look-out for other skiers and snowboarders.
- Observe adverse weather warnings.
- Use appropriate protective clothing, boots and safety equipment.
- Consider helmets for younger skiers and snowboarders.
- Learn to fall correctly and to release your ski stick before it causes 'skier's thumb'!

To minimise the risk of mugging

- Travel in groups.
- Avoid remote areas after dark.
- Use a torch.
- Keep on the move.
- Carry an alarm or an anti-personnel spray (may be illegal in some countries).
- Wear modest clothing – do not display wealth.

are usually well trained and well aware of the hazards. The risks remain very high indeed, for example, in high-altitude mountaineering, with a significant mortality and serious injury rate, which is amongst the highest of all the sporting and leisure activities.

Participants in all of these winter sports activities should read expert guides relating to their particular activity and to be fully conversant with basic survival techniques in cold climates.

Comprehensive insurance is essential and should include provision for repatriation in the event of serious injury – otherwise, it may cost the equivalent of several future holidays to get home.

Other accidents

VIOLENCE

All travellers must be fully aware of the possibility of becoming victims of crime or violence. Regular reports of tourists being mugged and even killed perhaps exaggerate the real risk. In some countries like Scandinavia, the Arabian Gulf and Japan, the risk is very small, but in parts of South and Central America, USA, Africa and South-East Asia, once off the beaten track, the risks can be quite high.

Where there is civil war and terrorism or a potential for it, the traveller is always at risk. Stray bullets or explosions may hit an innocent bystander. In modern wars, 75% of those killed and 90% of those wounded are civilians. In exceptional circumstances, the traveller may be taken hostage.

Currently, high-risk areas include Somalia, Ethiopia, Sudan, Mozambique, Angola, Rwanda, Burundi, the Middle East, Afghanistan, Cambodia and southern states of the former Soviet Union.

In areas where human rights are not respected, any encounter with the law should be avoided. Torture, beatings, rape, severe deprivation and hypothermia are all possible consequences.

DISASTERS

Travellers may become inadvertently involved in natural disasters such as volcanic explosions, earthquakes, hurricanes, floods or bush fires.[17–20] Visitors may be at more risk than local residents because they are more likely to be visiting remote areas. They will also be less familiar with the local hazards. Some travellers take a vicarious pleasure in climbing to the rims of active volcanoes or witnessing the ravages of hurricanes and floods. For most people these natural events are so terrifying that they do not go out of their way to get involved.

On active volcanoes people are overwhelmed by lava flows, and are killed by volcanic rocks, by burns and scalds, and by toxic fumes. In hurricanes, deaths are caused by the sheer force of the wind, by flying objects, by loss of boats at sea, and by flooding. The danger in floods stems from the physical force of the water, causing people to drown and later the spread of infection resulting from disruption to water supplies and sewerage services. As well as causing objects to fall, and buildings to collapse, earthquakes can spark off fires that are started by electrical faults and leaking gas supplies. Deaths from suffocation are common. Tidal waves (tsunamis) which follow may also cause drowning. People die in bush fires from direct burning and smoke inhalation.

When overwhelmed by natural disasters, it is remarkable how often people can survive by sheltering under cover, for example, during hurricanes. After earthquakes, specialist teams have found survivors by means of heat-seeking devices and sniffer dogs after up to 2 weeks. People have survived in open boats and life-rafts with the minimum of water and rations for several weeks.

During bush fires, there comes a time when it may be safer to lie under a non-flammable shelter (possibly a car or lorry, but there could be a risk of petrol explosion) or to jump into a watertank or pond than to be overwhelmed by fire. The fire moves so quickly that as long as one has enough oxygen, it is possible to survive and wait for the flames to pass over.

Following any major disaster, all the emergency services are put to full stretch and people with minor injuries will have to fend for themselves. The most useful action travellers can take is to keep calm, offer help to others where necessary and tend their own wounds. For days and sometimes weeks after a disaster, especially if there is massive disruption of the public utilities (water, gas, electricity, telephones and sewage), there is high danger of looting and violence, and also of epidemic diseases like cholera and malaria. There is also a need for considerable physical and psychological support for the victims and their relatives.

KEEP CLEAR OF DISASTER AREAS ('ACCIDENTS WAITING TO HAPPEN')

Certain natural and man-made hazards have a greater potential to become 'disaster areas'. These include active volcanoes, dry forests, flood plains and ravines, avalanche areas and all earthquake and hurricane zones. They also include certain forms of mass transportation, very large crowds, high-rise hotels with poor emergency escape routes, power stations, chemical plants and any area of civil, military or terrorist conflict.

Although many an adventurer will find it exciting and challenging to face these hazards, and

some do it as an extreme sport (like climbing active volcanoes), the more prudent will make serious attempts to avoid known or potential hazards areas wherever possible. However, even the best prepared can get caught out through no fault of their own. Here we are genuinely moving into the 'act of God' arena for which no amount of warning can prepare. Once caught up in the situation, individuals will have to use all of the survival skills they can command.

For the vast majority of tourists and travellers, the best cause of action is to distance themselves from possible disaster at the earliest opportunity. This may prove difficult as transport facilities may already be stretched or even disrupted. If this is the case, it may be better to stay put as long as you are not in or close to the disaster zone.

The only exception might be the individual with skills in the health or technical fields who could genuinely be of assistance to the authorities dealing with the disaster. Too often they are embarrassed by a plethora of advice and support and anything that is offered must be properly coordinated and controlled, ideally by trained and official organisations.

Concern is often expressed about liability although there are few medical professionals who would refuse to 'save a life' if in this situation. Some medical insurance companies will cover their clients in certain situations abroad such as when they are on aircraft of their national airline. Individuals should check this with their own insurer.

WARNING THE TRAVELLER

If a traveller is in any doubt about impending disasters, or indeed about travel information generally, they can tune in to one of the local 'Travellers' Information Systems' (TIS) radio stations. Information about these is typically found at state or international boundaries, especially in North and Central America.

IATROGENIC (OR DOCTOR-INDUCED) RISK

It is recognised that there is always a risk when undergoing any form of medical treatment. The risks vary greatly depending on the individual and the disease being treated, the method of treatment and the competence of those carrying out the treatment.

In many parts of the world, regrettably, we must retain a strong index of suspicion about the competence of many medical and nursing staff to make an accurate diagnosis and to carry out correct treatment. Minimal interest in health and woefully inadequate facilities often compound the problem. There may be poor training, supervision and sometimes incompetence.

> **Beware of the following when undergoing medical care**
>
> - Inhalation or spinal anaesthesia
> - Blood and fluid transfusions
> - Surgical operations
> - Serious bone and joint manipulations
> - Antibiotic treatment (possibility of side effects)
> - Unsterile injection needles and vaccinations.

The traveller in most of Europe, North America and Australasia will receive good treatment. In many other parts of the world there are very competent doctors and nurses practising often under very difficult circumstances. If you are at all unsure about your diagnosis or treatment, it is quite justifiable to ask for an interpreter or for another doctor. The embassy or consulate office, the university hospital, private hospitals and clinics or a church or missionary hospital will often be able to help. If there is still a lingering doubt, insist on repatriation. It helps if you have comprehensive insurance to cover this.

HOMICIDE AND SUICIDE

Homicide

In most assaults or muggings from robbery or rape, the attacker does not intend to kill the victim. However, in some circumstances, notably in parts of the USA – and most typically in Florida – the attacker may be on drugs or mentally ill and therefore of 'diminished responsibility', or just so criminal that the taking of life is merely part of the overall robbery. The average tourist will be most unfortunate to be involved but it does happen.

Suicide

Suicide is a different matter since this is a deliberate attempt by the person to take his or her own life. The majority of people who are at risk of taking their own lives are not likely to be travelling. However, it is always possible. These are situations for which no special rules apply in relation to travel. They are the same as for other circumstances where suicide is likely.

ACCIDENTS IN THE 'DISADVANTAGED' AND THOSE WITH EXISTING MEDICAL CONDITIONS

Disadvantaged people or those with existing medical conditions – including older people, pregnant women, the physically disabled, those with sensory disabilities, the mentally ill, people with learning difficulties and those dependent on drugs and alcohol– all have higher risks of accidents and this also applies when they are travelling.

Rather than expect the disadvantaged person to be aware of, or necessarily capable of dealing with the many problems experienced by travellers, there is often a responsibility on the attendants or carers to be fully aware of the risks and to take the necessary precautions. This is not to say that disadvantaged people should not travel, often they will not want to anyway. But if they do wish to travel, they should be afforded every opportunity, always bearing in mind their special needs and vulnerability are taken into account. Many of the organisations that regularly take disadvantaged people abroad, for example on the pilgrimages to Lourdes, will be fully equipped for this purpose so that the risks of accidents can be reduced to a minimum.

Summary of measures to prevent serious accidents

SAFETY AND SECURITY

All companies and organisations that regularly send staff abroad are strongly advised to make contact with one of the specialist organisations that can advise on security and safety precautions. These organisations have a very effective intelligence network which is constantly kept up to date about 'hot spots', high-security-risk areas and terrorist activity. In addition, they prepare pamphlets and bulletins and carry out training programmes designed to help anyone who is travelling abroad to the more high-risk areas.

Safe travellers are the ones who are as fully prepared as possible for all contingencies. They are psychologically and culturally well adjusted and physically fit. They are aware as possible of all the hazards that they will face. They will have fully prepared themselves with as much information as possible from their travel agent, from embassies and from specialist organisations. They will have taken all the necessary health advice from their doctor or a travel medicine clinic which will include being up to date with tetanus and rabies vaccinations if post-exposure vaccine is not likely to be available.

INSURANCE

For the majority of travellers it is wise to get as comprehensive an insurance policy as possible. Many policies specifically exclude certain, high-risk activities, so studying the 'small print' is important. Others can be comprehensive but at a prohibitive price. It is important to check to see just exactly what kind of treatment is covered and what type of repatriation, if any, is allowed. If not fully covered, travellers may find themselves incurring very heavy repatriation fees, which are beyond their means. Equally, in certain countries, but most notably the USA, they can find themselves incurring astronomical medical fees.

THE INITIAL RESPONSE TO AN INJURY

If an injury is sustained abroad travellers are usually more concerned about how they will be treated than when they are at home in familiar surroundings. Sometimes their fears will be justified. In general terms, the more developed the country concerned, the better will be the standards of medical care but there are exceptions. Carrying and understanding how to use a first aid kit[21] is essential.

MINOR INJURIES

Cuts, grazes and burns should be treated with respect since infection is more common in countries where heat, dust and poor hygiene are the norm. They should normally be covered after careful cleaning. If there is an open wound, the possibility

Possible contents for a first-aid kit for injuries
All to be kept in a compact, plastic (or heavy-duty nylon), zip-up, waterproof bag (or bags). *Note:* The contents will vary according to the needs of the traveller but the smaller the better.

Equipment
Thermometer – mercury or 'fever scan' skin strip
Scissors and tweezers, possibly as part of Swiss army knife
Safety pins, micropore tape, surgical gloves, gauze swabs

Wound dressings
Cotton wool (cotton buds), antiseptic wipes (alcohol)
Bandages – light, adhesive plasters
Plaster sutures 'Steristrips'
Crepe bandages

Special equipment for 'high-risk' areas (all pre-packaged and sterile)
Intravenous fluid kit, sterile needle drip set, plasma expanders
Suture kit, or needles and holder

Bottles – small
Oil of cloves – for toothache
2% tincture of iodine

Tablets to be considered
Antibiotics for wound infections
Analgesics of varying strengths
Anaesthetic (local 'spray on')
Anti-emetics

Ointments and creams
Eye ointment (e.g. chloramphenicol)
Antibiotic ointment for skin (e.g. Fucidin or chlortetra-cycline)
Burns (e.g. Flamazine)

Protective agents
Mosquito net, insect repellent
Sunscreen cream, lipsalve
Compeed for blisters

Documentation
First-aid instruction book
Details of blood group (chronic illness and regular medication, if any)
Official letter explaining kit is for personal use only
Immunisation records (e.g. for tetanus and rabies)

of a foreign body, any sign of infection or if the injury was due to a bite, urgent professional advice should be sought. Large and deep cuts will probably need to be sutured. Sprains and strains may sometimes be self-treated with initial rest, analgesics and then mobilisation. If a fracture is possible, the injury should be properly diagnosed and correctly treated. You can treat fractures of fingers and toes as long as they are not displaced or compound by strapping two or more digits together.

PRACTICE POINTS

- Although they receive wide publicity, accidents in the air or at sea are very rare.
- Being aware of the possible risks and taking steps to avoid injuries should always be the first priority.
- Common accidents include sports injuries (skiing, cycling), swimming accidents (slipping around pools and getting out of depth or carried away by current at sea), and road accidents, especially when using motorbikes (traffic on opposite side of the road, poorly maintained road surfaces, poor vehicle servicing).
- Foot injuries on the beach, for example, are common in those not wearing shoes.
- Unfamiliar sea creatures (e.g. fish or molluscs) and caterpillars may be unexpectedly venomous.
- Dogs in many countries run wild and will respond aggressively when approached.
- All travellers should be insured to cover accidents as well as other illness, and cover for repatriation is also important.

REFERENCES

1. Paixio MJ D'A, Dewar RD, Cossar JH, et al. What do Scots die of when abroad? Scottish Medical Journal 1991; 36: 114–116.
2. Baker TD, Hargarten SW, Guptill FS. The uncounted dead – American civilians dying overseas. Public Health Reports 1992; 107: 155–159.
3. Hargarten SW, Baker TD, Guptill K. Overseas fatalities of United States citizen travellers: an analysis of deaths related to international travel. Annals of Emergency Medicine 1991; 20: 622.
4. Steffen R. Travel medicine – prevention based on epidemiological data. Transactions of the Royal Society for Tropical Medicine and Hygiene 1991; 85: 156–162.
5. Fairhurst RJ. Accidents and the traveller. Travel Medicine International 1996; 1: 33–44.
6. Prociv P. Deaths of Australian travellers overseas. Medical Journal of Australia 1995; 163: 27–30.
7. Carey MJ, Aitken ME. Motorbike injuries in Bermuda: a risk for tourists. Annals of Emergency Medicine 1996; 28: 424–429.
8. Petridou E. Epidemiology of road traffic accidents during pleasure travelling: the evidence from the island of Crete. Accident Analysis and Prevention 1997; 29: 687–693.
9. Bladin C, McCrory P. Snowboarding injuries: an overview. Sports Medicine 1995; 19: 358–364.
10. Crisp T. Ski trauma: prevention and treatment. Practitioner 1995; 239: 88–94.
11. Deibert MC, Aronsson DD, Johnson RJ, et al. Skiing injuries in children, adolescents, and adults. Journal of Bone and Joint Surgery 1998; 80A: 25–32.
12. Harlow T. Factors predisposing to skiing injuries in Britons. Injury 1996; 27: 691–693.
13. Kocher MS, Dupre MM, Feagin JA Jr. Shoulder injuries from alpine skiing and snowboarding. Aetiology, treatment and prevention. Sports Medicine 1998; 25: 201–211.
14. Macnab AJ, Cadman R. Demographics of alpine skiing and snowboarding injury: lessons for prevention programmes. Injury Prevention 1996; 2: 286–289.
15. Pigozzi F, Santori N, Di Salvo V, Parisi A, Di Luigi L. Snowboard traumatology: an epidemiological study. Orthopaedics 1997; 20: 505–509.
16. Salminen S, Pohjola J, Saarelainen P, et al. Alcohol as a risk factor for downhill ski trauma. Journal of Trauma 1996; 40: 284–287.
17. Alexander D. Natural disasters. London: UCL Press; 1993.
18. Auf den Heide E. Disaster response. Principles of preparation and co-ordination. St Louis: CV Mosby; 1989.
19. Bouma MJ, et al. Global assessment of El Nino's disaster burden. Lancet 1997; 350: 1435–1438.
20. Coburn A, Spence R. Earthquake protection. Chichester; Wiley; 1992.
21. First aid manual – The authorised manual of St John Ambulance, St Andrew's Ambulance Association, The British Red Cross Society. London: Dorling Kindersley; 1995.

BIBLIOGRAPHY

Alexander D. Natural disasters. London: UCL Press; 1993.

Auf den Heide E. Disaster response. Principles of preparation and co-ordination. St Louis: CV Mosby; 1989.

Coburn A, Spence R. Earthquake protection. Chichester: Wiley; 1992.

Hargarten SW. International travel and motor vehicle crash deaths; the problem, risks and prevention. Travel Medicine International. 1991; 9: 106–110.

Illingworth RM. Expedition medicine. A planning guide. Oxford: Blackwell Scientific; 1984.

Keatinge WR. Survival in cold water. The physiology and treatment of immersion hypothermia and of drowning. Oxford: Blackwell; 1969.

Noji EK. The public health consequences of disasters. New York: Oxford University Press; 1997.

Martin J. Accidents Abroad. Healthy Practice. 1997; 10: 46–47.

McIntosh I. Accidental trauma and the vacationer. Travel Medicine International 1997; 15: 15–18.

Wilkerson J. Medicine for mountaineering and other wilderness activities. 4th ed. Seattle: The Mountaineers; 1992.

Wilson E. Personal risks for foreign travellers. Practice Nurse. 1996; 11: 599–605.

Swimming and sub-aqua diving

Eleanor Wilson

Introduction

This chapter considers hazards associated with swimming and deep sea diving. Most of the material is taken from studies and safety practice in the UK but the principles of prevention are universal. In many, particularly developing, countries, standards may be very different from those to which the traveller is accustomed. In the same way as 'water from the tap' may not be safe, water in swimming pools and even the sea may be heavily contaminated. Cost and equipment may limit the attention given to filtration and sterilisation. Legally required environmental controls may not be present or may be disregarded in many less developed countries.

Swimming

Swimming is a recreation enjoyed by many of all ages. Indeed, second only to walking, it can be an ideal, all-round sport, giving freedom to many who by reason of disability are denied participation in many other activities. The majority of those actively involved do so throughout the year in well-supervised facilities at sports centres, swimming baths and in smaller, sometimes less well-supervised, hotel pools. In the summer, beaches, rivers, lochs, canals and reservoirs provide alternative locations.

SAFETY MEASURES

In the UK, a guidance booklet, *Safety in Swimming Pools*, prepared and published as a joint venture by the Health and Safety Commission and the Sports Council[1] is the main source of reference on safety.

This booklet covers all pools used for swimming and leisure except:

- pools used for medical and therapeutic purposes (while in use for such purposes)
- private swimming pools in domestic premises
- paddling pools.

Regional environmental health departments are responsible for these pools. The guidance notes also have limited application to pools that consist of segregated areas of rivers, lakes and sea.

The Health and Safety Executive is the enforcing authority for local-authority-run pools, school premises and other pools (including leisure complexes) except where the main activity is the provision of residential accommodation. At pools that form part of residential accommodation (hotels and holiday camps), enforcement is the responsibility of the local authority, usually the environmental health department.

The purpose of the guidance notes is to provide an authoritative starting point for swimming pool operators and managers to assess requirements for safe operation at their premises as is required by the Health and Safety at Work Act 1974.

Relevant regulations are numerous and directed at many aspects of pool safety, including but not exclusively:

- the safe design of pool structure, systems and equipment
- maintenance requirements and safe systems of work
- pool water purification and sterilisation system
- supervision arrangements to safeguard pool users
- equipment for use by swimmers.

There are nine appendices to the document, one of which imposes upon swimmers, responsibility for their own safety. Recognised as the 'swimming pool users' safety code', the six points identified therein were the outcome of collaboration with the Royal Society for the Prevention of Accidents (RoSPA).[2]

In the introduction to *Safety in Swimming Pools*, it is estimated that 3–5% of drowning occurs during the 150 million visits per year to swimming pools. While each of these is a personal tragedy, it nevertheless indicates that safety is much more secure within the confines of a supervised and controlled swimming pool environment than it is in the sea, river or other open waterway. RoSPA reported 317 drownings in outdoor water settings in 1996–7. Greater attention, however, is now being directed to water safety outdoors. Advisory notes for local authorities and others pertaining to this are available from RoSPA.

'ILLNESS AND INJURY' ASSOCIATED WITH SWIMMING ARISE FROM BOTH RISKY ACTIVITIES AND ENVIRONMENTAL PROBLEMS

Personal failings

Young males tend to overestimate their swimming ability, even when in unfamiliar territory, swim irrespective of previous eating and drinking, and ignore safe swimming areas. These statements are supported by figures appearing in the press, themselves drawn from official UK statistics, and in a report by RoSPA[2] which stresses that the majority of *accidents* involve young males between the ages of 15 and 24 years and alcohol consumption plays a major role.

Water contamination

The Scotsman newspaper of 2 October 1998 stated that:

> Almost half of bathing beaches in Scotland failed to reach minimum standards of hygiene this summer (1998), equalling the worst ever year on record. High levels of sewage and other pollutants mean that eleven favourite holiday

spots around the country are more of a health hazard than places of recreation.

Perhaps the greatest testimony to the degree of convergence on water contamination has been the willingness on the part of the World Health Organization expert group to create guideline values for recreational water quality based on epidemiological evidence.

Infection from drinking water while swimming

As steps towards the global eradication of poliomyelitis achieve success, it is expected that the transmission of polio by water contamination will continue to decline. However, hepatitis A, typhoid and cyst-borne infections remain possible. Microorganisms, which could give rise to gastrointestinal infections, are usually rapidly diluted and dispersed, thereafter being removed by filtration systems. Enterovirus infections have occurred.[3] *Giardia lamblia* has been identified in an outbreak in a swimming class.[4]

Where illness is the sequel to ingestion, the most probable causes are swimming in untreated pools or in contaminated river or pool water, particularly if close to sewage discharge pipes. The degree of infection will be proportional to the level of contamination and length of exposure. Individual levels of resistance will determine the severity of any ensuing illness.

Skin infection

The human skin and mucous membranes are covered with a variety of non-pathogenic organisms which, given certain conditions, can become pathogenic.

This can occur in several ways:

- bathers, and to a lesser extent, mains water or treatment plants, concentrating microorganisms in the pool water
- contaminated floor surfaces, furnishings and fomites
- direct contact with other more vulnerable members of the public
- atmospheric aerosols.

The microorganisms from bathers that pollute a swimming pool, surrounds and atmosphere are those of the upper respiratory tract, stool, urine, skin, hair and scalp. Viable organisms from infected open cuts and wounds may also be present.

Two of the most common skin infections, well established as foot infections spread particularly in changing rooms, are tinea pedis (athlete's foot) and verruca (plantar warts).[5]

Additionally *Escherichia coli*, *Pseudomonas aeruginosa* and *β-haemolytic streptococci*, all of which are associated with wound infections have been implicated in cases of swimming-pool-acquired infections.[6]

Apart from the possibility of bacterial skin sepsis, hookworms and *Strongyloides* may gain entry as may also the Schistosoma cercaria.

Ear infections

Otitis externa is often caused by *Pseudomonas aeruginosa* when contracted in a swimming pool setting[5] while Gram-positive bacteria such as *Staphylococcus aureus* have been frequently implicated in cases of swimming-pool-contracted otitis externa.[7]

Otitis media is more likely to be due to upper respiratory tract organisms. Differences in pressure, owing to submersion in pool water, may force infected mucus into the middle ear, and respiratory and nasal discharge, expelled by other bathers, may gain access to the Eustachian tube via the outer ear.[5]

Eye infections and irritation

Conjunctivitis may be due to infection with microorganisms or caused by chemical or physical irritation. The water in swimming pools needs to be isotonic otherwise severe irritation can ensue. Freshwater, which is hypotonic, and seawater, which is hypertonic, readily give rise to irritation-induced conjunctivitis. Chlorine compounds in high concentrations or exposure over prolonged periods and chemicals such as algaecides predispose to excessive lachrymation, blurred vision and irritation.

Central nervous system

Prior to the introduction of poliomyelitis vaccination in 1956 and treatment of swimming pool water, polio was a serious risk. At the 1948 Olympic Games in Monte Carlo, the British breaststroke swimming champion developed and died from swimming pool contracted poliomyelitis.

Naegleria fowleri, a free-living amoeba inhabiting warm, muddy environments, has been associated with rare cases of fatal meningo-encephalitis further to swimming in polluted waters,[5] while several outbreaks of amoebae-related meningitis have been reported from New Zealand and Czechoslovakia.[7]

Human immunodeficiency virus

The risk of becoming infected by this virus, as a result of participating in swimming pool activities, is considered to be unlikely,[7] but occupational exposure of personnel in life-saving situations merits different considerations. Although, under laboratory conditions, the virus is capable of survival for a period of 14 days in water, it is readily de-activated by the addition of 0.5 mg of free chlorine per litre of water.

OCCUPATIONAL HAZARDS FOR SWIMMING POOL ATTENDANTS

Occupational exposure of employees to health risks within swimming pool areas is greater than that to the general pool user. Although the main risks are slips, trips and falls, additional hazards exist. Work in confined spaces, the use of electrical equipment and storage and handling of chemicals are required work activities. Uncontrolled escapes of chlorine gas have occurred. Disinfectants are strong, oxidising agents thereby increasing the flammability of many materials. Many, when mixed, give off highly toxic vapours, therefore care is essential to ensure that those used as water disinfectants are not mixed with those used for cleaning surrounds. Sodium hypochlorite, commonly handled by attendants, is highly corrosive to skin, eyes and clothing.

Extrinsic alveolitis or hypersensitivity pneumonitis[8] as a result of inhalation of organic or inorganic particulates by sensitised persons has been reported from the UK and elsewhere. Affected employees were chiefly those working in enclosed 'flume areas' for extended periods of time prior to the realisation of there being a potential problem.

Accidents related to swimming

While most accidents follow slips on the wet surrounds of swimming pools, the presence of sea snakes (especially in the coastal waters around Asia and the Western Pacific), jelly fish, spined flat fish and submerged rocks contribute to potential hazards of swimming in the sea in these areas.

A report in *The Glasgow Herald* (July 1998) related an incident in which a 15-year-old boy swimming from a boat during a sailing holiday in the Western Pacific died. Death was presumed to have resulted from a bite and envenoming by a sea snake.

Unfortunately, each year also brings cases of hypothermia and drowning.

UK AND EUROPEAN SURVEILLANCE OF ACCIDENTS

The Leisure Accident Surveillance System (LASS)[9] run in tandem with the Home Accident Surveillance System (HASS)[10] is a monitoring system within the UK. Data are collected by the Consumer Safety Unit of the Department of Trade and Industry with reference to the essential characteristics of outdoor product accidents, the LASS reports falling within the international definition of 'leisure accidents'. Accidents are classified according to the cause, circumstance and outcome, and records from the unit are entered into the leisure accident database. From this information, the proportions and national estimates for each accident type can be calculated.

Data collection and processing are a cooperative effort between NHS Hospital Trusts and the Department of Trade and Industry. Conforming to set criteria, 18 hospitals throughout the UK participate in the scheme. Accident interviewers, working with medical and reception staff in the participating hospitals, record accident details in casualty departments, then transmit this information to the central database. For the LASS, only 11 of the 18 hospitals are used. The amassed information is supplied to the Commission of the European Community for inclusion in the European Home and Accident Surveillance System (EHLASS).[11] A classification system, common to all of the European Community countries, is then used, so enabling inter-country comparisons to be made.

The database records only a small number of fatal accidents. Since relatively few deaths occur during or after treatment in accident and emergency units, these cases are not considered representative of fatal cases as a whole.

In the 20th Annual Report from the Consumer Safety Unit, namely the 12-month period commencing January 1996, LASS analysed all accidents occurring within a multitude of categories, one of which was the recreation environment site. The swimming environment accounts for a further six sub-divisions as follows:

- outdoor swimming pool
- indoor swimming pool
- unspecified swimming pool
- water slide/flume
- other swimming equipment
- diving board.

A cumulative total of 1052 swimming-related accidents appear within the report. Sustained injuries are numerically greater than the number of accidents, and the majority are capable of being categorised as relatively minor. Affecting mainly the upper and lower limbs as a result of body or equipment clashes, there are, nevertheless, reports of more serious injuries to head and neck, mainly as an outcome of water entry or foolhardiness.

Overseas accident figures are difficult to estimate since information is not readily available. However, in a paper presented at the Asia Pacific Conference in Hong Kong in 1996, Dr Richard Fairhurst (Chorley and South Ribble NHS Trust) reported on his study of 7934 consecutive incidents to travellers from the UK who attended his own hospital. The study covered a 12-month period in 1994 and although, numerically, swimming-and-diving-related accidents were small, they were significant because of the severity of injuries sustained.

According to a report from RoSPA in 1997, figures for death by drowning totaled 440, but not all were swimming accidents. Of those that were, locational settings of inland waterways proved to be the main danger areas. RoSPA has an area of responsibility extending to a water area distance of 5 miles outward from the shoreline.

International comparisons for mortality rates in respect of accidents can be obtained in figures published by WHO, and for those within the European Community, data are provided by the Eurorisc Project, Peach Unit, Royal Hospital for Sick Children, Yorkhill, Glasgow.[12]

Eurorisc findings

Eurorisc data in Table 8.5 show the population totals, the number of accidental drownings and submersions and the rate per 100 000 population for 14 European Community member states. Generally, 1993 data is used, but the data for Ireland and Spain are from 1992. Belgium is excluded because the last available mortality data is for 1989. Luxembourg has been included in the table, although it is excluded from the more detailed Eurorisc work because of its small population size.

TABLE 8.5 Data for drownings and submersions in Europe 1992–3

Country	Year	Population	Drowned	Rate per 100 000
Austria	1993	799 200	117	1.46
Denmark	1993	518 900	37	0.71
Finland	1993	506 700	119	2.35
France	1993	5 765 400	583	1.01
Germany	1993	8 147 200	655	0.80
Greece	1993	1 036 800	279	2.69
Ireland	1992	354 900	60	1.69
Italy	1993	5 685 900	582	1.02
Luxembourg	1993	39 900	10	2.51
Netherlands	1993	1 529 100	90	0.59
Portugal	1993	987 600	81	0.82
Spain	1992	3 900 500	682	1.75
Sweden	1993	871 900	119	1.36
UK	1993	5 819 200	229	0.39

HYPOTHERMIA

Hypothermia follows immersion in cold water and particularly affects children who have a greater relative surface area and small subcutaneous fat and energy stores. A fall in body temperature follows immersion, the body response to which is, initially, an increase in heat production by shivering and an attempt to reduce heat loss by vasoconstriction

As the body temperature drops below 35°C:

- shivering stops
- there is a reduction in ventilation prior to ventilatory arrest
- body metabolism slows
- cardiovascular involvement gives rise to hypotension, sludging of blood, myocardial electrical instability with arrhythmias and arrest
- metabolic acidosis.

Further deterioration accompanies falling body temperature. At between 35°C and 32°C, hypothermia is considered to be moderate.

In severe hypothermia (below 32°C), victims appear to be dead but can survive, and every effort should be made to continue resuscitation efforts until rewarming procedures have returned body temperature to normal. Children, especially, have a good chance of survival. 30% of children with fixed, dilated pupils on rescue recover neurologically intact.

NEAR-DROWNING

As would be expected, most drowning out-of-doors occurs in summertime whether it is in the UK or abroad.

Pathophysiology

Unlike most other emergency situations, respiratory arrest precedes cardiac arrest. It is often associated with hypothermia

A highly influential factor is the 'cold challenge': the colder the temperature, the longer the heart can remain stopped without major problems. Limitation is dictated by the development of ventricular fibrillation.

In cold water drowning (i.e. temperature 10°C or below)

The victim's initial response is an inspiratory gasp followed by hyperventilation. This can precipitate death by inhalation of water and wet drowning. It may also precipitate sudden hypertension, severe cardiac arrhythmias and arrest.

In the short-term (up to 15–20 minutes), there is inability to cope with cold shock. As hyperventilation, continues, both swimming and breathing become uncoordinated, leading to water inhalation and wet drowning. In the longer-term, there is hypothermia, wet drowning, and ventricular fibrillation.

Lung injury

This is caused by water inhalation. 10% of drowning cases have not got water in the lungs and only rarely is there more than 1.5 L.

Brain injury

Hypoxia results in cerebral oedema and the lower the temperature, the less the injury. Cerebral oedema may increase as the patient warms up.

It is important to remember that, when a rescue is achieved:

- During immersion, the hydrostatic pressure of water lends support to an otherwise compromised circulation.
- As the victim is removed from the water, this support is withdrawn and this may cause catastrophic circulatory collapse (similar to suddenly deflating a pneumatic antishock garment).
- This effect may be exacerbated by over-rapid warming.

THE FUTURE

An optimistic outlook is contained within RoSPA's review of 1996–7,[2] where the following paragraph appears:

Drownings reported in the UK for last year were the second lowest on record according to statistical analyses, and although the figure remains high, it reflects the possibility that many people may, at last, be beginning to heed the warnings.

A word of caution

RoSPA in respect of water and leisure safety, has identified the need for a consensus on package travel safety abroad. Working on an estimate of 10–14 million UK citizens who holiday abroad each year and who may not enjoy the same safety standards as in the UK, it is continuing to work with the travel industry to encourage and improve high standards of safety in package travel abroad.

A word of optimism

Equal optimism for future, hotel, swimming pool safety abroad is portrayed in a review article in *Holiday Which?* (September 1996) further to an inspection of 39 hotels at favourite holiday destinations (20 pool hotels in Turkey and 19 in Gran Canaria). Although, scathing in its criticism of the lack of safety standards at the majority of inspected sites, a reply from 10 of the 11 to which a letter outlining deficiencies was sent, was received within a 2-week period from date of issue. Contrary to ideas commonly promulgated by some tour operators that there is a resistance to improve standards abroad, the replies indicated not only a willingness to comply, but evidenced that in some, work had already commenced, the remainder having plans drawn up for imminent action.

Sub-aqua diving

Diving can be viewed as either recreational or occupational.

RECREATIONAL DIVING

- Near flat dives from the side of pools.
- Dives from varying heights above the water surface as in the use of springboards and diving platforms.

The above can be considered as a means of water entry after which very little time is spent below the surface. Clearly, accident potential exists and accidents occur but facts are not readily available. In Dr Fairhurst's paper at the Asia Pacific Conference in 1996, injuries to head, neck, limbs and spine featured prominently in the section, covering water sports but injuries specific to diving were not recorded.

Scuba diving

The use of self-contained, underwater, breathing apparatus allows participants to remain below the water surface at varying depths for varying periods of time depending on training, experience and ability.

Injuries can be sustained, for example, as a result of poor technique, faulty equipment or shark attack, but illness rather than injury is the main hazard.

In the UK, the Diving Regulations, which set the minimum standards of fitness required, impose a level of control. Nevertheless, annually there are reports of between 150 and 200 cases of serious dysbarism in civilians. As many travellers holiday outside the UK to pursue their hobby, it is to be expected that some incidents will take place overseas.

OCCUPATIONAL DIVING

People who enjoy diving may be attracted to particular occupations where the hobby can be used professionally. Arising out of and in the course of employment, others are required to become divers either as a means of travel to a destination for carrying out operational procedures, for example in the deep sea oil industry, or for more prolonged duties. General groupings can be considered under the headings of installation and commissioning, salvage and reclamation, and maintenance and repair and rescue work. The Health and Safety at Work Act 1974 (p. 181) and the delegated legislation of the Diving Regulations set standards and controls for employers and employees. Those working at depths greater than 50 m and saturation divers (i.e. where a diving bell is in use and with workers remaining submerged for many days) usually have their own occupational health services and medical back-up offshore. These situations are beyond the scope of this chapter.

PROBLEMS OF DESCENT

Dysbarism

- As a diver descends, the surrounding water pressure increases by 1 bar every 10 m (33 ft).
- As pressure increases, gases become compressed.
- Human tissues are compressible but hollow spaces (e.g. sinuses and lungs) are not. Unless gas can enter these spaces, either the space will collapse (abdomen, chest, lungs) or extra fluid or tissue will be drawn into the spaces (e.g. sinuses). Termed as compression barotrauma (compression dysbarism), a variety of body parts can be affected.

Ear compression barotrauma

This is a relatively common problem, especially in inexperienced divers. It arises when there is general, unequal pressure on one side of the tympanic membrane. Injury to the membrane may result in either haemorrhage or rupture. Although the incidence of round window rupture is rare, the only management is urgent assessment by a specialist in ear, nose and throat care. Symptoms of both problems are very similar:

- tinnitus
- disorientation
- giddiness.

Sinus compression barotrauma

If the openings to the sinuses are blocked because of catarrhal swelling or polyps, then pressure equalisation between sinuses and upper respiratory tracts cannot take place and the following can result:

- on descent, the volume of air in the sinus decreases. Owing to the rigidity of the bone in the sinus, a negative pressure develops, thereby drawing transudate in.
- there will be damage to the mucosal lining of the sinus.
- if large vessels are involved, haemorrhage may be severe.
- rarely, there may be facial nerve neuropraxia.

Pulmonary compression barotrauma

This occurs only in breath holding divers and is rare.

- On descent, the volume of gas in the lung decreases and becomes more dense. (At a depth of 30 m (99 ft), the pressure has increased to 4 atmospheres.)
- The lung volume gets smaller until it nears residual volume thus changing the chest configuration to one of expiration. Further descent and ever-increasing pressure give rise to 'chest squeeze' where there is haemorrhage into the alveoli.
- Signs are dyspnoea with respiratory distress, cyanosis, ventilatory insufficiency and pulmonary oedema.

Management is aimed at redressing the balance by: careful evacuation to the surface (in the horizontal position), oxygen administration (100% where possible) and if necessary, artificial ventilation using positive end expiratory pressure (PEEP).

PROBLEMS OF ASCENT

Decompression illness and decompression barotrauma

This occurs on return to atmospheric pressure following significant exposure to increased pressure (depth- and time-related). It is usually a consequence of expanding gas and inert gas bubble formation but it may also occur after any dive in which air is breathed from a self-contained, underwater, breathing apparatus.

Usually it follows poor, diving discipline, equipment failure, accidents and/or panic. It has also, rarely, occurred during ascent, as gases expand. If this pressure reduction is over rapid, problems for the body arise in two ways:

Systemic decompression barotrauma. Gases, normally dissolved in the blood, form bubbles. These may be either intra- or extravascular and, depending on which, can cause either a mechanical effect blocking arterioles or a reaction at the bubble/tissue interface which can result in protein denaturation, lipid emboli, red cell sludging, platelet aggregation, activation of clotting mechanisms and histamine release.

Pulmonary decompression barotrauma and air emboli

During ascent as the air in the lung expands, the diver should breathe out. Failure to do so, or in a situation where a mucous plug may obstruct an alveolus, increasing intra-alveolar pressure causes rupture. This rupture may extend through the visceral pleura to cause pneumothorax. It may also extend anteriorly to cause pneumopericardium, mediastinal emphysema and subcutaneous emphysema or into the pulmonary veins causing air embolism, leading to arterial air embolism which usually affects the brain or limbs but can affect any body part.

Mild and serious decompression

In practice, decompression illness has a wide spectrum of symptomatology, often making it difficult to differentiate between the two types:

Mild decompression illness. Symptoms usually begin within the first hour of surfacing but can be delayed for up to 24 hours (very occasionally longer). Complaints are usually of unexplained fatigue, malaise and anorexia, transient pruritus, especially of the ears, hands and wrist, and musculoskeletal pain around synovial joints (limb or joint bends).

'The bends' are usually of an aching character to begin with, often attributed wrongly to recent physical exertion. Initially, this ache may flit from joint to joint, but, later, the pain becomes more severe and localised. The most common sites are knee and shoulder. It is extremely rare for there to be any associated tenderness and, if present, another cause should be considered.

Skin rashes appear on the trunk and abdomen owing to cutaneous venous stasis; the limbs, owing to cutaneous and subcutaneous oedema or on any body part owing to bubble formation in the lymphatics.

Serious decompression illness. Appearance is usually within a few minutes of surfacing. However, it can be delayed for several hours. Neurological effects are the most common and involve brain, spinal cord and rarely the peripheral nerves.

Cerebral decompression illness results in unconsciousness, visual disturbance (particularly peripheral vision), migraine-like headache, behavioural changes (e.g. personality, cognitive and mood) and symptoms or signs mimicking a cerebral vascular accident

Pulmonary decompression ('the chokes') may develop slowly and cause pneumothorax, retrosternal pain on inspiration, dyspnoea and hypoxia in severe cases.

Circulatory effects are due to a rise in capillary permeability resulting in hypovolaemia, haemoconcentration, hypotension and peripheral circulatory failure.

Important warning

Any symptoms presenting within 36 hours of a dive should be considered as being caused by dysbarism until proven otherwise. Diving dysbarism may be complicated by other associated conditions such as near-drowning, hypothermia and carbon monoxide inhalation.

Advice on medical diving problems

The Royal Navy provides a 24-hour emergency advice service. This gives information on:

- the location of nearest, medical, diving-problem treatment facility (recompression chamber)
- the emergency management of diving-related illness.

The telephone number is: 0831 151523 (cell phone). If there is difficulty in obtaining a reply, use Portsmouth 01705 822351, ext. 41769 during the day or 01705 818888 out of hours.

State clearly that there is a diving problem.

PRACTICE POINTS

- Ignoring the risks from currents, both undercurrents near the shore and tidal currents, are common causes of accidents at sea. In developing currents, coastguard warnings can be absent or unreliable.
- Various sea snakes, jellyfish, and poisonous spiny fish are potential hazards when swimming at sea although minor injuries to feet from discarded glass and metal objects on the beach are more common.

PRACTICE POINTS (cont'd)

- Hypothermia can kill very quickly, within minutes, both at sea and in cold, inland lakes.
- In swimming pools, diving and slipping on wet surroundings are common causes of accidents.
- Sub-aqua diving is very dangerous for the inexperienced – training and qualified supervision are essential.

REFERENCES

1. Health and Safety Commission and the Sports Council. Safety in swimming pools. A guidance document. London: HMSO.
2. The Royal Society for the Prevention of Accidents (RoSPA) Review 96–97. Birmingham: RoSPA.
3. Lenaway DD. An outbreak of an enterovirus-like illness at a community wading pool: implications for public health inspection programmes. American Journal of Public Health 1979; 7: 889–890.
4. Harter L, Frost F, Grunenfelder G, et al. Giardiasis in an infant and toddler swim class. American Journal of Public Health 1984; 74(2): 155–156.
5. Emslie J. Infections associated with swimming pools and spas, Stirling Seminar Paper 1984. Environmental Health in Scotland 1984; 1(5): 8–10.
6. Ross PW, Peutherer JF. Clinical microbiology. Edinburgh: Churchill Livingstone; 1987.
7. Storey A. Microbiological problems of swimming pools. Environmental Health 1989; 7(10): 260–262.
8. Lynch DA, Rose CS, Way D, et al. Hypersensitivity pneumonitis diagnosed in a population of swimming pool employees. American Journal of Roentgenology 1992; 156(3): 469–472.
9. Department of Trade and Industry. 20th Annual Report, 1996. London: HMSO.
10. Department of Trade and Industry. 19th Annual Report, 1995. London: HMSO.
11. Department of Trade and Industry. EHLASS UK Report, 1996. London: HMSO.
12. Eurorisc Newsletters 1 and 2. Eurorisc Project, Peach Unit, Royal Hospital for Sick Children, Glasgow.

FURTHER READING

Kizer KW. The scuba diving traveller. Travel medicine advisor. Water Activities 24.1–24.7.
Newmann K. Illness from water-related recreational activities. Travelling Health 1995; 8:4.
Pruss A. A review of epidemiological studies on health effects from exposure to recreational water. International Journal of Epidemiology 1997; 27: 1–9.
Royal Society for the Prevention of Accidents. Drownings in the UK. 1997. Birmingham: RoSPA.

CONTACT INFORMATION

Health and Safety Commission, Rose Court,
    2 Southwork Bridge, London, SE1 9HS.
Royal Society for the Prevention of Accidents: Rospa.co.uk

The effects of altitude on health

Andrew J. Peacock

Synopsis

Increasing numbers of Westerners are travelling to the high altitude regions of the world. As these regions have sparse medical care, it is essential for both travellers and their general practitioners to understand the possible consequences of high-altitude travel and how to prevent and treat those syndromes that are either caused by or made worse by high altitude.

This chapter describes the effects of altitude on human physiology, the process of acclimatisation to altitude, the diseases specifically associated with altitude and also those diseases that are made worse by altitude or commonly occur in high-altitude areas of the world. A comprehensive understanding of this chapter should allow the practitioner to advise adequately anyone proposing to travel to altitudes of up to 5500 m (18 000 ft).

Introduction

Increasing affluence and thirst for adventure lead many lowlanders to travel to the high-altitude regions of the world such as Tibet, Nepal, Northern India, Chile and Peru. It is no coincidence that these regions also happen to be amongst the poorest, and as a consequence the medical facilities and the transport necessary for urgent medical evacuation may be virtually non-existent. Thus anyone wishing to travel to these regions should have a working knowledge of the problems associated with altitude, how to prevent them and how to treat them.

The inhabitants of the affluent Western countries live mostly at fairly low altitudes, indeed Leadville, Colorado at 3048 m (10 000 ft) is the highest town in either Europe or North America where people live continuously. It is a long tradition in Western countries to travel to high altitude regions for the purpose of skiing holidays but in most instances participants in winter sports sleep at low altitude and only travel briefly to a high altitude before skiing down. This has meant that the incidence of high-altitude illness amongst recreational skiers has remained very low; low enough that little interest has been taken in diseases associated with altitude. In recent years however, trekking and mountaineering have increased enormously. It is estimated that approximately 30 000 Britons will travel to Nepal each year and may well travel to altitudes of up to 5500 m (18 000 ft), the height of Everest base camp. When trekking, the altitude exposure is prolonged and the trekker is unable to sleep low and therefore unable to follow the old mountaineering adage: climb high but sleep low. Undoubtedly it is the continuous 24-hour exposure to high altitude that causes the problems.

The principal reason that altitude can be harmful to health is the relative decrease in partial pressure of oxygen as one goes higher. This hypoxia has many effects that will be described below and is also the principal cause of potentially fatal, high-altitude illnesses, such as acute mountain sickness, high-altitude pulmonary oedema and high-altitude cerebral oedema.

What is high altitude?

Traditionally high altitude is considered to be altitudes between 2400 and 4300 m. These are the sort of altitudes encountered in ski resorts. It is generally believed that 2400 m is the threshold for altitude sickness and therefore people travelling to altitudes below this should not fear altitude-related problems.

Very high altitude is 4300–5500 m. This is the altitude of many high-altitude base camps such as Everest and K2. At this height, altitude-related illness is common, particularly if the travellers ascend quickly. In 1975, a study by the Himalayan Rescue Association at Pheriche in Nepal showed that 69% of trekkers who flew into 2825 m and then hiked to Everest base camp at 5350 m suffered from mountain sickness.[1]

Extreme altitude exists between 5500 and 8848 m (the summit of Mount Everest). At these altitudes, not only are there risks of altitude-related illness but there is also high-altitude deterioration in the form of progressive dehydration, weight loss and possible cerebral damage.

This chapter focuses on altitudes up to 5500 m, since altitudes above this will only be experienced by mountaineers who necessarily will need specific advice and will usually have medical support as part of their expedition team.

Why does high altitude cause problems?

The principal reason why humans travelling to high altitude suffer from pathophysiological consequences is exposure to hypoxia. The fraction of oxygen in the air remains unchanged at 20.9% but as we ascend, the atmospheric pressure falls and with it the partial pressure of oxygen. As a rule of thumb, the atmospheric pressure is one-half of normal at 5500 m thus the partial pressure of oxygen is also one-half of normal. At the summit of Everest it is one-third of normal. Until recently, it was believed impossible that man could climb to that altitude without oxygen. In fact, Rheinhold Messner and Peter Habeler did climb Everest without oxygen in 1978 and since then a further 38 climbers have made it to the summit without the addition of bottled oxygen. These heroic physiological feats are rare, and are possible only for perfectly acclimatised supermen. The reason why some people can cope with these extraordinary altitudes and others cannot remains unclear.

Figure 8.1 shows graphically the sorts of altitudes experienced in different situations with corresponding % oxygen available compared with sea-level.

It should be noted that the cabin altitude of commercial aircraft is between 1830 and 2430 m (6–8000 ft) which is not a problem for healthy individuals but could of course cause difficulties for those with chronic lung disease. Apart from Leadville, Colorado, there are people in other parts of the world, notably South America, who live continuously at altitudes of 4860 m (16 000 ft). Despite the fact that these populations have lived in these areas for a long period they still suffer the consequences, and have an increased incidence of chronic mountain sickness, miscarriage and pulmonary hypertension.

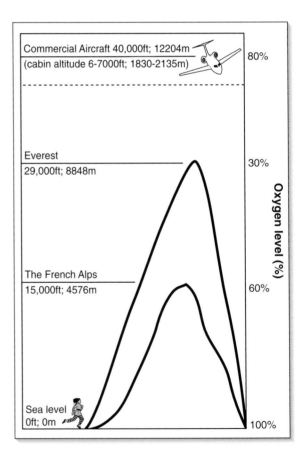

Fig. 8.1 Oxygen-level availability at varying altitudes (reproduced by kind permission of the British Lung Foundation).

There are two other main environmental insults associated with high altitude: low temperatures and dehydration. These are important because acute mountain sickness is more common when the subjects are also cold and dehydrated. Furthermore, hypoxia reduces metabolic heat production, making frostbite and hypothermia more common at higher altitudes than at sea-level for a given temperature insult.

Dehydration occurs because humidity in the air falls at higher altitudes and, since all the air that we breathe is warmed and saturated with water vapour, we can lose huge amounts of water in the expired air. In addition, it is often difficult to maintain hydration when trekking through deserted, unpopulated areas. Everyone travelling to altitude should be told to take adequate, warm clothing and a flask of at least 1 L in capacity to replenish water loss and plan to drink 3 L per day.

Effects of altitude on human physiology

LUNGS

Adequate oxygenation depends on central respiratory drive, an intact chest wall to provide the negative pressure pump, unobstructed airways and adequate gas exchange across the alveolar capillary membrane. Each part of this system may be affected by high altitude.

High altitude affects the lung in different ways

- Ventilation
- Airway function
- Gas exchange

Ventilatory control

The most obvious change is that in ventilation. It is well known that the principal control of ventilation at sea-level is provided by the CO_2 response curve. As arterial CO_2 rises, chemoreceptors switch on ventilation to keep PaCO_2 at a normal level of about 5 kPa. The CO_2 response curve is linear, unlike the hypoxia response curve which is non-linear. Hypoxic ventilatory response commences in most people when the inspired PO_2 falls to less than 12 kPa (equivalent altitude 3100 m). This is the point at which the oxygen dissociation curve steepens and the purpose of the reflex is to preserve the partial pressure of arterial oxygen above 8 kPa such that haemoglobin saturation remains more than 90%. As the inspired PO_2 falls further below 12 kPa there is an exponentially steep rise in the ventilatory response and it has been thought in the past that an inadequate ventilatory response to hypoxia is responsible for mountain sickness. The evidence for and against this hypothesis remains controversial[2] but the most recent studies suggest that there is a poor correlation between the hypoxic ventilatory response and the incidence of mountain sicknesses such as high-altitude pulmonary oedema.

Another effect of hypoxia on control of breathing is the prevalence of periodic breathing or Cheyne–Stokes breathing at altitude. This occurs particularly during sleep and is very disruptive to sleep quality. It can be a frightening experience to spend the night in a mountain hut with a group of other climbers or skiers in the typical dormitory arrangement. Nearly all of them will be 'Cheyne–Stoking' and to a trained medical practitioner this can be very unnerving since we normally associate this symptom with severe left ventricular failure or central nervous system damage.

Ventilatory control seems to be even more affected at night. Normally at sea-level there is a slight decrease in arterial oxygen saturation and increase in partial pressure of carbon dioxide during sleep. These are insignificant physiologically. At altitude, these effects are worsened, for example at 4300 m the normal sea-level value for oxygen saturation of 96–98% will be reduced to 86%, but this will fall a further 10–76% during the night. There is some evidence that the carbonic anhydrase inhibitor acetazolamide will prevent the desaturation. Acetazolamide works by making the cerebrospinal fluid more acidic. This has a consequence of driving the medullary respiratory centre and preventing deoxygenation. The role of this drug in prevention and treatment of acute mountain sickness will be discussed later.

Airways/parenchyma

The airways are fairly resilient to altitude but patients with asthma may get worse. This is because they are inhaling large volumes of cold, dry air that is a bronchial irritant. They need to be warned to take extra prophylactic medication. Interestingly, though there are no formal studies, there is little evidence of significant deterioration in asthma, which may be due to the decreased allergen exposure at altitude.

- There is little evidence of deterioration of asthma at altitude.

On the whole, gas exchange at the peripheral diffusion barrier is well maintained at altitude; indeed, the alveolar arterial gradient for oxygen may in fact narrow. This is so unless high-altitude pulmonary oedema develops when the alveoli are flooded with high protein oedema, gas diffusion is severely impaired and the alveolar–arterial gradient widens.

There is no reported effect of hypoxia on the respiratory muscles but at altitude there is catabolism of all muscular protein and it would not be surprising if there was also loss of respiratory muscular power. This however remains unstudied.

HEART

The Operation Everest II studies in which a group of fit, young men were decompressed in a chamber over 40 days to the 'altitude' of the summit of Everest showed that cardiac function is remarkably well preserved at altitude.

- Cardiac function is well preserved at altitude.

It is known that acute exposure to altitude raises cardiac output and initially the ratio of cardiac output to work rate is inefficiently high. However, with acclimatisation cardiac output falls to sea-level values as does heart rate which initially rises but later falls providing altitude is less than 4500 m. At altitudes above 4500 m, heart rate stays persistently raised. It is apparent that stroke volume is unchanged and left ventricular ejection fraction is actually increased, suggesting that myocardial contractility is preserved. Systemic blood pressure does not seem to change with altitudes up to 4600 m and after a year at altitude may actually fall. Indeed the incidence of systemic hypertension is lower in lowlanders living at high altitude. The principal effect of hypoxia on the cardiovascular system is on the pulmonary circulation. Unlike systemic arterioles that dilate, pulmonary arterioles contract when faced with low levels of oxygen.

- Principal cardiovascular effect of hypoxia is on the pulmonary circulation: pulmonary vessels contract whereas systemic vessels dilate.

The reason for this reflex is thought to be twofold: first to close down the pulmonary circulation while the fetus is in utero because oxygenation is provided by placental blood flow and, second, in the adult to preserve ventilation perfusion matching in the lung when there are isolated ventilatory defects. This may be beneficial for patients suffering from localised lung disease but for a subject going to altitude where generalised hypoxia is experienced, the effects are a rise in pulmonary artery pressure and a strain on the right ventricle. This can be catastrophic and the pulmonary vasoconstrictive response reflex is likely to be at least partially responsible for the syndrome of high-altitude pulmonary oedema which will be discussed later.

RENAL AND ENDOCRINE FUNCTION

The effects of high altitude on salt and water balance are complex. They are important because excessive fluid retention that occurs with poor acclimatisation

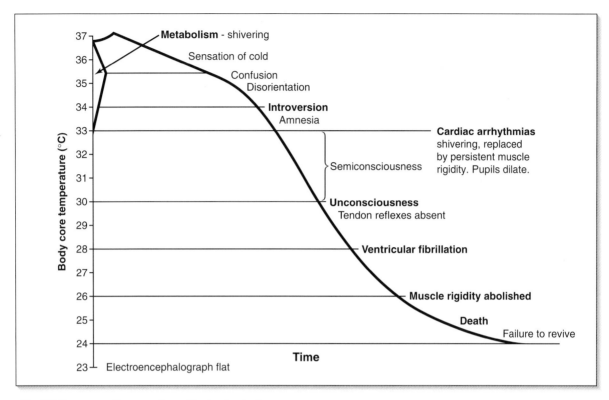

Fig. 8.2 Symptoms of 'exposure' to cold related to body core temperature.

may be an additional factor responsible for mountain sickness and high-altitude pulmonary and cerebral oedema. It is likely that the principal hormones responsible for salt and water balance, namely the hypothalamic–pituitary–adrenal axis and atrionatriuretic peptide levels are disturbed in hypoxic conditions but the exact changes that occur are still the subject of intense research. It is known that antidiuretic hormone does not change. Aldosterone levels initially fall but are normal after 15–20 days at altitude. However, there is a decreased response of aldosterone to renin. Aldosterone and plasma renin activity rise on exercise. Atrionatriuretic peptide is increased in hypoxic conditions and increases further when the subject exercises at altitude. It should be noted that acute mountain sickness often occurs following a bout of exercise at high altitude. As far as adrenal activity is concerned, there is a rise in plasma noradrenaline but plasma adrenaline remains unchanged. These adrenal hormone shifts are accompanied by an increase in heart rate initially but, as stated above, this falls back to sea-level

values after 5–7 days. Thyroid function is relatively undisturbed. Thyroid stimulating hormone remains unchanged but thyroxine levels may rise, possibly because of movement of the hormone from the extravascular to intravascular compartments. Control of blood sugar is maintained but acute hypoxia will raise blood sugar by almost 2 mmol. Chronic hypoxia is associated with a mild rise in blood sugar level, a decrease in insulin level and a diminished insulin response during the glucose tolerance test.

Renal function is relatively undisturbed but there is an increase in proteinuria by a factor of two for reasons that remain unclear.

CENTRAL NERVOUS SYSTEM

Preservation of central nervous system (CNS) activity is the primary function of the cardiopulmonary axis. CNS tissue does not regenerate once it is damaged and hence recovery may not occur following hypoxic damage to the brain.

- Hypoxia damages CNS function and this may not recover.

Factors that are important for cerebral function are:

- the degree of hypoxia
- the state of the cerebral circulation.

The principal control of cerebral circulation is by the arterial partial pressure of carbon dioxide ($PaCO_2$). This regulates the relationship between arterial blood pressure and cerebral blood flow, which is a sigmoid relationship rather like the oxygen dissociation curve. Over a limited range of fall in pressure, there is no fall in flow but below a critical mean pressure of approximately 50 mmHg, there is a steep fall in cerebral blood flow. Since blood pressure does not change a great deal at altitude, it is likely that the principal effects are due to a shift of this curve by change in CO_2 and O_2. Hypoxia causes dilatation of cerebral blood vessels and they may increase in size by up to 500%. However, the hypoxia is often accompanied by a fall in arterial PCO_2 and $PaCO_2$ which has the opposite effect. Measurements have been made at 3800 m where it was found that the combination of hypoxia and hypocapnia caused an increase in cerebral blood flow of about 24% at 6 hours. This had fallen to 13% at 3–5 days. It is worth pointing out at this stage that cerebral blood flow is further compromised by a rise in packed cell volume, a necessary consequence of hypoxia-driven erythropoietin secretion and erythropoiesis. It is reasonable to say that the relationship between cerebral blood flow, cerebral function and high-altitude cerebral oedema is at present uncertain.

There has been concern over a number of years that cerebral function can be disturbed by hypoxia. Certainly at altitudes above 4500 m (very high altitude), there is a decrease in arithmetic and writing ability and eye–hand coordination worsens. Of greater concern is that some of these abnormalities may persist long after return to sea-level altitude. The American Medical Research Expedition to Everest showed that 1 year after subjects had been to altitudes above 8000 m there were significant decrements in verbal learning and memory, verbal expression and finger tapping

speed. It should be remembered that these subjects were using oxygen for their ascent of the mountain. The cause of this neurological damage remains uncertain but since retinal haemorrhages are very common at very high altitude, it is possible that it is due to a combination of diffuse intracerebral haemorrhage, hypoxia and changes in cerebral blood flow. The effects on sleep have been described above. At altitudes over 2500 m (high altitude), sleep is disturbed, subjects will awake unrefreshed and may actually be awoken during the night by the periodic breathing. At these altitudes, between 60 and 90% of sleep is periodic and during the apnoeic periods there is profound desaturation. This is apparently all related to loss of central control of breathing and is probably significant because the nocturnal hypoxaemia may be responsible for some or all of the responses to the hypoxia of high altitude.

One of the problems of the high packed cell volume and hence sluggish cerebral circulation is the higher incidence of thrombotic stroke. This occurs particularly where there is dehydration and, not surprisingly, the accompanying hypoxia makes any damage sustained worse. Prevention and treatment of stroke will be discussed below.

GASTROINTESTINAL SYSTEM AND NUTRITION

One of the more obvious features of travelling to high altitude is that nearly everyone loses weight. This may not be of great significance to trekkers and may even be welcomed by some, but for mountaineers it can be disastrous. Profound loss of weight during walk-ins to mountain base camps means that the climber is already debilitated before getting to the stage of the serious technical aspects of climbing the mountain. The initial weight loss, which occurs very rapidly, is fluid loss. Following the fluid loss there is progressive loss of body tissue, especially muscle. The cause of this weight loss is multi-factorial. Appetite is poor, there is relative malabsorption and basal metabolic rate rises. It was found that above 5000 m there is definite anorexia and most people will become increasingly selective about what they eat, preferring easily digestible carbohydrate to protein and fat. Basal metabolic rate may rise about 10%, especially if the weather is cold. Weight loss is proportional to body fat but protein is also lost. At high and very high altitudes the weight lost is about 25% lean but at extreme altitudes above 6300 m the reverse is true and 75% of the loss is lean. Obviously there are important consequences for high-altitude climbing where muscle bulk is necessary for the technical aspects of difficult climbs. Muscle wasting appears to be in the smaller fibres and is associated with an increase in capillary density.

It has been found that there is no important malabsorption up to very high altitudes of 4800 m but above that level there is decrease in xylose absorption and fat absorption of between 25 and 50%.

There is considerable interest in the composition of diet and its effect on gas exchange. Theoretically, an increase in the carbohydrate component of the diet would increase the respiratory quotients (CO_2 evolved divided by O_2 consumed). The effect of this is to increase the number of alveolar oxygen molecules (PaO_2) for a given number of alveolar CO_2 molecules ($PaCO_2$). This has the effect of promoting absorption of oxygen and hence PaO_2. Perhaps fortunately, most climbers at high altitude prefer a high carbohydrate diet.

BLOOD AND CIRCULATION

The effects of hypoxia are an increase in haemoglobin and increase in the number of muscle capillaries. Of these the most important is the increase in haemoglobin. This increase is caused by two different mechanisms. Initially, on exposure to altitude, there is loss of intravascular volume and, as a consequence, the haemoglobin concentration rises though the total haemoglobin remains constant. However, shortly after arrival at altitude, the effect of hypoxia in the kidneys is to switch on erythropoietin and hence increase erythropoiesis. This results in a sustained increase in haemoglobin and levels between 18 and 20 g/dL may be found in those spending time at very high altitudes. This rise in haemoglobin is a two-edged sword. Clearly, it promotes oxygen carriage because the oxygen content of the blood is directly related to haemoglobin concentration. However, the increase in packed cell volume also results in

more sluggish circulation with an increased incidence of pulmonary embolism, peripheral thrombosis and stroke. All of these are made worse by the accompanying dehydration that can occur particularly amongst climbers at very high and extreme altitudes. This will be discussed further below.

Acclimatisation to altitude

Acclimatisation to high altitude involves a complex series of physiological changes, including changes in ventilation, changes in pulmonary artery pressure, changes in cardiac output, changes in red cell number, changes in the number of capillaries in muscle and altered control of fluid balance. If the subject is well acclimatised then the risk of high-altitude illness is considerably reduced. Thus the medical practitioner must ensure that travellers going to altitudes above 2400 m are considering acclimatisation and have included an acclimatisation schedule in their programme. With the advent of easy access to remote regions of the world it is all too common for people to fly into high-altitude areas, then attempt to climb further with often disastrous effects. It is important to remember that high-altitude acclimatisation is quickly lost. In 1 or 2 weeks, physiology is returned to sea-level values and thus people who are initially well acclimatised and then descend are at risk of re-entry high-altitude illness.

The rate of acclimatisation depends very much on the altitude at which travellers start and the altitude at which they plan to finish. A reasonable schedule below 4300 m is to climb at a rate of no more than 400 m per day. Above 4300 m, this should be reduced to 150–300 m per day and with every third day a rest day. It is very important that the acclimatisation schedule is set for the weakest member of the party and not the strongest.

- Acclimatisation schedule should be set to the weakest member of the party.

If travellers suffer from the effects of altitude, they should ascend no further until these disappear. Simple headache relieved by paracetamol is acceptable but symptoms of nausea, persistent headache and dyspnoea should be taken seriously. Travellers should climb no further until the symptoms have remitted. If they do not remit within 24 hours, then the travellers should descend 300 m and wait until they do.

Diseases specifically related to altitude

SYNDROMES OF ALTITUDE ILLNESS

- Acute mountain sickness
- High-altitude pulmonary oedema
- High-altitude cerebral oedema
- Retinal haemorrhages
- Systemic oedema
- Clotting.

Acute mountain sickness

Acute mountain sickness is a syndrome comprising headache, dizziness, dyspnoea, drowsiness, yawning, poor appetite often associated with nausea and poor sleep related to Cheyne–Stokes breathing described above. On physical examination, there may be few important abnormalities but it is important to exclude crackles in the lung, which might suggest the onset of high altitude pulmonary oedema, and evidence of cerebral oedema. At present we are unable to predict who will develop acute mountain sickness but there is no doubt that individuals vary in susceptibility. One person can travel at the same rate, workload and altitude as another but can manage the climb without any difficulty, while others are prostrate with mountain sickness. There is no doubt, however, that the onset of mountain sickness is related to the rate of climbing, the elevation achieved and the amount of work being done while climbing. A survey in 1975 showed that when trekkers flew in to Lukla at 2825 m and then hiked to Everest base camp at 5350 m, 70% developed some symptoms of mountain sickness.

Thus it is very unlikely that anyone is completely unaffected but some are more resistant than others.

Once the symptoms of mountain sickness develop, the climber should go no higher but should rest at the altitude achieved for at least 24 hours. Providing the symptoms settle down completely, they can then recommence climbing at a slow pace. If the symptoms do not remit with simple measures such as paracetamol and rest at that altitude, then the climber should descend as fast as possible and wait until they do.

> - If symptoms of altitude illness develop, then ascend no further until they remit. If in doubt, **descend!**

The treatment of acute mountain sickness is supportive but there is good evidence that prophylaxis can be achieved by giving acetazolamide 125–250 mg bd. This drug, a carbonic anhydrase inhibitor, probably works by making the CSF acidic and hence drives respiration which in turn has the effect of improving oxygenation.

High-altitude pulmonary oedema

This condition, which is often fatal, has been known about for thousands of years but was only properly described in the 1960s. The symptoms are those of acute mountain sickness accompanied by cough, often productive of frothy, sometimes blood-stained sputum and severe breathlessness. The symptoms are unrelieved by change of posture and there are no accompanying symptoms of infection. In the past it has often been misdiagnosed as pneumonia. In fact, it is a condition where there is leak of high protein fluid into the lungs caused probably by a combination of leaking at the endothelial cell junction and the very high pulmonary artery pressures caused by hypoxic vasoconstriction.

The causes of high-altitude pulmonary oedema are a fascinating subject and are worthy of a whole chapter of their own. It is important to say here that it must be recognised quickly and treated appropriately. The signs are cyanosis, crackles in the lung, high heart rate and high respiratory rate. The immediate treatment is the administration of oxygen if available, sublingual nifedipine 20 mg and then further nifedipine on a 6-hourly basis. These measures however, are only supportive and the most important action is to descend. The patient should be got down as fast as possible, often only 300 m will make a significant difference. If it is impossible to get the patient to a lower altitude, then a substitute is to place the patient in a Gamov bag which can be inflated to artificially raise apparent atmospheric pressure and hence inspired Po_2.

High-altitude cerebral oedema

Like high-altitude pulmonary oedema, the cause of this condition remains an enigma. Even more interesting is that the two do not always go together, although hypoxia is definitely the common link. In this condition there is brain injury then swelling which worsens the injury. The symptoms are headache, poor cerebral function, hallucinations, psychotic symptoms and ataxia. There is obvious loss of cerebral function, inappropriate behaviour is common and retinal haemorrhages are evident on fundoscopic examination. It is important to exclude hypothermia which can cause similar symptoms. This can be excluded by simply measuring body temperature. Immediate treatment is dexamethasone 8 mg IV and 4 mg 6-hourly. Once again, however, the most important action is descent. The patient should be got down the mountain as quickly as possible. An alternative, as indicated above, is to place the patient in a Gamov bag.

Other conditions

Retinal haemorrhages. These are common at more than 4300 m and occur in 30–100% of climbers ascending above 5400 m. They probably represent cerebral injury but do not in themselves cause visual problems. However, they can be very alarming for the expedition doctor.

Systemic oedema. Widespread oedema is fairly common, particularly in those who are acclimatising poorly. It is not in itself an indication of the onset of cerebral or pulmonary oedema but should make the observer watch out for other evidence of a high altitude illness.

Clotting. Initially on ascent to altitude there is loss of plasma volume with a rise in red cell volume and hence packed cell volume. This has the effect of increasing the likelihood of clotting and thrombosis may occur. Particularly worrying are pulmonary emboli or cerebrovascular stroke. The best treatment for these conditions is prophylaxis. It is very important to maintain adequate hydration but in addition many doctors would give 150 mg aspirin daily to all those ascending above 4300 m.

Diseases common in high-altitude areas or made worse by altitude

INFECTIONS

Many infections, particularly gastrointestinal infections, are common in the high-altitude areas of the world. The problem is they respond very poorly to antibiotics at high altitude and often it is necessary to take the patient down 300–600 m in order to treat effectively infections that do occur. The most common problems are acute bronchitis, skin infections and gastrointestinal infections which are nearly always bacterial or protozoal in origin.

LUNG DISEASE

Anyone with lung disease is clearly going to suffer at high altitude. Indeed, they may suffer at the cabin altitude of commercial aircraft. If there is any doubt at all about respiratory function of a trekker, the individual should have a full respiratory assessment in a respiratory clinic before departing.

HEART DISEASE

Heart disease can cause problems in exactly the same way and the same degree of caution and assessment prior to travel are necessary.

Conclusions

There are special syndromes associated with travelling to high altitude, which are a consequence of the hypoxia of altitude. Since many travellers go to altitudes where significant hypoxaemia can be expected, it is necessary for advising medical staff to know what severity of hypoxia to expect at the altitude to which the traveller is going and what likely effects this might have on their cardiac, pulmonary and renal function. Specific syndromes associated with altitude, namely high-altitude pulmonary oedema, high-altitude cerebral oedema and acute mountain sickness can be prevented if sensible precautions are taken. Travellers should also have adequate emergency therapy to treat these syndromes while ensuring that they are brought down to a lower altitude as fast as possible.

PRACTICE POINTS

- Hypoxia, hypothermia, dehydration and accidents are serious risks for mountaineers – careful planning and appropriate equipment are essential to deal with them.
- The excitement of the challenge must be balanced against the danger to both the mountaineers and their potential rescuers.
- The symptoms of acute mountain sickness such as headache, dizziness and drowsiness may not be recognised for what they are and can occur in ski resorts, high-altitude airports and tourist resorts.
- Advance planning should always allow time for slow ascent; there is nothing heroic about struggling on placing both those affected and their companions in serious danger.
- Common high-altitude tourist destinations include the Himalayas in Nepal, Mount Kilimanjaro in Tanzania and the Andes in South America.

REFERENCES

1. Hackett PH, Rennie D, Levine HD. The incidence, importance and prophylaxis of acute mountain sickness. Lancet 1976; 2: 1149–1154.
2. Peacock AJ. High altitude pulmonary oedema: who gets it and why. European Respiratory Journal 1995; 8: 1819–1821.

BIBLIOGRAPHY

Heath D, Williams DR. High altitude medicine and pathology. 4th ed. Oxford: Oxford University Press; 1995.

Houston CS. Mountain sickness. Scientific American 1992; October: 34–39.

Milledge J, Beeley JM, Broome J, Luff N, Pelling M, Smith D. AMS susceptibility. European Respiratory Journal 1991; 4: 1000–1003.

Pollard AJ, Murdoch DR. The high altitude medicine Handbook. New York: Radcliffe Medical Press; 1997.

Vallotton J, Dubas F. Colour atlas of mountain medicine. 3rd ed. London: Wolfe; 1991.

Ward MP, Milledge J, West JB. High altitude medicine and physiology 2nd ed. London: Chapman and Hall; 1995.

Wilkerson J. Medicine for mountaineering. Seattle: The Mountaineers; 1985.

Health risks from the sun and solar skin damage (including heatstroke and heat exhaustion)

Colin Fleming   Rona MacKie

Introduction

Radiation from the sun has been responsible for the birth and development of life on earth for billions of years. Excessive radiation can be damaging, and animals have evolved mechanisms for solar protection. One adaptation obvious in humans is the production of the dark pigment, melanin, in the skin. Fair-skinned individuals have little melanin in the skin. Darker coloured, for example Asian, skin expresses proportionally more melanin, and negroid skin contains relatively large quantities of melanin. It has been proposed that humans originated in equatorial regions where possession of deeply pigmented skin conferred a selective advantage. Light-skinned races are thought to have evolved when humans migrated to temperate regions with relatively little sunlight. Sunlight is needed for production of vitamin D in the skin, and it is suggested that individuals with lightly-pigmented skin metabolised vitamin D more efficiently and thus gained a survival advantage.

In the 20th century, there has been a huge change in the relationship between humans and sunlight. This has partly resulted from cheap global travel. Millions of fair-skinned individuals have been able to visit and live in sub-tropical and tropical climates, and have become accustomed to living with the effects of strong sunlight. There has also been a major change in attitudes to suntanning. The popularity of suntanning has been attributed to Coco Chanel, the French fashion designer, and from the 1930s to the 1970s suntanning became a social norm in light-skinned populations. There is now evidence of a reduction in suntanning in some countries,[1] but sun worshipping is still commonplace in Western cultures and most foreign holidays from countries such as the UK are to sunny destinations.

This increasing exposure to strong sunlight in fair-skinned populations has resulted in changes in the incidence and presentation of sunlight-related diseases. Prevention of these conditions will depend on raising awareness of the effects of excessive sunlight exposure.

The most important effect of solar radiation in humans is in the initiation and promotion of skin cancer. The three main types of skin cancer are:

- basal cell carcinoma
- squamous cell carcinoma
- malignant melanoma.

At present, the most important factor in the development of these cancers is excessive exposure to sunlight.[2] In the last 20 years, there has been a significant rise in the incidence of all three diseases, with a doubling between 1980 and 1990.[3] Around 50 000 basal and squamous cell cancers were treated in the UK in 1993, and there is a 5% annual increase in incidence in these tumours at present.[4] This rise in skin cancer is worldwide[5] and associated with considerable morbidity and increasing mortality.[6] Skin cancer increases with age and is likely to continue to rise in incidence in countries with ageing populations.

Chronic sun exposure is associated with skin thickening, wrinkling, pigmentation, textural change and loss of elasticity, known as photo-ageing. A $12 billion industry has developed in the USA to mask the signs of skin ageing, 90% of which is caused by photoageing.[7]

A number of skin conditions are triggered or exacerbated by exposure to strong sunlight, and may first present when travelling in warm climates. Another group of skin diseases, known as photodermatoses, are characterised by excessive sensitivity to sunlight. Knowledge of solar protection is essential for health specialists preparing such patients for travel to hot countries.

Basic skin biology

A basic knowledge of skin biology is necessary to understand the effects of solar radiation. The skin is the largest organ in the body. It is involved in protection from the external environment, heat regulation, touch, fluid balance, drug and vitamin metabolism and sexual function.

The skin comprises the external layer, the **epidermis**, the supporting tissue of the epidermis, the **dermis** and the **skin appendages** (Fig. 9.1).

The epidermis consists of four main types of cell, the **keratinocyte**, the **melanocyte**, the **Langerhans cell** and the **Merkel cell**.

Keratinocytes produce the protein keratin and are arranged in distinctive layers. Keratinocytes divide in the layer of the epidermis furthest

from the surface, the **basal layer**, and either remain in this layer or migrate towards the surface into the adjacent layer, the **germinative** or **prickle cell layer**. This layer contains most of the living epidermal keratinocytes. Keratinocytes in the germinative layer move towards the surface and slowly die. The next layer from the basal layer is the **granular layer**, which contains dying keratinocytes with disintegrating nuclei. The **horny, or cornified, layer** lies nearest to the surface. It contains compressed, dead keratinocytes which form a strong protective coat.

Melanocytes are found in the basal layer. They produce melanin through the process of **melanogenesis**. Langerhans cells are derived from bone marrow and are found in the dermis and epidermis. They are important in the skin immune system. Merkel cells contain catecholamines and the function of these cells is not well understood at present.

The dermis is the supporting tissue of the epidermis. It contains blood vessels, lymphatics, nerves, collagen and elastic fibres. The dermis also has immune cells such as macrophages and mast cells. These cells release various immune and inflammatory mediators, such as histamine.

The skin appendages consist of hair follicles, and sebaceous and sweat glands.

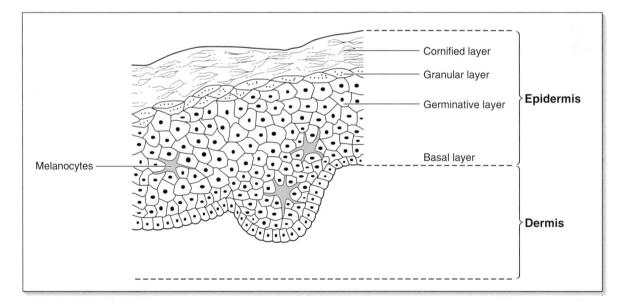

Fig. 9.1 Layers of the skin.

Terms used to describe skin lesions

It is neccessary to have some knowledge of the clinical terms used to describe different types of skin lesions. A list of descriptive terms is shown in Box 9.1.

Solar radiation

Radiation results from energy emitted when an electron moves from a more excited to a less excited state. The energy released has a specific velocity and wavelength, and multiple emissions result in a wavefront of radiation. The electromagnetic spectrum is a term used to describe the spectrum of radiation of different wavelengths, varying from short-wavelength cosmic rays and gamma rays to long-wavelength radar and television waves. Ultraviolet radiation (UVR), visible light and infrared radiation form a small part of the electromagnetic spectrum.

The commonest source of UVR is natural sunlight, but UVR can be emitted from man-made sources such as sunbeds. UVR consists of radiation of wavelength 100–400 nanometres (nm). It is subdivided into UVC (around 100–280 nm), UVB (around 280–320 nm) and UVA (around 320–400 nm).

UVC is potentially very damaging to humans but is normally absorbed by ozone in the earth's atmosphere. If ozone depletion continues, it is possible that UVC will penetrate the earth's atmosphere in sufficient quantities to cause skin cancer and damage to simple life forms essential in food chains.

UVB is important in sunburn, carcinogenesis, photoageing and vitamin D synthesis. UVA is responsible for tanning and photoageing, and recent evidence suggests it also may be involved in carcinogenesis. The amount of UVA reaching the surface of the earth is about 10 to 20 times that of UVB. UVA may also cause sunburn, but only at doses of energy much higher than UVB. UVA is the main type of radiation produced from sunbeds. Visible light generally causes little damage, but some skin conditions may be caused or exacerbated by visible light.

The greater the amount of UVR transmitted to the skin, the greater the risk of damage to the skin. A number of factors will determine the amount of UVR in a given location. Intensity of sunlight increases with decreasing latitude and increasing altitude. Solar radiation is greatest around noon, at the zenith of the sun. UVR is reflected by water, snow, sand and man-made structures (e.g. white walls, glass) and sunburn is therefore made more likely at the sea, at the beach and during winter sports. It is common to confuse the strength of sunlight with the warmth of sunlight, and the burning potential may be underestimated when individuals are cooled by wind or water.

Box 9.1 Definitions of terms used to describe skin lesions	
Macule	Flat, circumscribed alteration in colour or texture of the skin
Papule	Localised elevation of the skin, usually less than 0.5 cm
Nodule	Solid mass in the skin, either projecting above the skin or palpable beneath the skin
Plaque	A flat-topped, elevated area of skin, usually greater than 2 cm
Vesicle	A fluid-filled elevation of the skin, usually less than 0.5 cm
Bulla	A fluid-filled elevation of the skin, usually greater than 0.5 cm, also referred to as a blister
Telangectasia	Multiple, small blood vessels on skin surface
Scale	Flakes of silvery white layers of the corneal layer of the skin
Crust	Dried serum and other exudates
Erythema	Redness of the skin produced by increased blood perfusion

Effects of UVR in normal individuals

SUNBURN

Sunburn is the result of acute, excessive UVR exposure, and is an important risk factor for development of cutaneous malignant melanoma. Although sunburn usually causes only mild

TABLE 9.1 Classification of skin types based on responses to sunlight

Skin type	Response to sunlight
1	Always burns, never tans
2	Usually burns, sometimes tans
3	Sometimes burns, usually tans
4	Very rarely burns
5	Mediterranean-type skin
6	Darkly pigmented skin

symptoms, it appears to be a very common condition, despite recent public sun awareness campaigns. In one report, 38% of children in one area of the UK suffered sunburn in the preceding year,[8] and in a separate study of 2025 British adults, 37% of respondents reported sunburn in the previous 12 months.[9] There has been little research into sunburn in travellers, but in a study of 48 Scottish adolescents,[10] 60% of subjects reported sunburn while on holiday.

Individuals can be categorised according to their tendency to develop sunburn (Table 9.1). This can be useful in assessment of individual susceptibility to UVR, although individuals may be influenced by recent experience of sunburn when reporting their skin type.[11]

Sunburn occurs when UVR penetrates through the skin and causes damage to DNA and cell proteins. Inflammatory mediators are released and an inflammatory response develops. Even mild UVR exposure, sufficient to cause slight skin redness, can cause considerable damage to keratinocytes and melanocytes.[12] Mild sunburn is characterised by erythema, warmth and pain. In more severe sunburn, there is swelling, blistering and weeping of affected skin, with nausea, weakness and fluid loss.

Treatment of sunburn is not usually necessary, but topical steroids, oral fluids, analgesics and non-steroidal anti-inflammatory drugs may be helpful. In very severe cases, hospital admission may be required.

SUNTANNING

Suntanning is due to melanin production in response to UVR stimulation. It may be immediate or delayed. Immediate tanning is due to darkening of existing melanin and delayed tanning results from synthesis of new melanin. Recent evidence suggests tanning is a direct consequence of DNA damage induced by UVR, and therefore tanned skin should be regarded as damaged skin.[13]

One common misconception is that a suntan protects the skin against further UVR damage. Suntanning may prevent further episodes of burning but does not protect against skin carcinogenesis. Evidence for this comes from an Australian study of people who have type 4 skin, that is, those with fair skin but who never burn and always tan in strong sunlight. The rate of non-melanoma skin cancer in these individuals still occurs at the high rate of 400 cases per 100 000 people per year.[14]

SKIN THICKENING AND PHOTOAGEING

One of the early consequences of UVR exposure is thickening of skin. All layers of the skin are affected but most prominent thickening is seen in the cornified layer. These changes are reversible but with prolonged light exposure the skin develops signs of photoageing.

Ageing of skin results from chronological, or intrinsic, ageing and chronic exposure to UVR, or photoageing. Intrinsic ageing produces diminished epidermal turnover and dermal thinning. There are also changes in skin functions such as wound repair and heat regulation. Photoageing produces an exaggeration of all the changes of intrinsic ageing. In addition, large quantities of abnormal elastic and collagen fibres are deposited in the dermis, melanogenesis is increased and the dermal blood vessels become dilated and twisted. The difference between intrinsic ageing and photo-ageing is appreciated when skin is examined in light-exposed and light-spared areas of the body in the elderly. In severe photoageing, the skin becomes dry, rough, leathery, loose, wrinkled and sallow with patchy brown discolouration, black-heads and an increased risk of skin cancer.

Photoageing may be at least partially prevented by regular use of topical sunscreens. Some of the unwanted cosmetic changes of photoageing may be reversed by topical preparations containing retinoid or alpha-hydroxy acid formulations.[15]

Skin malignancy

UVR plays a role in the development of all main forms of skin cancer and several premalignant skin conditions. Travel medicine specialists need to be aware of the aetiology of skin cancer to counsel travellers appropriately about the risks of excessive UVR exposure. It is also important to have some knowledge of the clinical features of skin cancer as early diagnosis and treatment are curative.

Premalignant conditions

SOLAR KERATOSIS

Solar or actinic keratosis is a common dermatosis seen in sun-exposed skin. There is a strong relationship with exposure to UVR and maximum prevalence of the condition is found in the light-skinned population of Queensland, Australia. They are important as an indicator of UVR damage to the skin and as a predictor of development of cutaneous squamous cell carcinoma.[16,17]

Microscopic examination of solar keratoses reveals loss of the normal maturation pattern of the keratinocytes in the epidermis and signs of photoageing in the dermis. The abnormalities in the keratinocytes may progress and develop into the type of cells seen in squamous cell carcinomas.

A solar keratosis usually starts as a small collection of skin capillaries or a persistent area of adherent yellowish, dirty-brown scale on sun-exposed skin. They are usually seen in the middle-aged or elderly. The lesions are often multiple and there is often evidence of sun damage in surrounding skin. Solar keratoses may resolve spontaneously, persist unchanged, ulcerate, or become thicker with a horny surface.

Management of the traveller with a solar keratosis consists of full skin examination to exclude skin malignancy, and sun-avoidance education. Further solar keratoses may be prevented with regular sunscreen use.[18] Superficial lesions are treated with rapid freezing by liquid nitrogen. Large, indurated or multiple lesions may require referral to a dermatologist for treatment.

ACTINIC CHEILITIS

Actinic cheilitis can be regarded as a form of actinic keratosis of the lip. The lower lip is predominantly affected and there is often a history of recurrent sunburn of the lips.

Malignant conditions

BASAL CELL CARCINOMA

Basal cell carcinomas, also known as rodent ulcers, are the commonest form of skin cancer. They are composed of cells similar to those in the basal layer of the epidermis. They present most frequently as slowly growing papules or nodules on the head and neck of middle-aged and elderly individuals. The growth characteristically has a translucent, pearly rolled edge, often with small superficial blood vessels. These tumours rarely metastasise, but can cause extensive local destruction.

Basal cell carcinomas may be caused by skin damage from physical injury or radiotherapy, but UVR is the most important aetiological factor. The relationship with UVR is complex.[19,20] Development of basal cell carcinoma correlates with excessive childhood sun exposure, severe childhood sunburn, degree of freckling and fair skin. There is no clear correlation with recreational or occupational sun exposure in adult life, however, and many tumours appear on body sites sheltered from light, such as behind the ear. Basal cell carcinomas should be referred for treatment by a dermatologist or plastic surgeon (Fig. 9.2).

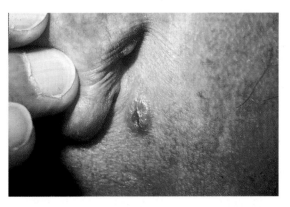

Fig. 9.2 Basal cell carcinomas behind the ears are often overlooked.

CUTANEOUS SQUAMOUS CELL CARCINOMA

Cutaneous squamous cell carcinomas are malignant tumours derived from keratinocytes.[21] They are the second commonest form of skin cancer in whites and are increasing in incidence. The tumours typically arise as firm, indurated nodules in sun-damaged skin. The tumours may be warty, ulcerated or plaque-like, and associated with regional lymphadenopathy. Aggressive types of squamous cell carcinomas will metastasise and lead to death unless treated early.

Squamous cell carcinomas may result from contact with carcinogens such as arsenic, but the most consistent, causal relationship is with UVR exposure.[22] The tumours arise in body sites most exposed to sunlight, such as hands, lips or ears, and are commonest in fair-skinned populations living in tropical climates such as Queensland, Australia. There is also a high prevalence in albinos of dark-skinned families. The chance of development of the tumour increases linearly with the amount of sun exposure, so outdoor workers and sun-worshippers are at particular risk. The tumours are very common in immunosuppressed patients, for example transplant recipients.

CUTANEOUS MALIGNANT MELANOMA

Cutaneous malignant melanoma (CMM) is a tumour of the epidermal melanocytes and is the most serious form of skin cancer. It is the cause of 1 in 12 cancers between the ages of 15 and 34 years in the UK. The incidence of and mortality from CMM have been steadily increasing in fair-skinned populations around the world in the past few decades,[23] although there is some early evidence that this rise may be stabilising.[24] Studies of the pathology of melanomas have demonstrated that this rise is a real effect and not related to an artefact in tumour reporting.

Four main variants of the tumour are recognised:

- superficial spreading melanoma
- lentigo melanoma
- nodular melanoma
- acral lentiginous melanoma.

The commonest type is superficial spreading melanoma. This presents as a changing, irregularly shaped, irregularly pigmented macule or plaque. Nodular melanoma is the most aggressive type. It presents with a rapidly enlargening nodule which may be irregularly pigmented or lacking pigment. Lentigo malignant melanoma is usually seen as a slow growing, deeply pigmented lesion on the face in the elderly. Acral lentiginous melanoma is a rare form found on the palms and soles.

There are many risk factors for cutaneous malignant melanoma. These include a family history of the disease, skin types 1 and 2, multiple benign moles or naevi and irregular moles, known as atypical naevi. The most important preventable risk factor for malignant melanoma is exposure to excessive UVR, but the relationship is more complex than for squamous cell carcinoma.

ROLE OF UVR IN MALIGNANT MELANOMA[25,26]

The role of UVR in development of CMM is not yet entirely clear, but it seems likely that intermittent, strong sun exposure and sunburning are critical in increasing risk in genetically susceptible individuals, and that excessive sun exposure is particularly important in children and adolescents. Thus healthcare specialists working in travel medicine can play a pivotal role in prevention of malignant melanoma, through targeting sensible sun exposure advice to those embarking on annual summer holidays to sunny destinations.

The evidence suggesting sunlight is a major cause of CMM in susceptible populations is as follows:

1. Case control studies from Europe have identified intermittent, strong sun exposure, sunburn, indoor occupation, high social class and sunbathing holidays as risk factors for CMM.
2. The incidence of the disease increases with proximity to the equator in regions with essentially similar populations, such as Australia and New Zealand. In Europe, the opposite appears to be true, in that there is a higher prevalence of melanoma in northern than southern regions of some countries. This 'conundrum' is at least partly due to

differences in pigmentation within populations in the same country – natives of Southern Italy, for example, tend to have darker skin than those of Nothern Italy, and much darker skin than Scandinavians.

3. Strong evidence comes from studies of individuals migrating from countries with low ambient UVR to areas of high ambient UVR. Fair-skinned individuals born in Australia and New Zealand have approximately double the incidence and mortality from CMM compared with recent immigrants to Australia from the UK. Similar findings have been reported from Israel and Hawaii. The age at migration is important. Children who migrate to Australia before age 15 years acquire the same risk of CMM as native Australians.[27]

4. Melanoma is very rarely found in sun-spared areas, such as the buttocks. It is most commonly seen on the upper back in men, and on the upper back and lower legs in women, all sites of intermittent, intense, 'summer holiday' type of sun exposure. Sites of maximal exposure to UVR, such as the head and neck, are less frequently involved, with the exception of lentigo malignant melanoma. These observations suggest intermittent UVR exposure is of more importance than chronic UVR in melanoma development.

Prevention of skin cancer

Primary prevention of cancer is prevention of the development of cancer. Secondary prevention is prevention of death resulting from a cancer. The most important aspect of primary prevention of skin cancer is reduction of exposure to excessive UVR. The most important aspect of secondary prevention is early diagnosis and surgical removal of CMM, as early forms of CMM do not metastasise if excised. It has not yet been demonstrated that reduction in sun exposure produces fewer deaths from skin cancer, but campaigns to encourage early detection of CMM may save lives.[28]

Awareness of skin cancer is increasing[29] and there is evidence of improvements in suntanning attitudes and behaviour in some countries.[30,31]

These improvements may explain the stabilisation of the death rate from CMM reported from some countries.[32] These findings should be viewed cautiously, however, as there is plentiful evidence of continuing widespread, inadequate, sun protection behaviours.[33–35]

Primary prevention of skin cancer also includes reducing UVA exposure from artificial sources. Sunbeds have become popular in Northern European countries and excessive use of sunbeds is a risk factor for CMM. Use of sunbeds should therefore be discouraged.[36]

Skin conditions triggered or exacerbated by excessive sunlight

Many skin diseases may commence or worsen after exposure to strong sunlight. Patients with such conditions may need to be particularly cautious when travelling to sunny climates. Individuals involved in travel clinics do not need an exhaustive knowledge of dermatology, but it is important to be aware of skin conditions which may worsen in sunlight. A list of these is provided in Table 9.2.

TABLE 9.2 Skin conditions which may worsen in strong sunlight

Conditions exacerbated by sunlight (photodermatoses)	Conditions regularly exacerbated by sunlight	Conditions occasionally caused by sunlight
Polymorphic light eruption	Lupus erythematosus	Acne vulgaris
Solar urticaria	Dermatomyositis	Acne rosacea
Actinic prurigo	Porphyria	Erythema multiforme
	Herpes simplex	Atopic eczema
		Lichen planus
		Seborrhoeic eczema
		Psoriasis

Photodermatoses

The photodermatoses are skin conditions characterised by marked sensitivity to sunlight, or photosensitivity. These conditions usually present with a skin eruption on light-exposed sites. The face, neck and back of the hands are most frequently involved. There is often sparing of photoprotected sites such as the upper eyelid, behind the ear-lobes and under the chin.

A large variety of these disorders have been described but most are rare, and should be referred to a dermatologist. One condition, however, called polymorphic light eruption (PLE), is very common and worth recognising. Travel medicine specialists should also be aware that certain drugs may induce photosensitivity (Fig. 9.3).

POLYMORPHIC LIGHT ERUPTION

This condition occurs in up to 20% of females exposed to strong sunlight, and in a smaller percentage of males. It usually is seen in spring with the onset of good weather. It presents with non-scarring, itchy, pink papules, vesicles and plaques. These are seen on the dorsum of hands, arms and other light-exposed sites. The condition usually occurs within a few hours of exposure to sunlight and may last for several hours to several weeks.

PLE is diagnosed on the basis of history and clinical findings. The differential diagnosis of the condition includes drug-induced photosensitivity and cutaneous lupus erythematosus, and difficult cases may require referral to a dermatologist. The

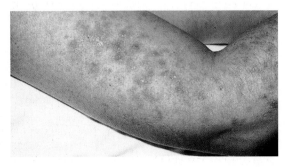

Fig. 9.3 Polymorphic light eruption: note sparing above T-shirt sleeve line.

condition can be treated in the short-term with moderately potent or potent topical steroids. In the longer-term, patients may require sun protection, or gradual introduction to increasing amounts of UVR under supervision of a dermatologist.

Drug-induced photosensitivity

Drug-induced photosensitivity is relatively common. It most often affects the middle-aged and elderly. Travel medicine specialists should consider the possibility of drug-induced photosensitivity in any individual on regular medication travelling to a sunny destination. Diuretics, non-steroidal anti-inflammatories and antibiotics are all common culprits.

A number of drugs may induce photosensitivity, through either phototoxic or photoallergic mechanisms. In a photoallergic reaction, light absorption causes the drug to produce an allergic reaction in the skin. Prior exposure to the drug is required and the skin eruption occurs within 24 hours of re-exposure to the drug in the presence of light.

Phototoxic reactions are caused by a variety of non-immunological mechanisms. They are more common than photoallergic reactions and will occur in almost any individual given a high enough dose of the drug in the presence of strong sunlight. The phototoxic reaction does not require prior exposure to the drug and may occur within 4–24 hours of first exposure. Many drugs act through both mechanisms, and in practice it is difficult to distinguish clinically between phototoxic and photoallergic reactions.

Photosensitive drug eruptions may present with red, weeping, blistered, painful skin, eczema, a rash similar to lichen planus, or with hyper-pigmentation. The rash may persist for years after the offending drug has been withdrawn and diagnosis depends on eliciting a careful drug history, including medications taken before the onset of the condition. Drugs which most frequently cause photosensitivity include thiazide diuretics, phenothiazines, azapropazone, nalidixic acid, tetracyclines, sulphonamides, retinoids and amiodarone. Photosensitive drug eruptions may only present after exposure to strong sunlight and therefore individuals taking any of these medications need to be aware of the risk of a reaction before travelling.

Treatment of drug-induced photosensitivity consists of drug elimination, topical or systemic drug therapy for the skin and sensible sun avoidance.

Prickly heat

This condition can occur in those staying in tropical and sub-tropical areas during the hot summer season. It is thought to be due to stasis in the sweat glands and affects any part of the body but most usually the scalp and skin flexures. Itch and tingling can be intense. A papular rash occurs and secondary infection may be present.

It is more common in children and as it takes time to develop, it is not very common in short-term tourists.

Treatment can be difficult and in severe cases a period in a cooler environment such as a hill station may be necessary. Air-conditioning may also prevent the condition developing and can help it to resolve more rapidly.

Simple, 'soothing' lotions such as zinc and castor oil cream or calamine lotion may relieve symptoms.

Benefits of UVR

The main physiological benefit of UVR is stimulation of the production of vitamin D, cholecalciferol, in the skin. UVB penetrates into the skin and causes conversion of 7-dehydrocholesterol to precholecalciferol, which is subsequently converted into vitamin D. Casual exposure to sunlight is adequate to provide daily vitamin D requirements in most children and adults.[37] There is therefore little risk of causing vitamin D deficiency through sun protection advice.

UVR may be useful in the treatment of skin conditions, such as psoriasis and eczema. In temperate climates, UVR is administered in specially-designed cabinets where the dose is closely monitored. In warmer climates, people often treat themselves with natural sunlight. Many people are now travelling to the Dead Sea for treatment of psoriasis and there is some evidence that the combination of salts in the Dead Sea and natural sunlight may be helpful. There are also pyschological benefits from UVR exposure. It is common to experience a feeling of well-being in good weather and it is important to take this into account when giving sun-avoidance advice.

Sun protection

Travel medicine specialists need to be able to provide sensible advice about sun protection for travellers. It is important for all fair-skinned individuals to have a rudimentary understanding of the hazards of excessive sun exposure, but clearly some travellers are at greater risk than others (Box 9.2). These higher risk individuals, or their parents, will require stronger messages about the risks of sun damage, and may need to practise more assiduous sun protection.

The ability of health personnel to change sunbathing behaviours depends on many factors. The most important of these are the persuasive powers of the counsellor, the knowledge and beliefs of the counsellor about sun awareness and the knowledge and attitudes of the individual

---

Box 9.2 Sun-awareness advice should be reinforced in the following groups:

- Fair-skinned children and adolescents (and/or parents).
- Travellers with a family or personal history of skin cancer.
- Travellers with type 1 or 2 skin or a history of previous, excessive, sun exposure or frequent sunburning.
- Travellers from temperate regions intending to spend long periods in tropical or sub-tropical regions.
- Travellers on long-term, immunosuppressant therapy, for example renal transplant patients.

receiving advice. It is important to have some understanding of the views of the traveller before attempting to give sun advice. Any attempt at changing sunbathing behaviour which does not consider the traveller's viewpoint is unlikely to succeed. Simple measures, such as administration of sun-awareness leaflets, are unlikely to influence travellers.[38]

The UK Skin Cancer Working Party has recommended a four point approach to sensible sun avoidance which provides a good basis for discussion with patients and travellers:[39,40]

- avoidance of the midday sun
- use of natural shade
- protection with clothing and hats
- use of sunscreens with a sun-protection factor of 15 or greater.

AVOIDANCE OF MIDDAY SUN

The amount of UVR from sunlight is maximum around noon, although many people believe the sun is strongest in the mid-afternoon.[41] It is therefore important to stress this point. It can be helpful to suggest travellers organise activities in the morning and later afternoon, and adopt the midday break practised in many warm countries.

USE OF NATURAL SHADE

Individuals should be encouraged to use shade such as provided by trees, umbrellas or buildings. Shade alone may provide insufficient protection in tropical sun, as there is risk of skin damage from scattered UVR. 5- to 10-fold more UVB radiation is scattered than visible light. In a recent study, it was suggested that a fair-skinned person sitting in the shade in a tropical country could suffer sunburn in under 1 hour.[42] Light is reflected from sand, water, snow and white or light-coloured objects, and the presence of these will increase the risk of UVR damage.

PROTECTION WITH CLOTHING AND HATS

Travellers should be encouraged to wear comfortable, loose, long-sleeved shirts and long trousers, made with a tightly weaved fabric which will prevent penetration of UVR. Certain fabrics provide little UVR protection, for example the most popular type of ladies stocking in the UK has a sun protection factor of less than two.[43]

Wide-brimmed hats and legionnaire-style caps provide good protection for the head and neck. Clothing has been produced which changes colour when a certain amount of UVR is absorbed. This may encourage safe sun behaviour in children, but caution is advised, as it is not possible at present to define a safe level of UVR exposure.

SUNSCREENS

There are two main types of sunscreen: physical and chemical. Physical sunscreens usually consist of zinc oxide or titanium dioxide. They are very effective in blocking UVA and UVB, but are highly visible on the skin, and therefore often cosmetically unacceptable. Chemical sunscreens are derived from the chemical *p*-aminobenzoic acid or newer chemicals such as cinnamates, and are effective in protection against UVB. They are cosmetically more acceptable than physical sunscreens, and are used in some facial cosmetics to protect against photoageing. Chemical sunscreens may cause allergic or irritant reactions on the skin, and only the more recently developed compounds are adequately effective against UVA.

The ability of a sunscreen to protect against sunburn is measured by the sun-protection factor (SPF). This is calculated by comparison of the time taken to develop mild sunburn, in skin covered with sunscreen, and in unprotected skin. The SPF is a measure of sunburn, and thus largely a measure of UVB damage. At present there is no widely agreed measure of UVA protection in sunscreens, but it is likely new measures of sunscreen efficacy will come into use.[44]

Although sunscreens may be very effective in prevention of sunburn, there is concern that they do not prevent skin cancer, and it has been suggested that use of sunscreens may even lead to increased risk of skin cancer.[45-47]

The studies incriminating sunscreen use as a cause of melanoma have all involved sunscreens available up to the mid-1990s. Prior to that time, available sunscreens were effective against UVB, but the newer, broad-band sunscreens with addditional UVA screening capacity only became available from 1992. Thus these reports could be interpreted to indicate that UVB sunscreening which prevents the biological warning of sunburn allows greater exposure to UVA. Alternatively, it could be argued that the observation that sunscreen users appear to have a higher incidence of melanoma is a reflection that those with skin types 1 and 2 find it is necessary to use sunscreens. Thus sunscreen use may be a confounding factor rather than an aetiological agent in these case control studies.

At present, the best policy is to advise use of sunscreens only in addition to other methods of sun protection.

Box 9.3 Points to remember about sunscreens

- Use high SPF (>factor 15) with both UVA and UVB protection.
- Apply sunscreen every 2–3 hours.
- Sunscreens may increase the risk of skin cancer, so should be used only in conjunction with other sun protection.

PRACTICE POINTS

Although sunbathing may be enjoyable it must be remembered that excessive sun exposure is a health hazard owing to the effect of ultraviolet radiation on the skin.
- Ultraviolet A (UVA) and Ultraviolet B (UVB) radiation are known to cause premature cancers. UVB also causes sunburn.
- Sun damage is more likely when the light is also 'reflected' from water (swimming pools or the sea), white sand or snow.

Particularly vulnerable groups include:
- babies and children
- fair-skinned people who often also have red hair or blue eyes
- those with certain medical conditions such as albinism or previous skin cancer
- those on certain medications such as tetracyclines or diuretics.

General precautions
- Babies under 9 months should be kept out of direct sunlight.
- Children should wear long-sleeved shirts, hats and high-factor, waterproof sunscreen.
- Everyone should avoid the midday sun, usually around noon until 14.00 hours (15.00 in tropical regions).
- Adults should wear a broad-brimmed hat, long-sleeved shirts and sunglasses.

Sunscreens
- The sun-protection factor (SPF) refers to the protection against UVB. (e.g. 'SPF 8' allows approximately 8 times longer sun exposure without burning than without protection).
- There is a voluntary star system denoting UVA protection; more stars indicating greater protection.

Heat exhaustion and heatstroke

J. Gordon Avery

Heat exhaustion occurs following heavy sweating and excessive fluid loss with inadequate replacement. This occurs particularly in hot climates when unaccustomed exercise is taken during acclimatisation. Symptoms include malaise, headache, light-headedness and fatigue. The symptoms partly depend on whether loss of salt or loss of water is the main component.

- Water loss results in thirst and clouding of consciousness.
- Salt loss does not cause so much thirst and the person remains rational. The person does, however, become lethargic, have severe muscle cramps and may vomit.

The emergency treatment of heat exhaustion with predominantly water loss consists of fluid replacement with water and/or fruit juice, and cooling by cold water and fans.

The treatment of the salt loss component consists of giving salty fluids such as soup or Bovril. A popular and quite refreshing Far Eastern treatment is salt in lime juice with soda.

The far more dangerous **heat stroke** may develop if there is serious damage to the sweating mechanism with an excessive rise in body temperature, irrational and hyperactive behaviour and, eventually, loss of consciousness and death. Rapid cooling by spraying the body with water and fanning is ideal. Using ice is a less rapid alternative. Emergency fluid and electrolyte replacement is usually also required by intravenous drip.

Prevention of heat exhaustion and heat stroke is particularly important during the early stages of acclimatisation in hot climates when every opportunity should be taken to keep cool, drink extra fluids and add salt to meals.

PRACTICE POINTS

Causes of heat exhaustion
- Water loss due to heavy sweating
- Salt loss causing lethargy and muscle cramps

Treatment
- Fluid replacement
- Salty fluids e.g. soup

Heat stroke
- Dangerous condition with excessive rise in body temperature and irrational behaviour

Treatment
- Cool the body
- Replace fluid and electrolytes.

REFERENCES

1. Hill D, White V, Marks R, Borland R. Changes in sun-related attitudes and behaviours and reduced sunburn in a population at high risk of melanoma. European Journal of Cancer Prevention 1993; 2: 447–456.
2. IARC monographs on the evaluation of carcinogenic risks to humans. IARC Scientific Publications 1992; 55.
3. Devesa SS, Blot WJ, Stone BJ, et al. Recent cancer trends in the United States. Journal of the National Cancer Institute 1995; 87: 175–182.
4. Bowers PW. Skin cancer in Cornwall 1980–1990. British Journal of Dermatology 1993; 129(Suppl. 42): 50–51.
5. Boyle P, Maisonneuve P, Dore J-F. Epidemiology of malignant melanoma. British Medical Bulletin 1995; 51: 523–547.
6. Office of Population, Censuses and Surveys. Cancer statistics registration, England and Wales 1993. London: HMSO; 1995 (series DH2 No. 20).
7. Rossi JS, Blais LM, Redding CA, Weinstock MA. Preventing skin cancer through behaviour change. Dermatology Clinics 1995; 3: 613–622.
8. Jarrett P, Sharp C, McLelland J. Protection of children by their mothers against sunburn. British Medical Journal 1993; 306: 1448.
9. Melia J, Bulman A. Sunburn and suntanning in a British population. Journal of Public Health Medicine 1995; 17: 223–229.
10. Sutton H. Scottish adolescents and sun exposure on holiday abroad. MSc Thesis, University of Glasgow; 1997.
11. Blizzard L, Dwyer T, Ashbolt R. Changes in self-reported skin type associated with experience of sunburn in 14–15 year old children of Northern European descent. Melanoma Research 1997; 7: 339–346
12. Young AR, Chadwick CH, Harrison GI, et al. The in situ repair kinetics of epidermal thymine dimers and 6–4 photoproducts in human skin types 1 and 2. Journal of Investigative Dermatology 1996; 106: 1307–1313.
13. Eller MS, Yaar M, Gilchrest BA. DNA damage and melanogenesis. Nature 1994; 372: 413–414.
14. Marks R, Staples M, Giles GG. Trends in non-melanocytic skin cancer treated in Australia: the second national survey. International Journal of Cancer 1993; 53: 585–590.
15. Gilchrest BA. A review of skin ageing and its medical therapy. British Journal of Dermatology 1996; 135: 867–875.
16. Frost CA, Green AC. Epidemiology of solar keratoses. British Journal of Dermatology 1994; 131: 455–464.
17. Marks R, Rennie G, Selwood T. The relationship of basal cell carcinomas and squamous cell carcinomas to solar keratoses. Archives of Dermatology 1988; 124: 1039–1042.
18. Thompson SC, Jolley D, Marks R. Reduction in solar keratoses by regular sunscreen use. New England Journal of Medicine 1993; 329: 1147–1151.
19. Gallagher RP, Hill GB, Bajdik CD, et al. Sunlight exposure, pigmentary factors, and risk of non-melanocytic skin cancer. 1. Basal cell carcinoma. Archives of Dermatology 1995; 131: 157–163.
20. Marks R. An overview of skin cancer: incidence and causation. Cancer 1995; 75: 607–612.
21. Marks R. Squamous cell carcinoma. Lancet 1996; 347: 735–738.
22. Preston DS, Stern RS. Non-melanoma cancers of the skin. New England Journal of Medicine 1992; 327: 1649–1662.
23. Boyle P, Maisonneuve P, Dore J-F. Epidemiology of malignant melanoma. British Medical Bulletin 1995; 51: 523–547
24. MacKie RM, Hole D, Hunter JAA, et al. Cutaneous malignant melanoma in Scotland: incidence, survival, and mortality, 1979–94. British Medical Journal 1997; 315: 1117–1121.
25. Langley RGB, Sober AJ. A clinical review of the evidence for the role of ultraviolet radiation in aetiology of cutaneous melanoma. Cancer Investigations 1997; 15: 561–567.
26. Elwood JM, Jopson J. Melanoma and sun exposure: an overview of published studies. International Journal of Cancer 1997; 73: 198–203.
27. Khlat M, Vail A, Parkin M, Green A. Mortality from melanoma in migrants to Australia: variation by age at arrival and duration of stay. American Journal of Epidemiology 1992; 135: 1103–1113.
28. MacKie RM, Hole D. Audit of public education campaign to encourage earlier detection of malignant melanoma. British Medical Journal 1992; 304: 1012–1015.
29. Melia J, Ellman R, Chamberlain J. Investigating changes in awareness about cutaneous malignant melanoma in Britain using the Omnibus survey. Clinical and Experimental Dermatology 1994; 19: 375–379.
30. Robinson JK, Rigel DS, Amonette RA. Trends in sun exposure knowledge, attitudes and behaviors: 1986 to 1996. Journal of the American Academy of Dermatology 1997; 37: 179–186.
31. Baade PD, Balanda KP, Lowe JB. Changes in skin protective behaviors, attitudes, and sunburn: in a population with the highest incidence of skin cancer in the world. Cancer Detection and Prevention 1996; 20: 566–575.
32. Melia J. Changing incidence and mortality from cutaneous malignant melanoma. British Medical Journal 1997; 315: 1106–1107.
33. Hall HI, May DS, Lew RA, et al. Sun protective behaviours of the US population. Preventative Medicine 1997; 26: 401–407.
34. Kakourou T, Bakoula C, Kavadias G, et al. Mothers' knowledge and practices related to sun protection in Greece. Paediatic Dermatology 1995; 12: 207–210.
35. McGee R, Wiliams S, Glasgow H. Sunburn and sun protection amongst young children. Journal of Paediatics and Child Health 1997; 33: 234–237.
36. Autier P, Dore J-F, Lejeune F et al. Cutaneous malignant melanoma and exposure to sunlamps or sunbeds: an EORTC multicenter case-control study in Belgium, France and Germany. International Journal of Cancer 1994; 58: 809–813.

37. Holick MF. Environmental factors that influence the cutaneous prroduction of vitamin D. American Journal of Clinical Nutrition 1995; 61(suppl): 638s–645s.

38. Dey P, Collins S, Will S, Woodman CBJ. Randomised controlled trial assessing effectiveness of health education leaflets in reducing incidence of sunburn. British Medical Journal 1995; 311: 1062–1063.

39. MacKie RM. Melanoma prevention and early detection. British Medical Bulletin 1995; 51: 523–547.

40. United Kingdom Skin Cancer Prevention Working Party. Consensus statement. London: British Association of Dermatologists; 1994.

41. Fleming C, Nicolson C, Toal F. Sun awareness in schoolteachers. British Journal of Dermatology 1988; 139: 280–284.

42. Parsons PG, Neale R, Wolski P, Green A. The shady side of solar protection. Medical Journal of Australia 1998; 168: 327–330.

43. Sinclair SA, Diffey BL. Sun protection provided by ladies stockings. British Journal of Dermatology 1996; 135: s119.

44. Davenport V, Morris JF, Chu AC. Immunologic protection afforded by sunscreens in vitro. Journal of Investigative Dermatology 1997; 108: 859–863.

45. McGregor JM, Young AR. Sunscreens, suntans, and skin cancer. British Medical Journal 1996; 312: 1621–1622.

46. Naylor MF, Farmer KC. The case for sunscreens. A review of their use in preventing actinic damage and neoplasia. Archives of Dermatology 1997; 133: 1146–1154.

47. Autier P, Dore JF, Schifflers E et al. Melanoma and use of sunscreens: an EORTC case-control study in Germany, Belgium and France. International Journal of Cancer 1995; 61: 749–755.

TRAVEL-RELATED RISKS: SEXUAL

Sexual risks related to travel, including HIV infection

Brian Mulhall

Introduction

Sexually transmissible diseases (STDs) continue to be the most common, notifiable infectious conditions worldwide. Their unacceptably high incidence is underlined by the recent emergence of a (presently) incurable and lethal STD – human immunodeficiency virus (HIV) infection – which merits its description as a pandemic, and with which other STDs interact in an epidemiological synergy. Data that quantify the association between STDs/HIV infection and travel are difficult to obtain; nevertheless figures are presented that reveal the lower limit to be large enough to be of considerable concern. Studies from around the world show, overall, although knowledge of STDs is increasing amongst travellers, the level of knowledge has little to do with actual behaviour, with a modest increase in the use of condoms, but abundant evidence that a wide variety of sexual behaviours take place among travellers and with local inhabitants. Certain travellers, by virtue of their behavioural interactions with 'core-groups' of efficient transmitters, may have a high risk of acquisition of an STD/HIV. Worldwide, sexual health promotion for travellers is in its infancy; indeed, it could more accurately be merely described as 'sexual education'. A fresh approach is recommended, which includes comprehensive programme planning and outcome, impact, and process evaluations, and which is based on a behavioural rather than an informational paradigm.

1. Global epidemiology of sexually transmissible diseases

STDs are a group of communicable diseases that are transferred predominantly by sexual contact, and are thus to a large extent 'behavioural diseases'. They are now the commonest group of notifiable infectious diseases in most countries. Despite some fluctuations, their incidence remains unacceptably high; in 1995, there were over 333 million cases of the four major curable STDs in adults between the ages of 15 and 49 –12 million cases of syphilis, 62 million cases of gonorrhoea, 89 million cases of chlamydia, and 170 million cases of trichomoniasis.[1,2] Many pathogens are known to be spread by sexual contact and these are shown in Box 10.1 (the agents in parentheses are considered to be either less strongly associated with sexual contact except in certain circumstances, or to have less epidemiological importance in the context of this review). Some, like *Chlamydia trachomatis* and viral agents, were tending to replace the classical bacterial diseases (syphilis, gonorrhoea and chancroid) in importance and frequency, until the recent realisation that not only are the latter diseases incriminated in transmission of HIV (see section below on the interaction of STDs and HIV) but also that the number and variety of antibiotic-resistant strains have increased markedly.[3] However, these agents, which may be regarded as the second generation of STDs, are frequently more

Box 10.1 Classification of sexually transmissible agents

Bacterial agents
Chlamydia trachomatis
Haemophilus ducreyi
Neisseria gonorrhoeae
Treponema pallidum
Calymmatobacterium granulomatis
(*Mycoplasma hominis*)
(*Mycoplasma genitalium*)
(*Ureaplasma urealyticum*)
(*Shigella* spp.)
(*Campylobacter* spp.)
(Group B streptococcus)
(Bacterial vaginosis-associated organisms)

Viral agents
Human papilloma viruses
Hepatitis virus B
Human herpes virus 1 or 2
Human immunodeficiency viruses HIV-1, HIV-2
Human herpes virus 5 (formerly cytomegalovirus)
(Hepatitis virus C)
(Hepatitis virus D)
(Hepatitis virus A)
(Human herpes virus 6)
(Human T lymphotropic virus type 1 (HTLV-1))
(Human herpes virus 8)

Protozoal agents
Trichomonas vaginalis
(*Entamoeba histolytica*)
(*Giarda lamblia* (intestinalis))

Fungal agents
(*Candida albicans*)

Ectoparasites
(*Pthirus pubis*)
(*Sarcoptes scabiei*)

difficult to identify, treat, and control, and can cause serious complications resulting in chronic ill-health, disability and even death. Data on frequency of various STDs, are largely dependent on the accuracy of reporting. The most comprehensive data available on incidence are from a few industrialised countries. In most developing countries, the data is prevalence data derived from ad hoc surveys in population groups that are not necessarily representative of the total population. Although these surveys provide useful estimates, they must be interpreted with caution.

In the following sections, the epidemiology of most of the common STDs is considered (though not necessarily in order of frequency). Broad guidelines for treatment are indicated, though other clinical data are not provided, except for those diseases that Western-trained physicians may not have encountered.

Syphilis

DEVELOPED COUNTRIES

After the large peak during the Second World War, the number of cases of primary and secondary syphilis dropped to a low level in the late 1950s with a slow but steady increase since that time. However, from 1986–90 there was an epidemic of primary and secondary syphilis in the USA with increases ranging from 10 to 200% in 25 cities.

The most notable trends were the substantial increase in cases involving black heterosexuals, changes in geographical distribution and the association with 'crack' cocaine use. This enormous increase was attributed to several factors, the most important being the exchange of drugs for sex, the widespread use of spectinomycin rather than penicillin for the treatment of gonorrhoea and the shifting of resources from syphilis to AIDS. By 1996, however, rates had dropped precipitously, leaving an endemicity (>4.0/100 000) concentrated in less than 15% of all counties.

DEVELOPING COUNTRIES

Most available data are prevalence figures; in addition, seropositivity can be due to venereal syphilis (infectious or non-infectious), or to previous infection with non-venereal treponematoses. Nevertheless, prevalence rates are high, varying from 5 to 20% in women attending antenatal clinics to 70% in certain groups, for example prostitutes. A few studies report incidence data showing an increase in cases of infectious syphilis.

All strains of *Treponema pallidum* worldwide are sensitive to penicillin, which remains the treatment of choice. Second-line treatments include, amongst others, the tetracycline group of antibiotics.

Gonorrhoea

DEVELOPED COUNTRIES

The trends show a clear increase from 1957 onwards, reaching a peak in the early 1970s and decreasing since, although not as steeply as syphilis. There was an increase in rectal gonorrhoea in the 1970s in homosexual men which has since declined; however, both the number and variety of antibiotic-resistant strains have increased markedly. In the 1950s strains partially resistant to penicillin emerged which were soon found to be prevalent throughout the world. Fortunately, these (chromosomally-mediated) resistant strains proved sensitive to a step-wise increase in therapeutic levels of penicillin, until penicillinase-producing *Neisseria gonorrhoeae* (PPNG) strains were isolated in 1976, simultaneously in England and the USA, containing plasmids probably originating from West Africa and Asia respectively. These strains with plasmid-mediated resistance have spread worldwide. In addition, partial resistance to quinolones is becoming more frequent, and although resistance to ceftriaxone has yet to be reported, the genetic flexibility of the gonococcus is such that it is never entirely unexpected when resistance to newly introduced antimicrobial agents appears. Fears are held even for third generation cephalosporins as minor changes would see PPNG become 'expanded spectrum' beta-lactamase producers. In some developed countries, heterosexually acquired gonorrhoea in males is predominantly acquired from foreign prostitutes, overseas, or from working in the host country.

DEVELOPING COUNTRIES

The available incidence figures are unreliable but estimates for large cities in Africa suggest an annual incidence rate for gonorrhoea of 3000–10 000 cases per 100 000 inhabitants.

Chlamydial infections

(Lymphogranuloma venereum is discussed separately.)

DEVELOPED COUNTRIES

Genital infection caused by *Chlamydia trachomatis* has been the most common bacterial STD in the USA and the UK since the early 1980s.

Non-gonococcal urethritis (NGU) in men is caused by *Chlamydia trachomatis* in at least 40% of cases. The female counterpart to NGU, mucopurulent cervicitis, is also increasing, as is its major complication, pelvic inflammatory disease. It is estimated that chlamydia causes 4–6 million infections per year in the USA. It is not known how much of this increase may be due to the recording of 'epidemiological treatment'; certainly efforts to control chlamydia have been hampered by the relative difficulties, compared with gonorrhoea, of diagnosis and treatment. *Chlamydia trachomatis* is sensitive to most tetracycline and macrolide antibiotics, and conveniently, to a single dose of the new macrolide antibiotic, azithromycin.

DEVELOPING COUNTRIES

Until recently, the spectrum of STDs commonly identified in developing countries was limited to the classical, 'venereal' diseases. However, sexually transmitted pathogens of the second generation have started to be identified. In general, the prevalence of *Chlamydia trachomatis* infections is higher, especially in sub-Saharan Africa.

Genital herpes virus infection

DEVELOPED COUNTRIES

Genital herpes is the most common cause of genital ulceration in the developed world. More than 20 000 cases of genital herpes are reported annually from STD clinics in the UK, and 500 000 new cases are estimated each year in the USA. Recent sero-epidemiological surveys have shown widespread exposure (usually asymptomatic); however, nucleic acid amplification techniques have demonstrated viral shedding in symptom-free, herpes simplex virus-infected individuals.

DEVELOPING COUNTRIES

There is virtually no published data on clinical herpes, probably reflecting the fact that individuals do not present to health services, and more importantly, the difficulties in differential diagnosis with other genital ulcer diseases which are common, and the absence of laboratory facilities for virus culture. One report, from Durban, South Africa, found herpes virus to be an aetiological agent in 18% of all genital ulcers (mixed infections were common). Moreover, in a review of sero-epidemiological surveys, evidence of exposure was high, or even higher (than developed countries) in the countries for which results are available (Costa Rica, Jamaica, Zaire, Rwanda, Congo, and Senegal). This may be particularly important in those countries in which genital ulcer disease is thought to be important in facilitating acquisition and spread of HIV infection.

Genital human papillomavirus (HPV) infection

DEVELOPED COUNTRIES

The epidemiology of genital HPV infections is similar to that of genital herpes, except for its magnitude, which is three times higher, and the fact that its key consequence, cervical cancer, is more severe. Even more than for genital herpes, genital warts represent only the symptomatic tip of the iceberg of HPV infections. Sub-clinical papillomavirus infections of the male and female genital tract are becoming more commonly recognised. At present, no reliable serological test is available, and the virus cannot be recovered

through tissue culture. Sub-clinical infection may be diagnosed by the presence of koilocytes on a cytological smear or tissue biopsy, HPV DNA sequences detected by hybridisation studies, HPV antigen detected by immunoperoxidase stains, or certain morphological features on colposcopy. All of these remain controversial with respect to management.

However, using these techniques, about 50% of sexually active women are infected with HPV types that have the potential to progress to malignancy. Thus, HPV infections of the genital tract are probably the most prevalent STD. No specific wart treatment has been shown clearly to be superior to any other; podophyllin should not be used in pregnancy.

DEVELOPING COUNTRIES

No reliable data are available, but it seems unlikely that a ubiquitous virus such as HPV does not exist with similarly high prevalence rates. In view of the lack of access to healthcare facilities, it is probable that patients do not present for treatment, since lesions are usually painless, if unsightly. The facilities to diagnose sub-clinical infections are almost totally absent in most developing countries.

Chancroid

The global incidence of chancroid greatly exceeds that of syphilis. Chancroid is caused by *Haemophilus ducreyi*. The disease starts with a painful papule at the site of infection, resulting in a single or in multiple ulcers. Inguinal lymphadenopathy may be present in up to 50% of patients. Accurate diagnosis of chancroid depends on the ability to culture *Haemophilus ducreyi*. Different isolation media have been used with varying success. Chancroid lesions are highly infectious.

DEVELOPED COUNTRIES

In the UK fewer than 100 cases have been reported annually for the last 15 years. However, in the USA there have been repeated outbreaks with frequent prostitute contact repeatedly implicated. In 1985, the number of reported cases rose above 2000 for the first time since 1956, and in 1987 almost 5000 cases were reported.

DEVELOPING COUNTRIES

Chancroid is endemic in many developing countries, particularly in South East Asia, Eastern and southern Africa and Papua New Guinea. Prostitutes play an important role in its spread. In Africa, even in areas where syphilis is highly prevalent, most genital ulcers are due to chancroid, though mixed infections are common.

Owing to the unreliability of clinical diagnosis and the frequent presence of the two agents in the same genital ulcer, appropriate chancroid treatment combined with syphilis therapy has been recommended. Multi-dose therapy with erythromycin for 7 days and single-dose treatment regimens with azithromycin and ceftriaxone are now recommended as the treatments of choice for chancroid, at least in the USA. Unfortunately, in other parts of the world where such regimens are impractical, resistance to other previously useful antibiotics is increasing. In addition, in patients with concurrent HIV infection, extensive and persistent genital ulcers may be present without bubo formation, and they heal less frequently after short-course treatment and often fail to respond to longer antimicrobial courses.

Trichomonas vaginalis

Despite the fact that *Trichomonas vaginalis* receives less attention in the world literature than *Neisseria gonorrhoeae* and *Chlamydia trachomatis*, it is not a benign condition. The presence of *Trichomonas vaginalis* may predispose to premature rupture of membranes, premature labour, and low birthweight, and its potential in HIV transmission is of great concern. It affects an estimated 3 million American women annually, and although the incidence of trichomoniasis is believed to have decreased in the UK in recent years, it is still the most commonly diagnosed STD worldwide and affects an estimated 170 million people annually.

Metronidazole remains the drug of choice for treatment of trichomoniasis and is the only agent approved by the US Food and Drug Administration for the infection.

Lymphogranuloma venereum

Lymphogranuloma venereum (LGV) is caused by *Chlamydia trachomatis*. Three serovars (L1, L2, L3) are responsible for the vast majority of cases. LGV is a chronic disease with acute and late complications. A primary stage causing a small genital lesion is seen in a minority of patients. Most common is the secondary stage characterised by acute inguinal (and femoral) lymphadenitis with bubo formation. Late complications may occur in the anogenital area, such as ulcers, fistulas, strictures and elephantiasis. The laboratory diagnosis of LGV may be based on positive chlamydial serology, isolation of *Chlamydia trachomatis* from the infected site, and histological identification of chlamydia in infected tissue. In the differential diagnosis, syphilis, chancroid and herpes should always be considered.

LGV has a worldwide distribution, although few reliable data are available. It is sporadic in North America, Europe, Australia, most of Asia and South America. It is endemic in Eastern and Western Africa, India, parts of South-Eastern Asia, South America and the Caribbean. Since 1950, no country in Europe has reported more than a few dozen cases of LGV annually, and the average for the USA has been 595 cases per year, with slight increases during the wars in Korea and Vietnam. In contrast, one municipal clinic in Ethiopia reports several thousand cases of LGV annually. In general, this infection accounts for 5–10% of cases of STDs seen in developing countries. LGV is sensitive to tetracycline and macrolide antibiotics.

Donovanosis (granuloma inguinale)

Donovanosis is a chronic infection of the genital region caused by *Calymmatobacterium granulomatis*. The disease starts with a subcutaneous nodule at the site of infection. This nodule enlarges and erodes through the skin to reveal a red granulating ulcer. This disease may spread haematogeneously, resulting in cutaneous lesions at extragenital body sites. The diagnosis and treatment of donovanosis have recently been comprehensively reviewed. Diagnosis requires the careful collection of smears or biopsies for demonstration of the pathognomonic Donovan bodies within histiocytes.

Donovanosis has an unusual geographical distribution; it is rare in most developed countries but it is among the most prevalent STDs in some developing countries. It is endemic in the southern states of India, especially along the eastern coast, and to a remarkable degree in Papua New Guinea. Additional foci are found in the Caribbean and neighbouring parts of South America, Zambia, South Africa, Vietnam and Japan and among Australian aboriginals.

Antibiotics reported as showing good activity against donovanosis include streptomycin, chloramphenicol, erythromycin, co-trimoxazole and the tetracyclines. Good results have also been reported with norfloxacin and thiamphenicol. More recently, azithromycin has been shown to be very effective in early studies.

Hepatitis virus infections

HEPATITIS B

Viral infections, principally affecting the liver, are among the STDs with the highest incidence worldwide. The most important of these is infection with hepatitis B virus (HBV), which is estimated to be responsible for chronic infection in at least 300 million individuals, and is the ninth major cause of premature mortality. 75% of these carriers live in Asia and the Far East. Soon after the first description of the 'Australia antigen', its discoverer speculated that sexual partners of an infected carrier had an increased probability of also being infected. With increasing experience it became more apparent that sexual activity (rather than vertical or horizontal transmission during childhood) may be one of the most common forms of HBV transmission, particularly in regions of moderate or low endemicity of HBV. Most studies of transmission have been performed in developed countries. The strongest epidemiological association between sexual behaviour and HBV infection is among homosexual men, with markers of previous exposure in 50–75%, and HBV carrier rates of 1.5–4%.[4] The major risk factor for transmission in homosexual men is unprotected, anal intercourse.

Prevalence studies among heterosexual persons attending STD clinics, and case control studies of acute HBV infection suggest that heterosexual transmission is common, although there is wide geographical variation. Fortunately, HBV is the first hepatitis virus against which a vaccine has been developed, and indeed the first STD against which there is an effective vaccine. Recommendations for the control of HBV infection in general, and sexual transmission in particular, must take account of the widely varying prevalences in different countries.

In one review of retrospective and follow-up studies in travellers visiting developing countries, it was suggested that 1 in 2500 develops symptomatic HBV infection after returning home. Vacationers were rarely affected, whereas persons working in developing countries frequently seroconverted. However, none of these studies controlled adequately for asymptomatic infections, and more importantly, sexual activity. The author concluded that vaccination against HBV was advisable for people working in developing countries, and for those travellers who might engage in high-risk activities (such as sexual intercourse).

Recently, preliminary evidence has been forthcoming to suggest that a hitherto-unsuspected route of transmission, via bedbugs, may be important, and intervention studies involving vector control are currently in progress in Gambia to further investigate this possibility. If proven, this would represent a (semi-) sexual route of transmission.

HEPATITIS A

Hepatitis A virus (HAV) is spread by the faecal–oral route, and sexual transmission is thought not to be a major mode of transmission, although there has been evidence for some time of an increased risk among homosexual men. The recent increase in the number of cases of hepatitis A among homosexual men is possibly due to the increased prevalence of oro–anal intercourse being adopted as a 'safer' practice with respect to HIV transmission, which still permits transmission of HAV.

HEPATITIS D (delta)

The group most affected by hepatitis D virus (HDV) are injecting drug users. Studies in Europe and the USA have found surprisingly little HDV infection among homosexual men, although a recent study in France showed a prevalence of 14% among 42 homosexual HBV carriers who did not have a history of being injecting drug users (IDUs).

HEPATITIS C

In an epidemiological study, Alter et al.[5] showed that sexual contact was a risk factor for acute non-A, non-B hepatitis. However, the evidence is not conclusive, and hepatitis C virus infection is much more efficiently transmitted by needle-sharing than sexual intercourse.

OTHER HEPATITIS VIRUSES

Hepatitis E virus (HEV) has recently been characterised, and is transmitted by the faecal–oral route like HAV. Outbreaks of HEV infection have been described, particularly in Asia. There is no evidence yet of sexual transmission of HEV; however, the possibility of oro–anal transmission among homosexual men, as has been documented for HAV infection, cannot be discounted.

Evidence of sexual transmission exists for cytomegalovirus (CMV). Studies of homosexual men have found a high prevalence of antibodies to CMV (90–95%), compared to age-matched, heterosexual controls (50–60%). CMV, however, is a rare course of acute hepatitis, most infections being asymptomatic.

HIV/AIDS

The acquired immunodeficiency syndrome (AIDS) was first described in 1981[6] but it has since reached pandemic proportions; as of June 1998, the World Health Organization estimates that there are approximately 30.6 million people living with HIV/AIDS, of which 1.1 million are children under 15 years of age.[7] Moreover, HIV infections have been documented in virtually all countries.

Medical and scientific progress has been remarkably rapid, including: the isolation of the aetiological agent human immunodeficiency type 1 virus (HIV-1) in 1983–4; the development of sophisticated, diagnostic, screening tests; rapidly expanding knowledge of the modes of transmission (see below), molecular biology and immunopathogenesis of disease; and considerable experience in treatment and prophylaxis, at least in developed countries. Until recently, the disease was thought to be completely irreversible with a variable, latent period between infection with HIV, and progression to the opportunistic infections, tumours and other conditions that variously satisfy the case-definitions of AIDS.

In the past 5 years, a better understanding of HIV pathogenesis has led to the development of new concepts such as early therapeutic intervention, combination antiviral therapy and complete suppression of viral replication that have had a major impact on the clinical management of HIV disease – in particular, decreasing progression to AIDS and prolonging survival – at least in industrialised countries.[8–10] Public interest and political commitment in the quest for an AIDS vaccine have dwindled in most parts of the developed world, partly because of a perceived lack of progress. In fact, although the obstacles to development, production and delivery of an effective and safe vaccine for HIV remain formidable, there is a large and growing body of sound scientific data indicating that vaccination against lentivirus infection is feasible and attainable.

Extensive epidemiological investigation has affirmed the principal means by which HIV-1 is spread: through blood, by sex, and from mother to child. Sexual transmission of HIV accounts for about three-quarters of all infections worldwide. The majority have been through heterosexual transmission. Homosexual transmission also occurs in most parts of the world, and is predominant in some developed countries. American and European studies suggest that male-to-female transmission is more efficient than vice versa. The probability of female-to-male transmission per sexual contact in Thailand has been estimated as 0.031, while the estimate in North America was about 0.001. Moreover, per-contact risk from rectal sex is relatively greater than vaginal intercourse. Perinatal transmission includes transmission during pregnancy, during delivery and through breast-milk. Prospective cohort studies reported that the range of perinatal transmission rate was approximately between 15 and 30%. Even though breast-feeding may be an additional and important route of transmission, it is still recommended where infectious diseases are a common cause of death in childhood, despite the additional risk of HIV transmission. Infected blood or blood products is another transmission route. Besides IDUs, improper use of needles and syringes in the medical setting has been noted to cause transmission of HIV in Africa, Romania, and Russia. Contaminated instruments such as inadequately sterilised needles and syringes, skin-piercing instruments and ritual scarification tools account for only a small proportion mainly in Asia and sub-Saharan Africa.

Although HIV-1 is found in low concentration in saliva, this transmission route is not thought to be frequent. The following pieces of evidence indicate that HIV is *not* transmitted via insects; the age-specific rates of HIV infection and disease do *not* fit the pattern for arthropod-borne diseases (which have high attack rates in young children); rates of HIV infection in Africa are higher in urban than rural areas; serological studies of humans have failed to show a relationship between the presence of antibody to HIV and antibody to arboviruses; and HIV does not replicate in cell lines derived from arthropods. Finally, 'casual' transmission has not been reported.

During the past decade, it seemed possible to distinguish three broad, yet distinct, geographical patterns of HIV-1 infection. *Pattern 1* is pre-dominant in North America, Western Europe, Australia and New Zealand. In Pattern 1, sexual transmission occurs principally among homosexual and bisexual men, but heterosexual transmission also occurs and appears to be increasing. Transmission through blood occurs principally as a result of injecting drug use. Perinatal infection is less common because relatively few women in these areas have been infected thus far. *Pattern 2* is found in sub-Saharan Africa, and increasingly in Latin America and the Caribbean. Sexual transmission is predominantly heterosexual, while transmission via contaminated blood transfusion continues in areas where the screening of blood is not yet routine, and perinatal transmission is a major problem since, in some cities, at least 5–15% of pregnant women are infected. *Pattern 3* areas include North Africa, the Middle East, Eastern Europe, Asia (but see below) and the Pacific. These areas accounted until recently for only a small proportion of AIDS cases reported. Initial cases resulted from contact with people in Pattern 1 or 2 areas, or from exposure to imported blood. However, indigenous transmission of HIV-1 infection is increasing, especially among prostitutes and IDUs. Indeed, it is becoming apparent that India and South-East Asia are in the middle of a major epidemic, at least of the same order of magnitude as sub-Saharan Africa. In these areas, a 'fourth' pattern has been suggested, created by rapid spread among IDUs and female prostitutes, followed by rebound waves in male clients of prostitutes, and then in their wives. There are major features distinguishing Pattern 4 from other patterns (1 and 2), namely faster spread with more rapid and widespread transmission into the general population. This exceptionally rapid spread makes for a large, infected, but not yet actively sick, population (larger iceberg and smaller tip).

It is possible that these so-called epidemiological 'patterns' are spurious, or at least misleading, and they are described here simply because most national surveillance systems still utilise them when referring to cases thought to be acquired outside their national boundaries.

The increasing epidemic in Asia, but encouraging signs in some African countries have been recently extensively reviewed.[11,12] Other recent, epidemiological trends have been a relative stabilisation of new cases of HIV infection in homosexual men, and in IDUs (in the cities where harm-reduction policies are in place), but an alarming epidemic among IDUs and heterosexuals in countries of the former Soviet Union.

Finally, a closely related virus, HIV-2, was described in 1985 in asymptomatic West African prostitutes. It appears to be endemic in West Africa but rare elsewhere, to be transmissible in identical ways to HIV-1 but perhaps is less pathogenic than HIV-1. Differentiation from HIV-1 by serological tests is problematic but feasible.

Transmission of STDs and HIV via blood products and inadequately sterilised instruments

Excess mortality of international travellers, especially tourists, is commonly due to traffic accidents; in addition, pregnant travellers suffer the extra risk of obstetric complications, and in both of these situations blood transfusion might be necessary as a life-saving measure. In the USA, approximately 1 million persons are transfused annually, with each person receiving an average of 2.9 units of blood. If these figures were applied to a typical international trip, the number of persons requiring transfusion would be 1.3 per 10000 per 2-week period. The first indication that HIV may be transmitted by blood products came in 1982 in three haemophiliacs, and Amman reported the first case thought to be transfusion-related in April 1983. Efficient screening techniques for HIV antibodies were implemented in most industrialised nations by 1985–6, and, in addition, improved techniques for preparation of blood components, which can maintain their biological activity for days, weeks or months, have been developed over the last 10 years. Using data from over 17 million American Red Cross donations, it was estimated that the probability of contracting HIV infection in 1987 was 1:153 000 per unit transfused. Sadly, this is not the case in the developing world, especially Africa, where blood transfusion carries a high risk to the recipient of acquiring HIV, and other infections such as hepatitis B, hepatitis C, syphilis and malaria. Indeed, in Africa, blood transfusion has become the third most important mode of HIV transmission, after heterosexual and perinatal transmission.

A number of factors contribute to unsafe operation and limited screening of donated blood and the WHO Global Blood Safety Initiative was formed to address these important concerns. It has issued a number of recommendations, including the development of rapid screening tests, use of plasma expanders and the testing of HIV antibody on serum pools. In certain situations, autologous blood transfusion including pre-operative deposit, perioperative haemodilution and intra-operative blood salvage may be appropriate and feasible. However, all possible steps should be taken to avoid unnecessary blood transfusion and to encourage alternative treatment modalities using saline, plasma expanders and albumin solutions for acute hypovolaemia. Anecdotal reports suggest some diplomatic communities make provisions for their own programmes of homologous blood transfusion. Finally, it should be noted that even in countries where blood screening is routine and efficient, but where HIV seroprevalence is increasing rapidly, for example Thailand, the theoretical risk of transfusing blood from an HIV-seronegative but viraemic donor in the 'window period' of infection has increased greatly; in these countries, screening for p24 antigen has been suggested.

Improper use of needles and syringes has also been noted to cause transmission of HIV in Africa, Romania and Russia. This is unnecessary since HIV is easily inactivated by standard methods of sterilisation or disinfection, such as autoclaving or boiling for 20 minutes. International travellers should also be warned of the dangers of unnecessary injections; some travel clinics provide sterile syringes, needles and intravenous infusion sets for this reason.

The inequities between the developed and developing world with regard to access to a safe blood supply have recently been comprehensively reviewed.

2. Epidemiology of STDs and HIV in the context of travel and travellers

The association between travel and STDs has been known for centuries, particularly for syphilis, and it has been traditional to blame foreigners, usually sailors and armies. For example, Christopher Columbus's sailors allegedly brought syphilis to Europe, having acquired the infection during their first trip to America in 1492 after intercourse with Haitian women, and Captain James Cook was concerned with the spread of venereal disease, especially during his third voyage (1776–9), when almost half the ship's company had been affected.[13] Today's international travellers are a heterogenous group which includes holidaymakers, business persons, students, refugees and migrants. It has been stated[14] that migrants and travellers provide two fairly different questions, mirror images of each other when seen from the point of view of an individual country. Immigrants come to a specific country, and travellers leave for more or less brief periods. The notion of time is fundamental. The United Nations, WHO and the International Organization for Migration define travellers as people entering a country for 3 months or less. This section concentrates more or less on 'travellers', rather than 'immigrants'; studies showing the influence of migration on the spread of STDs/HIV have been presented by others.[15–18] Two special features of modern travel are that the largest group are now tourists; there were 341 million in 1986, and that the mode of transport is shifting increasingly towards air-travel. One consequence of the latter observation is that there is a greater chance now than before for a traveller to return within the incubation time of many STDs.[19]

Concepts of STDs/HIV interactions

Three relationships between STDs and HIV have been postulated:

1. increased transmission of HIV in the presence of other STDs, possibly because of disruption of the genital mucosa, or to recruitment of HIV-susceptible or HIV-infected lymphocytes or macrophages.
2. alteration in the natural history, diagnosis, or response to therapy of other STDs in the presence of HIV-induced immunosuppression.
3. accelerated progression of HIV disease in the presence of other STDs, for example by repeated immunostimulation.

Most studies have suffered from serious problems of confounding by differing sexual behaviours, co-infection with other STDs, lack of HIV-seronegative controls, or because they have been case control or cross-sectional in design. However, Wasserheit has recently conducted an extensive analysis of previously available data from observational studies.[20] 163 studies on the interrelationships between HIV infection and other STDs were examined. Of 75 studies on the role of STDs in HIV transmission, the 15 analyses of clinical or laboratory evidence of STDs adjusted for sexual behaviours showed that both ulcerative and non-ulcerative STDs increase the risk of HIV transmission approximately three- to five-fold. Owing to limited data, the role of STDs in progression of HIV disease remains unclear. However, data from 83 reports on the impact of HIV infection on STDs suggest that, at a community level, HIV infection may increase the prevalence of some STDs, especially genital ulcers. If co-infection with HIV prolongs or augments the infectiousness of individuals with STDs, and if the same STDs facilitate transmission of HIV, these infections may greatly amplify one another. This 'epidemiological synergy' may be responsible for the explosive growth of the HIV pandemic in some populations. Randomised controlled trials are the most effective way of proving a causal relation and estimating the magnitude of effect. They are, however, difficult to conduct, especially where the unit of randomisation is the community rather than the individual. Nevertheless, two such studies are being evaluated. In the first, improved STD case-management over two years in Tanzania has reduced HIV incidence by about 40%, and is the clearest evidence thus far of the interaction of STDs and HIV.[21] The second trial, whose results are awaited, involves an intervention of mass treatment for STDs in the Rakai district of Uganda.

Relationships between STDs and HIV and sexual behaviour and sexual networks

One fundamental, theoretical tenet of STD epidemiology, that of 'core-groups', was developed for gonorrhoea.[22] It is based on the observation that this infection is 'endemic' among a small sub-population of highly sexually active individuals, from whom it spreads in mini-epidemics to the population at large (Fig. 10.1).

Thus, the epidemic behaviour of STDs is related to the heterogeneity of the sexual behaviour of the population. This concept can be applied to all STDs, including HIV. This theory has been re-visited recently, using principles of mathematical ecology to give core-group theory biological plausibility. This work has been very influential in designing control programmes for controlling STDs and HIV and is discussed further here.

The ecological success for any infectious disease is described by its basic reproductive rate (R_0). To achieve long-term persistence, the effective R_0 must equal or exceed 1. For STDs including HIV, R_0 is determined by the product of the probability of infection transmission given contact between infective and susceptible individuals ($), the contact rate between infectives and susceptibles (c), and the duration of infectivity (D). Thus: $R_0 = \$cD$. A small sub-population of highly sexually active individuals forms a mixing sub-set which exceeds the threshold of the value of 'c', and thus becomes the reservoir for endemic persistence in a community, and is the site from which most infections in the community originate. This reservoir is termed 'core-group'. Core-groups are defined by their sexual behaviour and connectivity. By definition, R_0 exceeds unity only in the core, and is less than 1 in the non-core population. Thus in theory, only within the core-group are productive chains of infection sustained. Although many infections exit the core and enter adjacent populations, infection chains ultimately extinguish in these adjacent populations; thus the endemic persistence is entirely dependent on the core group.

$$R_0 = \$cD$$
R_0 = basic reproductive rate
$ = infectivity per contact
c = rate of contact change
D = duration of infectivity

Despite this probability-based biological theory, personal risk and mixing patterns, which include specific behaviour and social diffusion, are other important factors. Personal behaviour is embedded in a social and geographic context which may provide the link between behaviours which place individuals at risk, and sustain transmission of HIV in the community. Selection or preference of partner, self-perception and connection with the 'highly infective component' which form the social network, contribute to the dynamics of transmission of many STDs, including HIV. This may explain different transmission dynamics of HIV and other STDs such as gonorrhoea, syphilis, and *Chlamydia trachomatis* infection, and different patterns among specific sub-population groups, as well as providing insights into the demographic impact of STD/HIV. In summary, the core-group concept has a major impact on STD/HIV control

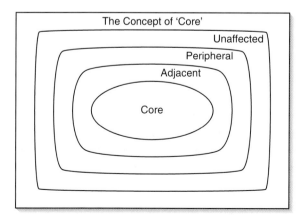

Fig. 10.1 The concept of core.

and surveillance programmes. If core-group members could be kept free of STD/HIV, infection should, in theory, disappear from the entire population.

Finally, it should be noted that R_0 can be decreased by decreasing infectiousness (by use of condoms) or decreasing duration of infectivity (access to effective healthcare).

Prostitutes and their clients are not the only type of 'core-group' for HIV and STDs but it should be apparent how important they may be in continued transmission of these pathogens. The usual composition of core-groups in Africa seems to comprise a few women and a large number of men. The opposite situation, a large number of women having sex with a small number of men would probably be similarly efficient; two such situations of male core-groups are seafarers and long-distance truck drivers. These groups will be discussed below under travellers.

STDs and HIV and travellers

Travelling may be difficult to recognise as an obvious epidemiological component. In addition, people can return home and have several sexual contacts before symptoms are obvious. Accurate contact-tracing is occasionally feasible; an often quoted example is that of a Californian prostitute, nicknamed 'syphilis Mary', who had secondary syphilis; she kept a diary which helped trace 168 long-distance truck drivers among her 310 male consorts spread over 34 American states, Canada, and Mexico. In England and Wales, during the year 1976 (the last year for which these data are available), 14% of cases of early syphilis were believed to have been contracted abroad, and in Sweden the percentage of new cases of syphilis contracted abroad was 20% in 1986 and 32% in 1987, implying that the impact of travel on STDs is not diminishing.

Geographical tracing for STDs is perhaps easiest for gonorrhoea because it is usually a symptomatic and acute infection. It can be done by the taking of an accurate history and/or microbiological techniques that take advantage of the fact that different strains of the gonococcus can be classified according to nutritional requirements (auxotype), reaction with a monoclonal antibody to the major outer membrane protein (serovar) and antibiotic-resistance patterns, including plasmid profiles. The most complete example of geographically accurate history-taking is available from six policlinics of dermatology in Switzerland. In the six Swiss clinics, among 1988 heterosexuals who were not IDUs, 25% of patients reported that they had acquired their STD abroad. Casual sex and sexual contacts with prostitutes played an important role in the acquisition of the STDs abroad, particularly in developing countries. In Sweden, using a combination of several of these techniques, there were 665 cases of gonorrhoea in 1991, 536 in 1992 and 417 in 1993. More than half the patients had been infected abroad, mostly during vacation; women predominantly in the southern parts of Europe, and men in East Asia and southern parts of Europe. Almost all PPNG infections could be traced from abroad (there are no endemic PPNG infections in Sweden).

In Singapore, a country in which the reporting system is particularly robust, 88.9% of gonococcal infections in heterosexual men 1981–9 were thought to have been acquired abroad (Goh A., personal communication, 1992).

In Sydney, Australia, an increasing proportion of heterosexually acquired gonorrhoea in males in the years 1981–9 was an Asian strain of PPNG, and was acquired either outside the country, or from Asian prostitutes working in Australia on short-term visas.[23, 24] In another study in Kenya, 6% of tourists reporting sick presented with urethritis. The attitudes, knowledge and behaviour of the largest group of international travellers (tourists) will be discussed later, but there are certain other groups of travellers, by virtue of their strange living and working conditions, that could be at increased risk with respect to STDs/HIV. These core-groups are seafarers and long-distance truck drivers. Seafarers all over the world acquire venereal diseases 5–20 times more frequently than the male population living on land. An epidemiological study in an unselected population of seamen from all over the world attending for check-ups in an outpatient clinic in Hamburg from 1967–87 showed that 3.1% had venereal disease.

British seafarers still have a relatively high incidence of STDs; infection rates have been shown to be between 17% and 23%. Long-distance truck drivers will be discussed in the context of HIV.

Although travel is not a risk factor for HIV per se, the importance of travellers in the spread of HIV from one population to another is undeniable. Present in the minds of many is the image of 'Patient Zero', implanting HIV in one country after another in Europe and North America.[25] It is possible that HIV left Africa at least a few times over the last few decades. From Africa, HIV spread to Haiti among Haitian guestworkers returning from Zaire in the 1970s, and then from Haiti to the USA, the Caribbean and South America, particularly among homosexual men and Hispanic IDUs. There was also early spread from Central Africa to Europe, among African students and among returning Europeans. The excess of HIV from pattern II countries[26] and several case-clusters[27] reflects in many cases the longstanding links certain African countries have with the European ex-colonial powers. Nearly all cases had histories of multiple sexual partners, local African contacts, and contact with prostitutes. In the late 1970s, HIV moved from the USA to Europe and Australia via homosexual men. In the Mediterranean, spread was initially among IDUs, and then into populations of homosexual men. In Norway and Sweden, reliable reporting systems reveal that up to 1993, the proportion of 'imported' HIV infections were 27% and 20% respectively (Hasseltvedt V. and Ramstedt K., personal communications). HIV has entered Asia (India, Thailand, Myanmar, Southern China) through changing patterns of drug trafficking and widespread female prostitution. In the view of the present author, the last two risk-factors, when found in close association, represent the most explosive means of spreading HIV.

It is possible that in certain instances advances in molecular epidemiology may prove enlightening. It is recognised that HIV DNA sequences from different geographic regions vary; the spread of variants to other locations has been used to suggest origins of HIV and how it has spread throughout the world.[28]

As mentioned previously, certain core-groups are pre-eminent – female prostitutes, truck drivers, seafarers and migrants. Rates of infection among prostitutes may be seen as a watershed for the importance of heterosexual transmission of HIV in any area in the world and infection rates from 6–90% have been recorded among female prostitutes in urban areas of central, eastern and southern Africa, and 0–60% (median 15%) in Thailand. In all cases, the 'lowest class' prostitutes (who service the most customers) have the highest rates of infection. Prostitutes who travel internationally have higher rates of infection than their domestic counterparts. They also have higher rates of STDs; this has become an increasingly serious epidemiological problem in Europe. This can be ascribed in part to socio-economic differences between the countries of the former socialist bloc and the countries of Western Europe. These differences have led to a great increase in the traffic of sex-workers and of their clients across the frontiers between these two previously separated parts of the continent.[29] Foreign bar-hostesses in Vienna, when offered a special health service in 1991, had an infection rate with gonorrhoea of 50%, dropping to 18% in 1992 (Stary A. and Kopp W., personal communication 1994). In the same city, the overall rate of STDs among illegal, 'female sex-workers' was 38 times higher than the infection rate among the licensed prostitutes (Schmidt A., personal communication, 1994). 90% of the window prostitutes in the red-light district of Amsterdam are not native to the Netherlands; a similar proportion applies to 'go-go' girls in Switzerland (Lebert M., personal communication, 1994).

Women from the former Eastern bloc are also vulnerable because of low levels of knowledge; a study of Romanian sex-workers in Istanbul revealed that 28% of the girls were first-time prostitutes. They had either very little or no knowledge about STDs or the means to protect themselves against them. Immigration in Europe of prostitutes from areas such as Africa, the Caribbean, South America and Thailand, where the prevalence of HIV is much higher than in Europe, seems to constitute an underestimated epidemiological phenomenon that could accelerate the spread of HIV-1 and HIV-2. In Asia, there is mobility of sex-workers from Nepal to India, Myanmar to Thailand and Thailand to Japan.[30] International sex-workers in Sydney who attend dedicated clinics in the largest STD facility (mostly from Thailand and Malaysia) have much higher rates of gonorrhoea, chlamydial infection and hepatitis B carriage, as well as much lower condom usage, than their local counterparts.

Long-distance truck drivers, by virtue of their travel within countries and across borders, are an important example of a male core-group. In fact, the epidemiology of much of the African HIV epidemic can be directly traced along the major highways.[31] Three studies have examined the prevalence of HIV infection in seafarers; in Valencia in 1987, seven of 290 (2.4%) seafarers were infected, a prevalence much higher than in the general population. In another study of seafarers working with Belgian shipping companies, 15 of 336 screening tests (4.5%) yielded a positive result, compared to an average, estimated prevalence among Belgians of 0.062%. A third study conducted between 1985 and 1987 in 2000 seamen revealed nine HIV infections (0.5%); in this sample, general knowledge about AIDS was very poor.

A final core-group might be 'sex-tourists'; they are discussed below along with the sexual attitudes and behaviour of tourists in general.

Calculation of rates of infection, relative risks and trends in HIV prevalence in various groups of travellers requires that accurate numerators and denominators are available. This is rarely the case. Moreover, only a few studies have estimated the *relative risk* of HIV infection associated with travel, by comparing travellers with a group of non-travelling controls. One difficulty with these investigations is that the relationship between HIV and travel may be confounded by differences between travellers and their controls in other factors (Elford J., personal communication, 1993). Among Danish homosexual men, HIV seropositivity in 1981 was strongly associated with travel to the USA (relative risk 3.5, $p < 0.007$). In 1987, 20% of people with Ugandan or Rwandan links had HIV infection, compared with only 2.2% of those who had never left Tanzania – a nine-fold difference in risk ($p < 0.01$). Using surveillance data, the risk of AIDS to heterosexual UK residents travelling abroad was estimated as

being 300 times greater than their risk of acquiring AIDS in the UK. However, changing the assumptions as to whether those 'presumed to be infected abroad' were travellers, immigrants or returned expatriates reduced the risk estimate to 6.0.[32] IDUs who share needles while travelling may also face a risk of HIV-infection. In a study conducted in Victoria, Australia, IDUs who had travelled to Sydney were more likely to be infected with HIV.[33]

3. Sexual behaviour of international tourists and sexual health promotion

Knowledge, attitudes and perceptions of risk in intending travellers

In two early studies[34,35] of several hundred new attendees at a travel clinic in London, there was mostly correct knowledge about general risk factors for AIDS, but only 25% requested more information, even if 30% did not know AIDS was present in the country they were visiting, and only 10% said they would purchase condoms abroad. An important conclusion emerged that has since been confirmed many times, that despite adequate knowledge of sexual transmission of HIV, there was no perceived *personal* risk of acquisition. In Korea,[36] intending male travellers were misinformed about many aspects of AIDS. In Canada, as recently as 1991, 14% of 331 travellers did not think that avoiding sexual intercourse was protective, and many thought that condoms were more effective if used with fellow travellers than with locals. In a cross-sectional study by the present author of young Australians travelling alone to Thailand (n = 213, mean age 26 years), only 34% of the sample reported a definite intention not to have sex.[37] More males than females said they would have sex with a Thai national, while more females than males said they would choose an

Australian traveller; 18% of men said they would have sex with a bar-girl. 82% of the sample reported they would use condoms 100% of the time, but there were significantly more females than males who expressed this intention. However, a larger number of females reported that they did not intend taking condoms with them. Once again, travellers did not perceive a higher personal risk of acquisition of AIDS in Thailand than Australia, even though they were aware of the magnitude of the difference in prevalence. An alarming misclassification was made between female Thai nationals and 'bar-girls', and this group of travellers were not obviously 'sex-tourists' (see below).

Sexual behaviour identified during travel

To the knowledge of the present author there are only five published studies; this probably reflects (methodological) problems of access.

In a study in Copenhagen in the late 1980s[38] 21% of male and 6% of female tourists (n = 1229, mean age 22.5 years) were carrying condoms, but only 19/40 males who had sex used one, compared to 0/4 females. A sample of 105 Japanese men (55 tourists and 50 businessmen) were interviewed in 1993 in Bangkok, using in-depth interviews and focus group discussions, facilitated by the Japanese Chamber of Commerce.[39] Both groups made extensive use of commercial sex-workers (71%), though 76% saw this as risky behaviour. Condoms were used by at least 95% of respondents, but only 51% used condoms all of the time. The same authors performed a situational analysis of young Japanese women tourists on the island of Phuket in Thailand[40] (and Vorakitphokatorn S., personal communication, 1994). The study started with interviews with tour company managers, then with Thai tour guides, Thai beach boys and last with Japanese female tourists. Absolute figures were not supplied. Nevertheless, beach boys reported that 70% of their tourist lovers were female Japanese. The sexual initiation was made mutually by 35%, by beach boys 30% and by tourists 13.6%. The

author concluded that these young women tourists are culturally and socially naive, and yet willing to take risks with the local service boys, who quickly develop a casual sexual relationship with them. Condom use was sometimes requested by the women, but the place and the frequency of sex acts did not lend themselves to any effective preventive behaviour. In the UK resort of Torbay, another group of 386 tourist industry workers were surveyed; only 7% had not engaged in intercourse in the last year; nearly half the male workers had engaged in intercourse with four or more tourists. Levels of condom use were low, with only 40% using a condom during their last intercourse; levels of condom use were lower still among those respondents reporting the most partners. The last two studies, of German visitors to Thailand and other destinations, are presented below, under the sub-heading 'sex-tourists'.

Sexual behaviour identified post-travel

The only national sex survey to ask specifically about partner change while on holiday was a Swiss telephone survey conducted in 1990. Among 1220 men aged 17–45, 66% had holidayed abroad in the first 9 months of 1990, and 7% of the sample reported that they had sexual relations with a person in the holiday country in that year. In a postal survey of returning travellers in the UK, 17/353 had sex with a new partner, but only 12 had been carrying condoms, and only 9 had used them. In Switzerland, in an unusual study, travel physicians claimed to be able to correctly identify (by dress and manner) travellers who were likely to be promiscuous; when interviewed post-travel 60% of this group had had casual sexual contacts while travelling (mean age 33 years) vs 3.6% of an unselected control group. In a study[41] of 782 attendees at the largest travel clinic in London (probably a mixture of tourists, expatriates and migrants) over a 6-month period in 1991–2, 141 (18.6%) had had new sexual partners during their most recent trip abroad. Almost two-thirds of those having sex abroad did not use condoms with a new partner, and 5.7% had contracted an STD during their most recent trip. 26% of men who had new sexual partners abroad paid for sex. 16 out of 731 (2.2%) participants were HIV-positive. The authors concluded that high-risk behaviours were found in both male and female international travellers. Men had more new partners abroad, but were more likely to use condoms.

In theory, STD/sexual health clinics should be ideal venues for establishing the risk of STDs attributable to travel, investigating past and recent sexual behaviour (e.g. use of condoms) when travelling, and identifying sub-groups of travellers who might be considered core-transmitters. They should also be able to highlight the opportunity for health education about sexual health risks in any geographical location, which can be incorporated into the counselling of attenders at sexual health clinics. Up to August 1996, there have been six published and one unpublished study of travellers in STD clinics.[42-46]

At the Melbourne Sexual Health Centre in a 6-month period in 1990, 111 men who had sex in South-East Asia were studied. 66 had evidence of an STD (not HIV or syphilis); all of these had sex with at least one prostitute, 28% without a condom, and 43% had sex with a partner after return to Australia. In Bergen, Norway, 245 (41%) of 606 consecutive patients reported having a sexual partner abroad in the previous 5 years; and, in three English STD clinics, 25–52% of heterosexual males and 18–20% of heterosexual females who had travelled in the previous 3–6 months had new partners during their trips. In the most thorough of these investigations, the authors estimated the proportion of infections stemming from travel abroad at 11.6%. They also identified risk factors such as being male, single and having visited an STD clinic previously.

There are several important limitations with these studies. First, the patients studied were probably not representative of the travelling public as a whole, or even of all STD clinic attenders; however, the number of visits made abroad by members of the public is high. Thus, even if the sexually active proportion of the total number of travellers is low, the absolute numbers of people at risk may be considerable. Second, in few of these studies have the demographic and behavioural

characteristics of travellers who attend STD clinics been compared with STD attendees who have not travelled, that is with non-travelling controls. This is the only way that behaviour and disease can be properly attributed to travel, in a quantifiable way, information that could form the basis for a prevention campaign that is amenable to evaluation. Third, comparison of previous studies is difficult because of differences in the questionnaires and reporting biases because of different time-lags.

Most of the information presented above has been quantitative, but researchers are beginning to realise that more qualitative research is needed as a means of placing this information within its social context.[47]

'Sex-tourists'

It can be safely assumed that there are some who travel abroad with the primary intention of having sexual encounters (in 1987, the Committee of Ministers of the Council of Europe identified the group of 'sex-tourists' as a special target group for AIDS/HIV-prevention activities). It is probable however, that the distinction between a person who has sex while travelling and a 'sex-tourist' is not only difficult and arbitrary, but also potentially misleading. Certainly men and women do travel specifically for the purpose of sex; men are said to prefer Thailand, the Philippines, Sri Lanka and some of the Caribbean and Latin American countries, and women (considered by some to account for 10% of 'sex-tourists') have a slight preference for Kenya and Haiti (Inquiry Commission of the Federal Republic of Germany, 1990). Sexual encounters take place in sociocultural contexts that vary as widely as their geographical ones. Thailand will be taken as an illustration.

Men do travel to Thailand specifically for the purpose of sex, but they are a difficult group to identify, at least in their country of origin, since 'sex-tours' are usually officially banned by tourist organisations. One study interviewed 152 German tourists in the company of Thai prostitutes at well-known ('girlie'), tourist spots such as Pattaya, Patong village in Phuket and the Patpong area of Bangkok. Even these 'sex-tourists' may not have been easily identified at their place of departure; the share of business travellers or men travelling with a club or group was low (3.4%); indeed, 66.2% travelled as so-called 'individual tourists'. They were generally older men (median 38 years), two-thirds of whom were regular visitors to Thailand, and just under half were married, widowed or divorced. 61% of their sample had brought condoms with them, although only 28% used them regularly, compared to 50% of those who also visited prostitutes in their own country. The study of returning male travellers from South-East Asia who presented at an STD clinic in Melbourne[44] found that the mean age was older than their usual clinic population (33.6 years vs 24 years), and that there was a low frequency of use of condoms (28%). In addition to age, other factors may distinguish so-called 'sex-tourists' from other travellers, for example length of stay. It is possible that the former group generally stay for a shorter time. In the German study, the median length of stay was 4 weeks; in the Melbourne group, the median figure was not provided, but 70% of 97 men stayed less than 5 weeks. Both studies found the number of partners in Thailand to be high; 25% of the Australians and 12% of the Germans had more than five partners during their holiday.

'Sex-tourists'
- Difficult and arbitrary definition
- Men – Thailand, Philippines, Sri Lanka, Latin America
- Women – Kenya, Haiti, Bali
- Difficult to identify at place of departure
- Sociocultural contexts vary widely.

The German study group later extended their findings in a series of interviews between 1991–3[48] (Kleiber D. and Wilke M. personal communication, 1994). Since this is the largest, and as far as is known, only, detailed study of 'sex-tourists' (defined as individuals who had commercial sex with local partners), performed in situ, it is reported here. 766 interviews were carried out in selected countries: Kenya (n = 136), Brazil (n = 112), Thailand (n = 204), Philippines (n = 78),

and Dominican Republic (n = 236), with male heterosexual (n = 661) and homosexual (n = 105) 'sex-tourists'. Only the results for the heterosexuals are reported here. The instruments used were a standardised questionnaire, face-to-face interviews and in-depth, personal interviews. The average age was 35 (range 19–74), and the level of educational attainment was poor (45% junior high school, 25% high school graduate, 13% pre-college, 9% college graduate). 70% were single (vs 51% German population census data). They were largely not participants in package tours. Only 40% of those questioned were first-time visitors to the respective countries; many had previously vacationed or travelled in other non-European countries, where the majority reported having had sexual intercourse (visitors to the Dominican Republic were an exception). The majority were travelling with the explicit intention of engaging in sex, and had an average sexual contact with four women.

Since the previous study by the same authors, condom use in Thailand had increased ('always' increased from 28% to 50%, 'never' decreased from 45% to 30%), and there was high rate of use ('always', 75%) in the Dominican Republic. However, overall, only 45% of the whole sample regularly used condoms, and one-third never used them. The average age of the female partners was reported to be around 23, while the youngest was 13. There was little mention of explicit child prostitution; sex with partners younger than 11 years was a priority for 2.8%. 23% reported having had sexual contacts with prostitutes in Germany in the previous 12 months, with the number of such instances showing a very skewed distribution (median – 3 times, mean – 10 times). In the view of the present author, this almost certainly reflects a small 'core' of very frequent visitors to prostitutes. One-third reported having had an STD at least once (mostly gonorrhoea, 22.9%); about half had been tested for HIV at least once. Finally, on the coast of Kenya, the same group interviewed 81 German women (average age 36 years); nearly one-third reported sexual contact with local males. With one exception, all the women interviewed reported having had only one sexual partner; however, 13 (68%) had never used a condom.

A smaller study of German 'sex-tourism' in the Philippines by a different author (and Weiler G., personal communcation, 1995) suggests a dichotomy between short- and long-term 'sex-tourists', and therefore that different health promotion messages are probably needed for each group.

The interactions between tourists and commercial sex-workers vary from country to country depending on the sociocultural context. This has been most extensively studied in Thailand.

Certain aspects about prostitution in Thailand are important to emphasise. First, it is widespread. Commercial sex is illegal, but it is nevertheless condoned, and estimates of the number of sex-workers in Thailand range from 100 000 to 800 000 individuals, mostly in the upper range. Thai men of all ages and all social classes, whether single or married, frequently visit sex-workers. Thai male customers have been estimated to number between 3 and 8 million in total. Therefore, Thai women working (full-time, or occasionally) as sex workers are ubiquitous; the proportion catering especially to tourists is small in comparison, concentrated in a few, well-known tourist spots.

Second, with regard to encounters between Thai sex-workers and foreign ('fareng') customers, there is little in common with prostitution in Western society. For example, in the first German study, 63% of the men spent several days together with their last Thai date, many of them regarding themselves as being 'in love'. Other authors have described these encounters as 'open-ended', that is, a mixture of pecuniary interest and emotional attachment (by the Thais), and 'romantic interludes' (by foreigners).[49]

Third, pre-marital or extra-marital sex is uncommon among Thai women, though common among Thai men. Therefore, most (if not all) of the 'Thai nationals' identified by male subjects in the previous study as potential sex partners are probably commercial sex-workers, even if not obviously 'bar-girls', an alarming misclassification. The newcomer 'fareng', unable to grasp this culture-specific category, a vaguely defined grey area lying between 'full-fledged prostitution' and 'straight' sexuality, initially refuses to label the girls as 'prostitutes'. Although no figures are available on how many young, single, male tourists pass through Thailand without a sexual encounter with

a Thai female, it is possible that the number is small. Therefore, the intention of female participants in the previous study to have sex with fellow tourists (and indeed Thai males) is also alarming. Although only one study of homosexual 'sex-tourism' to Thailand has been identified, there is evidence that an increasing number of 'bar-boys' are infected with HIV. Many of the latter also have Thai and 'fareng' girlfriends.

In summary, while 'sex-tourists' should be specifically targeted if possible, particularly as they may act as so-called 'core-transmitters' of STDs and HIV, they are usually difficult to identify. Therefore, it is vital that all sexually active persons should be warned forcefully of the dangers of casual sex, particularly if they are young, travelling without spouse or partner and going to countries where the sociocultural context is conducive to risky behaviour.

Sexual health advice from the travel industry and other agencies

Although travellers have been identified as being important targets for sexual health promotion, regrettably, there have been until recently remarkably few attempts to educate the travelling public, and to bridge the obvious gap between knowledge and changes in sexual behaviour. A certain proportion of this inaction has been due to attempts by various governments to play down the problem of STDs, and especially HIV, particularly in those countries heavily dependent upon tourist revenue for foreign currency.

Efforts to influence the sexual behaviour of travellers can be sub-divided into the passive provision of health information (by healthcare providers, travel agents and public health authorities), and active health promotion interventions, aimed at specific groups of travellers on location. These will now be considered in more detail.

Only one study, by the present author, has attempted to collate global knowledge, information and health promotion initiatives by an important core-group of healthcare providers, namely travel physicians (unpublished data).

The conclusion from this pilot survey is that although travel is widely recognised as an epidemiological factor by STD clinicians, there appears to be insufficient awareness or emphasis among workers in the field of travel medicine. This is particularly evident in North America and needs to be urgently remedied.

A Canadian survey[50] revealed that 60% of all travellers relied to some extent on their travel agent to provide them with information on diseases and health hazards. However, a telephone survey of 30 travel agents in Leeds, UK revealed that although 19 recognised the risk of HIV infection in Bangkok, only 4 advised customers of that risk. Booklets containing health advice either did not mention HIV, or were distributed only sporadically. Two noteworthy projects of travel agents taking an active stance were identified. The famous chain of 'Club Mediterrane' holiday resorts, with 98 holiday villages in 26 countries, and more than 8 million overnights per year, has a programme for its staff (1700 in the villages) whereby oral, written and video information is given. Condoms are available in the village shops, which are also accessible to holiday guests.[51] In Scarborough, Ontario, Canada, travel agencies distributed condoms with sunscreen oil and lip balsam; the reaction from travellers was, in general, very favourable.

In response to an overwhelming need, the National Committee on AIDS of the Netherlands (with support from the Commission of the European Communities, the Ministry of Welfare, Health and Cultural Affairs of the Netherlands, and from the Regional Office for Europe of WHO) has embarked on an ambitious project, named 'AIDS and mobility – The impact of international mobility on the spread of HIV, and the need and possibility for AIDS/HIV prevention programmes.' This project continues to be the single biggest resource in Europe and produces bibliographies, educational materials and annual reports.[52] In September 1994, WHO designated 'AIDS and Mobility' as a 'special project' of the WHO Global Program on AIDS.

The most commonly used means of information are the so-called 'AIDS/HIV holiday campaigns,' with accompanying posters, brochures and television advertisements. These campaigns probably fail to reach a significant number of travellers.

In Australia, sexual health promotion aimed at travellers (Travel-Safe) began in 1991, and has consisted of the passive provision of convenience advertising, billboards and pamphlets to an indiscriminate group of travellers, and is mostly concerned with provision of information, rather than any attempt to change behaviour. In addition, evaluation has been minimal, consisting mostly of process evaluation. New initiatives have included a cooperative agreement with Thailand to advertise at well-known entertainment venues in Bangkok, the distribution to general practitioners of a 'Travel-Safe' kit, and the development of a corporate policy on travel health for the Australian Chamber of Commerce and Industry. As the 'AIDS and Mobility' project notes, it is somehow embarrassing that no information materials have been identified which are exclusively directed towards female travellers. What is the use of encouraging men to use condoms without making a similar effort towards women, for example to help women insist that their male partners use a condom?

Several Swiss organisations have adopted a different approach, aiming at 'sex-tourists,' and particularly those involved in child prostitution. Their actions are coordinated with the International Campaign to End Child Prostitution in Asian Tourism (ECPAT), which emerged in 1990, and which drew heavily on earlier work by others.[53] The Federal Department of Equal Rights between women and men convened a working group in 1992, and prepared a leaflet 'Wenn einer eine Reise tut'/'A vous qui partez en voyage' for the purpose of providing sensitising information on the situation of women in developing countries, particularly with regard to child prostitution. 100 000 have been distributed to places where travellers prepare their holidays, and the campaign is presently being evaluated (Pluss C., personal communication, 1995).

Several countries, following the example of Germany in 1992, have attempted to provide a more powerful deterrent to 'sex-tourism' involving child prostitution. For example, the Child Sex Tourism Act was ratified in the Australian parliament in July 1994 (and later adopted by New

Zealand), essentially making it an offence for Australians to engage in sex with children overseas. However, with the exception of the discovery of incriminating evidence on Australian soil, the greatest problem is that the child sex trade in Asia is a crime normally without an official complainant. Recently, the Philippine government has been enraged by reports by women's groups which claimed that Australians were dominant in the country's sex industry, including 80% of the sex bars in Angeles City. This figure was disputed by the Australian Embassy in Manila.

In general, although they would be very useful but expensive, attempts to involve airline carriers in AIDS prevention, for example, by including messages in in-flight magazines, have been unsuccessful. An appeal to all major European airlines failed, with the exception of LOT, the Polish carrier (Broring G., personal communication, 1994).

Finally, more active intervention programmes are hard to identify. In Torbay, UK, a pilot project in 1990 involved fun-nights, local taverns and competitions, and was so successful that a 3-year HIV/AIDS Prevention Project 1993–5 was launched – 'Happy Health Holiday Campaign' with the slogan 'Sea, Sand and Safe Sex' – whose central strategy was to recruit and train peer-educators (age 11–25) for the summer holiday season (Inman M., personal communication, 1995). A less ambitious programme took place at a Norwegian resort in Mallorca in 1992 (Amundsen N., unpublished data). In Berne, Switzerland, the Federal Office of Public Health is endeavouring to target various sub-groups within the extremely heterogenous group of travellers by training travel professionals (tour leaders, flight attendants, resident managers) as mediators of AIDS prevention.

Conclusions on sexual health promotion efforts in travellers

1. The provision of information on modes of transmission of HIV/AIDS/STDs during international travel has recently increased (with the exception of North America), but may be insufficient to change sexual behaviour. More vigorous interventions are probably required.
2. The reluctance of the travel industry, especially international air carriers, to promote safer sex to travellers, needs to be addressed.
3. Behavioural research, particularly situational and contextual analysis of the different sexual behaviours of travellers is urgently needed, the results of which should be incorporated into health messages. These should include culturally specific information relating to the effects of 'sex-tourism', with special emphasis on child prostitution.
4. While not fully understood, the factors that link travel to STD/HIV risk probably include:
   - the higher prevalences of infections in other countries
   - situational or contextual factors such as the relative availability of sex, different cultural expectations, and the relative unavailability of condoms
   - psychological disinhibition (the 'traveller's head-space').
5. Appropriate methodology is needed to evaluate sexual health promotion interventions in travellers. A completely fresh approach is recommended, including comprehensive programme planning and evaluation.

The purpose of programme planning is to devise an intervention or series of interventions that are appropriate to the health problem and the identified target groups, within the resources available, and which will have the best chance of bringing about the desired change. In the present context, this might include:

Programme goal: To minimise the incidence of STDs/HIV in travellers.
Outcome evaluation: minimisation of reported cases of HIV/STDs attributable to travel.

Programme objective: To reduce risk taking behaviour by travellers.
Impact evaluation: reduction in self-reported risk-taking.

Strategy objectives

1. To increase awareness of personal risk by particular groups of travellers.
   Process evaluation: measurement of the reach of elements of the programme among the target groups.
2. To increase awareness and develop the skills to address the risks to travellers of STDs/HIV among travel and health professionals.
   Process evaluation: acceptability and evaluation of training modules and materials.
3. To establish ongoing surveillance mechanisms for risk behaviours and STD/HIV morbidity among travellers.
   Process evaluation: generation of timely and meaningful reports.

The central message

Obviously, existing educational materials will continue to be available and distributed. Most governmental strategies have been informational, concentrating on the speed of spread of HIV/AIDS and protection through the use of condoms. However, as a number of behavioural studies have shown, many travellers are fully informed but do not personalise the risk.

The central message of future campaigns should be to deliver the idea that many travellers behave differently while away from home and to confront individuals with the notion that they might also behave differently whether they intend to or not. This represents a fundamental shift, from an *information* paradigm to a *behavioural* one.

Program evaluation

CONSTRAINTS

The overriding problem for evaluating health promotion programmes is to ascribe positive (or negative) measurable outcomes to the program itself. Numerous examples abound. For example,

was the minimisation of HIV/AIDS among Australian IDUs a result of the needle and syringe exchange programme or other factors? The biggest difficulty is ascribing, in an hierarchical fashion, successes demonstrated for impact and process evaluation to programme/goal successes. Process evaluation is usually relatively straightforward, but translating that to impact (behaviour) or to outcome (reduction in STDs/HIV) is much more problematic. The last two may have to be reasonably inferred rather than epidemiologically proven.

PROCESS EVALUATION
(i.e. message penetration)

In essence, process evaluation assesses the numbers in various target groups, who have seen, remembered, or have an opinion on the message delivered. The last two elements can be measured regularly using well-established, intercept techniques.

IMPACT EVALUATION
(i.e. reduction in risk-taking behaviour)

Self-administered questionnaires can be designed, piloted and distributed to representative community-derived samples from each group of interest (e.g. business travellers, backpackers). A baseline survey would be required, followed by regular, follow-up surveys, taking care to ensure that the demographic features of each cross-sectional sample were as similar as possible to the baseline. While recognising the inherent biases of the sample, longitudinal behavioural trends (e.g. proportion using condoms when having sex overseas) will also be accessible from sexual health service databases.

OUTCOME EVALUATION
(i.e. minimised STD/HIV infection)

The true number of cases of STDs/HIV attributable to travel is unknown, and the methods of estimating the number will remain imperfect. Any effect on outcome may have to be inferred in part from measures of impact.

Personalising the risk

A central message of future programmes should be to deliver the message that many travellers behave differently while away from home, and to confront individuals with the notion that they might also behave differently whether they intend to or not. This represents a fundamental shift from an informational paradigm to a behavioural one.

4. From epidemiology to clinical practice

Practical conclusions and advice for travellers and their physicians

The risk of acquisition of STDs or HIV infection can be virtually eliminated by avoiding penetrative sexual intercourse with casual partners, especially IDUs and persons who have had multiple sexual partners (such as prostitutes), or reduced by the use of condoms. The risk of parenteral exposure to these agents can be reduced by avoiding parenteral drug use and behaviour that is likely to lead to injury (with its attendant risk of requiring blood transfusion), and by seeking facilities with adequate capabilities to screen blood donors and to sterilise instruments.

Post-travel checks for STDs (except HIV) are usually unnecessary and impractical in most asymptomatic persons. However, if travellers have been exposed to high-risk individuals/behaviours and request assessment, this is best done at centres specialising in genitourinary medicine. If patients are symptomatic, this is even more important for the following reasons:

- the patient may have had multiple exposures, making history-taking more complex
- the patient may have been partially treated, altering the natural history, and making special investigations more difficult
- knowledge of patterns of antibiotic resistance and interpretation of serological tests for syphilis are usually limited to a few centres

- facilities such as selective media, and dark ground microscopy are not usually available in travel clinics.

With respect to choice of testing centre for exposure to HIV-1 or HIV-2, this is a matter for individual clinicians to decide; it should be remembered that pre- and post-test counselling requires considerable skill, is time-consuming and is recommended by most Departments of Health in developed countries. If there is a possibility of exposure to HIV-2, this should be emphasised to the laboratory, so that appropriate tests are performed and difficulties in interpretation are taken into account.

PRACTICE POINTS

Travellers at greater risk of sexually transmitted diseases
- Travellers to highly endemic areas.
- Those who have casual and multiple sexual partners.
- Those travelling for long periods away from home, for example truck drivers.
- Expatriate workers travelling without partners.
- Commercial sex-workers travelling to work in foreign countries.
- 'Sex-tourists'.

Prevention of sexually transmitted diseases in travellers
- Be aware of the risk.
- Practise safer sex.
- Carry condoms.
- Realise alcohol can release inhibitions and lead to unprotected casual sex.
- Remember the inexperienced may be unprepared for the temptations offered by professional sex-workers.
- Identify higher risk groups so that sex education can be focused.

REFERENCES

1. Gerbase AC, Rowley JT, Heymann DHL, et al. Global prevalence and incidence estimates of selected curable STDs. Sexually Transmitted Infections 1998; 74(Suppl. 1): S12–S16.

2. Gerbase AC, Rowley JT, Mertens TE. Global epidemiology of sexually transmitted diseases. Lancet 1998; 351(Suppl. 111): 2–5.

3. Ison CA, Dillon J-AR, Tapsall JW. The epidemiology of global antibiotic resistance among *Neisseria gonorrhoeae* and *Haemophilus ducreyi*. Lancet 1998; 351(Suppl. 111): 8–12.

4. Gilson RJC. Sexually transmitted hepatitis: a review. Genitourinary Medicine 1992; 68: 123–129.

5. Alter MJ, Coleman PJ, Alexander WJ, et al. Importance of heterosexual activity in the transmission of hepatitis B and non A, non B hepatitis. Journal of the American Medical Association 1989; 262: 1201–1205.

6. Centers for Disease Control. Pneumocystis pneumonia–Los Angeles. Morbidity and Mortality Weekly Report 1981; 30: 250–252.

7. UNAIDS/WHO. Report on the global HIV/AIDS epidemic, June 1998. Geneva: WHO.

8. Carpender CCJ, Fischl MA, Hammer SM, et al. Antiretroviral therapy for HIV infection in 1997: updated recommendations of the International AIDS Society–USA panel. Journal of the American Medical Association 1997; 77: 1962–1969.

9. Pantaleo G, Perrin L. Can HIV be eradicated? AIDS 1998; 12(Suppl. A): S175–S180.

10. Stott J, Hu S-L. Overview: vaccines and immunology. AIDS 1998; 12(Suppl. A): S95–S96.

11. Kaldor JM, ed. AIDS in Asia and the Pacific. (2nd ed.) AIDS 1998.

12. Laga M, ed. AIDS in Africa. (2nd ed.) AIDS 1998.

13. Watt J. Lettsonian lectures. Medical perspectives of some voyages of discovery. Transactions of the Royal Society of London 1979; 95: 61–91.

14. Haour-knipe M. Assessing AIDS prevention among migrant populations. In : Paccand F, Vader JP, Gutzwiller, eds. Assessing AIDS Prevention. Basel: Birkhauser; 1992.

15. De Schryver A, Meheus A. Sexually transmitted diseases and migration. International Migration 1990; 29(1): 13–22.

16. Quinn TC. Population migration and the spread of types 1 and 2 human immunodeficiency viruses (review). Proceedings of the National Academy of Science 1994; 91(7): 2407–2414.

17. Mabey D, Mayaud P. Sexually transmitted diseases in mobile populations. Genitourinary Medicine 1997; 73: 18–22.

18. Decosas J, Adrien A. Migration and HIV. AIDS 1997; 11(Suppl. A): S77–S84.

19. De Schryver, Meheus A. International travel and sexually transmitted diseases. World Health Statistical Quarterly 1989; 42: 90–99.

20. Wasserheit JN. Epidemiological synergy. Interrelationship between human immunodeficiency virus infection and other sexually transmitted diseases. Sexually Transmitted Diseases 1992; 19(2): 61–77.

21. Grossfurth H, Mosha F, Todd J, Mwijarubi E, et al. Impact of improved treatment for sexually transmitted diseases on HIV infection in rural Tanzania: randomised controlled trial. Lancet 1995; 346: 530–536.

22. Yorke JA, Hethcote HW, Nold A. Dynamics and control of transmission of gonorrhoea. Sexually Transmitted Diseases 1978; 5: 31–36.

23. Donovan B, Bek M, Pethebridge AM, Nelson MJ. Heterosexual gonorrhoea in central Sydney: implications for HIV control. Medical Journal of Australia 1991; 154: 175–180.

24. Donovan B, Harcourt C, Bassett I, Philpot CR. Gonorrhoea and Asian prostitution: the Sydney Sexual Health Centre experience. Medical Journal of Australia 1991; 154: 520–521.

25. Shilts R. And the band played on. New York: St Martin's Press; 1987.

26. Noone A, Gill ON, Clarke SE, Porter K. Travel, heterosexual intercourse and HIV-1 infection. Communicable Disease Report 1991; 1: R39–R43.

27. Vitteroq D, Rove RT, Mayand C, et al. Acquired immunodeficiency syndrome after travelling in Africa: an epidemiological study in seventeen Caucasian patients. Lancet 1987; i: 612–615.

28. Weniger BG, Takebe Y, Ou CY, Yamazaki S. The molecular epidemiology of HIV in Asia. AIDS 1994, 8(Suppl. 2): S13–S28.

29. Mardh PA, Genc M. Migratory prostitution with emphasis on Europe. Journal of Travel Medicine 1995; 2(1): 28–32.

30. Brown T, Mulhall B, Sittitrai W. Risk factors for HIV transmission in Asia and the Pacific. AIDS 1994; 8(Suppl. 2): S173–S182.

31. Mbugua G, Hearst N, Linden C, Waiyaki PG, et al. Risk factors associated with HIV infection among long distance truck drivers in Kenya.Abstract PoD 5367, (Western Journal of Medicine 1987; 147: 694–701).

32. Feachem RG, Phillips-Howard PA. Risk to UK heterosexuals of contracting AIDS abroad. Lancet 1988; ii: 394–395.

33. Crofts N, Hay M. Entry of human immunodeficiency virus infection into a population of injecting drug users, Victoria, 1990. Medical Journal of Australia 1991; 155: 378–382.

34. Porter JDH, Phillips-Howard PA, Behrens RH. AIDS awareness among travellers. Travel Medicine International 1991; 28–32.

35. Behrens RH, Porter JDH. HIV infection and foreign travel. British Medical Journal 1990; 301: 1217.

36. Choi KH, Catania J, Coates TJ, Hearst N. International travel and AIDS risk in South Korea (letter). AIDS 1992; 6(12): 1555–1557.

37. Mulhall BP, Hu M, Thompson M, Lin F, et al. Planned sexual behaviour of young Australian visitors to Thailand. Medical Journal of Australia 1993; 158: 530–535.

38. Worm AM, Lillelund H. Condoms and sexual behaviour of young tourists in Copenhagen. AIDS Care 1989; 1(1): 93–96.

39. Vorakitphokatorn S, Cash R, Elliot ST. Heterosexual behaviour related to the risk of HIV infection among Japanese men in Bangkok, Thailand. Xth International Conference on AIDS/International Conference on STD, Yokohama 7–12 August 1994. Abstracts, Volume 1, PD0367.

40. Vorakitphokatorn S. Sexual behaviour of young Japanese women tourists in Southern Thailand and risk for HIV infection. Xth International Conference on AIDS/International Conference on STD, Yokohama 7–12 August 1994. Abstracts, Volume 1, 066D.

41. Hawkes SJ, Hart G, Johnson AM, Shergold C, et al. Risk behaviour and HIV prevalence in international travellers. AIDS 1994; 8: 247–252.

42. Rowbottom J. Risks taken by Australian men having sex in South East Asia. Venereology 1991; 4(2): 56–59.

43. Treit KS, Nilsen A, Nyfors A. Casual sexual experience abroad in patients attending an STD clinic and at high risk for HIV infection. Genitourinary Medicine 1994; 70: 12–14.

44. Daniels DG, Kell P, Nelson MR, Barton SE. Sexual behaviour amongst travellers: a study of genitourinary medicine clinic attenders. STD & AIDS 1992; 3: 437–438.

45. Mendelsohn R, Astle L, Mann M, Shahmanesh M. Sexual behaviour in travellers abroad attending an inner-city genitourinary medicine clinic. Genitourinary Medicine 1996; 72: 43–46.

46. Hawkes S, Hart GJ, Bletsoe E, Shergold C, Johnson AM. Risk behaviour and STD acquisition in genitourinary clinic attenders who have travelled. Genitourinary Medicine 1995; 71: 351–354.

47. Hawkes SJ, Hart GJ. Travel, migration, and HIV. AIDS Care 1993; 5(2): 207–214.

48. Kleiber D, Wilke M. Sexual behaviour of German (sex) tourists. IXth International Conference on AIDS, Berlin, June 6–11,1993, Abstract Volumes, WS-D10-2.

49. Ford N, Koetsawong S. The socio-cultural context of the transmission of HIV in Thailand. Social Science and Medicine 1991; 33(4): 405–414.

50. Zutis A. Travel project. Scarborough Health Dept, Scarborough, Ontario, August 1989 (unpublished).

51. Binder M. Collective protection measures in distant Club Med villages. In: Pasini W, ed. Tourist health. WHO Collaborating Centre for Tourist Health and Tourist Medicine, Rimini, 1990.

52. AIDS and mobility. A manual for the implementation of HIV/AIDS prevention activities aimed at travellers and migrants. Amsterdam: National Committee on AIDS Control; 1993.

53. Caught in modern slavery. Tourism and child prostitution in Asia. Ecumenical Coalition on Third World Tourism, Bangkok, 1990.

TRAVEL-RELATED RISKS: INFECTION (excluding malaria)

Diseases spread by food, water or soil

Philip Welsby

Introduction

This chapter considers the infection hazards which travellers may face through exposure to contaminated food, water or soil. This is usually by contamination from human or animal excreta. Brucellosis contracted through contaminated milk is also included.

An introduction to the diseases is given here and further details can be found in Section 7 on perspectives in Africa, Asia and South and Central America, and in the discussion on travellers' diarrhoea (pp. 273–286).

As there are no available vaccines or appropriate chemoprophylaxis for many of these diseases, other methods of prevention are very important. Management of the illnesses is considered, including the occasional need for repatriation. Often and more realistically, travel to local centres with good facilities, is the main course of action and advice is highlighted in Practical travel issues, boxes.

vomiting of sudden onset affecting groups of people are almost always food- or water-borne.

Contamination of drinking water with living organisms is a major cause of illness amongst travellers. In the UK, we drink water straight from the tap and rarely consider it may be a source of disease. Hepatitis A and E, enteric fever and cholera may all be contracted through drinking contaminated water.

Many of the diseases considered in this section can be spread via food and water, but for the purpose of this review they will be categorised according to the most likely vehicle of transmission. Most food-related illness is caused by either infection, or a change in the amount or type of food consumed. Infection may originate in the food (e.g. tapeworm or toxoplasmosis) or be introduced by dirty hands or through washing foods and utensils in unclean water. (See pages 276–281 for details on ETEC travellers' diarrhoea, *Shigella*, *Campylobacter* and *Salmonella* infection, amoebic dysentery and giardiasis.)

Introduction

Intercontinental travel becomes more common each year. It is now possible to be anywhere in the world within 36 hours.

In developed countries, there are stringent regulations regarding food and drink preparation and sewage disposal. In developing countries, such regulations may be poor or totally lacking and problems may arise if food or water is contaminated with animal or human faecal pathogens. For example, most cases of diarrhoea are caused by faecal–oral spread of infection, and diarrhoea and

Bacterial diseases contracted through ingesting food and water

Enteric fevers

These are caused by the faecal–oral spread of *Salmonella typhi* and *Salmonella paratyphi* A, B, or C. Enteric fevers, especially typhoid fever, are septicaemic illnesses with fever, headache, impaired mentation, vague abdominal pain and

1. Do not drink local water without boiling, chemical sterilisation or using a reliable filter, unless you are sure of the purity of the local water supply (see Box 11.2).
2. This also applies to water used for making ice cubes and cleaning teeth.
3. Bottled water is usually safe, as are hot tea, coffee, beer and wine.
4. Plates, cutlery and other utensils may have been washed in contaminated water.
5. Unpasteurised milk should be boiled. Cheeses and ice cream are often made from unpasteurised milk and when in doubt these should only be bought from larger firms when quality can be assured.
6. All meat should be thoroughly cooked and eaten hot whenever possible. Avoid leftovers.
7. At certain times of the year, certain fish and shellfish can be hazardous, even if well cooked. Take local advice about seafood, but when in doubt it is best to avoid them.
8. Eat only cooked vegetables and avoid green leafy salads.
9. Peel all fruit, including tomatoes.
10. Wash hands thoroughly with soap and clean water **before** eating or handling food, and always **after** using the toilet.

constipation (rather than diarrhoea which tends to occur in the third week of illness) being main features. Occasionally, there may be a brief episode of vomiting after the circumstantial time of infection (as occurs in a typical gastroenteritis, from *Salmonella*). Embolic 'rose spots' may occur.

TYPHOID FEVER

Salmonella typhi organisms are ingested, reach the small intestine and, without multiplication, penetrate the intestinal mucosa and proliferate in the lymphoid tissue before entering the bloodstream to cause systemic illness. This invasion of the bloodstream marks the end of the incubation period.

The organism circulates to all bodily tissues to cause various manifestations. In the meninges and brain: headache or confusion; in the non-pigmented skin: the famous 'rose spots'; in the gall bladder: symptomatic or asymptomatic infection; and in the chest: a cough. Patients may not have diarrhoea at the onset of symptoms; indeed, they may be constipated as a result of fever-induced dehydration, but diarrhoea often develops once the organisms have relocalised to the ileum and is more common in children. Later, the organism relocalises in the Peyer's patches of the ileum and these, at the end of a prolonged, febrile illness, may be the site of haemorrhage or perforation or both. Without antibiotics, the mortality rate is about 15%.

Paratyphoid fever, caused by *Salmonella paratyphi* A, B or C, is a milder illness than typhoid and 'rose spots' may be more common.

Diagnosis

This is by isolation of the organism in blood (in 90% of those untreated), urine or stool cultures. Widal's serology test may be misleading, especially in those vaccinated or infected with certain other non-typhoidal salmonellae.

Treatment

The treatment of choice is an 8-aminoquinolone such as ciprofloxacin, especially in areas where chloramphenicol-, β-lactam- and co-trimoxazole resistance is present.

Prevention

Disease risks reflect carriage rates in the areas to be visited and also the traveller's lifestyle. Again, adhering to general food and water precautions and those detailed under hepatitis A infection (p. 247) will help protect the traveller against the enteric fevers. Vaccination against typhoid but not paratyphoid is available.

CHOLERA

The cholera vibrio is usually transmitted by water contaminated with faeces. It is an uncommon, and always imported, infection in the UK.

A survey of reported cholera in travellers indicated that the risks of infection are low, even allowing for under-reporting and illness occurring while in the country visited. However, many infections are probably mild and do not result in investigations.

Vibrio cholerae, of which man is the only known host, is a classical enterotoxin-mediated, small-bowel type of diarrhoea which lasts for 1–7 days unless death supervenes. Neither the vibrio nor its toxin invades the gut wall, bacteraemia and associated fever do not occur, and red blood cells and leukocytes are not usually present in the stool.

After incubation of 6–72 hours, there may be illness ranging from the trivial to fulminant dehydration with up to 20 L of fluid being passed within 24 hours. Antibacterial therapy, usually with a tetracycline, is used in conjunction with rapid and adequate fluid replacement.

Cholera immunisation provides only poor, short-lived protection. Although new, more effective, oral vaccines are becoming available, the prevention of cholera depends upon good food, and particularly water hygiene.

BRUCELLOSIS

Brucellosis is a zoonosis with a near-worldwide distribution. Acquisition is usually by ingestion of infected milk or milk products although occasionally entry is via the respiratory tract or via the sexual route. Vets can acquire infection through abraded skin in contact with infected material.

Human brucellosis, when caused by *Brucella abortus*, is a disease which is usually acquired from milk of cattle. *Brucella abortus* has been eradicated in several parts of the world by eradicating the disease in cattle. *Brucella mellitensis* is acquired from goats or sheep (possibly camels) and *Brucella suis* from pigs. Brucellosis, once established, may persist for life in affected animals.

The incubation period of acute brucellosis is usually 1–3 weeks.

Symptoms

Acute brucellosis is often dramatic with fever, sweats, aches and pains and severe malaise. Fever may be undulant with days of feverishness separated by weeks without fever. There may be lymph node enlargement, hepatomegaly or splenomegaly. Skeletal problems include arthritis, spondylitis and osteomyelitis, but the organism can also localise in testes, meninges or heart valves. Some patients with acute brucellosis progress to chronic brucellosis, but other patients insidiously develop the chronic form with persisting foci of infection in the bone, liver or spleen with a number of non-specific symptoms including malaise, fatigue and depression.

Diagnosis and treatment

Diagnosis is by culture of the organism from blood, bone marrow or other biopsy specimens. Serological tests are available.

Treatment is difficult because the organisms reside intracellularly in reticuloendothial tissues. In 1986, WHO recommended 6 weeks of doxycycline and rifampicin for uncomplicated brucellosis although other regimens may be equally as effective.[1] Treatment for 6 weeks suppresses symptoms but may not eradicate the organism and relapses may occur necessitating long-term, suppressive therapy while the host's immune system eradicates the organism. Other regimens include streptomycin or co-trimoxazole.

There is no vaccine available for humans. Prevention relies upon avoidance of unpasteurised dairy products.

LEPTOSPIROSIS

There are fewer than 100 cases of leptospirosis notified in the UK each year so significant disease, indigenous or imported, is uncommon. Leptospirosis is essentially a disease of animals which is transmitted to humans by the infected urine of a wide range of domestic and wild animals. Urinary excretion in animals may be of long duration, with or without clinical illness. Humans usually acquire infection because of occupational exposure to infected urine but travellers may become infected in the course of water sports or river expeditions.

Leptospira spirochaetes gain entry to humans via skin abrasions, mucous membranes or the conjunctivae. After entry the organisms particularly affect capillary epithelium and, in severe infections, cause capillary damage, hypoxia and haemorrhages into various organs. Illnesses caused by leptospires may be biphasic, with initial symptoms related to leptospiraemia and a second element several days later associated with the host's immune responses to the infection.

Possible syndromes include abrupt onset of a feverish illness with muscular pains, marked constitutional upset and haemorrhages, nephritic features, jaundice, meningitis and a fever which may persist for up to 4 weeks. Isolation is not necessary as person-to-person spread is negligible.

Blood cultures may be positive in the early stages, but some leptospires resist standard culture techniques and the diagnosis is usually made serologically. Cerebrospinal fluid culture may be positive and usually there is cerebrospinal fluid lymphocytosis with essentially normal biochemistry. Dark ground illumination may also demonstrate the organism in cerebrospinal fluid or urine.

The pathogenic leptospires are sensitive to several antibacterial agents including penicillin and erythromycin but if the disease has entered its immunological phase, then antibacterial agents cannot be expected to have a dramatic effect.

Viral diseases caused by ingestion

HEPATITIS A

Hepatitis A is a common infection in which less than 10% of those infected develop jaundice. Epidemics occur especially when water supply systems are contaminated with enteric organisms. Travellers to

---

Practical travel issues

No vaccine is available. Infection is usually through skin or mucous membranes. Muscle pain can be marked. Treatment with antibiotics needs to be prompt or else they are of little help.

---

developing countries from the UK are at risk because less than 50% of the population are immune by virtue of previous (mostly sub-clinical) infection. The incubation period is usually 3–6 weeks. Infection occurs from faecally contaminated water or food, especially water-filtering shellfish.

Symptoms

There is a prodromal period with mild fever, gastrointestinal upset and sometimes a rash. Symptoms in diagnosed cases include nausea/vomiting and diarrhoea (both more common in children), abdominal pain in about half, and fever in less than a half. Notably up to three-quarters of children may be asymptomatic whereas most adults develop symptoms. Jaundice is less likely to be a feature of hepatitis A in childhood.

The diagnosis is usually only suspected if jaundice develops. Importantly, once jaundice is established, patients should feel better and be afebrile: if they are not feeling better and remain febrile, then they have hepatic necrosis or the diagnosis is wrong (a febrile, unwell patient with jaundice from the tropics or sub-tropics has malaria until proven otherwise). The duration of jaundice is usually 7–10 days.

Most patients make an uneventful recovery. Fulminant hepatitis is rare (less than 1%). Occasional patients show prolonged cholestasis or have a minor relapse about 4 weeks after the initial illness resolves[2] and interestingly the virus is present in the stool again in these patients.[3] Although a few patients may relapse, all patients who do not die in the acute episode make a complete recovery.

Diagnosis

The diagnosis of hepatitis is confirmed by finding raised alanine transferase (ALT) or aspartate transaminase (AST) levels with only a minor elevation of the alkaline phosphatase. As the liver enzymes fall, a cholestatic phase often develops. Hepatitis A is confirmed by finding hepatitis A IgM in the serum. This will be positive if the patient is symptomatic and can persist for up to about 3 months after the hepatitis has resolved. Both the specificity and sensitivity of the IgM test are very high.

Treatment

This is symptomatic. Bedrest is not indicated unless the patient desires it, and dietary fat restriction is unnecessary unless the jaundiced patient develops symptoms of fat intolerance or complains about steatorrhoea. Isolation is not necessary for jaundiced patients – by the time jaundice has developed, the virus is not present in infective amounts.

Prevention

Travellers can further protect themselves against hepatitis A by following the simple rules related to water and food hygiene (see Boxes 11.1 and 11.2). They should avoid drinking tap water and should stick to bottled or boiled water, hot drinks, fruit juices and canned or packaged beverages. Obviously, not all hotel tap water abroad is unsafe and if it smells of chlorine, it is probably safe. Ice is only as safe as the water from which it is made and freezing will not sufficiently sterilise water, so ice in drinks should be avoided.

When visiting individual remote areas, or going to countries where drinking water is not readily available, travellers should know how to render water safe. Boiling is the best method, although filtration works well when a good device is employed. Avoiding raw or inadequately cooked food, particularly vegetables and shellfish, can also help prevent infection with hepatitis A virus.

Highly protective, active vaccination is available and immunoglobulin gives short-lived protection.

HEPATITIS E

Before virological investigations (using immune electron microscopy and sophisticated serological techniques) in the 1970s were available, there were many outbreaks of hepatitis which were labelled as hepatitis A. Tests revealed that some of these

> **Practical travel issues**
>
> Travellers going to at-risk areas should consider vaccination. Hepatitis A is much commoner than typhoid except during outbreaks and the virus is more persistent. If hepatitis is confirmed then, unless a return to facilities with high technology care involves no physical exertion, patients who are jaundiced but otherwise well may be better to rest where they are. Beware that jaundice can be due to haemolysis from *Plasmodium falciparum* malaria.

outbreaks were not caused by hepatitis A but were caused by an enterically transmitted, non-A, non-B hepatitis which was subsequently labelled hepatitis E.[4]

Investigations of outbreaks of hepatitis have revealed that hepatitis E is probably the most common cause of hepatitis and jaundice in adults in poorer countries.

Hepatitis E is spread by the faecal–oral route, predominantly via contaminated water, and has an incubation period of 15–60 days (40 average). Hepatitis E has a low mortality (< 1%) but in pregnant women, the mortality rate can be up to 10% (in hepatitis A, B and C, the pregnant fatality rates are similar to the non-pregnant rates). There is no carriage of hepatitis E virus and it does not cause chronic liver disease.[5]

Outbreaks have been described in India, Pakistan, Russia, China, Africa, Peru and Mexico. No outbreaks have occurred in the UK or USA and sporadic cases in these countries are extremely rare.

The virus is present in the stool during the incubation period and early illness. Person-to-person spread is uncommon, probably because viral shedding in the stool is less than in hepatitis A. There is no known effective prophylaxis or specific treatment. Immune electron microscopy is a reliable means of confirming hepatitis E antigen and antibody.

There are no clinical distinguishing features between hepatitis A and E. In recognised hepatitis E, nausea and malaise are common (about 90%), jaundice in 90%, hepatomegaly in about 80% and splenomegaly in 25%. Children and patients over 50 years of age rarely developed jaundice.[6,7]

There is no vaccine available to protect against hepatitis E and it appears that pooled immunoglobulin does not offer significant protection.[8]

Similar precautions with water and food as described for hepatitis A apply.

Box 11.2 Methods of sterilising water (see also Ch. 19)

Boiling
Probably the most reliable and often the cheapest method, although stoves, kettles and heating coils may be inconvenient to use while travelling. Ideally boil the water for 5 minutes, especially if at high altitude when water boils at a lower temperature.

Chlorine and silver
Chlorine- and silver-based tablets are available from chemists and specialised, travel equipment shops. When used correctly, they destroy most bacteria (e.g. *Vibrio cholerae*), but are less effective for viruses and cysts (e.g. hepatitis A virus, *Giardia* and amoebic cysts).

Iodine
Iodine tincture, at a concentration of 8 mg/L and left for 10 minutes, destroys bacteria, viruses and cysts. As with all 'halogens', it is ineffective against *Cryptosporidia*. Adequate levels are normally achieved by using 4 drops of tincture of iodine to 1 L of water or one drop to a glass — wait 20 minutes if water is very cold or contaminated with organic material. Tablets and crystals are also available and the instructions should be followed carefully. Iodine is best avoided for long-term use, in pregnancy and in the very young.

Filters
A wide variety of filters are available. Filters remove sand, clay and other matter as well as organisms by means of small-pore-size membranes, adsorption, exchange resins and osmosis. They effectively remove bacteria, parasites and most viruses. Good filters are effective against *Cryptosporidia* and *Giardia*. Some versions have 'cores', which can be replaced.

Filtration + halogens
The removal of all enteric pathogens requires this combination. This is achieved by passing water usually through iodine exchange resins. When negatively charged contaminants contact the iodine resin, iodine is instantly released so killing the microorganisms without large quantities of iodine being in solution.

POLIOMYELITIS

WHO has given the year 2000 as the estimated date when poliomyelitis should be eradicated and so it is hoped that the following account will be largely of historical interest. Infection is usually spread by the faecal–oral route, through contaminated food or drink, although it may also be spread by droplets from the nasopharynx in the acute phase. In developing countries, poliomyelitis has caused much crippling disease but now widespread use of vaccine has virtually eradicated the disease. However, polio remains a hazard for non-immunised travellers to developing countries except the Americas which are polio-free. The incubation of the disease is on average 7–14 days and infection may have three different outcomes:

- asymptomatic illness (90% of cases) producing lifelong immunity to that particular serotype of virus
- mild, flu-like illness with pyrexia (8% of cases) leading to complete recovery
- major central nervous system illness (2% of cases) including flaccid, asymmetrical lower limb paralysis, bladder dysfunction and impairment of swallowing, breathing and speech (bulbar poliomyelitis) which may be life-threatening.

About two-thirds of those who develop the extreme form of the disease will be left with some residual paralysis of varying severity.

Polio virus is easily grown from stools (but will also be found in the stools of carriers), and in the initial stages from nasopharyngeal swabs. Virus may be isolated from cerebrospinal fluid, although this is rare. Diagnosis may also be confirmed by detecting high or rising poliovirus antibody titres in blood.

Treatment is mainly supportive and assisted ventilation may be required in severe cases. Meningitis alone is treated as for viral meningitis but with longer bedrest. After the acute stage, gradual physiotherapy is of great benefit.

Practising good hygiene and taking care with food and water will reduce the risk of infection, but cannot replace immunisation.

HANTAVIRUS INFECTION

Haemorrhagic fevers with renal involvement

comprise several diseases of varying severity that occur from the Far East to Western Europe. Far Eastern illnesses include Korean haemorrhagic fever which can cause fever, muscle pains, haemorrhagic manifestations and proteinuria: shock and renal failure may lead to death. In Europe, most notably Scandinavia, a milder illness, nephropathia epidemica, can occur without haemorrhagic manifestations. The incubation period is 2–3 weeks and illness tends to occur in late spring and late autumn. The virus is spread by the urine of rodents. An outbreak in the USA killed 26 people and respiratory involvement was a major feature.[9]

Practical travel issues

Hantavirus infection will only be suspected in those patients with unexplained fever and organ failure once other pathogens, notably malaria, have been excluded.

Helminthic (worm) infections caused through ingestion

Tapeworms (cestodes)

Tapeworms are contracted from ingesting contaminated meat, usually pork or beef. Most infections are asymptomatic but they may present to the horror of the traveller when segments of tapeworms are passed in the stool or when the patient is told of the diagnosis!

In general, niclosamide, which is poorly absorbed, is as effective as praziquantel and is less expensive. Praziquantel, which is well absorbed, is a broad-spectrum antihelminth which is useful for both cestodes and trematodes. It can be used as a single dose treatment in all tapeworms except *Hymenolepis nana* in which higher and longer duration therapy is required.

The beef tapeworm, *Taenia saginata*, (see below) resides in the human, upper small intestine, usually undetected, until segments are passed in the stools or emerge spontaneously from the anus. The infection is acquired by eating uncooked or undercooked beef. The infection is usually harmless and can be treated with niclosamide.

The dog tapeworm, *Echinococcus granulosus*, is acquired by ingesting dog faeces. Man is the accidental, intermediate host and hydatid disease follows with cysts in the liver (65% of diagnosed cysts) or in the lung (25% of diagnosed cysts) but cysts may develop in any organ. Treatment is with albendazole (praziquantel is not effective for treatment of hydatid cysts) and occasionally surgery.

The dwarf tapeworm, *Hymenolepis nana*, is found in tropical, semi-arid areas, and usually affects children. It is the only tapeworm that can be transmitted from person to person. Man is the sole host. Diagnosis is by finding eggs in the stool. Treatment is with niclosamide.

Man is the definitive host of the fish tapeworm, *Diphyllobothrium* and there are two sequential intermediate hosts. Classically, the infection is acquired from inadequately cooked fish in Scandinavia but infection is present elsewhere. Usually patients are asymptomatic but vitamin B_{12} deficiency may result as the worm selectively takes it up.

Infection with the pork tapeworm, *Taenia solium*, can be more serious. Larvae may develop from ingested eggs, invade tissues and form cysts in the muscles and brain (neurocysticercosis). The cysts in the brain may enlarge slowly and may cause epilepsy or mass effects. Cysts usually calcify which is diagnostically useful. Treatment of the intestinal worm is with niclosamide but neurocysticercosis requires long-duration praziquantel 50 mg/kg per day for 15–30 days. Albendazole is an alternative. Cyst death may be accompanied by local inflammation with exacerbation of neurological symptoms or signs that may require treatment in their own right. Prevention depends upon proper inspection of carcasses, and thorough cooking of meat.

Roundworms (nematodes)

GUINEA WORM (Dracunculiasis)

Transmission is by a crustacean (*Cyclops*) which is accidentally ingested by humans. Subsequently, Guinea worm larvae penetrate the human intestine and eventually mature into the adult form in the tissues. About 1 year later, there is ulceration, which is often multiple (usually on the feet where the adult female worm emerges, when the limb is exposed to cold water, to liberate larvae infective for *Cyclops*). Treatment is by gentle traction on the worm but thiabendazole or metronidazole may be useful prior to traction. Diagnosis is by observing the worms or by the X-ray appearances of calcified dead worms.

MUSCLE WORM (*Trichinella spiralis*)

This worm is of worldwide distribution and causes a clinical illness comprising fever, orbital oedema and myalgia. Eosinophilia is a reaction to migrating larvae. Infection is acquired by eating inadequately cooked meat, particularly pork, which contains encysted larvae. The larvae mature in the gut and the adult female liberates further larvae. These larvae then migrate to striated muscle (including heart muscle) and to the central nervous system where they may cause fits or encephalitis. After several years, cysts may calcify and be seen as small dots on X-rays. There is usually an eosinophilia and the diagnosis may be confirmed by serological tests or, less preferably, by muscle biopsy. Larvae may occasionally be found in the patient's stool.

ROUNDWORM (Ascaris)

Roundworm infection is found worldwide, particularly in countries where sanitation and hygiene are poor. The worms infect the small intestine of humans and are passed into the environment in the stool. Infection is commonly acquired by swallowing infective eggs, often present on vegetables.

Symptoms, if any, are caused by obstruction of the intestine or associated tubular structures, by allergic reactions as the larvae pass through the lungs (including pulmonary eosinophilia) or by malnutrition. Diagnosis is by identification of the worm or its eggs in the stool and treatment is with piperazine, thiabendazole or bephenium (the last two being useful as they are also effective against hookworm). If there are multiple infections with

worms, always treat the roundworm first: partial treatment can cause roundworm to become irritable and troublesome.

WHIPWORM (*Trichuris trichuria*)

This worm has a worldwide distribution but is most common in poor, rural communities in the tropics. If infection is heavy, especially in children, chronic diarrhoea and failure to thrive may result. Mild eosinophilia may be present. Diagnosis is by identification of the worms or their eggs in the stool. Treatment is with mebendazole.

Trematodes (Flukes)

SCHISTOSOMIASIS (Bilharziasis)

There are three major species of *Schistosoma* flukes: *haematobium*, *mansoni* and *japonicum*.

Schistosoma mansoni is mostly found in Africa, Arabia, eastern South America and the Caribbean; *Schistosoma haematobium* mostly in Africa and the Middle East, and *Schistosoma japonicum* in the Far East. There are two minor species, *Schistosoma mekongi* (in South-East Asia) and *Schistosoma intercalatum* (West and Central Africa). Notably, the Indian sub-continent is almost free of schistosomiasis.

Transmission

This depends on human faecal or urinary contamination of still freshwater, typically lakes, in which certain snails live. Humans excrete *Schistosoma mansoni* and *Schistosoma japonicum* eggs in the faeces or urine and *Schistosoma japonicum* in the urine. The eggs hatch to liberate larvae which then infect specific snails, in which multiplication occurs, and numerous parasites (miracidia) are liberated into the water: they then change into cercariae which can penetrate (intact) human skin of swimmers, occasionally causing 'swimmers' itch'. Less commonly larvae may be ingested. The parasites enter the venous system and are carried to the right side of the heart and arrive in the lungs between 4 and 7 days after skin penetration. They then migrate initially to portal and mesenteric veins. The (now adult) worms mature and migrate to various tissues (*Schistosoma mansoni* and *japonicum* via the mesenteric veins to liver and intestine, and *Schistosoma haematobium* to the bladder and to a lesser extent the large bowel). The larger adult female has a slit along her side (schistosomiasis = split body) in which the smaller male resides in a state of continual copulation. The eggs the female lays cause the pathology because of the granulomatous and fibrotic reactions they elicit.

Symptoms

These may occur when the cercariae penetrate the skin. First is 'swimmers' itch' and a week or so later, a multisystem, allergic illness (Katayama fever) may occur with fever, urticarial skin rashes, eosinophilia, aches and pains. Death may occur in massive *Schistosoma japonicum* infections. 'Swimmers' itch' may also result if non-human parasites (usually avian) penetrate the skin but systemic spread does not then occur. Pneumonic changes can appear as the larvae pass through the lungs. Diarrhoea and vomiting may occur at this stage as may generalised lymph node enlargement, mild hepatomegaly, and splenomegaly.

Subsequent illness may or may not occur, depending on the intensity of the infection and the egg load (*Schistosoma japonicum* eggs are particularly numerous), the host's allergic reaction to the eggs and the site of the reaction to the eggs.

Schistosoma mansoni may cause a typical, large-bowel, low-grade, chronic diarrhoea. Inflammation, fibrosis and strictures may occur and need to be distinguished from Crohn's disease, ulcerative colitis or amoebiasis. 'Pipestem' fibrosis within the liver may result in gross hepatomegaly, with portal vein fibrosis and portal hypertension leading to splenomegaly and formation of varices. Liver failure is uncommon but complications of portal hypertension are frequent.

Schistosoma japonicum may affect the liver and intestine, particularly the small intestine and proximal colon. Other organs that may be involved include the lungs and nervous tissue (where even single eggs can cause significant problems).

Schistosoma haematobium affects primarily the bladder. Chronic inflammation and fibrosis cause urinary frequency (especially if the bladder is fibrosed and thus small), dysuria and haematuria. Fibrosis elsewhere in the urinary tract may cause obstruction leading to hydronephrosis. There is a predisposition to carcinoma of the bladder.

Diagnosis

Identification of eggs in the stool, urine or biopsy of the rectum or other involved tissue confirms the diagnosis. The species involved may be identified by the appearances of their eggs. Eosinophilia is common. Serological tests are available and are often of most practical use in determining if there has been any infection after short visits to at-risk areas.

Treatment

This aims to reduce egg production by killing adult worms or by minimising tissue damage by the eggs. In endemic areas, attempts at curative treatment of those whose exposure will be continual is not realistic. In distinct contrast, treatment is definitely indicated for those whose future exposure will be minimal because the effects of even a few eggs might be significant (e.g. in the spinal cord).

Anti-*Schistosoma* drugs cause the worms to leave veins where they are relatively safe, to be destroyed by the host's defence mechanisms. Niridazole, although cheap, requires repeat courses of treatment and has troublesome central nervous system side effects. Praziquantel is, where affordable, the treatment of choice and is relatively free of side effects. It is given as a single dose of 40 mg/kg which cures about 90% of those infected with *Schistosoma mansoni* and *haematobium* but *Schistosoma japonicum* should be treated with a higher dosage of 60 mg/kg in divided doses over 1–2 days.

Prevention

There is no vaccine available to protect travellers against schistosomiasis. Individuals should avoid swimming in freshwater – streams, rivers and lakes – in endemic areas. This is often unrealistic and it may be encouraged by adverts and the media waxing eloquent about the joy of scuba diving in Lake Malawi without a mention of schisotosomasis. Chlorinated water in swimming pools should be safe.

Practical travel issues

At the earliest, egg laying only commences 6 weeks after infection. Therefore, it may be best to wait longer than this before collecting stool and urine specimens.

CLONORCHIASIS (Chinese liver fluke)

This fluke is a parasite of fish-eating mammals, mostly in China, Hong Kong, Vietnam and Korea. Humans are incidental hosts. Humans eat inadequately cooked fish, the parasite passes to the liver capillaries and eggs are subsequently passed in the stool which infect specific snails (in which they multiply profusely) and then are excreted into water to infect fish. Symptoms of heavy infections may include cholangitis produced by localised obstruction of bile ducts. Praziquantel is the treatment of choice.

OPISTHORCHIASIS

This infection is caused by common liver flukes of dogs and cats in South-East Asia and Eastern Europe. Praziquantel is effective.

FASCIOLIASIS

This is a common, worldwide infection of sheep. Man is an accidental host and acquires infection by eating vegetables on which the parasite has encysted. In human infection, there may be fever, right upper quadrant pain, hepatomegaly and marked eosinophilia. Diagnosis is by finding eggs in the stool and treatment is with bithionol.

FASCIOLOPSIASIS

Fasciolopsiasis is caused by an intestinal fluke (*Fasciolopsis buskii*). It lays eggs, which, on entering fresh water, develop and infect specific snails which liberate parasites which encyst on aquatic plants which are then eaten by humans. Infection is endemic in the Far East and South-East Asia. Infection is mostly asymptomatic but heavy infections affect the small intestine to produce diarrhoea, abdominal pain and malabsorption. Praziquantel is the treatment of choice.

PARAGONIMIASIS

Paragonimiasis is endemic in West Africa, the Far East and the Indian sub-continent. Humans eat fluke-infected crayfish and freshwater crabs and the parasites penetrate the gut and migrate to the pleural cavities and lungs where they lay eggs. Cough and haemoptysis may result although most infections are asymptomatic. Prevention is by ensuring that all food, particularly fish, shellfish and vegetables, is properly cooked as this will prevent infection in most cases. Praziquantel is the treatment of choice.

Other less common ingested infections which the traveller may rarely encounter

ANISKIASIS

The adult worms are found in the stomachs of marine animals. The eggs are shed into sea water and the larvae are ingested by crustaceans which, if ingested by fish, complete the life cycle by infecting their gut and muscles. Aniskiasis is thus essentially a disease of fish, which only accidentally infects humans. Eating raw or undercooked fish, notably herrings, typically infects humans, notably the Japanese for whom raw fish (sushi) is a delicacy. Symptoms of severe abdominal pain and vomiting usually occur within 48 hours of ingestion but are usually self-limiting.

CAPILLARIA PHILIPPINENSIS

As might be deduced from the name, *Capillaria philippinensis* occurs mostly in the Philippines. Freshwater fish contain the larvae which, if eaten, multiply in the human gut, become adults and lay eggs. With large numbers of worms, the small bowel may be severely affected and symptoms of pain, diarrhoea or malabsorption produced. Mortality rates have been as high as 30%. High-dose mebendazole or thiabendazole is effective.

Diseases acquired by ingestion of contaminated soil

TOXOCARIASIS

Soil sampling, especially of parks and playgrounds (in even the developed world), demonstrates widespread contamination with the eggs of *Toxocara canis*, the dog roundworm. Almost all puppies are infected at or soon after birth. Humans acquire infection by ingestion of the eggs. Pica is a risk factor. After ingestion of the eggs, the larvae migrate, particularly to liver, muscle (skeletal and cardiac), lungs and brain. Two main syndromes occur: ocular larva migrans and visceral larva migrans. Covert infection in which vague, non-diagnostic symptoms occur in childhood, is probably very common.

Visceral larva migrans causes fever, cough, bronchospasm, abdominal pain and, in children, failure to thrive. IgE levels are very high and eosinophilia is common. Ocular larva migrans usually occurs in older children and adults and is seldom associated with a raised IgE or eosinophilia. Penetration of an eye by a single larva can result in blindness. Fortunately, bilateral infection only occurs in about 3% of diagnosed cases. The current position has been well-detailed[10] and summarised.[11]

Practical travel issues

Keep young children away from areas that may be contaminated with dog faeces and avoid organically fertilised food and primitive catering establishments, particularly if the owner keeps dogs.

TOXOPLASMOSIS

Toxoplasmosis is a worldwide, protozoan infection. The traveller may contract infection by eating poorly cooked meats, particularly lamb and pork, although it can also be spread faecal–orally, usually from contamination of growing vegetables by cats. Most acute infections are asymptomatic but lymph node enlargement, fever, malaise, sweats, rash or hepatosplenomgaly may occur. Atypical lymphocytes may be found on blood film examination. In immunocompetent patients the acute illness is self-limiting. Diagnosis is often made after biopsy of lymph nodes but serological tests are available. Treatment in the immunocompetent patient is usually not required unless there are systemic features. Pregnant women should be treated (usually with spiramycin) because infection during pregnancy can result in spontaneous abortion or congenital infection.

Prevention requires insistence that meat should be thoroughly cooked and eaten hot wherever possible. Hands should be washed after contact with cat faeces, handling meat or gardening.

Diseases acquired by contact with contaminated soil

HOOKWORM

An estimated 450 million people are infected with hookworm, almost exclusively in the tropics and sub-tropics. Human hookworm are small (1 cm long) worms which attach themselves to the upper, small intestine mucosa where they cause bleeding. Eggs are passed in the stool, and under suitable soil conditions, hatch to liberate larvae that can penetrate intact human skin, usually of the feet. Larvae then enter the bloodstream, travel to the lungs, wriggle up the bronchi into the trachea, and then pass downwards to the small intestine where they mature, thus completing the life cycle.

Symptoms may arise at the time of skin penetration ('ground itch') or from allergic lung symptoms (pulmonary eosinophilia) as the larvae pass through the lungs. The main result is iron deficiency anaemia and/or hypoalbuminaemia if there is extensive blood loss. Occasionally, abdominal pain, diarrhoea or weight loss occurs if the worm burden is large. Diagnosis is by stool examination and treatment is with mebendazole 100 mg twice daily for 3 days.

Protective footwear should prevent transmission; sandal-type 'flip-flops' probably do not provide protection.

> **Practical travel issues**
>
> Wear shoes that avoid contact with soil whenever possible, but particularly when visiting bush latrines. The use of a beach towel when sunbathing is also sensible advice.

CUTANEOUS LARVA MIGRANS (creeping eruption)

Cutaneous larva migrans is caused by the intradermal migration of hookworm larvae from dogs, cats and other animals. The life cycle is similar to that of human hookworm except that the non-human larvae are unable to develop in humans and wander around in the skin for many weeks before they die. This produces an intensely itchy, skin eruption.

Prevention depends on the avoidance of barefoot walking on sand or soil contaminated by dog or cat faeces.

STRONGYLOIDES

Strongyloides is common in many tropical areas. Like hookworm, larvae are excreted in human faeces, develop in the soil and cause infection by penetrating the skin. The soil parasite penetrates unbroken skin, usually of the feet. The larvae then enter the bloodstream, travel to the lungs, wriggle up the bronchi into the trachea, and then pass downwards to the small intestine where they mature and produce larvae which pass in the stool to contaminate soil, thus completing the life cycle. However, intestinal larvae can penetrate the gut wall or peri-anal skin to enter the bloodstream. This later mechanism can lead to large worm burdens

and/or long-term persistence of the parasite: it is thus a chronic infection and illness may result many years after leaving an endemic area.

If patients become immunodeficient as with HIV infection (even decades after acute infection), then asymptomatic infection may become systemic and life threatening.

The actively migrating larvae travelling through skin (cutaneous larva currens), produce symptoms. The larvae travel relatively quickly, hence 'currens', and can cause allergic lung symptoms (pulmonary eosinophilia). Other symptoms include abdominal pain, diarrhoea with mucus or, if infection is severe, malabsorption.

Diagnosis is by demonstrating larvae in the faeces (examination of multiple stool specimens may be required to make a diagnosis) or duodenal aspirates. Eosinophilia is common because of the tissue invasion. As the parasite mostly lives in the duodenum and jejunum, stool examination is relatively insensitive and concentration techniques are necessary. Serological tests are available.

Treatment is with thiabendazole or praziquantel but the organism can survive in areas of stasis such as the appendix.

> **Practical travel issues**
>
> Wear shoes at all times, particularly when in rural areas and places likely to be contaminated with human faeces – underneath houses, roadsides, or bush latrines. The disease may have been contracted while travelling decades previously.

TETANUS

Tetanus is caused by the toxin produced by the anaerobe *Clostridium tetani*, which is harboured in the intestinal tracts of many vertebrates, including human. Spores of *Clostridium tetani* are widely distributed in the environment and infection usually follows inoculation of these spores into wounds at the time of an injury.

The incubation period of disease is between 3 and 21 days during which time muscle rigidity slowly increases. Trismus (inability to open the mouth wide), and rigidity of spinal and abdominal muscles develop. Painful spasms then become superimposed on the muscle rigidity resulting in facial grimacing and back arching. These spasms may be induced by sensory stimuli. Later in the disease, autonomic instability may cause arrhythmias and highly labile blood pressure.

Treatment involves giving human tetanus immunoglobulin (to neutralise circulating toxin) and benzylpenicillin (to treat any wound infection). An obvious wound should be opened and debrided. The spasms in mild cases can be controlled with diazepam, although more severe cases will require intensive nursing care, assisted ventilation and muscle relaxants. Recovery will take several weeks although death may result, usually caused by respiratory arrest or autonomic instability.

All travellers should have been immunised against tetanus since it is prevalent worldwide and correct treatment following injury may not be available in some countries.

PRACTICE POINTS

Additional practice points to prevent infection

- The term 'water-associated diseases' is used to contrast those contracted through contaminated drinking water and food and those contracted, for example, through skin penetration of organisms as in *Bilharzia* or hookworm infections. Leptospirosis, where contaminated water comes in contact with mucous membranes, and chemical injuries to the skin and conjunctiva also come into this category.
- Do not forget infections can also be spread through unpasteurised milk and milk products such as cheese.
- Freshly cooked rice, pasta, vegetables and bread are normally safe.
- Remember polluted water may have been used to wash dishes and cutlery.
- Hand-washing before meals is as important as hand-washing after defaecation in countries with poor hygienic facilities.

REFERENCES

1. Communicable Diseases Report. Brucellosis. Communicable Diseases Report. CDR Weekly 1991; 1:47.
2. Glickson M, Galun E, Oren R, et al. Relapsing hepatitis A: review of 14 cases and literature survey. Medicine 1992; 71: 14–23.
3. Sjogren MH, Tanno H, Fay O, et al. Hepatitis A virus in stool during clinical relapse. Annals of Internal Medicine 1987; 106: 221–226.
4. Purcell RH, Ticehurst JR. Enterically transmitted non-A, non-B hepatitis: epidemiology and clinical characteristics In: Zuckerman AJ, ed. Viral hepatitis and liver disease. New York: Alan Liss; 1988: 131–137.
5. Khuroo MS, Saleem M, Ramzan Teli M, et al. Failure to detect chronic liver disease after epidemic non-A, non-B hepatitis. Lancet 1980; 2: 97–98.
6. Zhuang H, Cao XY, Wang GM. Enterically transmitted non-A, non-B hepatitis in China. In: Shikata, Purcell RH, Uchida T, eds. Viral hepatitis C, D and E. New York: Excerpta Medica; 1991: 265–275.
7. Xue-Yi C, Xue-Zhong M, Yu-Zhang L, et al. Epidemiological and etiological studies on enterically transmitted non-A, non-B hepatitis in the south part of Xinjiang. In: Shikata, Purcell RH, Uchida T, eds. Viral hepatitis C, D and E. New York: Excerpta Medica; 1991: 297–312.
8. Joshi YK, Babu S, Sarin S, et al. Immunoprophylaxis of epidemic non-A, non-B hepatitis. Indian Medical Research 1985; 81: 18–19.
9. Advisory Committee on Dangerous Pathogens. Management and control of viral haemorrhagic fevers. London: HMSO (well summarised in Communicable Diseases Report CDR Weekly 1997; 7: 57–60).
10. Lewis JW, Maizels RM, eds. Toxocara and toxocariasis. Clinical, epidemiological and molecular prespectives. London: Birbeck; 1993.
11. Keer-Muir MG. *Toxocara canis* and human health. British Medical Journal 1994; 309: 5–6.

Diseases transmitted through the respiratory tract and skin-to-skin contact

Bibhat K. Mandal

Introduction

Other authors have dealt with infection risks to travellers from water, food, soil, animal contact and sex. This section reviews those infections that can be acquired through being in contact with other persons and their relevance to travel medicine. An introduction to the diseases is given here and further details can be found in section 7 on perspectives in Africa, Asia and South and Central America.

Contact with other people is inevitable during foreign travel – in airports, inside an aircraft, during transit to a hotel, inside the hotel and while conducting one's business in the country visited. The risk of an infection through contact depends very much on the closeness, duration and nature of the contact. Thus, the risks for business travellers flying first class, being met at the airport to be whisked away to a 5-star hotel, where they will stay for only a few days, differ enormously from a low-budget traveller staying close to local people or from immigrants visiting their homelands and staying with relatives. The infections that can be acquired through contact can thus be best categorised according to the nature of the contact.

Casual contact in public places

Only those infections which transmit through airborne transmission and are highly infectious can be acquired under these circumstances. Influenza, other respiratory viruses (common cold, adenoviruses, respiratory syncytial virus, para-

influenza viruses), mycoplasma, exanthemata, whooping cough and mumps are commonly transmitted in this way.

Infection is exhaled from a case or carrier by coughing, sneezing, speaking or even quiet breathing, is carried by air currents in invisible droplets of moisture and is inhaled by the new host. Droplet-spread is ineffective beyond a range of a few feet because drying through evaporation kills most organisms. However, some viruses (e.g. influenza) may survive in the dust which can transmit infection for longer distances (but rarely beyond several metres).

Respiratory viral and mycoplasma infections occur worldwide. However, there is frequent geographical and seasonal increase in prevalences. Thus, infection may be acquired by someone travelling from a low-prevalence area to a high-prevalence area. A good example is influenza.

INFLUENZA

Of the three types of influenza viruses (A, B and C), type A causes widespread epidemics and pandemics, type B causes regional or more widespread epidemics, whereas type C has only been associated with sporadic cases or minor outbreaks. The predominant mode of transmission is airborne, spread among crowded populations in enclosed places, but droplet spread and through direct contact with dried mucus also occurs. Elderly persons and persons with underlying health problems are at increased risk for complications of influenza and are usually advised to have annual influenza vaccinations.

The risk for exposure to influenza during foreign travel varies, depending on season and destination. Influenza can occur throughout the year in the tropics and in the Southern Hemisphere – mostly from April to September – whereas in the Northern Hemisphere, most activity is during November to March. Because of the short incubation period for influenza, a person can develop illness during travel which can cause considerable problems to a high-risk individual.

The Advisory Committee on Immunisation Practices (ACIP), USA, recommendations are as follows:

> Persons preparing to travel to the tropics at any time of year, or to the Southern Hemisphere from April through September should review their influenza vaccination histories. If they were not vaccinated the previous fall or winter, they should consider influenza vaccination before travel. Persons in the high risk categories should be encouraged to receive the most current vaccine. Persons at high risk who received the previous season's vaccine before travel should be re-vaccinated in the fall or winter with the current vaccine.

> Morbidity and Mortality Weekly Report 1995; 44(RR-3): 6

PNEUMOCOCCAL PNEUMONIA

Mode of transmission

Streptococcus pneumoniae are commonly found in the upper respiratory tract of healthy persons throughout the world. Infection occurs via droplet spread, by direct oral contact or indirectly through contact with freshly soiled (with respiratory secretions) articles.

Person-to-person transmission of the organisms is common, leading to colonisation of upper air passages but illness among casual contacts is rare.

Lower respiratory spread is necessary for pneumonia to develop and this is facilitated by anything which interferes with ciliary defence of the air passages (e.g. influenza), smoke inhalation, aspiration, alcoholism and also by chronic cardiorespiratory and other debilitating diseases.

Asplenia and immunosuppression increase the risk of bacteraemia and central nervous system involvement.

Geographical distribution

Pneumonia occurs worldwide. However, in recent years, penicillin and multi-drug-resistant strains have become increasingly common and their incidence is higher in certain countries like Spain and South Africa than in the UK. No reliable data are available from popular holiday destinations of India, South East Asia and East Africa.

Clinical manifestation

This is characterised by fever and chill of sudden onset, chest pain, cough and a rusty sputum. Signs of consolidation are present and there is usually a neutrophilic leucocytosis. Bacteraemia is common and pneumococcal meningitis may complicate the picture.

Diagnosis

Diagnosis is by clinical and radiological examination.

Demonstration of *Streptococcus pneumoniae* in sputum is corroborative and in blood confirmatory.

Treatment

In view of the rising incidence of penicillin-resistant pneumococcal infection, penicillin is no longer the recommended treatment for pneumococcal pneumonia, particularly if contracted abroad. A third generation cephalosporin should be used instead.

Prevention

Elderly, debilitated, asplenic and immunocompromised patients are more vulnerable to severe pneumococcal infections and should, ideally, be vaccinated with polyvalent pneumococcal vaccine. This will undoubtedly reduce their risks of contracting a resistant strain if they later travel to a high-incidence area. The vaccine is given once only in the immunocompetent, but in immunocompromised individuals may be repeated after 6 years or so in view of a more rapid decline in antibody level. It probably has an overall efficacy of 60–70% in preventing pneumococcal pneumonia but against other forms of pneumococcal infections (e.g. otitis media, meningitis), its efficacy is uncertain.

ACUTE DIARRHOEA OWING TO SMALL ROUND STRUCTURED VIRUSES (SRSVs)

SRSVs (Norwalk and Norwalk-like) have emerged as an important cause of non-bacterial gastro-enteritis outbreaks, often involving hotels and institutions. In recent years, many travellers have been affected in outbreaks involving hotels, holiday camps and cruiseships abroad.

Mode of transmission

This can be either person to person or food- and water-borne. Overall, person-to-person transmission is more common, involving either the faecal–oral route or inhalation of aerosols liberated by projectile vomiting, requiring close proximity for airborne spread. Rapid spread is characteristic. Community outbreaks are more often food- or water-borne. Often the outbreak grumbles along for weeks or longer through introduction of new susceptibles in the infected area (e.g. hotel or ship).

Clinical picture

The incubation period is 24–48 hours. The period of communicability lasts during the acute stage of the disease and up to 48 hours after diarrhoea stops. Abrupt onset of vomiting, diarrhoea, abdominal cramps, low grade fever with myalgia and headache are the usual symptoms, which usually subside within 48 hours.

Diagnosis

The nature of the outbreak and absence of positive stool bacteriology are presumptive evidence, whereas demonstration of viral antigen in faeces or vomitus is diagnostic.

Treatment/prevention

There is no specific therapy but hydration should be maintained. Isolation of the affected, environmental decontamination and closure of the premises to new intakes of visitors are important public health measures.

MEASLES, MUMPS, RUBELLA (MMR) AND WHOOPING COUGH

These infections, which are all transmissible through airborne route, have now become quite uncommon in the UK because of the success of the national immunisation policy. However, they are still highly prevalent in many countries of the world and can be contracted by a susceptible person from the UK travelling to an endemic country.

Such a person is likely to be an adult who:

a. did not receive immunisation against whooping cough, measles and rubella during the poor uptake years in the 1970s (mumps vaccine was not routine and rubella vaccine was given only to school girls), yet
b. escaped natural infection through partially successful herd immunity then prevalent
c. was too old for MMR when it was introduced in 1988 and for the measles and rubella vaccine campaign for 5–16-year-olds in 1994.

Can aircraft cabin air spread infectious diseases?

It is generally accepted that a passenger is no more likely to catch an infectious disease on a plane, through breathing air, than in an office or any other public place. In cases where passengers have been shown to fall ill, 'proximity' to other ill people rather than air-conditioning has been said to be responsible. However, there have been recent concerns over possible transmission of tuberculosis and SRSV diarrhoea within aircrafts via the airborne route ('We caught TB on flight to New York', *The Daily Telegraph*, 5 February, 1998).

In aircraft, the air-conditioning system takes in fresh air from outside. This is then heated by the engine, then cooled by an airpack, before it is piped into the front of the cabin. The air is then discharged at the back. Until recent times, all aircraft used 100% fresh air, but this is costly and many airlines now recirculate part of the used air. The UK Civil Aviation Authority requires not less than 50% of fresh air on planes at any time.

Although there is the possibility that bacteria and viruses may survive in the recirculated stale air, there is no hard evidence that the cabin air system is responsible for spreading infectious diseases. According to *The Daily Telegraph* report, the Federal Aviation Authority in the USA is carrying out long-term research.

Contact for prolonged periods

Some air-borne infections require a higher infecting dose that can occur only through prolonged contact. This allows transfer of sufficient number of infected droplets or of direct transfer of salivary/respiratory secretions to the host's air passages.

MENINGOCOCCAL INFECTION

Mode of transmission

Transmission is by close contact with an infected person or a carrier, facilitating spread by respiratory droplets. This is encouraged in overcrowded communities. Humans are the only reservoir.

Geographical distribution (p. 475)

The causative organism, *Neisseria meningitidis*, is the commonest cause of bacterial meningitis worldwide. Of the many pathogenic groups (A, B, C, D, X, Y, Z, W135), group A organisms cause epidemics in West Africa, Sudan, Ethiopia and East Africa as well as Nepal, India and the Middle East. Group B organisms predominate in Western countries followed by Group C. Asymptomatic carriage rate may be high (> 25%) in populations even in the absence of epidemics. Children and young adults are commonly affected.

Clinical manifestations

The usual incubation period is 1–3 days. The disease starts abruptly with fever, headache, irritability and restlessness, rapidly progressing to signs of meningitis. The illness may also present just as septicaemia with rapidly developing toxicity. A petechial purpuric rash is present in two-thirds of cases.

Diagnosis/treatment

Cerebrospinal fluid shows typical changes of pyogenic meningitis. The organisms can usually be seen in cerebrospinal fluid gram-smear and be cultured from cerebrospinal fluid/blood. Either iv penicillin or cefotaxime should be used.

Risk to travellers/prevention

Meningococcal disease in travellers to epidemic areas (see above) is rare. However, because of the lack of good surveillance and notification systems, it is difficult to have up-to-date knowledge of epidemic prevalence. Therefore, travellers to such areas who are likely to have prolonged contact with local people should receive meningococcal vaccine. In the UK, only the combined meningococcal A and C vaccine is available. The duration of immunity is uncertain but appears to be at least 3 years in children and 4 years in adults. Re-vaccination should be considered after 2 or 3 years in children below 4 years if they are at risk again from travel.

DIPHTHERIA

Mode of transmission

Humans are the only reservoir of *Corynebacterium diphtheria*, the causative organism of diphtheria. Transmission is by respiratory droplets or direct transfer of respiratory secretions from a case or carrier. Close contact of a household nature is usually necessary. Occasionally, direct contact is important in cases of cutaneous diphtheria. Immune persons may harbour organisms in their nose and throat for prolonged periods.

Geographical distribution

In Western countries, diphtheria has become rare through routine childhood immunisation. However, there has been a resurgence of the disease in former Soviet Union countries, particularly Russia, Ukraine, Azerbaijan, Belarus, Kazakhstan, Moldova, Tajikistan and Uzbekistan. The reasons for the resurgence of diphtheria epidemics in these countries seem to be low immunisation coverage among infants and children, a gap in immunity among adults, large population movements in recent years and changes in the organism or its toxin. Diphtheria remains prevalent in many areas of the tropics, in particular the Indian sub-continent. Inapparent cutaneous and wound diphtheria are common.

Clinical manifestations

The incubation period is usually 2–5 days. Symptoms depend on the site of infection and membrane formation caused by liberation of specific cytotoxin. In faucial or pharyngotonsillar diphtheria there is sore throat and low-grade fever, followed by development of an off-white, thick membrane affecting one or both tonsils which may then spread to the pharynx, palate or nasal passages. Marked enlargement of cervical glands is common. If the larynx is involved, there is rapid development of hoarseness, croupy cough and stridor. Myocarditis and polyneuritis are important complications. In the tropics, diphtheria organisms can secondarily infect wounds and impetiginous skin lesions even in immune persons who can then transmit infection to others. Thus, all indolent skin lesions in a returning traveller from the tropics should be investigated for cutaneous diphtheria.

Diagnosis/treatment

Diagnosis is initially on clinical grounds and then confirmation by the demonstration of toxin producing *Corynebacterium diphtheriae* in throat/ nose swabs. The major differential diagnoses are glandular fever and streptococcal tonsillitis. Laryngeal diphtheria requires differentiation from croup, epiglottitis and laryngeal foreign body. Antitoxin therapy and erythromycin are the mainstays of treatment.

Risk to travellers and prevention

Diphtheria is rare in the UK and the few cases seen in recent years are of imported origin (directly or indirectly). There is some evidence that immunity following a primary course of vaccination wanes in adulthood and a booster dose at school-leaving is the recommended policy in the UK. An antitoxin level of 0.01 unit/mL is considered protective. Vaccination is prudent for a person visiting a

highly endemic area (e.g. high density population areas in the former Soviet Union countries) who will come in prolonged close contact with local populace to ensure immunity. This will necessitate either a booster dose (in persons who only had childhood immunisation) or a primary course of adult diphtheria vaccine.

TUBERCULOSIS

Tuberculosis is commonly caused by *Mycobacterium tuberculosis* (reservoir primarily humans) and *Mycobacterium bovis* (primarily cattle).

Mode of transmission

Transmission is by exposure to bacilli in airborne droplets of respiratory secretions produced by an infected person with either open pulmonary or laryngeal tuberculosis, during coughing, singing or sneezing. Prolonged close exposure in a closed environment is usually necessary for contacts to become infected. Bovine tuberculosis results through ingestion of infected, unpasteurised milk.

Geographical distribution

Tuberculosis occurs worldwide with very high prevalence rates in the Indian sub-continent and sub-Saharan Africa. In many of the developed countries, the steady downward decline over the past few decades appears to have been halted in the 1980s or even increased, linked with the spread of HIV and increased homelessness. Bovine tuberculosis remains prevalent only in developing countries where cattle tuberculosis is a problem.

Clinical manifestations

It takes about 4–12 weeks to develop a demonstrable primary lesion in chest X-ray or significant tuberculin reaction. Many infections remain latent and in others the disease can present in a number of ways:

- primary tuberculosis of lung
- miliary tuberculosis
- tuberculous meningitis
- chronic pulmonary tuberculosis
- abdominal tuberculosis (peritonitis, ileocaecal tuberculosis)
- glandular tuberculosis

- genitourinary tuberculosis
- bone and joint tuberculosis.

The reader should refer to an appropriate textbook for a detailed description of these syndromes and their diagnoses and treatment.

Risks to travellers/prevention

Although tuberculosis is much more common in many of the developing countries that are popular holiday destinations for British tourists, risk is remote for ordinary, short-term travellers. To become infected a person usually has to spend a long time in a closed environment with an untreated patient with open pulmonary tuberculosis who is coughing. It is important to ensure that young persons of Indian sub-continent origin visiting their homelands where they will be spending prolonged periods with their relatives, should have had BCG immunisation.

Although there is controversy over BCG vaccine's efficacy because the protection conferred has varied markedly in different field trials, UK experience has consistently shown an efficacy of 70–80% against tuberculosis when given to schoolchildren. Studies have also demonstrated its protective efficacy in children less than 5 years old against tuberculosis meningitis and disseminated disease.

The risk of re-infection is very small in anyone with significant tuberculin reaction, but recrudescence can occur.

ENTEROVIRAL HAEMORRHAGIC CONJUNCTIVITIS (EHC)

This is usually caused by enterovirus 70 and occasionally by a variant of Coxsackie A24. Enterovirus 70 has caused large outbreaks of conjunctivitis in many areas of India, South-East Asia, Africa and Central and South America.

- The virus is transmitted by hands and contaminated towels from an infected person.
- The symptoms appear within 2 days of exposure to an infected person. Subconjunctival haemorrhage is common. Recovery is usual within 10 days.
- Travellers have contracted EHC while visiting epidemic areas.

- Prevention measures are personal: strict hygiene, no sharing of towels, avoidance of overcrowding.

Infections which require prolonged body contact

LEPROSY

This is a chronic granulomatous disease caused by *Mycobacterium leprae* and affects the skin, peripheral nerves and mucous membranes.

MODE OF TRANSMISSION

Prolonged close contact, usually in a household setting with an untreated lepromatous patient, is usually necessary. Such patients excrete millions of bacilli in their nasal and skin ulcer discharge. The organisms may remain viable for at least 7 days in dried nasal secretions. Transmission is probably through respiratory passages or through damaged skin. There is a high degree of natural resistance to the disease and 90% of exposed people show no sign of infection.

GEOGRAPHICAL DISTRIBUTION

Humans are the only proven reservoir for infection. The main endemic areas are South and South-East Asia (India, Bangladesh, Myanmar, Philippines, Indonesia, some Pacific islands), sub-Saharan Africa, and less commonly parts of Latin America.

CLINICAL MANIFESTATIONS

The earliest manifestations consist of a small, irregular, pale skin lesion anywhere on the body without any sensory loss, and this heals spontaneously. This is known as indeterminate leprosy and, pathologically, there is a non-specific inflammatory reaction. This stage may progress to three later types depending on the cell-mediated, immune response:

- *tuberculoid leprosy* occurs when immune response is vigorous, and is characterised by anaesthetic macules (depigmented in dark-skinned people, but reddish in pale-skinned) and thickened adjoining nerves with corresponding sensory and motor changes. The histology is of non-caseating, epitheloid granulomas without mycobacteria. This form of leprosy is probably not infectious.

- *lepromatous leprosy* occurs when there is no cell-mediated, immune response. There is infiltration of skin with foamy histocytes full of bacilli and typically ears, lips and nose swell. Nasal mucosal involvement leads to ulceration. Ulceration, disfigurement and deformity are common.
- *borderline leprosy* falls in between these two extremes.

Diagnosis

This is usually established by the clinical picture and histology of a skin lesion or thickened sensory nerve.

Treatment

Dapsone and rifampicin for 6 months for tuberculoid leprosy and triple therapy with rifampicin, clofazimine and dapsone for 2 years for other forms.

Risk to travellers

Chances of contracting clinical leprosy through travel are extremely remote, and there has been no report of leprosy among immigrants from the Indian sub-continent who visit their home country and live close to people for prolonged periods. BCG vaccination offers reasonable protection against development of tuberculoid leprosy.

Chemoprophylaxis with dapsone reduces incidence by 50% among close contacts, but requires close supervision. These measures have little relevance for travellers.

Other infections transmitted through direct or indirect contact

SCABIES

This is a skin infection caused by the scabies mite, *Sarcoptes scabiei*. It has a worldwide distribution.

Mode of transmission

Scabies is spread by close skin contact, typically by hand-holding or sharing beds. Contrary to popular belief, scabies is not spread by clothes or bedding. The mite burrows into the skin to the boundary between the strata corneum and the granulosum.

Clinical manifestation

The rash and itching of scabies are caused by sensitisation to the mite proteins, so symptoms may not start until infection has been present for 2 or 3 weeks, and may remain for the same time after the mites have been killed with insecticides. Enquiry may find that another person in the family, or a close friend, also has itching. The rash is usually symmetrical, on the fingers (especially on the webs), wrists, penis, around the waist and on the buttocks. Normally, the head and back are spared. The most common lesions are papular, with scratch marks, but the diagnostic lesion is the burrow, a pin-head-sized blister with a short line.

Diagnosis

The diagnosis of scabies can be confirmed by lifting the mite out of a burrow with a needle and examining it under a low-power microscope. Skin scrapings from a burrow or an unexcoriated papule will gather eggs and a mite to be examined in the same way.

Treatment

The whole family and sexual partners should be treated at the same time. A single application of lindane or malathion lotion should be sufficient. There is no need to wash clothes or bedding in any special way, because these articles do not harbour mites. Patients should be told that the itching may persist for some time, but can be relieved with calamine lotion.

Risk to travellers/prevention

The chances of coming into close skin contact with an infected person are not governed by travel alone. However, scabies is probably more endemic in developing countries and not infrequently British children of immigrant origin return home with scabies after a prolonged stay with their relatives on the Indian sub-continent, often in overcrowded, unhygienic settings. Backpackers living rough on a low budget also have a higher incidence. Prevention depends on increasing public awareness of how scabies is transmitted.

RINGWORM

These are skin infections caused by the dermatophyte fungi, the species *Microsporum, Trichophyton* and *Epidermophyton* and are clinically termed tinea capitis (scalp), tinea corporis (body), tinea cruris (groin), tinea pedis (foot) and tinea unguium (nail).

Mode of transmission

Transmission is by direct skin-to-skin or indirect contact, especially from theatre seats, barber's implements or clothing and hats of infected persons, communal showers or bathing areas. Animals are an occasional source.

Geographical distribution

Ringworm occurs commonly worldwide.

Clinical manifestation

This will depend on the site of infection: red scaling area with central clearing (body, groin); dull, discoloured and distorted nails; scaling patches with broken hair (scalp).

Treatment

Treatment is by topical or oral imidazole drugs.

Risk to travellers

All the infections described above have a worldwide distribution and acquisition depends on circumstances which are not greatly influenced by travel alone.

STREPTOCOCCAL SKIN INFECTIONS, WARTS AND MOLLUSCUM

These occur worldwide and travellers are not generally at greater risk. However, streptococcal skin infections are commoner in tropical, warm, humid climates. Visiting children staying with relatives may develop secondary infections of mosquito bites, presenting as impetigo.

DIRECT PERSON-TO-PERSON CONTACT MAY ALSO LEAD TO ACQUISITION OF THOSE INFECTIONS THAT ARE TRANSMITTED FAECAL–ORALLY, EITHER VIA INFECTED HANDS OR THROUGH OROGENITAL CONTACT

Giardia lamblia, Shigella sonnei, hepatitis A, hepatitis E and poliomyelitis are not infrequently acquired through direct bodily contact with an infected case or carrier. These have been described in detail on pages 243–248, 273–288.

PRACTICE POINTS

- Diseases of the respiratory tract are difficult to prevent except where an effective vaccine is available. Failure of vaccination programmes can result in epidemics as happened with diphtheria in the 1990s in Russia and the Ukraine.
- Outbreaks of respiratory infections frequently occur when people are crowded together in hotels and clubs at tourist resorts, at pilgrimage sites, at the start of college or university terms and in buses and trains.
- Diphtheria, meningococcal and tuberculosis vaccination or boosters should be considered for those going to endemic areas and who are likely to mix closely with the local population. This does not normally include package tourists staying in tourist hotels with other foreigners.
- Remember the influenza season in the Southern Hemisphere is during the summer and in the winter in the Northern Hemisphere, and offer immunisation to those in at-risk categories for complications.

BIBLIOGRAPHY

Benenson AS, ed. Control of communicable diseases in man. 15th ed. Washington: American Public Health Association. 1990.

Mandal BK, Wilkins EGL, Dunbar EM, Mayon-White RT. Lecture notes on infectious diseases. 5th ed. Oxford: Blackwell Science; 1995.

Diseases spread by insects and animals

Fiona Raeside

Synopsis

This section considers the more common or important insect- and animal-borne infections to which the traveller may be exposed. An introduction to the diseases is given here and further details can be found in Chapter 14 (malaria) and in Section 7 on perspectives in Africa, South-East Asia, the Indian sub-continent and South and Central America.

There is overlap between diseases spread by insects and animals and those spread by food, water or soil and through person-to-person contact. Description of further helminthic infections and certain other diseases with an animal reservoir can be found in other parts of this chapter.

Many of these infections have had a major effect throughout history on the patterns of human social and economic development – malaria, and plague are two well-known examples (see also Section 1).

Travellers, who may be exposed to these infections, as well as their advisers, should have a basic understanding of their natural history and so understand the basic principles of prevention and need for prompt management.

Introduction

Infections transmitted between animals and humans are termed zoonoses, and more than 150 zoonoses are recorded.[1-3] Some have been recognised for thousands of years e.g. in a Mesopotamian code from the 20th century BC, a fine was imposed on the owner of a rabid dog which transmitted the infection by biting another individual.[2]

Plague epidemics have been recorded for more than 3000 years; the animal reservoir resides in *Rattus rattus* and *Rattus norwegicas*. Bubonic plague has in fact exerted a major impact on human history.[4] In Europe, from the 14th to late 17th centuries, it is estimated that 25 million (one-quarter of the population) died from the Black Death.

Accurate descriptions of anthrax can be found in early Hebrew, Greek, Roman and Hindu scripts.

During the 18th and 19th centuries, yellow fever spread via shipping routes to most major ports of the Western Hemisphere.

In recent years, Lassa fever, and Marburg and Ebola diseases have become recognised as zoonotic diseases, small mammals forming reservoirs for human infection.

Infections conveyed by insects constitute a major health problem in tropical and sub-tropical countries.[5] The reservoir of infection may lie within the arthropod or alternatively the arthropod may act as the transmitting agent (vector), often from a zoonotic focus. For example, the reservoir of infection for *Yersinia pestis* (plague) lies in a wild rodent, but transmission to man is dependent on an infected flea.

Insect-borne hazards are likely to become more common and important in the future. For example, development of irrigation and hydroelectric projects inadvertently create environmental conditions ideal for mosquito-breeding, and visceral leishmaniasis (kala azar), spread by sandflies, is an opportunistic infection in AIDS and the number of cases worldwide is likely to escalate as the AIDS pandemic continues. Creation of wildlife and game reserves, with destruction of natural predators, can result in high tick populations, with propagation of tick borne diseases, such as Lyme disease, to humans.

The major infections reviewed in this section will be categorised according to the main vector responsible for transmission to humans.

Infections spread by mosquitoes

MALARIA

Four species of malaria parasite infect man. The most serious, and sometimes fatal, disease is caused by *Plasmodium falciparum*. These diseases are transmitted by the bite of an infected female *Anopheles* mosquito; they can also be acquired via a blood transfusion or contaminated needle, or rarely transmission is congenital.

The infection is confined to tropical and subtropical regions of the world although affected areas of the world are increasing; furthermore, parasites are developing resistance to a wide range of chemoprophylactic and chemotherapeutic agents. Prophylaxis is once again dependent on avoidance of mosquito bites.

The risk of malaria for travellers to endemic regions continues to assume a major significance and is discussed in greater depth in Chapter 13.

DENGUE

After malaria, dengue is the most common and serious mosquito-borne infection affecting travellers. Dengue is an arbovirus infection transmitted by the mosquito *Aedes aegypti*. It is endemic in tropical regions, especially in Asia, Africa and South and Central America (p. 474).

In recent years, it has spread and caused major outbreaks in India, Thailand, southern China, Vietnam, Indonesia, the Philippines and neighbouring countries. There has also been a large upsurge in mainland Central America.

Tourists have been affected, especially those staying for longer periods and living in rural areas with poorly screened accommodation. There is concern that the mosquito, particularly the 'Tiger mosquito' may be adapting to temperate climates and will spread the disease to southern Europe, further into China and to southern parts of North America.

Dengue has an incubation period of about 7 days, after which headaches and severe muscular pains occur. Typically, a fine maculopapular rash appears

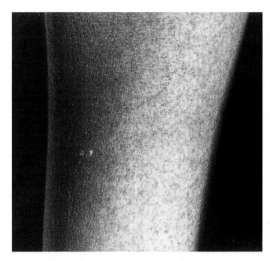

Fig. 11.1 The fine maculopapular rash of dengue.

around the 4th day of illness (Fig. 11.1). Most people recover within a week, but full convalescence may take considerably longer. A few patients, especially children, may suffer haemorrhagic complications and shock which are termed 'dengue haemorrhagic fever'. This is thought to be related to previous exposure to a different serotype. Treatment of dengue is symptomatic and includes intensive care measures if haemorrhage and shock occur.

Prevention of infection depends upon avoiding mosquito bites when travelling in infected areas by using appropriate clothing, repellents and mosquito nets. A vaccine against dengue is in the final stages of development.

YELLOW FEVER

Yellow fever is also caused by an arbovirus spread to humans by the bite of an infected mosquito. It is found in tropical Africa and South America, but does not occur in Asia even though the vector is present there. Two forms are recognised – jungle and urban.

Jungle yellow fever is transmitted among non-human hosts (mainly monkeys) via forest mosquitoes. It caused major morbidity and mortality among those constructing the Panama Canal, which is when the natural history of the disease was first discovered.

Spread to an urban area occurs when an infected monkey carries the virus to an area adjacent to the forest and is then bitten by a species of mosquito, usually *Aedes aegypti*, living in close association with humans. The infection is characterised by fever, jaundice, haemorrhage and renal failure. There is no specific anti-viral therapy and treatment is symptomatic. Mortality is high, up to 60%.

Although yellow fever still causes significant morbidity and mortality in indigenous populations, it is rare in travellers because an effective, live, attenuated vaccine (17D) has been available for more than 50 years.

JAPANESE B ENCEPHALITIS

Although Japanese B encephalitis is a disease endemic in South and South-Eastern Asia, epidemics of considerable magnitude emerge from time to time. It does not occur in other parts of the world (p. 476) including Africa and the Americas.

This arboviral infection is transmitted to man by the bite of an infected *Culicine* mosquito that normally breeds in rice paddies. The main reservoir is the domestic pig (Fig. 11.2), but other animals and some birds may also be carriers.

Disease prevalence has decreased during the last 25 years as a result of mass vaccination, antimosquito campaigns, use of agricultural pesticides and changes in agricultural practices of pig husbandry. However, annual epidemics still occur, for example, following the rains in low-lying parts of Nepal, the central river plains of China, northern Thailand, eastern and southern India.

Japanese B encephalitis can be a serious infection, causing a febrile illness with encephalitis, meningitis and paralysis. While many infections are asymptomatic, mortality is especially high in symptomatic children and can be up to 30%. Many who recover are left with disabilities and recovery can be very prolonged.

As with yellow fever, there is no effective antiviral therapy, and treatment is symptomatic.

An effective vaccine is available and can be used for those at higher risk, such as those staying for long periods in endemic, especially rural, areas or visiting epidemic regions during the Japanese B encephalitis season.

In Japan, the disease has been virtually eradicated since nationwide immunisation was introduced in 1965, and major inroads into eradication have been achieved in China.

The traveller should always employ anti-mosquito measures whether or not vaccination is considered appropriate.

FILARIASIS

The most common, systemic, helminthic or worm infection affecting humans is filariasis, caused by *Wuchereria bancrofti*.[5] It is spread by mosquitoes and is widespread in Asia, although it also occurs in Africa, South America and Oceania.

Adult worms live in the lymphatics of the groins or axillae, where females release microfilariae – the pre-larval stage – into the blood, especially at night. These microfilariae can be detected by microscopy. Fever, pain and initially transient lymphoedema are due to irritation caused by the presence of adult worms.

Repeated attacks can result in permanent oedema, usually of a limb, but sometimes affecting breasts or genitalia (Fig. 11.3). Travellers may be aware of the gross limb deformities (elephantiasis) caused by lymphoedema that can occur in chronic sufferers of filariasis. This complication usually occurs only in people who are repeatedly infected and is unlikely in short-stay tourists.

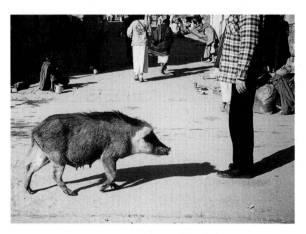

Fig. 11.2 The wild pig is a common scavenger in many parts of the world and is a natural reservoir of the Japanese B encephalitis virus.

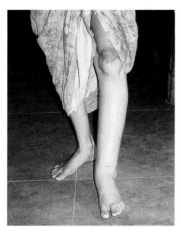

Fig. 11.3 Chronic lymphoedema as a result of Bancrofti filariasis.

So-called 'pulmonary eosinophilia' thought to be due to hypersensitivity to microfilaria can present like asthma.

Diethylcarbamazine is effective against microfilaria but needs to be given for up to 3 weeks in order to have any effect against adult worms. Ivermectin is a more recently introduced alternative.

Prevention depends on avoiding mosquito bites.

Infections spread by flies

ONCHOCERCIASIS

Onchocerciasis, which can cause 'river blindness', is caused by the helminth *Onchocerca volvulus* which is spread by a small blackfly (*Simulium damnosum*) (Fig. 11.4). This fly breeds in running water and is therefore endemic along river banks and in rain forests. Most cases of onchocerciasis are found in Central and West Africa (p. 477).

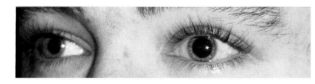

Fig. 11.4 Conjunctival infection in someone with onchocerciasis following a provocation test using diethylcarbamazine. This drug 'irritates' the microfilaria resulting in fever and inflammation at their site.

The fly injects larvae, which take about a year to develop into adult worms. The most serious pathology is caused in the eye but subcutaneous nodules and skin rashes and pruritus owing to the presence of microfilariae also result. Diagnosis may be suspected if there is otherwise unexplained eosinophilia in a patient who has been exposed, especially if associated with pruritus. Microfilariae may be detected in skin snips. Ivermectin is the treatment of choice but does not normally destroy adult worms so recurrence of symptoms can occur.

Prevention depends on avoiding bites. Sensible clothing and insect repellents should be used and travellers should be careful not to be unnecessarily exposed to blackflies, for example, by camping near rivers in endemic areas.

LEISHMANIASIS

Leishmaniasis is a protozoan infection spread by the female sandfly of the *Phlebotomus* species.[5] Sandflies normally bite from dusk until dawn and usually stay close to the ground, so sleeping in high hammocks or in upper storeys of buildings gives some protection. The flies can pass through an ordinary mosquito net, but are less likely to do so if the net is impregnated with an insecticide.

As well as human cases, there are various other reservoirs of the disease – usually canine or rodent – and this therefore is a zoonotic infection. Different *Leishmania* species are widely distributed in the Mediterranean coastal regions, Central Asia through to India and China, East Africa and parts of Central and South America (p. 473).

Leishmaniasis causes two major clinical sydromes as a result of systemic or visceral (kala azar), and skin (cutaneous) involvement. A local lesion at the site of inoculation may be the only sign of infection (Fig. 11.5), but a generalised infection can occur after an incubation of 3–18 months, especially when the immune system is compromised, as in AIDS. Onset is usually slow, with fever and sweating followed by lymphadenopathy, splenomegaly, which may be marked, and hepatomegaly. Anaemia, leucopenia and thrombocytopenia are usually present once the disease is established.

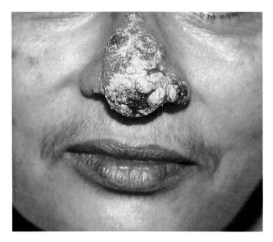

Fig. 11.5 The granulomatous lesion of cutaneous leishmaniasis which appears some weeks or months after the bite of an infected sandfly.

Diagnosis of leishmaniasis is based on identifying the typical amastigotes, the intracellular phases of the parasite, in bone marrow, spleen or lymph node biopsies. Serological tests are also available. Progress with chemotherapy has been slow, and pentavalent antimony compounds and pentamidine (which possess significant side effects) remain in widespread use. Amphotericin B, allopurinol and ketoconazole are alternatives.

Attempts at immunisation against kala azar have failed, although vaccination for cutaneous disease has been practised in Russia, Israel and Jordan. Improved sanitation and removal of sandfly breeding sites have reduced the incidence of urban, cutaneous disease. In areas where dogs form an important reservoir, destruction of sick dogs or strays is of value in prevention.

AFRICAN TRYPANOSOMIASIS

African trypanosomiasis ('sleeping sickness') is caused by *Trypanosoma brucei* species and is spread by the bite of the tsetse fly (*Glossina* species), which is found only in Africa, south of the Sahara and north of South Africa. There are two main types, Rhodesiense (East and Central Africa) and Gambiense (West and Central Africa), which produce similar illnesses, although the Rhodesiense form is frequently more acute. The former infection is zoonotic, various species of antelope and cattle forming the animal reservoir, and it is this disease which affects workers and tourists to the game parks of East and Central Africa. Gambiense is largely a disease of rural populations in West Africa.

A few days after the bite, which is usually painful, a chancre may develop that looks like a simple boil. At this stage, trypanosomes may be found in the chancre or in the blood. There may be lymphadenopathy and irregular or persistent fever with anaemia and splenomegaly. At a later stage, there may be a skin rash and generalised itch owing to involvement of the central nervous system. Dementia and other psychiatric features can occur, eventually leading to coma – hence the name 'sleeping sickness'.

Diagnosis is through identifying parasites, from blood or chancres initially, or from cerebrospinal fluid in the later stages. As with leishmaniasis, chemotherapy remains largely dependent on older agents: suramin and pentamidine, and melarsoprol if there is central nervous system involvement. Recently, eflornithine has proved valuable in treating the Gambiense form of the disease.

Travellers most at risk are those living for long periods in rural areas, particularly forests, as the tsetse fly requires shade and humidity to thrive. Early recognition of chancres and other symptoms is important in preventing serious illness.

MYIASIS

The larvae of certain tropical flies are able to burrow into human skin causing an infestation termed myiasis. One of the more common conditions is due to *Cordylobia anthropophaga*, or the tumbu fly.

Tumbu fly infection is mainly found in West and Central Africa. Eggs are laid on damp clothing which then hatch on contact with human skin. The larvae burrow into the skin, producing a characteristic 'blind boil' containing the developing maggot. The spiracles, or breathing apparatus of the larvae can usually be identified on the surface of the boil as a pair of black dots. The larvae can be removed by obstructing these spiracles with oil – petroleum jelly or liquid paraffin – and grasping the larvae as it emerges to the skin surface.

Prevention involves drying clothes indoors, away from flies, or using a hot iron on clothes dried outside to destroy any eggs which may be present.

Infections spread by ticks

BORRELLIOSIS (Lyme disease)

Lyme disease is caused by a spirochaete, *Borrelia burgdorferi*, spread through tick bites. It occurs mostly in temperate zones, including Europe, and especially in Scandinavia and North America. Philadelphia has a particularly high incidence. Farmers, forestry workers and those following recreational pursuits in the countryside are at the greatest risk of tick bites.

Ticks feed off many mammals, including sheep, deer and small rodents (Fig. 11.6). They may sometimes be carried into houses or urban areas by dogs and birds. Ticks usually crawl up grass or bracken then grasp onto clothing or skin. After finding a suitable moist site, such as the groin or axilla, they attach themselves and feed, thereby spreading the infection.

Lyme disease can present after a few weeks as a spreading erythematous rash at the site of the bite, sometimes reaching 10 cm or more in diameter. Acute or chronic arthritis, neurological features such as facial palsy, radiculitis, meningitis and rarely dementia have been recognised in untreated cases. The disease is probably under-diagnosed. Antibiotics such as penicillin, tetracyclines or cephalosporins are effective, and treatment should be started before permanent organ damage occurs.

Bites can be avoided by keeping to footpaths and by wearing long trousers tucked into socks. In severely infested areas, repellents can be used on clothing. People who believe they may have been exposed should inspect their skin for ticks and remove them before they begin to feed, using tweezers. If symptoms of Lyme disease occur, particularly a rash at the bite site, medical attention should be sought promptly.

TICK TYPHUS

This tick-borne infection is caused by a microorganism of the genus *Rickettsia* and is widespread in sub-Saharan Africa, especially in eastern and southern countries. The illness is usually mild with an ulcerated papule, or eschar, at the site of the bite, together with local lymphadenopathy and fever. A fine maculopapular rash after several days usually suggests the diagnosis (Fig. 11.7). Treatment, if necessary, is with tetracyclines.

As with Lyme disease, prevention depends on avoiding tick bites.

TICK-BORNE ENCEPHALITIS

Tick-borne encephalitis (TBE) is a flavivirus infection, which occurs in Central, Eastern, Northern Europe and Scandinavia and is particularly common in the Black Forest areas of Germany and Austria (p. 478). It occurs most

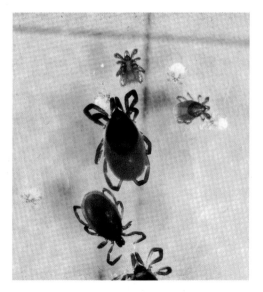

Fig. 11.6 A 'family' of ticks, showing the female (central), the male, the nymphs and larva. Ticks spread borrelia (the cause of Lyme disease), tick-borne typhus and encephalitis.

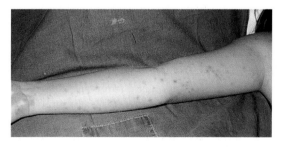

Fig. 11.7 The fine maculopapular rash of tick typhus.

commonly in early summer when ticks are active in warm, forested regions. The disease produces a flu-like illness after 7–14 days which can last for up to 1 week. About 30% of symptomatic patients develop neurological complications, including meningitis, encephalitis and muscular paralysis. There is no specific, antiviral treatment for the infection, although specific TBE immunoglobulin is available for post-exposure prophylaxis.

Travellers at risk of tick bites, for example, foresters, agricultural workers, scouts, campers and ramblers can be vaccinated against TBE. Routine childhood vaccination may be carried out in high risk areas. Tick bites should be avoided.

Infection caused by bugs

SOUTH AMERICAN TRYPANOSOMIASIS

South American trypanosomiasis (Chagas' disease) is caused by *Trypanosoma cruzi* which is transmitted by *Reduviidae* insects (assassin bugs or kissing bugs). They infect the walls and roofs of mud huts in extensive areas of South and Central America. They bite at night, transmitting infection by rubbing the organisms voided in their faeces into the bite wound during feeding. Infection may also be acquired via blood transfusion and congenitally.

The illness consists of an acute phase, which is usually asymptomatic, followed by chronic manifestations. These are usually life-long, consisting of cardiac involvement and damage to the neurological control of the intestinal tract, resulting in dilated oesophagus and large intestine.

Diagnosis is made by finding trypanosomes in blood films. In treatment, benznidazole and nifurtimox are of value in the acute form of the illness, but they have little or no impact on established or chronic disease. Cardiac and intestinal complications are managed by appropriate medication and surgery, respectively.

Prevention is dependent on elimination of vectors from houses. Argentina, Brazil and Venezuela have instigated national prevention campaigns. Impregnated bednets are helpful.

Infection caused by fleas

PLAGUE

Plague is an infection of wild rodents and is transmitted by fleas. It exists in many areas of Africa, Asia and the Americas, though most reported human cases are reported from Bolivia, Brazil, Madagascar, Tanzania, Uganda and Vietnam. During outbreaks many dead and dying rats are often observed (the fall). Fever, lymphadenopathy (bubo) and, rarely, a fulminant pneumonia can occur. Diagnosed early, plague is readily curable using tetracycline or chloramphenicol.

The risk to travellers is low and immunisation is not normally recommended. In enzootic areas, contact with rodents should be discouraged by preventing their access to food and waste, avoiding dead rodents and rodent burrows.

Fleas can be discouraged by use of insect repellents. Those entering known, high-risk areas and living in poor conditions can carry a course of tetracycline.

Infections spread by animals

There are many infections that can be contracted from animals, by eating animal products or drinking milk, or which have animals as intermediate hosts – the zoonoses. Examples include tuberculosis (milk), brucellosis (milk and close contact with body secretions), leptospirosis (urine), salmonellosis

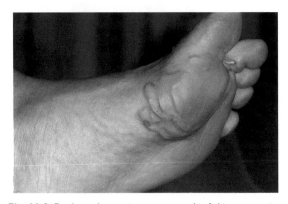

Fig. 11.8 Erythema larva migrans as a result of skin penetration of the animal hookworm.

(meat), Japanese B encephalitis (pigs), toxoplasmosis (cats and sheep), toxocariasis and erythema larva migrans (dog's faeces, see Fig. 11.8). Rabies and animal-related haemorrhagic fevers will be considered here.

RABIES

Rabies can infect many animals but the dog, fox and vampire bat are those most likely to come in contact with humans (Fig. 11.9). Infection usually occurs as the result of a bite by an infected animal; the virus is transmitted in the animal's saliva, usually by inoculation but occasionally by inhalation. The virus moves into the central nervous system and multiplies in nerve cells in the brain and peripheral ganglia. As a result, cells may become irritable (furious rabies) or depressed (dumb rabies). In the dog, the incubation period is usually between 2 weeks and 4 months, and in humans between 20 and 90 days.

Following a few days of prodromal, non-specific symptoms, hydrophobia or aerophobia may occur. Spasms involve the diaphragm and inspiratory muscles. Generalised convulsions and cardiac or respiratory arrest follow, usually within 1 week. Hypersalivation, lachrymation, sweating, fluctuating blood pressure and body temperature, and posterior pituitary symptoms suggest disturbances of hypothalamic and autonomic function. Only one case report of recovery from clinical rabies exists in the world literature. Human rabies can be diagnosed by immunofluorescence of skin or brain-biopsy material; in the clinical course of the disease, the virus can be isolated from saliva, brain, cerebrospinal fluid and urine.

Following the wound or bite, infected saliva should be thoroughly washed off with soap and water and the wound irrigated with an iodine solution or alcohol. Local treatment is very effective in removing virus from the bite site, providing it is prompt and thorough. Suturing should be avoided and tetanus prophylaxsis recommended. Specific post-exposure prophylaxis includes both active immunisation and passive immunisation with hyperimmune serum.

In South America, intensive vaccination of the dog population – including strays – has been highly effective in reducing canine, and hence human, rabies. In Switzerland and West Germany, use of oral, live attenuated vaccine in baits has reduced the prevalence of fox rabies.

Pre-exposure prophylaxis should be considered for high-risk individuals, such as veterinarians working in areas endemic for rabies, and for those staying in these areas who will be more than a day's journey away from a source of post-exposure treatment.

HAEMORRHAGIC VIRUSES

Lassa, Marburg and Ebola are examples of zoonoses which can also be transmitted from person to person, mostly in the hospital situation in conditions of very poor hygiene. In Lassa fever, a multi-mammate rat, found predominantly in rural West Africa is the reservoir and infection is thought to be mainly spread by its urine. In Ebola and Marburg, no animal reservoir has yet been identified although a non-human primate is likely.

While many cases of Lassa fever are mild, serious illness has a high mortality and as a result these illnesses have received much public attention, disproportionate to their public health importance. They pose little risk to travellers and the main risk is to those looking after viraemic patients in poor conditions.

Acknowledgement

Content of this section has been adapted from an original manuscript written by Dr Gordon Cook for the Glasgow University MSc/Diploma course in Travel Medicine.

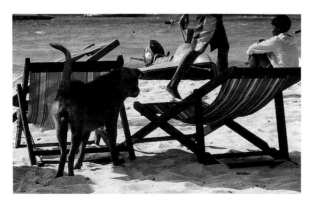

Fig. 11.9 Stray dogs are common in many countries and should be avoided, especially when rabies is present.

PRACTICE POINTS – PREVENTING BITES FROM MOSQUITOES, FLIES, BUGS AND TICKS

Mosquitoes (vector of malaria, dengue, yellow fever, Japanese B and St Louis encephalitis, Bancrofti filariasis)
- Wear clothing that covers as much of the body as possible. Use insect repellents on exposed surfaces. Many skin preparations are available, mostly containing diethyltoluamide (DEET). For those allergic to DEET, alternatives include eucalyptus or Neem tree oil.
- Use a mosquito net when sleeping in unscreened accommodation. Mosquito nets should ideally be impregnated with an insecticide. It can be helpful to practise erecting nets before departure.

Blackflies (vector of onchocerciasis), **tsetse flies** (vector of African trypanosomiasis), **sandflies** (vector of leishmaniasis)
- Avoid unnecessary work or sleeping in infested areas. Blackflies breed in fast flowing water.
- Clothing should cover as much of the body as possible.
- Sandflies can pass through bednets but impregnation with an insecticide may overcome this.
- Insect repellents should be used and local advice should be sought by those staying in rural infested areas for long periods.

Bugs (vector of South American trypanosomiasis – Chagas' disease)
- Bugs live in the walls of mud houses and only come out at night.
- Ideally avoid sleeping in these houses and sleep well away from walls.
- Mosquito nets, well-tucked in, can provide protection.

Ticks (vector of Lyme disease, tick-borne typhus, babesiosis and some other fevers such as Rocky Mountain spotted fever)
- Bites from these insects are unusual in organised tourist groups.
- Ticks normally become attached to skin or clothing after brushing against bracken and long grass and then migrate to warm, moist areas of the body such as groins or axillae to feed.
- Avoid unnecessary exposure in infested areas. Keep to paths.
- Clothing should especially cover the legs with 'socks outside trousers'. Insect repellents can be used to impregnate clothing.
- Ticks should always be removed as soon as possible, ideally with tweezers hooked under the tick's body. Applying grease such as Vaseline or butter to the site of attachment for 10 minutes may help to loosen their grip.

REFERENCES

1. Bell JC, Palmer SR, Payne JM. The zoonoses: infections transmitted from animals to man. London: Edward Arnold; 1988: 241.
2. Ruebush TK. Zoonoses. In: Strickland GT, ed. Hunter's tropical medicine. (7th ed. Philadelphia: WB Saunders; 1991: 959–962.
3. Cook GC. Zoonotic parasitic infections transmitted by food and drink: diagnosis and management. Health and Hygiene 1993; 14: 5–9.
4. McNeill WH. Plagues and people. London: Penguin; 1979: 330.
5. Cook GC. Insect-borne diseases: still the scourge of the tropics. Shell Agriculture 1993; 15 Nov: 20–23.

FURTHER READING

Bell DR, ed. Lecture notes on tropical medicine, 4th ed. Oxford: Blackwell Science; 1995.
Cook GC, ed. Manson's tropical diseases. 20th ed. London: WB Saunders; 1996.
Dawood R, ed. Travellers' health: How to stay healthy abroad. 3rd ed. Oxford: Oxford University Press; 1992: 15–53, 63–74, 80–160.
Dupont H, Steffen R, ed. Textbook of travel medicine and health. Hamilton, Ontario: Decker Publications; 1997: 78–108, 200–206, 235–252, 282–286.
Grist N, Ho-Yen D, Walker E, Williams G. Diseases of infection. 2nd ed. Oxford: Oxford University Press; 1994.
Howarth J. Bugs, bites and bowels. London: Cadogan Books; 1995: 20–39, 50–68.

Travellers' diarrhoea

Michael Farthing

Introduction

Diarrhoea is the most common ailment associated with travel. More than 30% of individuals travelling from developed to developing countries can expect to suffer an episode of diarrhoea during their visit or shortly after they return. A conservative estimate indicates that there are up to 10 million episodes of travellers' diarrhoea occurring each year.[1,2] Most episodes are mild, self-limiting and more inconvenient than medically hazardous. However, diarrhoea in travellers provokes considerable anxiety and may result in significant disruption of vacation, business or other travel plans.

There are considerable economic implications for the host country, since the threat of an illness may make some travellers disinclined to visit those high-risk regions of the world and thus reduce potential income from tourism. Health risks may also be a negative factor influencing decisions regarding foreign investment and business ventures in these locations. Occasionally, travellers' diarrhoea can be a serious and even life-threatening illness in a minority of travellers.

The cornerstones of management are appropriate self-therapy for mild or moderate illnesses, and a clear understanding by the traveller as to when it is necessary to seek medical advice. Avoidance strategies, although rational and intellectually satisfying, often seem to fail. Preventive measures will continue to play a relatively minor role until effective vaccines directed towards the organisms commonly responsible for travellers' diarrhoea are more widely available.

Definition

Travellers' diarrhoea is usually defined as the passage of three or more unformed stools in 24 hours occurring during or shortly after travel, or any number of loose stools when associated with fever, abdominal pain or vomiting.[3,4] Passage of any number of dysenteric stools (diarrhoea with blood) associated with travel is also included in the definition of travellers' diarrhoea. Although these definitions have been formulated to allow standardisation of research and communication, many travellers experience milder symptoms that do not satisfy these criteria. More than 25% of tourists in one study reported a change in stool consistency but passed only one to two motions each day.[5] Some recent, controlled, therapeutic studies in travellers' diarrhoea have modified the entry criteria by enrolling subjects who had had just a single watery stool. This has permitted the assessment of the effect of antimicrobial chemotherapy given early in the course of the illness, while allowing the placebo group to confirm that these individuals did go on to have an illness with the typical, natural history of travellers' diarrhoea.

Epidemiology

More than 300 million people cross international boundaries each year and at least 30 million of these travel from an industrialised country to a location in the developing world. About 30–50% of travellers will have an attack of travellers' diarrhoea depending on the country visited. Geographical locations can be classified according to risk.[6] Low-risk areas where attack rates are generally less than 8% include North America, Northern and Central Europe, Australia and New Zealand. Intermediate-risk areas include the Caribbean, the Northern Mediterranean, Israel, Japan and South Africa. High-risk areas with diarrhoea rates of 20–50% are found in Latin America, Africa and Asia.

As travellers' diarrhoea can usually be attributed to intestinal infection, it is now widely assumed that the geographical variation in prevalence relates to the likelihood of encountering a microbial enteropathogen in the environment. This will inevitably depend on local water quality, sewage disposal, asymptomatic carriage of enteropathogens by the local population, particularly food handlers, and catering standards in hotels, restaurants and other food and beverage outlets. The mode of travel also seems to be important in determining the risks in developing travellers' diarrhoea. Diarrhoea is less likely to occur in those who restrict themselves to the facilities of good quality hotels than in those who travel overland and eat in local restaurants where less attention may be paid to hygiene, water purity and food sources.[7] Previous travel to a tropical area during the preceding 6 months does offer some protection against travellers' diarrhoea although such protection is not long-lasting.[8]

The classic vehicles for infective diarrhoea include water, uncooked and unpeeled food and inadequately reheated food. Experimental studies in which microorganisms have been introduced into food heated to 50°C (a temperature which is uncomfortable to touch) have shown that a variety of enterovirulent bacteria can survive these temperatures and will multiply as the temperature decreases.[9] Enteropathogens in water can survive freezing in ice cubes and then multiply in soft and alcoholic drinks.[10] Even spirits such as whisky and tequila will not reliably 'sterilise' contaminated ice cubes.[11]

Person-to-person transmission of enteropathogens is relatively unimportant for travellers, although some viruses such as Norwalk virus and the other SRSVs may be spread by aerosol[12] which probably contributes to the high secondary attack rates that occur in families and in travellers on cruise ships. Some bacterial and protozoal enteropathogens are spread during sexual activity, particularly by intimate oro–anal contact.

There are a variety of host factors that appear to increase the risk of travellers' diarrhoea including the extremes of age, impaired gastric acid barrier and immune deficiency.

Acute infective diarrhoea predominantly affects pre-school children which reflects in part their immunological naiveté for these enteropathogens and the behavioural factors which make infants and young children more likely to acquire microbial enteropathogens from the environment and from each other.

Risk factors for travellers' diarrhoea

Environmental factors
- Prevalence of microbial enteropathogens
- Water quality, sewage disposal and other public health controls.

Host factors
- Residence in highly industrialised region
- No travel to tropical area in past 6 months
- Attitude to avoiding contaminated food and water
- Age (< 6 yr)
- Impaired non-immune defence mechanisms.

Immune deficiency.

Children of immigrants to developed countries who visit the parental homeland in the developing world may be particularly susceptible to severe travellers' diarrhoea.[13] These children presumably rapidly acquire the eating and drinking habits of their indigenous relatives, but are immunologically unprepared for the broad spectrum of enteropathogens they encounter.

Gastric acid is an important barrier to the transfer of orally acquired enteropathogens into the small intestine. Although in the past this was related to hypochlorhydria from gastric atrophy (pernicious anaemia) and gastric surgery,[14] more recently potent acid inhibitory drugs such as H_2-receptor antagonists and the proton pump inhibitors have been shown to increase the risk of infections, particularly in individuals more than 65 years of age.[15]

Acquisition of intestinal infection from food and drink does appear to relate to an individual's attitude towards dietary restriction. A study in Swiss travellers to Kenya and Sri Lanka showed a clear relationship between the number of dietary mistakes and the likelihood of experiencing travellers' diarrhoea and confirmed that only 2% of these individuals were able to consistently adhere to the strict dietary advice given.[7] Business travellers, diplomats and other VIPs may find it extremely difficult to comply with dietary advice because of social and professional pressures.

Certain leisure activities may also place an individual at increased risk of acquiring travellers' diarrhoea. Sea water in many coastal regions around the world is contaminated with sewage and faecal microorganisms.[16,17] A survey of a beach in the south-east of England confirmed that diarrhoea and other abdominal symptoms were more common in bathers than non-bathers and that the coliform count failed to achieve European standards on 12% of sampling occasions.[16] More recent surveys indicate that sea water on British beaches has improved markedly such that more than 80% comply with EU standards. Inland lakes and rivers are generally not approved for recreational swimming and are not routinely monitored. A recent survey, however, confirmed that more than 80% of freshwater locations tested in the UK were contaminated with cyanobacterial toxins, which is attributed to the increasing use of nitrate and phosphate fertilisers and unaccustomed warm summers.

Outbreaks of diarrhoea have been reported to emanate from swimming pools, particularly owing to infections with the protozoan parasites, *Cryptosporidium parvum* and *Giardia intestinalis*.[18,19] The cysts of these organisms are able to survive in cool, moist conditions outside the host and are relatively resistant to chlorination. Thus, there can be dissociation between coliform counts and the risk of acquiring an enteric, protozoal infection. Outbreaks of *Shigella* spp. and enterohaemorrhagic *Escherichia coli* dysentery have been reported in swimmers using a freshwater lake in Oregon;[20] the risk of acquiring infection in these individuals was clearly linked to a history of having swallowed lake water.

Clinical features

Symptoms of travellers' diarrhoea may begin at any time during travel or shortly after return. They most commonly start on the 3rd day with a second episode starting about 1 week after arrival in about 20% of cases.[6] Untreated, the mean duration of travellers' diarrhoea is 4 days with a median of 2 days. In a few cases symptoms persist for more than 1 month. Travellers' diarrhoea usually takes a mild course with most subjects having less than six bowel movements every 24 hours, although the symptoms frequently associated with travellers' diarrhoea may be more disruptive than the diarrhoea itself (Fig. 11.10).

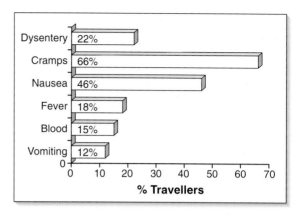

Fig. 11.10 Symptoms associated with travellers' diarrhoea.

The severity distribution of the diarrhoea is summarised in Figure 11.11. Almost 60% of those with travellers' diarrhoea have more than six bowel movements each 24 hours.[2] Abdominal cramps and nausea are commonly associated with the diarrhoea and 20–30% have the dysentery syndrome with fever and bloody diarrhoea. Less than 20% of patients have vomiting as a major symptom which is often due to ingestion of food containing preformed bacterial toxins (*Staphylococcus aureus* toxin and *Bacillus cereus* toxin), illnesses which generally have short incubation times (1–12 h) and a much shorter duration of illness, usually a few hours. This contrasts with the typical illness of travellers' diarrhoea that usually lasts for several days if untreated.

Travellers' diarrhoea can be classified into three clinical categories according to symptoms:

1. acute watery diarrhoea
2. dysentery (diarrhoea with blood)

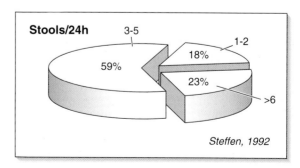

Fig. 11.11 Severity distribution of diarrhoea (bowel frequency) in travellers' diarrhoea.

3. persistent diarrhoea with or without intestinal malabsorption.

Complications

Reiter's syndrome, characterised by arthritis, urethritis, conjunctivitis and mucocutaneous lesions may sometimes complicate acute diarrhoeal infections, particularly those caused by *Campylobacter jejuni*, *Salmonella* spp., *Shigella* spp. and *Yersinia enterocolitica*. Clinical features vary, as not all afflicted individuals manifest all features of the syndrome. Although Reiter's syndrome may occur in any individual, there is a close association with HLA Haplotype B27.

A devastating complication of *Shigella dysenteriae* Type 1 infection is the haemolytic–uraemic syndrome which usually begins as bowel symptoms are starting to improve.[21] Enterohaemorrhagic *Escherichia coli* (EHEC) infection has a 2–3% mortality which again is related to the haemolytic–uraemic syndrome and thrombotic thrombocytopenic purpura. These serious complications are thought to be due to the systemic effects of shiga toxin and shiga-like toxins 1 and 2, the latter being produced by EHEC.

Infection with *Campylobacter jejuni* is now firmly associated with the Guillain–Barré syndrome.[22] Neurological symptoms have been documented to occur between 1 and 21 days after the onset of bowel symptoms and when associated with *Campylobacter jejuni*, the syndrome is predominantly a motor neuropathy and carries a poor prognosis.

Salmonellosis may disseminate widely from the gut and affect many other organs causing complications such as acute endocarditis, aortitis, septic arthritis and osteomyelitis and occasionally produce infections of the urogenital tract and lungs. Similarly *Entamoeba histolytica* trophozoites can penetrate the colon and enter the portal venous circulation, infecting the liver, to produce amoebic hepatitis and amoebic abscesses. Large abscesses, particularly those in the left lobe, may rupture into the pleural, pericardial or abdominal cavities.

ACUTE WATERY DIARRHOEA

Most cases of acute watery diarrhoea are mild and transient. However, the severity of the illness varies from mild looseness of stools to copious, high-volume, watery diarrhoea. Dehydration is rarely marked and systemic symptoms are usually mild or absent. Dehydration, sometimes accompanied by acidosis, may be clinically important in neonates and young children and in the elderly. There is usually a paucity of associated symptoms but when present they may include anorexia, nausea, vomiting, abdominal cramps, flatulence or bloating. Fever is unusual but when present is usually low grade. Recovery in most instances occurs within 2–3 days.

DYSENTERY

Although a dysenteric illness may begin with watery diarrhoea, the typical pattern of loose, small volume stools with blood and mucus, usually rapidly supervenes. Dysentery is a consequence of an invasive/inflammatory process in the colon and distal ileum. There may be a prodrome of constitutional symptoms, including headache, myalgia and general malaise. Abdominal pain, which may be severe, is usually present in the lower abdomen and is cramping in nature, particularly prior to defaecation. Pain, tenesmus and fever often accompany the diarrhoea but are not a reliable guide to aetiology. The illness is usually self-limiting but occasionally can be severe and prolonged. In fulminant cases, the dysenteric illness may be associated with toxic megacolon, colonic perforation, peritonitis and septicaemia, although fortunately for travellers these complications are exceptionally rare.

CHRONIC DIARRHOEA

Only a minority of travellers have protracted symptoms. Depending on the definition of chronicity, probably less than 1% of travellers suffer prolonged diarrhoea. After returning from abroad, persistent diarrhoea may have the clinical features of steatorrhoea, which is often accompanied by marked weight loss. Other associated symptoms include nausea, anorexia, dyspepsia, malaise and sometimes low-grade fever. Persistent infections in the small intestine can produce disaccharidase deficiency that may manifest as transient lactose intolerance.

Aetiology and pathogenesis

Travellers' diarrhoea has been attributed to many host and environmental factors, including a 'change in the water', travellers' nerves or over-indulgence in local food and wine. It is now clearly established that at least 80% of cases of travellers' diarrhoea can be attributed to an infective enteropathogen.[23–28] There is an extensive range of microbial enteropathogens that can cause travellers' diarrhoea, including bacteria, viruses and protozoa (Fig. 11.12). A convenient classification of aetiology can be based on the clinical patterns of disease, namely acute watery diarrhoea, dysentery and persistent diarrhoea. There is, however, considerable aetiologic agent overlap between these clinical syndromes, particularly with the organisms that are responsible for dysentery; the classic, invasive, bacterial enteropathogens such as *Shigella* spp., *Salmonella* spp. and *Campylobacter jejuni* do not always produce bloody diarrhoea. Thus one cannot make a confident microbiological diagnosis on the basis of symptoms alone, although the presence of blood would strongly suggest that an invasive microorganism was responsible for the illness.

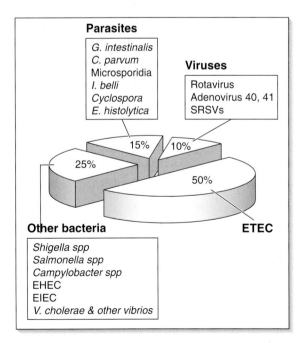

Fig. 11.12 Range of microbial enteropathogens responsible for travellers' diarrhoea.

ACUTE WATERY DIARRHOEA

The microorganisms commonly isolated from patients with acute watery diarrhoea are summarised in Table 11.1.

Enterotoxigenic *Escherichia coli* (ETEC) is by far the most common cause of diarrhoea in travellers and probably accounts for at least 40% of all cases. ETEC, like *Vibrio cholerae*, produce enterotoxins which promote a secretory state for fluid and electrolytes in the intestine without causing structural damage to the epithelium.[29–33] Human ETEC produce two major toxins, the heat labile toxin (LT) and the heat stable toxin (ST_a). LT closely resembles cholera toxin consisting of one A sub-unit and five B sub-units; the A sub-unit has two components (A_1 and A_2) linked by a disulphide bond. LT binds to a receptor on the enterocyte microvillus membrane, the GM_1 ganglioside which induces a configurational change in the membrane permitting entry of the enzymatically active A_1 sub-unit. The A_1 sub-unit is an ADP-ribosyl transferase which covalently links ADP ribose to G_s, the stimulatory component of adenylate cyclase, resulting in enzyme activation and increased intracellular concentrations of cAMP. Then, through a series of intracellular processes mediated by protein kinase C, a protein of the chloride channel is phosphorylated which results in active chloride ion secretion.

ST_a is a small polypeptide of about 2000 kDa which interacts with a specific receptor on the enterocyte apical membrane.[33] The receptor is closely linked to the enzyme guanylate cyclase and receptor occupancy results in a rapid increase of intracellular cGMP. This again promotes chloride channel ion secretion by phosphorylation of the chloride channel. Unlike LT, removal of ST_a from its receptor results in a reversal of the secretory process back to the basal state.

Although these intracellular mechanisms have been well characterised for LT and ST_a, there is increasing evidence that both toxins also promote intestinal secretion through neural reflexes in the enteric nervous system.[34] Unlike cholera toxin, however, these toxins do not appear to release 5-hydroxytryptamine (5-HT, serotonin) and are not inhibited by $5-HT_2$ and $5-HT_3$ receptor antagonists.

TABLE 11.1 Enteropathogens responsible for acute watery diarrhoea and dysentery in travellers

Enteropathogen	Acute watery diarrhoea	Dysentery
Viruses		
Rotavirus	+	–
Adenovirus (types 40, 41)	+	–
Small round structured viruses (SRSVs)	+	–
Bacteria		
Enterotoxigenic *Escherichia coli* (ETEC)	+	–
Enteroinvasive *Escherichia coli* (EIEC)	+	–
Enterohaemorrhagic *Escherichia coli* (EHEC)	+	+
Shigella spp.	+	+
Salmonella spp.	+	+
Campylobacter spp.	+	+
Yersinia enterocolitica	+	+
Vibrio cholerae (rare) and other vibrios	+	–
Protozoa		
Giardia intestinalis	+	–
Cryptosporidium parvum	+	–
Isospora belli	+	–
Cyclospora cayetanensis	+	–
Entamoeba histolytica	+	+

Acute watery diarrhoea also follows infection with rotavirus and the SRSVs. In this case, however, the viruses enter the villus epithelial cells, produce cytopathic changes which eventually result in enterocyte loss.[35] There is therefore acute villous atrophy during the first 24–48 hours of infection following which there is proliferation of crypt cells and subsequent recovery in villus morphology. Loss of enterocytes almost certainly accounts for the decrease in disaccharidase activity and the transient disaccharide intolerance that is sometimes associated with these infections.

DYSENTERY

The microbial enteropathogens that produce dysentery in travellers are listed in Table 11.1. These organisms express virulence factors that either permit direct invasion of the epithelial cell and/or liberate cytotoxins which produce cell death.[36,37] The classic invasive organisms, *Shigella* spp., *Salmonella* spp. and enteroinvasive *Escherichia coli* (EIEC), all express invasion plasmid antigens (Ipa) on their surface which trigger membrane-ruffling of the host epithelial cell with subversion of the cytoskeleton and formation of an endocytotic vesicle which transports the organism into the host cytoplasm. Lysis then invariably takes place and the organism multiplies and liberates cytotoxin intracellularly.

These organisms are also able to move 'horizontally' from cell to cell through the basolateral membrane, again subverting host cytoskeletal machinery to propel the bacterium through the cytoplasm. *Shigella dysenteriae* type 1 produces shiga toxin which is one of the most potent bacterial inhibitors of protein synthesis. EHEC intimately adhere to the apical enterocyte membrane producing the classic attaching/effacing lesion which is also characteristic of enteropathogenic *Escherichia coli* (EPEC) but in addition releases shiga-like toxins (SLT) 1 and 2 which have close sequence homology with shiga toxin and have similar effects on host cell protein synthesis. Although EHEC does not appear to directly invade epithelial cells, it is transported into the mucosa through M cells.

The invasion and cytotoxin virulence factors are only one component of the cascade of events that produces the inflammatory process in the distal ileum and colon. These invasive enteropathogens trigger IL-8 production by epithelial cells which, as a potent chemoattractant, produces a rapid influx of polymorphonuclear neutrophils (PMNs) which enhance the inflammatory cascade and also add to the secretory process by liberating the PMN secretagogue 5′ AMP which binds to adenosine receptors on the apical membrane of the epithelial cell to promote chloride secretion.

Entamoeba histolytica is an important cause of dysentery but is not strictly an invasive organism. Following lectin-mediated adherence to the epithelial cell, it liberates a variety of cytotoxic moieties which rapidly produce cell death.[38] One of these proteins, amoebapore, which is structurally related to the active components of bee venom, melittin, is a pore-forming protein which creates high conductance ion channels in the epithelial cell membrane, allowing rapid influx of calcium and other ions leading to disequilibrium and cell death. *Entamoeba histolytica* then phagocytoses the dead cell and moves on to penetrate further into the mucosa.

PERSISTENT DIARRHOEA

The major causes of persistent diarrhoea in the returning traveller are listed in Table 11.2.

Infectious agents are the most important causes, particularly the protozoal enteropathogens *Giardia intestinalis*, *Cryptosporidium parvum* and the recently described intracellular organism, *Cyclospora cayetanensis*. The mechanisms by which these organisms cause persistent diarrhoea is incompletely understood.[39] All are associated with varying degrees of villus architectural abnormality and an inflammatory response within the intestinal mucosa. Diarrhoea can occur in the absence of morphological changes suggesting that other mechanisms must also be operating. *Cryptosporidium parvum*, for example, has been associated with the presence of 'enterotoxic' activity in faecal filtrates which induces an increase in short-circuit current when introduced into an Ussing chamber containing mammalian intestine. However, intestinal perfusion studies in humans have failed to demonstrate a secretory state in the small intestine, suggesting that the diarrhoea relates either to a major abnormality of intestinal transit or to disease in the distal ileum or colon.

Persistent diarrhoea is sometimes associated with continuing bacterial infection, such as *Salmonella* spp. and *Campylobacter jejuni*. Tropical sprue still occurs in travellers but appears to be much less common than it was 10–15 years ago. Diarrhoea and malabsorption are thought to relate to villous atrophy and bacterial overgrowth in the proximal small intestine. In some patients, there is evidence of a 'colonopathy' which may contribute to the pathogenesis of diarrhoea.

Diarrhoea in the returning traveller may be the first presentation of non-specific inflammatory bowel disease; in one study, this accounted for 15% of patients attending a travel clinic with post-travel diarrhoea.[40] Finally, there is increasing evidence to suggest that acute intestinal infection may 'trigger' the onset of a functional bowel disorder such as irritable bowel syndrome. It is not entirely clear however, whether infection actually causes the functional disorder or whether it merely unmasks an established susceptibility to disordered bowel function.

Diagnosis

For individuals with acute watery diarrhoea which resolves without specific treatment, it is unnecessary to make a microbiological diagnosis. The majority of cases will be due to ETEC which cannot easily be identified in a routine laboratory and thus in practice, a specific diagnosis is never made.

In patients with bloody diarrhoea which does not resolve promptly, it is advisable to obtain faecal specimens for microscopy and culture. A fresh stool specimen, prepared as a saline wet mount, should be examined microscopically to search for the typical, motile trophozoites of *Entamoeba histolytica*. These can be distinguished from other non-pathogenic intestinal amoebae by the presence of red blood cells, since only *Entamoeba histolytica* is

---

TABLE 11.2 Causes of persistent diarrhoea in travellers

Protozoa	*Giardia intestinalis*
	Cryptosporidium parvum
	Cyclospora cayetanensis
Bacteria	*Salmonella* spp. infection*
	Campylobacter spp. infection*
	Intestinal tuberculosis
Helminths	*Strongyloidiasis*
	Colonic schistosomiasis
Miscellaneous	Inflammatory bowel disease
	Tropical sprue
	Post-infectious irritable bowel

*Mostly acute illness but may be prolonged

erythrophagic. *Balantidium coli* is extremely uncommon in travellers, but the large, highly motile, ciliated trophozoites can be identified by microscopy. Routine faecal culture will detect the classic invasive enteropathogens, *Salmonella* spp., *Shigella* spp., *Campylobacter jejuni* and *Yersinia enterocolitica*, although special conditions are required to isolate the latter two organisms.

Acute schistosomiasis occurs in travellers to endemic areas and although traditionally the ova are sought in rectal, mucosal biopsies, serology is now the standard screening test for this infection.

Individuals with persistent diarrhoea require more intensive investigation particularly to exclude chronic, intestinal, protozoal infection. High quality faecal microscopy by an experienced parasitologist using appropriate special stains is the standard approach to detecting *Giardia intestinalis*, *Cryptosporidium parvum*, *Cyclospora* and the *Microsporidia*. Unfortunately, many routine laboratories do not have extensive experience in identifying the intracellular protozoa; if these diagnoses are strongly suspected and faecal microscopy is persistently negative, then it would be worth while arranging for specimens to be examined by a specialised reference centre. These small intestinal parasites can be detected in mucosal biopsy specimens both by light microscopy and electron microscopy and thus if faecal microscopy is persistently negative, distal duodenal biopsy obtained at endoscopy may be an appropriate investigation to pursue.

Endoscopic examination of the large bowel either by rigid sigmoidoscopy or colonoscopy may be indicated if symptoms persist and microbiological examination is negative. This procedure has the advantage that it will not only identify any obvious macroscopic inflammatory changes in the colon but also provides an opportunity for obtaining multiple mucosal biopsies which can reveal the presence of infective microorganisms, notably *Cryptosporidium parvum*, *Entamoeba histolytica* and cytomegalovirus.

Treatment

As most attacks of travellers' diarrhoea are self-limiting, specific treatment is usually not required.

However, when (i) an attack of watery diarrhoea is severe and is causing marked disruption of travel plans, (ii) when bloody diarrhoea is due to amoebiasis or dysenteric shigellosis or when associated systemic symptoms such as fever are clinically important and (iii) when a specific cause for persistent diarrhoea is identified, then it is appropriate to intervene. Travellers are increasingly aware of the risks of a diarrhoeal illness and the culture of self-therapy is now well established; many individuals now routinely carry oral rehydration salts, antidiarrhoeal agents and a variety of antibiotics.

PRE-TRAVEL ADVICE ON TREATMENT

Travellers should be aware that the majority of episodes of travellers' diarrhoea are due to intestinal infection which will generally resolve without specific therapy and without causing any long-lasting harm to the intestine. Travellers should, however, be alerted to several clinical situations in which active intervention is advisable or necessary.[2,41–43]

SEVERE ACUTE WATERY DIARRHOEA

Morbidity and mortality associated with acute watery diarrhoea are invariably related to dehydration and acidosis. When faecal losses are high, oral fluid and electrolyte replacement should be started promptly either with a pre-packaged oral rehydration solution or by taking appropriate dietary supplements to ensure rehydration and maintenance of hydration while the illness resolves. Antidiarrhoeal agents may also be used in adults and older children although travellers should be aware that these agents do not 'cure' the illness and do not have a major impact on reducing faecal losses although they can be expected to reduce bowel frequency. It is now widely known that a broad-spectrum antibiotic can reduce the severity and duration of travellers' diarrhoea and some individuals who cannot afford to lose any time at all out of a business trip may wish to have the option of having the additional security offered by a broad-spectrum antibiotic. These individuals need to be advised as to when it might be appropriate to take an antibiotic and clearly warned about possible adverse affects such as photosensitivity, allergy and rarer complications such as the Stevens–Johnson syndrome and antibiotic-associated diarrhoea, particularly that owing to *Clostridium difficile*.

DYSENTERY

Travellers should be warned that the appearance of blood in the stool is indicative of an invasive and inflammatory diarrhoea and be alerted to the possibility that it might be due to amoebiasis which would require specific antibiotic therapy. Mild dysenteric illnesses can resolve spontaneously but travellers need to be prepared to seek medical advice if diarrhoea and bleeding are severe and if there are prominent associated symptoms such as abdominal pain, high fever and general malaise. Under these circumstances, it is reasonable to request a stool examination so that antimicrobial chemotherapy can be targeted towards a specific aetiological agent.

PERSISTENT DIARRHOEA

If diarrhoea has not resolved within 14 days, then it is appropriate to seek medical advice with a view to further investigation. Specific antimicrobial chemotherapy is available for many of the infective causes of persistent diarrhoea but if stool examination is negative, then it is reasonable to pursue additional investigations, particularly to exclude tropical sprue and non-specific inflammatory bowel disease.

An approach to treatment

Self-therapy of travellers' diarrhoea centres around the appropriate use of oral rehydration therapy, antidiarrhoeal agents, antimicrobial chemotherapy and non-antimicrobial therapy (Table 11.3).[2,41–43]

ORAL REHYDRATION THERAPY

Fluid and electrolyte losses should be replaced, especially in infants and young children and the elderly where losses have their greatest clinical impact. Thus, at the extremes of age, it is advisable to recommend formal oral rehydration therapy with a glucose electrolyte solution.[44,45] The simplest way to provide oral rehydration therapy is to advise travellers to take pre-packaged oral rehydration salts and to reconstitute these with bottled or boiled water. Oral rehydration therapy should be administered at the onset of diarrhoea to prevent dehydration and continued even in the presence of vomiting. Although the solution recommended by the WHO has been successfully used for more than two decades worldwide, hypotonic oral rehydration solutions with lower sodium concentrations are thought to be safer and possibly more effective in non-cholera diarrhoea (Table 11.4).[45,46] Infants should continue breast-feeding throughout the illness and children encouraged to eat as soon as their appetite returns.

Most adults will not require formal oral rehydration therapy but should be advised to increase their fluid intake, particularly fruit juices and salty soups (sodium and potassium replacement) accompanied by a carbohydrate source (bread, potatoes, rice, pasta) for the promotion of sodium–glucose co-transport (Fig. 11.13). Fasting should never be recommended.

ANTIDIARRHOEAL AGENTS

Drugs such as loperamide and a diphenoxylate–atropine combination are now widely available over

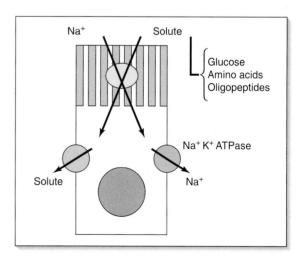

Fig. 11.13 Mechanism of sodium-solute-coupled co-transport in the enterocyte.

TABLE 11.3 Treatment options for travellers' diarrhoea

Treatment	Specific intervention	Impact on illness
Restoration and maintenance of fluid and electrolyte balance	Oral glucose–electrolyte solution (see Table 11.4)	No effect on duration but reduces morbidity and mortality
Antidiarrhoeal agents	Loperamide, lomotil	Reduce stool frequency
Antimicrobial chemotherapy	Co-trimoxazole Bicozamycin Furazolidone Doxycycline Pivmecillinam 4-Fluoroquinolones	Reduces average duration from 4.5 to 1.5 days
Non-antibiotic therapy	Bismuth subsalicylate Antidiarrhoeal agents	Reduce stool frequency No effect on duration of illness

For details of clinical trials see references 2, 42 and 43.

TABLE 11.4 Composition (mmol/L) of oral rehydration solutions available in the UK in 1998 (data from British National Formulary Feb./March 1998)

Oral rehydration solutions	Na	K	Cl	HCO$_3$	Citrate	Glucose	Osmolality (calculated)
Powders							
Oral rehydration salts							
WHO	90	20	80	–	10	111	311
Diocalm Junior	60	20	50	–	10	111	251
Dioralyte	60	25	45	–	20	90	240
Dioralyte Relief*	60	20	50	–	10	–	
Electrolade	50	20	40	30	–	111	251
Rehidrat**	50	20	50	20	9	91	336
Effervescent tablets							
Dioralyte	60	25	45	–	20	90	240

*Contains cooked rice powder 6 g/sachet (30 g/L)
**Also contains sucrose 96 mmol/L and fructose 1–2 mmol/L.

the counter. Many travellers routinely carry one of these preparations with them when they travel. In general, they are safe and moderately effective in decreasing stool frequency, although their most profound effects in modifying the duration and severity of the illness are apparent when combined with an antimicrobial agent. Antidiarrhoeal drugs are not recommended for use in infants and young children as there has been the occasional report of central nervous system depression,[47] and they are usually not advised when there is bloody diarrhoea and the possibility of infective colitis.

There is a continued search for antidiarrhoeal agents that have antisecretory activity. As stated previously, 5-HT has been implicated in the secretory state induced by cholera toxin and there is evidence that 5-HT$_2$ and 5-HT$_3$ receptor antagonists can inhibit secretion both in animal models and in a human model of cholera secretion.[34,48,49] The calmodulin antagonist, zaldride maleate, has also been shown to inhibit enterotoxin-induced secretion and clinical trials have demonstrated its efficacy in individuals with travellers' diarrhoea.[50] Another approach has been to use inhibitors of the enzyme enkephalinase such as acetorphan which enhances the activity of endogenous opioids in the intestine.[51] Again there is evidence that this agent is effective in model systems and preliminary data suggest that it may be useful in human diarrhoea.

ANTIMICROBIAL CHEMOTHERAPY

There is now unequivocal evidence that broad-spectrum antibiotics given for 3–5 days can significantly reduce the duration and severity of travellers' diarrhoea (Table 11.3).[2,42,43] Stool frequency is reduced on average by about 50% and the duration of illness limited to 12–24 hours. Recent studies of single dose or 1- or 2-day treatment regimens have shown that fluoroquinolone drugs have similar therapeutic benefits without the need for an extended course of treatment.[52–54]

It remains controversial, however, as to who should be supplied with an antibiotic for self-therapy. Many individuals now know the benefits of a short course of antibiotics for travellers' diarrhoea and are requesting a supply prior to travel. Doctors have known of these benefits for many years and have enjoyed the relief of terminating travellers' diarrhoea after a few hours. It is therefore reasonable to suggest self-therapy with an antibiotic if diarrhoea is severe (more than six stools per 24 hours) or when the severity is such that travellers are confined to their hotel room. Antibiotic self-therapy should also be considered in those individuals with moderate diarrhoea who cannot afford to lose 24 hours from their travel schedule. It must be understood however, that drugs used in this way would not normally be the responsibility of the National Health Service and therefore individuals requesting these drugs should be willing to cover the cost themselves, in the same way that travel vaccines and malaria prophylaxis are the financial responsibility of the user.

There are continuing concerns about the emergence of drug resistance and the point has been made on many occasions that 'indiscriminate' use of antibiotics for mild, non-fatal illnesses such as travellers' diarrhoea will only add to the resistance problem in future years. One can argue, however, that antibiotics are used for many other, mild, non-fatal respiratory, urinary and other

infections and occasional use in travellers' diarrhoea is unlikely to make a major impact on world resistance patterns. The ultrashort courses of antibiotics that are now known to be effective in travellers' diarrhoea may be less likely to produce drug resistance although to date this has not been studied extensively in the clinical setting.[55]

NON-ANTIBIOTIC THERAPY

Bismuth subsalicylate reduces stool frequency in travellers' diarrhoea and it has been demonstrated to have both antibacterial and antisecretory effects in the intestine.[56] Short courses are safe and there is no evidence that it leads to antimicrobial resistance. Overall, it is less effective than antibiotic and antidiarrhoeal agents.

Prevention

Despite widely available information for travellers, including the traditional dietary advice and the increasing sophistication of those who travel frequently, there is no convincing evidence that there has been a major decline in the prevalence of travellers' diarrhoea. Individual studies by highly motivated investigators and well-drilled experimental subjects will certainly demonstrate that such advice can have an impact on the prevalence of diarrhoea but even scrupulous care does not seem to be able to provide assured protection.[7] This has resulted in a search for other approaches to prevent travellers' diarrhoea (Table 11.5).

Chemoprophylaxis has been explored with antibiotics and bismuth subsalicylate. Immuno-prophylaxis in the form of enteric vaccines will probably be available within the next 5 years. Interest continues in the possibility that probiotics, such as *Lactobacillus* spp. or even prebiotics, such as administration of oligofructose, may be alternative approaches.

CHEMOPROPHYLAXIS

For more than 30 years, it has been shown that broad-spectrum, antimicrobial, chemotherapeutic agents can reduce the attack rate of travellers'

TABLE 11.5 Prevention of travellers' diarrhoea

Approach	Specific measures	Reduction in attack rate (%)
Minimise entry of enteropathogens	Avoid uncooked/unpeeled food, ice cubes and tap water Avoid reheated food left at room temperature Food should be > 65°C Beware swimming pools, lakes and sea water	Unknown
Antimicrobial chemoprophylaxis*	Sulphonamides Neomycin Doxycycline Co-trimoxazole 4-Fluoroquinolones (e.g. ciprofloxacin, norfloxacin ofloxacin, fleroxacin)	50 30 75 60 > 85
Non-antibiotic therapy	Bismuth subsalicylate* Lactobacillus spp. Vaccines	60 Unknown Unknown

*For details of clinical trials see references 2, 42 and 43.

diarrhoea.[2,41–43] Drugs shown to be effective by controlled clinical trial include sulphonamides, doxycycline, co-trimoxazole, trimethoprim, erythromycin, mecillinam, bicozamycin and several 4-fluoroquinolone antibiotics. Dosage regimens usually recommend approximately half of the usual therapeutic dose. The more recent studies with co-trimoxazole, doxycycline and the fluoroquinolones demonstrate efficacies of 70–> 90%. Thus the efficacy of antimicrobial chemoprophylaxis is not in doubt although whether such an intervention should even be used is highly controversial.

First, antimicrobials may cause adverse drug reactions, which are occasionally severe and include diarrhoea. There is thus considerable reluctance to place travellers at risk of potentially fatal complications for what, in the majority, is a mild, self-limiting illness; it will affect on average only 30% of travellers to intermediate- and high-risk areas. Second, there are also concerns that compliance decreases, the more complex the prophylactic regimen becomes, thus travellers might neglect malaria chemoprophylaxis if they were required to take agents against travellers' diarrhoea in addition. Finally, there is concern that the more widespread use of these antibiotics will lead to an increase in drug resistance and thereby decrease the usefulness of agents that would otherwise be effective in more serious conditions.

The decision as to whether individuals should be offered prophylaxis must be made on a case-by-case basis, but there are situations in which antimicrobial chemoprophylaxis may be appropriate. Chemoprophylaxis might be offered to a traveller who is making a very short tour (3–5 days) in which loss of even 12–24 hours would seriously impact on the success of the visit.[2] Similarly, a VIP on an official visit who finds it impossible to adhere to strict dietary practices because of official commitments might also seriously consider taking prophylaxis. Finally, patients with underlying medical disorders that would make their health grossly compromised by an acute diarrhoeal illness, with associated dehydration and acidosis, might also consider chemoprophylaxis as a reasonable option.

Bismuth subsalicylate is an effective, non-antibiotic approach to prevent travellers' diarrhoea with an overall efficacy of about 60%.[56–58] When only available in a liquid form, compliance was not easy as a 3-week supply of drug would add 5 kg to the travellers' luggage. A tablet formulation is now available and the best results are obtained when two tablets are taken 4 times daily at meal times and on retiring. Prophylactic action of the drug is thought to be related to an antibacterial effect of the bismuth moiety and possibly an antisecretory effect in the small intestine. There are concerns, however, about bismuth toxicity following long-term ingestion.

IMMUNOPROPHYLAXIS

As yet there are no widely available vaccines for acute diarrhoeal diseases. However, the cholera vaccine incorporating the B-subunit combined with dead, whole cell, cholera vibrios produce 52% protection against ETEC. Protection was short-lived but would be adequate for short-term travellers.[43] A variety of oral vaccines are under development which might be useful for travellers, and ultimately it might be reasonable to pursue a multivalent vaccine covering ETEC, *Salmonella* spp., *Shigella* spp., *Campylobacter jejuni* and possibly some of the protozoal parasites.

PROBIOTICS AND PREBIOTICS

The concept of colonising the gastrointestinal tract with a harmless but nevertheless protective microflora in the form of *Lactobacillus* spp. or bifidobacteria is an attractive 'natural' approach to the control of enteric infection. A number of lactobacillus strains have been developed and are able to colonise the human gastrointestinal tract. One isolate, *Lactobacillus* GG, has been shown to produce modest protection in travellers' diarrhoea[59,60] but recently *Lactobacillus acidophilus* and *Lactobacillus fermentum*, were shown to have no effect in a placebo-controlled study in Central America.[61] Further studies are required to determine whether this approach has any future.

There is some evidence that feeding preferred bacterial substrates, such as oligofructose, can increase the numbers of 'protective' microorganisms such as bifidobacteria. Again, further evidence is required to confirm that this approach will have clinical benefit.

Post-travel management

Although the majority of episodes of travellers' diarrhoea resolve without the need for intensive investigation, travellers who return with persistent diarrhoea which has continued for more than 14–21 days or bloody diarrhoea should be investigated further. A hierarchical approach to the clinical investigation of persistent diarrhoea and dysentery is suggested in Figures 11.14 and 11.15.

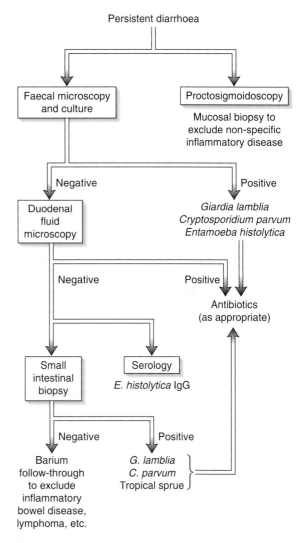

Fig. 11.14 An approach to the post-travel management of persistent diarrhoea in travellers.

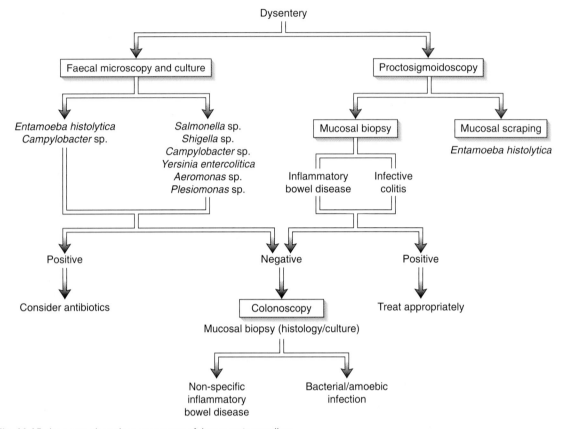

Fig. 11.15 An approach to the management of dysentery in travellers.

PRACTICE POINTS

- Travellers' diarrhoea is a term that does not imply a specific aetiology. There are many causes from viruses, bacteria and toxins to dietary change.
- Disabling diarrhoea may respond to a short course of antibiotics (e.g. an aminoquinolone) but rehydration must not be neglected.
- Giardiasis is very common in visitors to the Indian sub-continent and can present some time after return. Nausea, borborygmi and 'sulphurous'-smelling motions, often passed only in the mornings or after meals, are common, but profuse watery diarrhoea is not a normal feature.
- Chemoprophylaxis should not be routinely used but has a place, for example, when brief illnesses will seriously disrupt the reason for travel.
- Acute infective diarrhoea can 'unmask' inflammatory bowel disease.

REFERENCES

1. Handszuh H, Waters SR. Travel and tourism patterns. In: Dupont HL, Steffen R, eds. Textbook of travel medicine and health. Hamilton: Decker; 1997.
2. Farthing MJG, Dupont HL, Guandalini S, et al. Treatment and prevention of travellers' diarrhoea. Gastroenterology International 1992; 5: 162–175.
3. Merson MH, Morris GK, Sack DA, et al. Travelers' diarrhea in Mexico: a prospective study of physicians and family members attending a congress. New England Journal of Medicine 1976; 294: 1299–1305.
4. Sack DA, Kaminsky DC, Sack RB, et al. Prophylactic doxycycline for travelers' diarrhea: results of a prospective double-blind study of Peace Corps

volunteers in Kenya. New England Journal of Medicine 1978; 298: 758–763.

5. MacDonald KL, Cohen ML. Epidemiology of travelers' diarrhea: current perspectives. Reviews of Infectious Diseases 1986; 8 (Suppl. 2): 117–120.

6. Steffen R, Boppart I. Travellers' diarrhoea. In: KE Gyr (Guest editor) Tropical gastroenterology Vol 1, No. 2. London: Baillière Tindall; 1987: 361–376.

7. Kozicki M, Steffen R, Schar M. 'Boil it, cook it, peel it, or forget it' : does this rule prevent travellers' diarrhoea? International Journal of Epidemiology 1985; 14: 169–72.

8. Dupont HL, Haynes GA, Pickering LK, et al. Diarrhea of travelers to Mexico: relative susceptibility of United States' and Latin American students attending a Mexican university. American Journal of Epidemiology 1977; 105: 37–41.

9. Bandres JC, Mathewson JJ, Dupont HL. Heat susceptibility of bacterial enteropathogens. Archives of Internal Medicine 1988; 148: 2261–2263.

10. Sheath NK, Wisniewski TR, Franson TR. Survival of enteric pathogens in common beverages: an in vitro study. American Journal of Gastroenterology 1988; 83: 658–660.

11. Dickens DL, Dupont HL, Johnson PC. Survival of bacterial enteropathogens in the ice of popular drinks. Journal of the American Medical Association 1985; 253: 3141–3143.

12. Reid JA, Caul EO, White DG, et al. Role of infected food handler in hotel outbreak of Norwalk-like viral gastroenteritis: Implications for control. Lancet 1988; ii: 321–323.

13. Hutchinson P, Hindocha P, Phillips A, et al. Travellers' diarrhea with a vengeance in children of UK immigrants visiting their parental homeland. Archives of Disease in Childhood 1982; 57: 208–211.

14. Neal KR, Brij SO, Slack RCB, et al. Recent treatment with H_2 antagonists and antibiotics and gastric surgery as risk factors for salmonella infection. British Medical Journal 1994; 308: 176.

15. Neal KR, Scott HM, Slack RCB, et al. Omeprazole as a risk factor for campylobacter gastroenteritis: case-control study. British Medical Journal 1996; 312: 414–415.

16. Balarajan R, Raleigh VS, Yuen P, et al. Health risks associated with bathing in sea water. British Medical Journal 1991; 303: 1445–1455.

17. Walker A. Swimming – the hazards of taking a dip. British Medical Journal 1992; 304: 242–245.

18. Porter JD, Ragazzoni HP, Buchanon JD, et al. Giardia transmission in a swimming pool. American Journal of Public Health 1988; 78: 659–662.

19. Katelaris PH, Farthing MJG. Cryptosporidiosis – an emerging risk to travellers. Travel Medicine International 1992; 10: 10–14.

20. Keene WE, McAnulty JM, Hoesly FC, et al. A swimming-associated outbreak of hemorrhagic colitis caused by Escherichia coli 0157: H7 and Shigella sonnei. New England Journal of Medicine 1994; 331: 579–584.

21. Boyce TG, Swerdlow DL, Griffin PM. Escherichia coli 0157: H7 and the hemolytic–uremic syndrome. New England Journal of Medicine 1995; 333: 364–368.

22. Rees JH, Soudain SE, Gregson NA, et al. Campylobacter jejuni infection and Guillain–Barré syndrome. New England Journal of Medicine 1995; 333: 1374–1379.

23. Black ER. Pathogens that cause travelers' diarrhea in Latin America and Africa. Reviews of Infectious Diseases 1986; 8 (Suppl. 2): 131–135.

24. Taylor DN, Echeverria P. Etiology and epidemiology of travelers' diarrhea in Asia. Reviews of Infectious Diseases 1986; 8 (Suppl. 2): 136–141.

25. Taylor DN, Houston R, Shlim DR, et al. Etiology of diarrhea among travelers and foreign residents in Nepal. Journal of the American Medical Association 1988; 260: 1245–1248.

26. Wanger AR, Murray BE, Echeverria P, et al. Enteroinvasive Escherichia coli in travelers with diarrhea. Journal of Infectious Diseases 1988; 158: 640–642.

27. Synder JD, Blake PA. Is cholera a problem for US travelers? Journal of the American Medical Association 1982; 247: 2268–2269.

28. Taylor DN, Pollard RA, Blake PA. Typhoid in the United States and the risk to the international traveler. Journal of Infectious Diseases 1983; 148: 599–602.

29. Guth BE, Twiddy EM, Travulsi LR, et al. Variation in chemical properties and antigenic determinants among type II heat-labile toxins of Escherichia coli. Infection and Immunity 1986; 54: 529–536.

30. Gill DM, Clements JD, Robertson DC, et al. Subunit number and arrangement in heat-labile enterotoxin. Infection and Immunity 1981; 33: 677–682.

31. Gill DM, Richardson SH. Adenosine diphosphate-ribosylation of adenylate cyclase catalyzed by heat-labile enterotoxin of Escherichia coli: comparison with cholera toxin. Journal of Infectious Diseases 1980; 141: 64–79.

32. Field M. Intestinal electrolyte transport and diarrheal diseases. New England Journal of Medicine 1989; 321: 800–806.

33. Rao MC. Toxins which activate guanylate cyclase: heat-stable enterotoxins. In: Evered D, Whelan J, eds. Microbial toxins and diarrhoeal disease. Ciba Foundation Symposium 112. London: Pitman; 1985: 74–93.

34. Farthing MJG. Enterotoxins and the enteric nervous system. In: Rampal P, Boquet P, eds. Recent advances in the pathogenesis of gastrointestinal bacterial infections. Paris: John Libbey Eurotext; 1998: 191–203.

35. Salim AFM, Phillips AD, Farthing MJG. Pathogenesis of gut virus infections. In: Farthing MJG, ed. Virus infections of the gut and liver. Clinical Gastroenterology 1990; 4: 593–607.

36. Hale TL. Genetic basis of virulence in Shigella species. Microbiological Reviews 1991; 55: 206–224.

37. Acheson DWK, Donohue-Rolfe A, Keusch GT. The family of Shiga and Shiga-like toxins. In: Alouf JE, Freer JH, eds. Sourcebook of bacterial protein toxins. London: Academic Press; 1991: 415–434.

38. Ravdin JI. *Entamoeba histolytica*: from adherence to enteropathy. Journal of Infectious Diseases 1989; 159: 420–429.
39. Farthing MJG, Kelly MP, Veitch AM. Recently recognised microbial enteropathies and HIV infection. Journal of Antimicrobial Chemotherapy 1996; 37: (Suppl. B): 61–70.
40. Harries AD, Myers B, Cook GC. Inflammatory bowel disease: a common cause of bloody diarrhoea in visitors to the tropics. British Medical Journal 1985; 291: 1686–1687.
41. Dupont HL, Ericsson CD. Prevention and treatment of travelers' diarrhea. New England Journal of Medicine 1993; 328: 1821–1827.
42. Farthing MJG. Prevention and treatment of travellers' diarrhoea. Alimentary Pharmacology and Therapeutics 1991; 5: 15–30.
43. Caeiro JP, Dupont HL. Management of travellers' diarrhoea. Drugs 1998; 56: 73–81.
44. Farthing MJG. History and rationale of oral rehydration and recent developments in formulating an optimal solution. Drugs 1988; 36 (Suppl. 4): 80–90.
45. Farthing MJG. Dehydration and rehydration in children. In: Arnaud MJ, ed. Hydration throughout life. Paris: John Libbey Eurotext; 1998: 159–173.
46. European Society for Paediatric Gastroenterology and Nutrition Working Group. Recommendations for composition of oral rehydration solutions for the children of Europe. Journal of Pediatric Gastroenterology and Nutrition 1992; 14: 113–115.
47. World Health Organization. The rational use of drugs in the management of acute diarrhea in children. Geneva: WHO; 1990.
48. Farthing MJG. 5-hydroxytryptamine and 5-hydroxytryptamine-3 receptor antagonists. Scandinavian Journal of Gastroenterology 1991; 26: (Suppl. 188): 92–100.
49. Beubler E, Horina G. 5-HT$_2$ and 5-HT$_3$ receptor subtypes mediate cholera toxin-induced intestinal fluid secretion. Gastroenterology 1990; 99: 83–89.
50. Dupont HL, Ericsson CD, Mathewson JJ, et al. Zaldaride maleate, an intestinal calmodulin inhibitor, in the therapy of travelers' diarrhea. Gastroenterology 1993; 104: 709–715.
51. Turvill J, Farthing MJG. Enkephalins and enkephalinase inhibitors in intestinal fluid and electrolyte transport. European Journal of Gastroenterology and Hepatology 1998 (in press).
52. Salam I, Katelaris P, Leigh-Smith S, et al. Randomised trial of single-dose ciprofloxacin for travellers' diarrhoea. Lancet 1994; 334: 1537–1539.
53. Ericsson CD, Dupont HL, Mathewson JJ. Single-dose ofloxacin plus loperamide compared with single dose or three days of ofloxacin in the treatment of travelers' diarrhea. Journal of Travel Medicine 1997; 4: 3–7.
54. Steffen R, Jori J, Dupont HL, et al. Treatment of travellers' diarrhoea with fleroxacin: a case study. Journal of Antimicrobial Chemotherapy 1993; 31: 767–776.
55. Wiström J, Gentry LO, Palmgren AC, et al. Ecological effects of short-term ciprofloxacin treatment of travellers' diarrhoea. Journal of Antimicrobial Chemotherapy 1992; 30: 693–706.
56. Steffen R. Worldwide efficacy of bismuth subsalicylate in the treatment of travelers' diarrhea. Reviews of Infectious Diseases 1990; 12 (Suppl. 1): 80–86.
57. Steffen R, Dupont HL, Heusser R, et al. Prevention of travelers' diarrhea by the tablet form of bismuth subsalicylate. Antimicrobial Agents and Chemotherapy 1986; 29: 625–627.
58. Dupont HL, Ericsson CD, Johnson PC, et al. Prevention of travelers' diarrhea by the tablet formulation of bismuth subsalicylate. Journal of the American Medical Association 1987; 257: 1347–1350
59. Oksanen PJ, Salminen S, Saxelin M, et al. Prevention of travellers' diarrhoea by lactobacillus. Annals of Medicine 1990; 22: 53–56.
60. Hilton E, Kolakowski P, Singer C, et al. Efficacy of *Lactobacillus GG* as a diarrheal preventive in travelers. Journal of Travel Medicine 1997; 4: 41–43.
61. Salam I, Katelaris P, Leigh-Smith S, et al. A randomised placebo-controlled trial of single dose ciprofloxacin in treatment of travellers' diarrhoea. Lancet 1994; 344: 1537–1539.

Immunisation theory, practice and available vaccines

Jane Leese

Introduction

The most common health problems to affect travellers are largely not vaccine-preventable. Nonetheless, immunisation offers reliable, though not always complete, individual protection against certain infectious diseases. For diseases with the potential to spread, there may be an additional public health benefit through prevention of local spread or importation to another country. Decisions about which vaccines to recommend for an individual traveller depend on an assessment of the likely risks: on the one hand, the severity and consequences of the disease, the likelihood of the traveller being exposed to infection and any wider public health risk, and, on the other, the efficacy, contraindications and possible adverse reactions of the vaccine. Familiarity with the available vaccines and their use is essential.

Immunisation theory

IMMUNITY AND THE IMMUNE RESPONSE

The body's defence to infectious disease requires the recognition of antigens associated with pathogenic organisms, the ability to mount an appropriate immune response to eliminate the source of those antigens, and the ability to adapt to the different life cycles and pathogenic mechanisms of diverse pathogenic organisms. This defence is provided by the collection of tissues, cells and molecules known collectively as the *immune system*. It involves a complex interaction of cellular and soluble factors, part of which (the first, non-specific, line of defence) might be called 'innate' or 'natural' immunity, and part 'adaptive' or 'acquired', (i.e. specific for the infecting agent).

The adaptive immune response is of broadly two types: *antibody-mediated*, which is primarily directed against extracelluar microorganisms, and *cell-mediated*, mainly directed against intracellular pathogens. The two systems are, however, interdependent.

Antibodies are produced by B lymphocytes and can be demonstrated by their detection in serum. They recognise intact antigens which may be in solution (e.g. toxins), associated with microorganisms (e.g. surface antigens) or on the surface of infected cells (e.g. the haemagglutinin of influenza). They may act on their own, but more often depend either on phagocytes and neutrophils to phagocytose antigen–antibody immune complexes for their elimination, or on cytotoxic cells (eosinophils and large granular lymphocytes) to attack antibody-sensitised cells or parasites.

T lymphocytes are the main component of cell-mediated immunity. They recognise intracellular antigens by proxy, by recognising antigen fragments which are presented to them at the surface of infected cells. (The antigen has to be associated with histocompatibility antigens in a way which is still not fully understood.) There are two major types of T cell: CD8+ T cells which recognise and kill virus-infected cells; and CD4+ T cells which have a variety of functions in controlling immune responses, including by the release of soluble mediators of immunity called *cytokines*. The cytokine response depends on the cell type expressing the antigen the CD4+ cell recognises: if it is a macrophage, cytokines activate the macrophage to destroy intracellular pathogens; if it

TABLE 12.1 Contrasting properties of natural and acquired immunity

	Natural	Acquired
Specificity	Non-specific	Specific
Memory	Unaltered on repeated challenge	Improved by repeated challenge
Cells involved	Phagocytes Natural 'killer' cells	Lymphocytes
Other factors involved	Lysozyme Complement Acute phase Proteins Interferons	Antibodies Cytokines (from lymphocytes)

TABLE 12.2 Currently available vaccines by type

Inactivated vaccines

Inactivated organisms (whole cell)

Bacterial	*Viral*
Pertussis	Inactivated polio vaccine (IPV)
	Hepatitis A
	Rabies
	Japanese B encephalitis
	Tick-borne encephalitis

Inactivated toxins (toxoids)
Tetanus
Diphtheria

Immunogenic components of organisms

Capsular polysaccharide	*Subunit*
Haemophilus influenzae type b (Hib)	
Pneumococcal	Influenza
Meningococcal A and C	Hepatitis B
Typhoid capsular antigen vaccine (Typhim Vi)	

Live attenuated vaccines

Bacterial	*Viral*
BCG	Oral polio (OPV)
Oral typhoid	Measles
	Mumps
	Rubella
	Yellow fever

is a B lymphocyte, the B cell is activated to divide and differentiate, thus promoting the production of antibody.

Other important elements of the immune system are *neutrophils, eosinophils* and *macrophages*, whose primary function is to destroy antigens and pathogens, and *the complement system*. Complement is one of the main mediators of the inflammatory response and can be activated either by antibody in immune complexes or by the presence of various microbes. It is therefore involved in both innate and adaptive immunity.

An important feature of the 'adaptive' response, as well as being specific, is that it has *memory* by which a second challenge with the specific stimulus provokes a speedier and more vigorous immune response. Following natural infection, this may be lifelong (see Table 12.1).

IMMUNISATION

The terms 'immunisation' and 'vaccination' are often used interchangeably. Strictly speaking, vaccination applies only to immunisation with microorganisms or their components.

Immunisation is the induction in an individual, by either active or passive means, of an immuno-logically specific resistance to an infectious disease by the administration of a preparation of, or from, another organism – a vaccine.

The ideal vaccine should be safe, effective, able to give long-lasting immunity, stable and cheap. Vaccines currently available in the UK are listed in Table 12.2.

Active immunisation

Active immunity is induced by stimulation of the individual's own immune system using inactivated organisms, their inactivated products (e.g. toxins), immunogenic components of the organisms (e.g. capsular or surface antigens), or attenuated live organisms. Some inactivated vaccines contain an adjuvant, or are conjugated to proteins, to increase their immunogenicity. Toxoids alone, for instance, are weak antigens and are therefore adsorbed onto aluminium salts which act as adjuvants. The capsular polysaccharides of pneumococi and *Haemophilus influenzae* (Hib) are relatively weak immunogens which are ineffective in children under 18 months of age; Hib vaccines are linked to proteins such as diphtheria and tetanus toxoids to increase their immunogenicity so that they can be used in young children; conjugate pneumococcal vaccines are under development.

Passive immunisation

Passive immunisation involves the transfer to an individual of already formed antibodies. In the past, animals were used to raise the antibodies but the resulting antisera carried the risk of anaphylactic reactions. In the UK, all immune globulin preparations are now of human origin. They consist almost entirely of IgG. Human normal immunoglobulin (HNIG) is prepared from unselected, pooled, blood donations and contains antibodies against those infections which are common in the population. It gives adequate protection against hepatitis A. Specific immuno-globulins to diseases not prevalent in the general population (e.g. tetanus, varicella/zoster, hepatitis B and rabies) are prepared from pooled blood with known high titres or from the serum of convalescent patients.

THE IMMUNE RESPONSE TO VACCINES

Most vaccines produce their protective effect by the production of antibodies which can be measured in serum. The first injection of an inactivated vaccine (or toxoid) in a subject not previously exposed produces a slow antibody (or antitoxin) response of mainly IgM antibody – the primary response. Two injections may be needed to produce such a response. Subsequent injections lead to a more rapid, higher level and longer-lasting response of mainly IgG antibody – the secondary response. IgA antibodies may also be secreted across mucous membranes to provide protection in the gut or respiratory tract.

Following a full course of vaccine, antibody levels remain high for months or years. Without further boosting, however, antibody levels gradually fall over time. For common infections, this boosting may be provided by exposure to natural infection. For infections where exposure to natural infection is unlikely, as for most of those covered by 'travel' vaccines, a single booster dose of vaccine is usually sufficient to reinforce the response. Even if antibody levels fall below protective levels, subsequent exposure to infection should result in a more rapid immunological response than in a previously non-immune individual.

Polysaccharide vaccines are unable to induce memory in T lymphocytes in young children and therefore give only transitory protection in this age group.

TABLE 12.3 Advantages and disadvantages of live vaccines

Advantages	Disadvantages
Often single dose	Possible inclusion of other agents
Small amount of antigen in vaccine	Possible reversion to virulence
	Contraindicated if immunity impaired

Live vaccines promote cell-mediated immunity. Following BCG, this is usually demonstrable by a positive tuberculin skin test (Heaf or Mantoux). In many individuals, live attenuated virus vaccines such as measles, mumps and rubella, promote a full, long-lasting antibody response after one dose. Live oral poliomyelitis vaccine (OPV) requires three doses. Oral vaccines have the advantage of producing local gut immunity in addition to circulating antibodies. Advantages and dis-advantages of live vaccines are shown in Table 12.3.

Passive immunisation gives rapid onset protection (significant plasma levels occur within minutes of intravenous injection and 24–48 hours after intramuscular injection) but with a half-life for IgG of about 21 days, protection lasts at the most only 4–5 months.

CONTRAINDICATIONS TO VACCINES

1. Acute febrile illness on the vaccination day

In the event that an individual has an acute febrile illness on the vaccination day, vaccination should be postponed until the individual has recovered. Minor infections in the absence of fever or systemic upset are not contraindications.

2. History of severe local or systemic reaction to a previous dose of the vaccine

Re-immunisation is contraindicated if a previous dose of the vaccine caused severe or extensive local erythema, swelling or induration, or severe systemic symptoms (e.g. anaphylaxis, bronchospasm, laryngeal oedema, high fever).

3. Egg allergy

Anaphylactic hypersensitivity to egg products is a contraindication to influenza and yellow fever vaccines as the viruses for these vaccines are grown in hens' eggs.

4. Vaccines and pregnancy

Few published data are available, but in general all vaccines are best avoided in pregnancy because of a theoretical risk of an adverse effect on the developing fetus. If the risk of infection cannot be avoided, however, an inactivated vaccine can be administered.

Live vaccines should, if at all possible, be avoided in pregnancy. If yellow fever vaccination is required purely for entry purposes, exemption is normally allowed on production of an exemption certificate. This should be checked in advance with the relevant embassy. Where significant risk of exposure cannot be avoided, for example to poliomyelitis or yellow fever, the need for immunisation is likely to outweigh any risk to the fetus. The vaccine should then preferably be given during the second or third trimester. If a live vaccine is inadvertently given to a pregnant woman, she should be reassured that no fetal damage has been reported following yellow fever or oral polio vaccines.

5. Immunosupression due to disease or treatment

Inactivated vaccines may safely be given to immunocompromised patients, but their immunological response may be sub-optimal and may be inadequate to protect against infection. Where immunoglobulin is an alternative (e.g. for hepatitis A), it may be considered preferable to vaccine.

In individuals who are unable to mount a normal immune response, live vaccines may give rise to disseminated infection caused by the vaccine organism. Live vaccines should not therefore be given to patients who are immuno-compromised. This includes those with conditions such as lymphoma, leukaemia, Hodgkin's disease and other reticulo-endothelial tumours, HIV infection (although see also below), patients with impaired immunological mechanisms and all those currently receiving treatment with systemic corticosteroids or other immunosuppressive drugs, chemotherapy or general irradiation. For corticosteroids, the equivalent of an adult dose of prednisone 60 mg daily (for children prednisone 2 mg/kg/day) can be taken as the threshold for significant immunosuppression. If such a dose has been taken for a week or more, immunisation should be postponed until at least 3 months after the treatment has stopped. In individual patients, lower doses may be significant if the underlying disease, or other treatment, is causing immuno-suppression.

In general, 6 months should be allowed for recovery of the immune system following chemotherapy or generalised radiotherapy for malignant disease, although, if necessary, advice should be sought from the physician in charge of an individual patient's treatment.

The contraindication to OPV extends to close contacts of an immunocompromised patient because of the risk of transmission of the vaccine virus to that individual.

HIV-infected individuals may be given any inactivated vaccine and measles, mumps and rubella vaccines. OPV may be given to asymptomatic HIV-infected individuals, but they should be aware that they may excrete the virus longer than normal; inactivated polio vaccine is preferred for those who are symptomatic. BCG and yellow fever vaccines are best avoided in all HIV-infected individuals because of lack of firm data on their safety.

6. Vaccines and immunoglobulin

Live virus vaccines should not be given for 3 months following HNIG as the antibodies in the HNIG may inhibit the immune response to the vaccine. The exception is yellow fever vaccine since HNIG in the UK is unlikely to contain yellow fever antibodies. If there is a significant risk of exposure to poliomyelitis infection and time is short, polio vaccine should be given even if immunoglobulin has been given any time in the previous 3 months, accepting the response may be sub-optimal.

STORAGE AND RECONSTITUTION OF VACCINES

Vaccines should be stored according to the manufacturer's instructions in a refrigerator dedicated to the storage of medicinal products. A system should be in place to ensure strict rotation of stock.

The cold chain

Vaccines must at all times be stored within the recommended temperature range for that vaccine. Both too low and too high a temperature may cause deterioration of the vaccine and loss of potency. Refrigerators should have a maximum/minimum thermometer and the temperature should be regularly checked and recorded. Vaccines should be in the body of the refrigerator and the door should be opened as little as possible. Temperatures should also be maintained during any transport to maintain the 'cold chain'.[1] WHO has produced guidance.[2]

Reconstitution

The manufacturer's instructions should be followed when reconstituting vaccines. The vaccinator is responsible for checking that this has been done correctly and the preparation is within its expiry date.

TIMING OF IMMUNISATIONS

Individuals are capable of responding to multiple antigens administered simultaneously, but there is a period of 4–14 days after the administration of one when the response to a second may be impaired. The disadvantage is that attribution of adverse reactions, if they occur, may be difficult. If it is necessary to administer more than one live virus vaccine, they should in theory, either be given at the same time in different sites or at least 3 weeks apart. It is recommended that 3 weeks are allowed between administration of a live virus vaccine and tuberculin testing. The same applies to administration of BCG vaccine. No other vaccine should be given in the BCG arm for at least 3 months because of the risk of regional lymphadenitis.

For most vaccines requiring multiple doses, the optimal timing between the first and second doses is 4–8 weeks, and between the second and third, 4–6 months.

ROUTE OF ADMINISTRATION

Apart from the oral polio and typhoid vaccines, and BCG which is always given intradermally, most vaccines are administered either by deep subcutaneous or intramuscular injection. For some, either of these two routes is suitable, for others one or other route is specified. Some may be given intradermally as an alternative for some or all of the doses; this allows a smaller dose to be given. The techniques are described in more detail in the memorandum *Immunisation against Infectious Disease* (see Further Reading).

ADVERSE REACTIONS

Anaphylaxis is a rare event following immunisation, but no vaccination should be performed unless the vaccinator is trained and competent to recognise and treat it, and adrenaline, syringe, needle and an airway are immediately to hand. The time of onset of anaphylaxis varies; it may occur up to 72 hours following vaccination.

All significant adverse reactions should be reported on the yellow card system to the Committee on Safety of Medicines. This applies to established as well as new vaccines so that unexpected late events are detected.

RECORDS

All immunisations should be recorded in the patient's record with a note of the batch number of the vaccine and the name of the vaccinator. It is helpful if the patient also keeps a personal record card.

Available vaccines

Travel vaccines may conveniently be considered in groups:

1. Vaccines which are part of national recommendations and should be considered for

all travellers, for example diphtheria, tetanus, poliomyelitis (for children, a check should be made that the childhood immunisation schedule is up to date), or for certain risk groups, for example influenza, pneumococcal vaccines
2. Vaccines against diseases associated with poor hygiene and sanitation: poliomyelitis, hepatitis A, typhoid (there is currently no available vaccine against cholera)
3. Vaccines against diseases of close association: diphtheria, meningococcal infection, BCG (against tuberculosis)
4. Vaccines against arthropod-borne diseases: yellow fever, tick-borne encephalitis, Japanese encephalitis
5. Vaccines for longer-term, or remote, travel: hepatitis B, rabies.

1. Vaccines which are part of national recommendations

The distinction between vaccines for general use and 'travel vaccines' is an artificial one. Vaccines which are included in national immunisation programmes may be more important for travellers than some of the so-called 'travel vaccines'. A vaccine such as yellow fever vaccine which is a 'travel vaccine' for a UK resident may be part of a routine immunisation programme abroad. National vaccine recommendations for the UK are listed in Table 12.4.

Many people remain vulnerable to diseases which are covered in the national childhood immunisation programme. These diseases are now uncommon in the UK but may not be abroad. Serological studies in travellers from Scotland between 1977 and 1985 showed that:

- 13% had inadequate levels of tetanus antitoxin
- 20% had incomplete immunity to poliomyelitis
- 60% had inadequate levels of diphtheria antitoxin.

However, 64% had antibodies to hepatitis A.[3]

Tetanus in the UK is now mainly a disease of older people who have never been immunised or whose immunity has waned. Between 1985 and 1991 about half of all cases in the UK were in people aged over 65 years, two-thirds of them women.[4] Antibody levels in those aged 60–85 years have been found to be significantly lower than those in serving personnel aged 20–46 years.[5] In the USA, the risk of tetanus in those aged over 80 has been reported to be 10 times the risk in a person aged 20–29.[6]

A study of 1000 UK blood donors found that one-third were fully protected against diphtheria, one-third had partial protection and one-third had serum antitoxin concentrations which rendered them susceptible to diphtheria.[7] Immunity decreased with increasing age, just over half of those aged 50–59 years being susceptible compared with a quarter of those aged 20–29.

TETANUS

The disease. Tetanus is an infection of the nervous system characterised by muscular rigidity and spasms. It is caused by the toxin of the Gram-positive anaerobic bacterium, *Clostridium tetani* and contracted through the contamination of usually minor wounds.

Risk areas. Tetanus spores are universal in soil and the infection may be acquired through any contaminated cut or other injury in which the skin is breached, in any part of the world.

The vaccine. Tetanus vaccine is a toxoid vaccine, consisting of a cell-free preparation of tetanus toxin inactivated with formaldehyde and adsorbed onto either aluminium phosphate or aluminium hydroxide as adjuvant to increase its immunogenicity (plain vaccines are no longer available as they are less immunogenic and no less reactogenic). Tetanus toxoid is available in different combinations:

- *For all ages*
  Single antigen tetanus vaccine (T)
- *For children up to 10 years*
  With diphtheria and pertussis vaccines (DTP) for use in the childhood immunisation programme
  With diphtheria toxoid vaccine (DT) for use in children not receiving pertussis vaccine

TABLE 12.4 UK national immunisation recommendations

Age	Vaccine	Comments
Routine		
At 2, 3 and 4 months	Diphtheria	Primary course
	Tetanus	
	Pertussis	
	Haemophilus influenzae type B (Hib)	
	Poliomyelitis	
At 12–15 months	Measles Mumps Rubella (MMR)	1st dose
Aged 3–5 years	Diphtheria	Pre-school booster
	Tetanus	
	Polio	
	MMR	2nd dose
Aged 10–14 years	BCG	(Given in infancy for those at higher risk – see below)
Aged 13–18 years	Diphtheria	School leaving (and final)
	Tetanus	booster
	Polio	
For special risk groups		
Babies born to hepatitis-B-infected mothers	Hepatitis B	
Infants at higher risk of exposure to tuberculosis	BCG	At birth
Women seronegative for rubella	Rubella	
Those of any age with chronic respiratory, heart or renal disease, diabetes, or immunosuppression owing to disease or treatment, and all aged 75 years and over	Influenza	Given annually
Those who are asplenic, or have splenic dysfunction, chronic heart, lung, renal or liver disease, diabetes, or immunosuppression owing to disease or treatment	Pneumococcal	
Those with chronic liver disease, haemophiliacs	Hepatitis A	
Parenteral drug misusers, individuals who change sexual partners frequently, close contacts of a case or carrier, haemophiliacs, chronic renal failure on, or in anticipation of requiring, dialysis, healthcare (or other) workers likely to have direct contact with patients' blood, blood-stained body fluids or tissues, staff and residents in homes for people with learning disabilities	Hepatitis B	

- *For adults and children 10 years and over*
  With low-dose diphtheria toxoid (Td). This preparation is now given to school leavers, replacing the former school-leaving dose of tetanus alone.

Dose schedule. The primary immunisation course consists of three doses of 0.5mL of the appropriate preparation by intramuscular or deep subcutaneous injection, each 4 weeks apart. Children are given a pre-school booster and a further school-leaving dose; by then, they should have received five doses of vaccine and be protected for life. Adults should receive a booster if the primary course or a subsequent booster was more than 10 years previously. No further doses are necessary after a total of five doses has been received unless they are being given as part of the management of a tetanus-prone wound.

Contraindications. As for all inactivated vaccines.

Adverse reactions. Local reactions may persist for several days. General reactions are uncommon: acute anaphylaxis, urticaria and peripheral neuropathy are described but are rare.

Comments. Medical attention should still be sought for a tetanus-prone wound.

DIPHTHERIA

The disease. Diphtheria is an acute, upper respiratory tract infection spread by inhalation of infected aerosol droplets and characterised by a thick, grey membrane over the tonsils and pharynx which may cause respiratory obstruction. Diphtheria toxin may affect the myocardium, nervous system and adrenal glands.

Risk areas. Diphtheria is now mainly a disease of developing countries. It is likely where overcrowding and poor levels of vaccine uptake co-exist. In recent years, an epidemic in the Russian Federation and the Ukraine occurred because of a combination of low childhood immunisation uptake rates, waning immunity in adults and large-scale population movements. A number of cases were reported from other states of the former Soviet Union, and imported cases were described in neighbouring countries.

The vaccine. Diphtheria vaccine is a toxoid vaccine, consisting of a cell-free preparation of diphtheria toxin inactivated by formaldehyde and adsorbed onto aluminium phosphate or hydroxide as an adjuvant. It is available in different combinations:

- *For children up to 10 years*
  Adsorbed diphtheria/tetanus/pertussis vaccine (DTP/triple vaccine)
  Adsorbed diphtheria/tetanus vaccine (TD)
  Single antigen adsorbed diphtheria vaccine (D)
- *For adults and children 10 years and over*
  Adsorbed low-dose diphtheria vaccine for adults (d)
  Adsorbed tetanus/low-dose diphtheria vaccine for adults (Td). This preparation is now given to school leavers in place of the former school-leaving dose of tetanus toxoid alone.

Dose schedule. For primary immunisation, three doses of 0.5mL of a preparation appropriate for the age of the individual, each 4 weeks apart, are given by intramuscular or deep subcutaneous injection. If no suitable adult preparation is available, adults and children over 10 years may be given 0.1 mL, still by intramuscular or deep subcutaneous injection, of the single antigen preparation for children up to 10 years (see above). Children are given school entry and school-leaving booster doses of diphtheria toxoid vaccine. Adults at risk should be given a single booster if their primary course was more than 10 years previously.

Contraindications. As for all inactivated vaccines.

Adverse reactions. Local reactions are common. Transient headache, fever and malaise may also occur. Anaphylaxis and neurological reactions are described but are rare.

Comments. The Schick test was previously performed as a test for immunity to diphtheria. The materials for Schick testing are no longer available. All visitors to endemic or epidemic areas are advised to check that they have been immunised against diphtheria. Those who are likely to be in close contact by living or working with local people should be advised to have a booster dose, if appropriate, according to the dose schedule above.

POLIOMYELITIS

The disease. Poliomyelitis is an enterovirus infection of the nervous system, primarily affecting the anterior horn of the spinal cord and the motor nuclei of the pons and medulla. Most infections are asymptomatic or cause only mild gastrointestinal symptoms. About 1 in every 1000 infections is estimated to result in paralytic illness. Poliomyelitis is spread by the faecal–oral route, either person to person or through contaminated food or water.

Risk areas. Intensive immunisation campaigns, notably in South America and the Caribbean, have resulted in many countries, including the UK, being near to eliminating poliomyelitis. However, poliomyelitis is still endemic in most of Asia and Africa and can still be introduced into unimmunised pockets of the community, as occurred in The Netherlands in 1993.

The vaccines. OPV is a live virus vaccine prepared from attenuated strains of poliomyelitis types I, II and III, grown in monkey kidney or human diploid cell cultures. Inactivated polio vaccine (IPV) is a whole cell inactivated virus vaccine containing all three types of polio virus inactivated by formaldehyde.

Both vaccines may contain trace amounts of penicillin, streptomycin and neomycin and OPV may also contain polymyxin.

Inactivated polio vaccine is unlicensed in the UK but is available for named patients for whom OPV is contraindicated.

Dose schedule. The primary course consists of three doses, each 4 weeks apart. The dose of IPV is

0.5 mL by intramuscular or deep subcutaneous injection. Children are given booster doses at school entry and at 15–19 years. Adults require a reinforcing dose only if travelling to an endemic area and their last dose was more than 10 years previously.

OPV virus strains are excreted in the stools for up to 6 weeks following an oral dose.

Contraindications. OPV: as for all live vaccines. Vaccination with OPV should also be postponed if there is vomiting or diarrhoea and is contraindicated if a close family member is immunocompromised. IPV: as for all inactivated vaccines. Both vaccines are contraindicated if there is a history of extreme hypersensitivity to one of the trace antibiotics which may be in the vaccine.

Adverse reactions. Vaccine-associated poliomyelitis occurs rarely following OPV: it is estimated to occur in about one vaccine recipient, and one close contact of a recently vaccinated person, for over 2 million doses administered. The need for strict personal hygiene while vaccine virus is likely to be excreted should be emphasised.

Comments. Immunisation against poliomyelitis is still a universal recommendation although this is likely to be modified as elimination of poliomyelitis progresses. For the present, it is recommended that all travellers to countries outside Europe, North America, Australia and New Zealand have up-to-date polio immunisation.

INFLUENZA

The disease. Influenza is an acute, highly infectious, viral infection of the upper respiratory tract.

Risk areas. Influenza occurs every year in all countries, mainly during the winter months. In the Southern Hemisphere, the influenza season is therefore from May to October.

The vaccine. Influenza vaccines are inactivated, sub-unit vaccines prepared each year from virus strains or genetic reassortants similar to those considered most likely to be circulating during the forthcoming winter. The viruses are grown in embryonated hens' eggs.

Dose schedule. For adults and children aged 4 years and over, 0.5 mL is given by intramuscular or deep subcutaneous injection (0.25 mL for children aged 6 months–3 years). For children under 12 receiving influenza vaccine for the first time, a second dose is advised 4–6 weeks later.

Contraindications. As for other inactivated vaccines. Influenza vaccine is contraindicated in individuals with known anaphylactic hypersensitivity to hens' eggs.

Adverse reactions. In addition to mild local reactions, fever, malaise, myalgia and/or arthralgia lasting up to 48 hours may occur. Immediate allergic reactions are most likely to be due to hypersensitivity to residual egg protein. The Guillain–Barré syndrome has been reported very rarely following immunisation with influenza vaccine.

Comments. Annual influenza vaccine is recommended for certain risk groups as part of national policy and should be considered when such individuals travel during the winter months for the country being visited.

PNEUMOCOCCAL VACCINE

The disease. The pneumococcus is a major cause of morbidity and mortality as a result of pneumonia, bacteraemia and meningitis worldwide, especially among the elderly, the very young, and those with no spleen, splenic dysfunction or other cause of impaired immunity.

Risk areas. Pneumococcal infection is universal. The increased risk is for the individual rather than through travel itself.

The vaccine. Pneumococcal vaccine is a capsular polysaccharide vaccine containing components of the capsules of the 23 serotypes most commonly associated with serious infection.

Dose schedule. A single dose of 0.5 mL is given subcutaneously or intramuscularly.

Contraindications. As for all inactivated vaccines. Re-immunisation within 3 years is not recommended.

Adverse reactions. Local reactions and a low grade fever may occur. Re-immunisation with earlier 12- and 14-valent vaccines was reported to produce more severe reactions, especially when the interval between injections was less than 3 years.

Comments. Pneumococcal vaccine is recommended for those falling within the current national recommendations for pneumococcal vaccine, if they have not already been immunised.

2. Vaccines against diseases associated with poor hygiene and sanitation

Poliomyelitis (see above), **hepatitis A, typhoid** and **cholera** are all spread by the faecal–oral route, either person to person or via contaminated food and water, and are therefore a risk in areas of poor hygiene and sanitation. The order of risk varies, however. Hepatitis A is the most common, vaccine-preventable disease in returning travellers, occurring 40 times more frequently than typhoid and 800 times more frequently than cholera.[8] Immunisation against typhoid may therefore be less important than against hepatitis A, especially for those staying in first-class tourist accommodation. There is no currently available cholera vaccine although occasionally officials, acting unofficially, may still ask for evidence of vaccination (see p. 305).

Travellers should be aware that a large enough inoculum, especially for typhoid, may still cause illness: immunisation does not remove the necessity for scrupulous attention to personal, food and water hygiene.

HEPATITIS A

The disease. Hepatitis A ('infectious hepatitis') is a viral infection spread by the faecal–oral route, person to person or through contaminated food and water. Shellfish are notorious for transmitting infection. Asymptomatic infection is common, especially in children, but the virus is still excreted and asymptomatic children may therefore be the source of secondary cases. The severity of illness tends to increase with age. The illness can cause debility for several months, although long-term sequelae are rare.

Risk areas. Hepatitis A occurs worldwide. In a study of sporadic cases of hepatitis in the UK, travel was the single most important risk factor.[9] The Indian sub-continent and the Far East were

the highest risk areas, but risk extended to Eastern Europe. For most of Europe, North America, Australia and New Zealand, the risk of acquiring infection is likely to be no greater than in the UK.

The vaccine. Hepatitis A vaccine is a whole cell, inactivated virus vaccine prepared using a strain of hepatitis virus grown in human diploid cells and inactivated with formaldehyde. Three preparations are available: two for adults, with different dose schedules, and a paediatric version for children aged 1–15 years. All give very reliable seroconversion and are especially suitable for longer-term or frequent travel to endemic areas.

Passive immunisation with HNIG gives short-term protection against hepatitis A for up to about 4 months according to the dose. Fears that declining immunity to hepatitis A in the general population would lead to declining levels of hepatitis A antibodies in immunoglobulin have not yet been founded but this remains a concern for the future. HNIG is suitable for single trips of up to 4 months' duration.

Dose schedule. Vaccine: the original hepatitis A vaccine formulations for adults and children required a primary course of two injections of 0.5 mL by intramuscular injection in the deltoid region 2–4 weeks apart for protection for 1 year; these have been replaced by single, 'monodose' preparations for both adults and children which give equivalent immunity. All require a booster dose at 6–12 months to give immunity lasting at least 10 years.

HNIG: for travel lasting up to 2 months, 250 mg (125 mg or 0.02–0.04 mL/kg for children under 10 years) is given by intramuscular injection; for travel lasting 3–5 months, the dose is 500 mg (250 mg or 0.06–0.12 mL/kg for children under 10 years).

Contraindications. As for all inactivated vaccines.

Adverse reactions. Hepatitis A vaccine may cause transient, mild, local reactions; less commonly, fever, malaise, fatigue, headache, nausea and loss of appetite occur; transient erythematous rashes have been reported.

Comments. Vaccine is now the preferred protection against hepatitis A. Many older people in the UK will already have been exposed to hepatitis A infection and developed immunity. Where practicable, their antibody levels should be measured to assess their need for immunisation.

TYPHOID

The disease. Typhoid fever is a serious, systemic illness caused by the Gram-negative bacillus *Salmonella typhi*. Spread is by the faecal–oral route, either person to person, or through contaminated food or water. All patients with typhoid excrete the organisms at some stage during their illness, about 10% excrete organisms for a further 3 months, and 2–5% become permanent carriers.

Risk areas. Typhoid is endemic in areas of poor hygiene and sanitation, especially in Asia, Africa and Central and South America. About 200 cases a year are notified in the UK, almost all imported, mainly from the Indian sub-continent.

The vaccines. Two typhoid vaccines are available in the UK. *Typhoid Vi polysaccharide antigen vaccine* contains the Vi antigen from the capsule of *Salmonella typhi* preserved with phenol. *Oral typhoid vaccine* contains a live attenuated strain (Ty21a) of *Salmonella typhi* in an enteric coated capsule. It has the theoretical advantage of stimulating local gut immunity, but this has not been proven to confer clinical advantage. The vaccines have roughly equivalent efficacy of 70–80% in field trials in endemic areas. Few data are available concerning their efficacy in travellers. The old, *whole cell, inactivated typhoid vaccine* is no longer available.

Dose schedules. *Vi capsular polysaccharide antigen vaccine:* a single dose of 0.5 mL by intramuscular or deep subcutaneous injection confers immunity for at least 3 years. The dose is repeated after 3 years as necessary. This vaccine is not suitable for children under 18 months of age.

Oral vaccine. One capsule is taken on alternate days for three doses (four doses are recommended in the USA). They must be taken on an empty stomach, with a cool, not hot, drink, and the capsules must be stored in a refrigerator at 2–8°C until taken. The full course is repeated after 1 year as necessary.

Oral typhoid vaccine is not suitable for children under about 6 years of age, or for anyone else who may bite the capsules.

Contraindications. The different lower age limits for the two preparations should be noted. The general contraindications to inactivated vaccines apply to the polysaccharide antigen vaccine. The general contraindications to live vaccines apply to the oral vaccine. The oral vaccine should not be taken during persistent diarrhoea or vomiting nor administered to people taking sulphonamides, or within 12 hours of a dose of mefloquine. It is usually advised that the oral vaccine is not given concurrently with OPV because of possible interference with the development of gut immunity. A gap of at least 2 weeks is usually recommended.

Adverse reactions. Both local and systemic reactions to the Vi polysaccharide antigen vaccine appear to be less common than to the old, whole cell, parenteral vaccine. The oral vaccine may cause transient, mild, gastrointestinal symptoms and an urticarial rash.

CHOLERA

The disease. Cholera is an acute infection characterised by profuse watery diarrhoea caused by the enterotoxin of *Vibrio cholerae* bacteria which have colonised the gut. Severe fluid and electrolyte loss can lead to severe dehydration and hypovolaemic shock. The disease is mainly water-borne and acquired through the ingestion of contaminated food or water, but person-to-person spread may also occur. The infecting dose can be very small.

Risk areas. Cholera is endemic or epidemic in most of the Indian sub-continent and South-East Asia and in many countries in Africa and Central and South America. Epidemics regularly follow natural disasters. The disease is, however, relatively rare in travellers, a few cases a year being imported into the UK. The new serotype, 0139, which emerged in Bangladesh, has spread to neighbouring countries.

Vaccine. Although traditionally regarded as a vaccine-preventable disease, the whole cell vaccine which contained heat-killed Inaba and Ogawa serotypes of *Vibrio cholerae* had an efficacy of, at the most, 50% and of short duration (up to 6 months). It was not effective against the 0139 serotype. WHO has long discouraged its use and it is now no longer available in the UK.

No country now officially requires cholera vaccination as an entry requirement.

Comment. Prevention of cholera is by scrupulous personal, food and water hygiene precautions.

3. Vaccines against diseases of close association

Diphtheria (see above), **meningococcal infection** and **tuberculosis** are all spread by infected aerosol droplets. Spread generally requires close association with an infected person or carrier. The risk is mainly for longer-term travellers who are to have close contact (usually living or working) with local people in risk areas.

MENINGOCOCCAL INFECTION (A AND C)

The disease. Meningococcal meningitis and septicaemia are systemic infections caused by the Gram-negative diplococcus *Neisseria meningitidis*. They can be rapidly fatal, with a fatality rate of up to 30%. Five antigenic groups of *Neisseria meningitidis* occur, most commonly – A, B, C, Y and W135. Group B, for which a vaccine is not yet available, is the commonest cause of infection in the UK. Group A is uncommon in the UK but commonly the cause of epidemics in other parts of the world. About 10% of the population carry meningococci in the nasopharynx; the proportion is higher in young adults, about 25% of whom may be carriers at any one time.

Risk areas. Broadly, the risk areas for travellers are: Africa between the equator and 15°N, parts of the Middle East and parts of the Indian sub-continent. Epidemics have occurred in Kenya, Nepal, India and Saudi Arabia (p. 475). However, the overall risk to most travellers is small. The highest risk is when conditions are crowded, hot, dirty and dry, all of which favour aerosol transmission.

The vaccine. Meningococcal vaccine contains a purified extract of the polysaccharide outer capsules of *Neisseria meningitidis* serogroups A and C. The vaccine affords about 95% protection to the vaccine serogroups in adults, but protection in children under 18 months is poor. The vaccine does not protect against other serogroups.

Dose schedule. A single dose of 0.5 mL by deep subcutaneous or intramuscular injection gives immunity starting 5–10 days after the injection lasting 3–5 years (immunity may be of shorter duration in young children).

Contraindications. Meningococcal vaccine is not recommended for children under 2 months of age.

Adverse reactions. Generally mild, local, injection site reactions occur; systemic reactions are less common.

Comments. Meningococcal A and C vaccine is recommended for longer stays (generally more than 1 month) in endemic areas during the risk season, especially for those intending to live or work with local people. However, the risk season may vary from year to year and from place to place and some latitude should be allowed. Meningococcal vaccine is recommended for all visits of more than a few days to Nepal and Bhutan. Since an epidemic in 1987, pilgrims on the Haj in Mecca have been required to carry a valid certificate of vaccination (see p. 305).

BCG

The disease. Tuberculosis is an infection caused by acid-fast bacteria of the *Mycobacterium tuberculosis* complex (*Mycobacterium tuberculosis, bovis* or *Africanum*). It can affect many parts of the body but most commonly affects the lungs or lymph nodes. It is usually acquired by respiratory droplet spread from a person with sputum-positive pulmonary tuberculosis, or, in endemic areas, through the ingestion of unpasteurised, infected milk. The interval between acquisition of infection and developing disease may be prolonged, and apparently quiescent, old infection may reactivate later in life as a result of age or immunocompromising disease or treatment.

Risk areas. Tuberculosis is endemic in the whole of Asia, Africa and South America and in many countries is increasing because of inadequate control measures fuelled by the HIV/AIDS epidemic. Increasing numbers of cases are also being reported from several Eastern European countries. Increasing drug-resistance is a concern in many of these countries.

The vaccine. BCG (*Mycobacterium bacille Cal-mette-Guerin*) is a live attenuated variant of *Mycobacterium bovis* in a freeze-dried preparation. Although the efficacy of the vaccine has varied considerably between studies in different parts of the world, in British schoolchildren efficacy has been shown to be 70–80%, protection lasting for at least 15 years.

Dose schedule. A single dose of 0.1 mL is administered *intradermally* after confirmation of a negative, tuberculin skin test. The standard site, over the insertion of the left deltoid, should be used as this is the only validated site and so that the resulting scar is easily detected. Most, but not all, UK schoolchildren will have been immunised as part of the national immunisation programme between the ages of 10 and 13 years. Re-immunisation is only recommended if the immunisation history is in doubt, no characteristic scar is detected *and* the tuberculin skin test (Heaf or Mantoux) is negative.

Infants and very young children may be given BCG percutaneously using a multiple puncture device with 18 to 20 needle points. A special 'percutaneous' vaccine preparation which is approximately 10 times the strength of the intradermal preparation is available and must be used.

Contraindications. As for all live vaccines. In the UK, BCG is not recommended for HIV-infected individuals at any stage in their infection.

Adverse reactions. The normal reaction to intradermally administered BCG is a small blister which may take several weeks to heal. More severe, local reactions are uncommon if the immunisation technique is correct; they are usually due to the injection being given too deep or to an individual already sensitised to tuberculoprotein. Keloid in the scar is an uncommon complication which is more likely if the injection is given too high up the arm. Regional lymphadenopathy is rare.

Comments. BCG immunisation is recommended for travellers spending longer (1 month or more) in endemic areas, especially if they are planning to live or work with local people.

4. Vaccines against arthropod-borne diseases

Vaccines are available against three viral infections which are transmitted to man via an intermediate arthropod vector: **tick-borne encephalitis** is spread by ticks and occurs in Central, Eastern and Northern Europe; **yellow fever**, which is endemic in tropical Africa and South America, and **Japanese encephalitis** which occurs in most of South-East Asia, are spread by infected mosquitoes. Vaccination against yellow fever is recommended for all visitors to endemic areas, whereas for tick-borne encephalitis and Japanese encephalitis, although the infections may be widespread, the risk is largely confined to certain types of travel and in most areas varies according to the season the vector is most prevalent. Mosquitoes, for instance, are likely to be most active during and just after the wet season; ticks emerge in warm weather.

Measures to prevent being bitten should be advised whether or not vaccine is being recommended. These include covering arms, legs and ankles at the appropriate times, and the use of insect repellents.

TICK-BORNE ENCEPHALITIS

The disease. Tick-borne encephalitis is a meningoencephalitis caused by a *Flavivirus*. In Sweden, the case fatality rate is about 1%; 10–15% of adults develop paresis during the acute phase of the illness and recovery may be slow. The virus is maintained in nature in small mammals, domestic livestock and certain species of birds. The disease is transmitted to man by the bite of an infected tick or, less commonly, by ingestion of unboiled milk from infected animals, especially goats.

Risk areas. Tick-borne encephalitis is endemic in Austria, Germany, Scandinavia, the Czech and Slovak republics, Romania and western states of the former Soviet Union, in heavily forested areas. Morbidity in Latvia is reported to have increased sharply in recent years and is highest in occupationally exposed groups. The high risk period is June to September. Travellers most at risk are those camping or walking in heavily forested areas in the spring and summer (July and August are the peak seasons).

The vaccine. Tick-borne encephalitis vaccine is an inactivated whole cell virus vaccine containing a suspension of purified tick-borne encephalitis virus, grown in chick embryo cells and inactivated with formalin. It contains thiomersal as preservative.

Dose schedule. Two doses of 0.5mL (irrespective of age) 4–12 weeks apart give protection for 1 year. A third dose 9–12 months later gives 3 years protection and a single booster can be given up to 6 years later for longer protection. The vaccine must be administered intramuscularly.

Contraindications. As for all inactivated vaccines. Allergy to the preservative thiomersal and to egg protein are relative contraindications.

Adverse reactions. Local reactions and local lymphadenopathy may occur. Febrile reactions in children are described after the first dose. General reactions lasting up to 24 hours, and a transient pruritic rash may rarely occur.

Comments. The vaccine is not licensed in the UK but is available for named patients. It should be considered for travellers who are to walk or camp in late spring and summer in warm, forested parts of Europe, especially if there is heavy undergrowth. Covering arms, legs and ankles and the use of insect repellents gives good protection and should be advised whether or not vaccine is given.

YELLOW FEVER

The disease. Yellow fever is an acute viral infection spread by the bite of an infected mosquito and ranging in severity from non-specific symptoms to a severe haemorrhagic disease with jaundice. Fatality rates of up to 50% have been reported in non-indigenous individuals and in epidemics. Urban and jungle forms exist – the host of the former is humans while the latter is primarily a zoonosis transmitted incidentally to humans.

Risk areas. Yellow fever occurs in tropical Africa and South America.

The vaccine. Yellow fever vaccine is a live attenuated virus vaccine containing the 17D strain of yellow fever grown in leucosis-free chick embryos and freeze dried. The vaccine may contain very small amounts of neomycin and polymyxin.

Dose schedule. A single dose of 0.5 mL (irrespective of age) by deep subcutaneous injection gives immunity for at least 10 years.

Contraindications. The usual contraindications to all vaccines and to a live virus vaccine apply. Infants under 9 months of age should only be immunised if the risk of exposure to yellow fever is unavoidable as there is a very small risk of encephalitis (see below).

Adverse reactions. Mild local and systemic reactions may occur. Immediate allergic-type reactions such as urticaria and, rarely, anaphylaxis have also been reported. Encephalitis has been documented in infants immunised under 9 months of age (all recovered without sequelae).

Comments. Yellow fever vaccination is recommended for all visits to endemic areas whether or not it is an official requirement for entry (the latter requirements are listed, and updated each year, in the WHO handbook *International Travel and Health*). Vaccination can only be given at centres designated by the national health authority (WHO keeps a record of these) and must be with a vaccine approved by WHO. The International Vaccination Certificate becomes valid 10 days after immunisation and lasts for 10 years.

JAPANESE B ENCEPHALITIS

The disease. Japanese B encephalitis is a *Flavivirus* infection (related to St Louis encephalitis), spread via the bite of an infected mosquito. Illness ranges from asymptomatic infection to a severe encephalitis with a high mortality and a high rate (about 30%) of residual neurological sequelae in survivors. Approximately 1 in every 200 infections is estimated to lead to invasive neurological disease.

Risk areas. Japanese B encephalitis occurs throughout South-East Asia where it is the leading cause of viral encephalitis – about 50000 cases (1–10/100000 population in endemic areas) are estimated to occur each year. It is endemic in rural areas, especially wet areas such as rice fields, where mosquitoes flourish and where pig-farming occurs (pigs and wading birds are the most common hosts). Epidemics occur in both urban and rural areas. Highest transmission rates are when mosquitoes are most active, that is during and just after the wet season. In temperate regions, this is normally approximately May to September; in tropical and sub-tropical areas, seasonal patterns vary both within individual countries and from year to year.

The risk for travellers of acquiring Japanese B encephalitis is extremely low, but travel during the transmission season and exposure in rural areas contribute to the risk. It is estimated that fewer than 3% of the vector mosquitoes are infected.

The vaccine. Japanese B encephalitis vaccine is an inactivated, whole cell virus vaccine grown in mouse brains and inactivated with formaldehyde. It has been shown to have about 90% efficacy.

Dose schedule. Although two doses 1–4 weeks apart are used in many parts of Asia and are said to give short-term immunity in 80% of vaccinees, studies in the USA and among British subjects have shown that three doses (at days 0, 7 and 30) are needed to provide protective levels of neutralising antibody in most vaccinees.[10] The recommended primary course is three doses of 1 mL (0.5 mL for children aged 1–3 years) by deep subcutaneous injection on days 0, 7 and 30. Full immunity takes up to 1 month to develop. The vaccine is not recommended for children under 1 year of age unless the risk of infection is unavoidable.

The duration of protection is not known. Neutralising antibody persists for at least 2 years after a three-dose primary course. A booster may be given after this time.

Contraindications. As for all inactivated vaccines. Any history of anaphylactic hypersensitivity is a contraindication.

Adverse reactions. There is a small (< 1%) risk of urticaria and angio-oedema which can occur within minutes to up to 2 weeks after receiving the vaccine. It is recommended that people given Japanese B encephalitis vaccine are kept under observation at the vaccination centre for about 30 minutes, and that the course is completed at least 10 days prior to departure.

Comment. Japanese B encephalitis vaccine is not licensed in the UK but is available for named patients. It is **not** recommended for all travellers to

South-East Asia. In general, vaccine should be offered to those spending a month or longer in endemic areas during the transmission season, especially if travel will include rural areas (more detail is in reference[11] and in *Health Information for Overseas Travel*). Occasionally, it should be considered for shorter trips if there is a high risk of exposure, (e.g. extensive outdoor activities in endemic areas). Travellers should be advised to take personal precautions against mosquito bites.

5. Vaccines for longer-term and/or remote travel

HEPATITIS B

The disease. Hepatitis B is an acute viral infection of the liver, often of insidious onset. 5–10% of infected adults develop a chronic carrier state (chronic carriage is even more common in children) and approximately 25% of carriers eventually die of cirrhosis of the liver or primary liver cancer. Spread is blood-borne via sexual intercourse, needle-sharing, blood transfusion and injections or other invasive procedures (including acupuncture and ear-piercing) using contaminated, inadequately sterilised equipment.

Risk areas. Hepatitis B is highly endemic in Africa and much of South America, Eastern Europe, the eastern Mediterranean and South-East Asia. In some of these areas 5–15% of the population may be chronic carriers of the virus.

The vaccine. Two preparations of hepatitis B vaccine are available in the UK. Both are sub-unit virus vaccines containing hepatitis B surface antigen prepared from yeast cells by recombinant DNA technology and adsorbed on aluminium hydroxide as adjuvant. They differ in the amount of antigen per dose, but the recommended schedules are the same.

Dose schedule. Three doses of 1.0 mL (0.5 mL for children aged 0–12 years) are given intramuscularly in the deltoid region (anterolateral thigh for infants), the first two a month apart and the third 6 months later, to give immunity lasting at least 10 years. Antibody titres should be checked 2 months after completing the course – 10–20% of people have an inadequate response to the vaccine; this is more common in people aged over 40 years of age.

For travellers, the third dose can be brought forward and given 1 month after the second but a further booster should then be given at 12 months.

Contraindications. As for all inactivated vaccines.

Adverse reactions. In addition to local reactions, fever, rash, malaise, an influenza-like syndrome, arthritis, arthralgia, myalgia and abnormal liver function tests have been reported following hepatitis B vaccine. Neurological syndromes, such as the Guillain–Barré syndrome and demyelinating disease, have rarely been reported following hepatitis B vaccine, although a causal relationship has not been established.

Comments. Hepatitis B vaccine is recommended for people planning to live or work in areas of high endemicity, where there may be a risk of acquiring infection through contaminated medical or dental equipment. If the full course cannot be completed prior to travel, as many doses as possible should be given and the course completed during the stay or on return.

RABIES

The disease. Rabies is an acute viral infection of the central nervous system characterised by an encephalomyelitis with hydrophobia. It is invariably fatal once symptoms have developed. It is spread through a bite or scratch from a rabid animal. The incubation period varies from 2–8 weeks but may be even longer.

Risk areas. Canine rabies is endemic throughout most of Asia (especially Thailand, India, Nepal and Pakistan), Africa and Latin America: worldwide, more than 33 000 people die of rabies each year, most of them in China and India. The disease is also maintained by foxes in Europe and racoons, skunks and bats in North America, although in Europe mass immunisation campaigns have considerably reduced the numbers of reported cases of animal rabies in recent years and human cases are rare.

Vaccine. Rabies vaccine is an inactivated, whole cell virus vaccine grown in human diploid cells, inactivated by propiolactone and freeze dried. The

vaccine contains traces of neomycin. In some parts of the world, brain-derived vaccines are still in use.

Dose schedule. For full protection, three doses of 1.0 mL should be given by deep subcutaneous or intramuscular injection in the deltoid region on days 0, 7 and 28. The vaccine also appears to be effective when given as 0.1 mL intradermally at these time intervals, but this is not covered by the data sheet. The intradermal route should not be used in individuals taking chloroquine.

Two doses of rabies vaccine 4 weeks apart can be expected to result in seroconversion in about 98% of recipients and may be considered for travellers since all will, if bitten, still require post-exposure prophylaxis.

Reinforcing doses for those at continued risk should be given after 2–3 years.

Contraindications. As for all inactivated vaccines.

Adverse reactions. Local reactions occur. Systemic symptoms such as headache, fever, muscle aches, vomiting and urticarial rashes have been reported and may become more severe with repeated doses. If this occurs, antibody levels should be checked before administering further doses as they may still be protective. Anaphylactic shock and the Guillain–Barré syndrome have rarely been reported.

Comments. Pre-exposure prophylaxis is recommended only for people travelling to remote areas of rabies-endemic countries who are likely to be more than 24–48 hours away from urgent medical attention, and for people exposed to possibly rabid animals in the course of their work abroad. The vaccine may also be considered for some trips where there is a high risk and doubt about whether human diploid cell vaccine or rabies-specific immunoglobulin would be available should urgent post-exposure prophylaxis be required.

Post-exposure treatment for rabies. Fully immunised travellers require two further 1.0 mL doses of rabies vaccine intramuscularly in the deltoid region at days 0 and 3–7.

Unimmunised individuals require:

(i) 5 doses of 1.0 mL of rabies vaccine by deep subcutaneous or intramuscular injection in the deltoid region on days 0, 3, 7, 14 and 30

(ii) if the bite occurred in a high-risk country, rabies-specific immunoglobulin 20 iu/kg body weight, up to half infiltrated in and around the wound and the rest by intramuscular injection.

Advice should be sought about the need for immunoglobulin. The course of vaccine can be stopped if the animal concerned is confirmed not to have rabies.

Immunisation for International Health Regulations

The International Health Regulations were adopted by the 22nd World Health Assembly in 1969 to ensure the maximum security against the international spread of disease with the minimum interference with world traffic. A country could, until recently, require an international certificate of vaccination against smallpox, yellow fever and/or cholera. The Regulations were amended in 1973 so that no country should require a certificate of vaccination against cholera. Smallpox was deleted from the diseases subject to the Regulations in January 1982 following eradication of the disease. Yellow fever is currently the only disease for which an international certificate may be required.

CHOLERA

There has been widespread misunderstanding about the cholera regulations, and a belief still widely prevails that a certificate is required for visits to endemic or infected areas. There was some considerable delay in the new regulations being implemented by all countries and until recently there was evidence that border officials, acting unofficially, were sometimes asking for evidence of vaccination against cholera. This now appears to be limited to a few remote borders in infected areas. For visits to such areas, travellers may wish to carry a statement to the effect that vaccination is not indicated, since no cholera vaccine is currently available.

YELLOW FEVER

Yellow fever vaccine can be given only at a centre designated by the national health administration. A record of such centres is kept by WHO and by the Department of Health. WHO must also be assured that the vaccines used are of suitable quality.

In the UK, the vaccine and certificates are supplied only to designated centres. General practitioners, health authorities and private clinics may apply to become designated centres; details are available in the UK Health Department's 'Green Book', under the section on yellow fever.

The named doctor at the designated centre may authorise another doctor or nurse working at the centre to administer the vaccine and sign the certificate provided he/she has assured him- or herself that the authorised person has the appropriate training and competence.

The International Health Regulations are concerned with public health rather than individual protection. The requirement for yellow fever vaccination under the Regulations is a measure to stop the importation of yellow fever into countries with the climate to support the vector. Not all countries in which yellow fever is endemic and for which the vaccine would be recommended for personal protection require a yellow fever vaccine certificate for entry.

MENINGOCOCCAL MENINGITIS

Since an outbreak of meningococcal infection among pilgrims in 1987, Saudi Arabia has required all pilgrims to carry proof of immunisation against meningococcal meningitis A and C during the annual pilgrimage to Mecca (the Haj). The vaccine should have been given not less than 10 days and not more than 3 years before arrival in Saudi Arabia.

Which vaccines to recommend – balancing the risks

It will be apparent from the preceding information that several factors need to be taken into account in assessing the vaccine recommendations for an individual traveller. These will include:

- the whole itinerary – yellow fever vaccination, for instance, may not be required for a traveller arriving in a particular country direct from the UK, but may if entry is from another country
- the parts of each country to be visited
- the type of holiday/travel and accommodation
- the season
- the length of stay
- the age, health and previous vaccination history of the traveller, including if pregnant or travelling with children
- the available vaccines, their type (e.g. live or inactivated), known efficacy and adverse reactions, and whether any egg products or small traces of antibiotics they may contain are relevant in the individual circumstances.

REFERENCES

1. Hawarth EA, Booy R, Stirzaker L, Wilkes S, Battersby A. Is the cold chain for vaccines maintained in general practice? Bristish Medical Journal 1993; 307: 242–244.
2. World Health Organization. Immunisation in practice: a guide for health workers who give vaccines. Oxford: Oxford University Press; 1989.
3. Cossar JH, et al. A cumulative review of studies on travellers, their experience of illness and the implications of these findings. Journal of Infection 1990; 21: 27–42.
4. Public Health Laboratory Service. Communicable Disease Report 1993; 3: 73.
5. Cumberland NS, Kidd AG, Karalliedde L. Immunity to tetanus in United Kingdom populations. Journal of Infection 1993; 27: 255–260.
6. Prevots R, Sutter RW, et al. Tetanus surveillance – United States, 1989–90. Morbidity and Mortality Weekly Report 1992; 41(SS-8): 1–9.
7. Maple PA, Efstratiou A, George RC, Andrews NJ, Sesardic D. Diphtheria immunity in UK blood donors. Lancet 1995; 345: 963–965.
8. Steffen R. Hepatocyte. International hepatitis update. Chester, UK: Adis International; 1991(7): 1–3.
9. Maguire HC, Handford S, et al. A collaborative case control study of sporadic hepatitis in England. Communicable Disease Report 1995; 5: R33–40.
10. Japanese encephalitis – inactivated Japanese encephalitis virus vaccine. WHO Weekly Epidemiological Record 1994; 69: 113–120.
11. Centers for Disease Control. Inactivated Japanese encephalitis virus vaccine. Recommendations of the ACIP. Morbidity and Mortality Weekly Report 1993; 42 (RR-1): 3–4

FURTHER READING

Health information for overseas Travel. UK Health Departments with the PHLS Communicable Disease Surveillance Centre. London: HMSO; 1995.
Immunisation against infectious disease. UK Health Departments. London: HMSO; 1996.
Kassianos GC. Immunization: Precaution and contraindication. 2nd ed. Oxford: Blackwell Scientific; 1994.
Staines N, Brostoff J, James K. Introducing immunology. St Louis: Mosby; 1993.
World Health Organization. International travel and health – Vaccination requirements and health advice. Geneva: WHO; 1999 (revised annually).

SECTION 6

MALARIA

Malaria: the parasite, the disease and management

Eric Walker

Introduction

When advising travellers on malaria prevention, it is important to understand some of the basic natural history and epidemiology of the disease. This can help to convince the traveller of the life-threatening nature of the illness and make clear, for example, why compliance with prophylaxis is so important. Many travel advisers also see patients on return and so some knowledge of diagnosis and treatment is important. When emergency, stand-by treatment is prescribed, clear instructions as to its use must be given to the traveller.

Transmission

Malaria is spread by the bite of the female anopheline mosquito (Fig. 13.1). This was discovered as recently as 1897 when Ronald Ross reported pigmented bodies, later shown to be oocysts, in the stomachs of mosquitoes which had fed on patients with malaria.

There are numerous species of anopheline mosquitoes, and their feeding habits (some prefer animals), breeding sites and flight ranges vary, all of which can influence control measures. However, most anopheline species prefer to feed between dusk and dawn which is when most transmission of malaria occurs.

It is important to remember that malaria is only one of a number of infections spread by mosquitoes. Others include yellow fever, dengue, Bancrofti filariasis and Japanese B encephalitis.

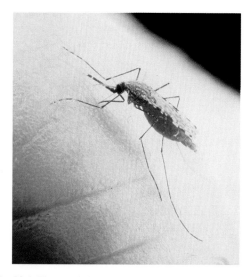

Fig. 13.1 The anopheline mosquito, the vector of malaria.

Distribution

Malaria is now predominantly a disease affecting Africa, South and Central America, Asia and the Middle East.

Travellers from non-endemic countries can contract the disease when visiting these areas and become ill while abroad or present with symptoms on return home. When malaria is patchy within a country, those living in non-malarious parts can become infected when travelling to malarious areas. **In both these instances local physicians may not consider the diagnosis as they are unaware of the risk.**

Prior to the 20th century, malaria was endemic in North America, Southern Europe and Russia.

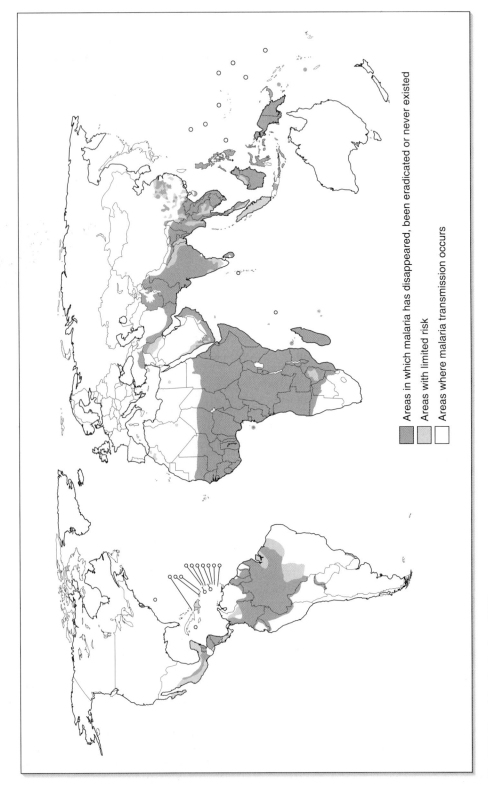

Fig. 13.2 Map of distribution from WHO.

Areas in which malaria has disappeared, been eradicated or never existed

Areas with limited risk

Areas where malaria transmission occurs

More recently, the disease has declined in the Middle East, China and in much of Thailand, especially in urban areas. In the Indian sub-continent, after control programmes in the 1950s had largely confined the disease to the north east, malaria has now spread back into all states although it is uncommon in the far south. In South America, the Amazonian, rainforest region is most affected (see Fig. 13.2).

In most of sub-Saharan Africa, expect for regions in the far south, the disease is holo- or hyper-endemic with an estimated 1–2 million deaths each year, mostly in children. There are parts of Africa where it is estimated that people are likely to be bitten by an infected mosquito several times each year. If those affected survive, these repeated infections eventually result in a degree of immunity, which minimises symptoms, although chronic anaemia and splenomegaly often persist.

In some malarious areas, for example in parts of South-East Asia, there is a seasonal pattern of transmission. Development of the parasite in the mosquito only takes place when the ambient temperature is between 16°C and 33°C and also, since mosquitoes like a humid atmosphere and breed only in freshwater, their numbers usually increase after periods of heavy rainfall or monsoons. Unusual rainfall can lead to temporary spread of the disease into areas where it is normally uncommon, as happened during 1997 in the north-east, coastal regions of South Africa.

Migration can also result in the disease occurring in neighbouring areas where it is unusual; Calcutta experiences seasonal outbreaks thought to be due to workers commuting into the city from rural areas. Transmission has occurred in Europe, when infected mosquitoes have been brought in on aircraft, resulting in so-called 'airport malaria'.

Travellers need to know not only whether malaria is likely to be present at their intended destination(s) but also whether the risk is substantial enough to warrant chemoprophylaxis. If the risk is limited, bite-avoidance measures and prompt attention for febrile illnesses may be sufficient for personal protection.

Whether the predominant species in a particular area is malignant or benign and the proximity of good emergency medical care can also influence the decision on whether to advise chemoprophylaxis.

Many common destinations have only a limited risk of serious disease, especially when travellers are staying in good accommodation. These include most tourist areas and cities in Turkey, Morocco, Egypt, Saudi Arabia, United Arab Emirates, Mexico, Thailand and China. WHO publishes these details, with maps of endemic areas, in its annual 'Yellow Book' publication called *International Travel and Health*, and includes regular updates in the WHO Weekly Epidemiological Record. This information is also available in some of the detailed, 'on-line' databases of healthcare advice for travellers (see Ch. 2).

The parasites

There are four different species of human malaria parasite. *Plasmodium falciparum* causes 'malignant' disease and is the predominant species in sub-Saharan Africa, Papua New Guinea and in the Amazon rainforests of South America.

The other species cause less serious, so-called benign disease. *Plasmodium vivax* predominates in the Indian sub-continent and is rare in sub-Saharan Africa where the predominant benign form of disease is caused by *Plasmodium ovale*. *Plasmodium malariae* occurs rarely in all malarious areas but may be found in Africa.

LIFE CYCLE

The mosquito inoculates 'sporozoites' through its salivary ducts as it feeds. These enter the circulation and within a few minutes settle in hepatic parenchyma cells. Asexual reproduction takes place and the hepatic cells then rupture releasing into the blood up to 40 000 'merozoites' for every sporozoite inoculated (see Fig. 13.3).

This takes 5–7 days for *Plasmodium falciparum*. *Plasmodium vivax* and *Plasmodium ovale* can cause illness after a similar period but these species can form 'hypnozoites' which persist in the liver and may not become active for many months, sometimes for more than 1 year. The reason why these hypnozoites develop is not clear but it

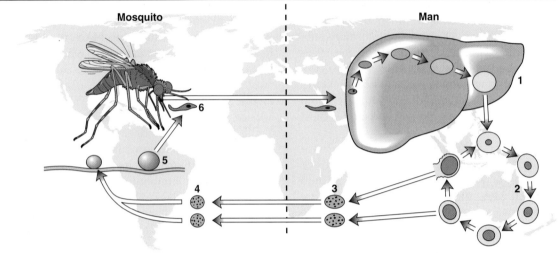

1. Merozoites develop from sporozoites in the human hepatocytes and are released into the blood.
2. Merozoites form trophozoites within the red blood cells (erythrocytes). They develop into schizonts, the red cells rupture and as merozoites the parasites are released into the plasma (this is when fever occurs).
3. Male and female gametocytes form in some erythrocytes to be ingested by the mosquito.
4. Sexual gametes develop in the mosquito and fertilisation takes place.
5. The resulting oocysts form in the mosquito's stomach wall.
6. Mature oocysts rupture releasing sporozoites which migrate to the mosquito's salivary glands.

Fig. 13.3 Malaria parasite life cycle.

appears to be seasonal. Chemoprophylaxis with chloroquine or mefloquine, during exposure and for the usual 4 weeks afterwards, may not prevent these delayed illnesses since they only destroy the *post-hepatic*, erythrocytic forms of the parasite. Primaquine (often used after treatment of illness to eradicate hypnozoites), and to a lesser degree proguanil, can destroy these hepatic forms.

The merozoites invade red blood cells and develop into ring forms or 'trophozoites' (Fig. 13.4). These destroy the contents of the erythrocytes, which eventually rupture releasing parasite and red cell debris plus 6–36 new merozoites (depending on the species), which rapidly invade new erythrocytes. This is when the typical fevers of malaria occur. The number of infected cells increases rapidly as the process repeats itself. Each erthyrocytic cycle takes around 48 hours to complete for *Plasmodium falciparum*, *vivax* and *ovale* and 72 hours for *Plasmodium malariae*.

Especially with *Plasmodium falciparum*, fevers may not be at regular intervals since several cycles can occur simultaneously. Red cell destruction with

Plasmodium falciparum is much more rapid and severe than with the other species, which is why it causes more serious, life-threatening disease. Death can occur within days.

After several cycles, if the patient survives, a sub-population of sexual forms of parasite called

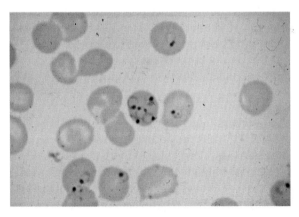

Fig. 13.4 Numerous trophozoites of *Plasmodium falciparum* about to rupture as merozoites from the red blood cells, causing extensive capillary and multi-organ damage.

'gametocytes' appear which are ready to be ingested by further mosquitoes. The male and female gametes fuse and develop in the gut wall of the mosquito. These 'oocysts' eventually rupture releasing sporozoites, which find their way to the mosquito's salivary glands, completing the life cycle.

Clinical features (see Box 13.1)

INCUBATION PERIOD

Plasmodium falciparum has a short development phase within the human host and illness usually begins within 2–4 weeks of the infected bite. This period can be prolonged if partially effective or irregular chemoprophylaxis has been used, and is caused by the persistence of small numbers of parasites that multiply after prophylaxis is discontinued.

This early development phase in *Plasmodium vivax* and *ovale* infection may be similar but is often longer due to the formation of hypnozoites as described above. This phase in *Plasmodium malariae* infection lasts up to 35 days.

THOSE AFFECTED

People of all ages can contract malaria and *Plasmodium falciparum* causes the most severe illness. Infants under 6 months may not develop such severe malaria if their mother has transferred to them a degree of temporary immunity, and also because fetal haemoglobin retards parasite

---

development. This does not apply to the non-immune visiting from a non-endemic country. Repeated infections may eventually result in less serious illness. Malaria in pregnancy frequently results in fetal loss or premature labour.

PRODROME AND FEVER

Sometimes there is a prodrome of malaise, headache and muscle pains, but the first major symptom is usually fever, irregular in *Plasmodium falciparum* malaria but usually occurring every 2nd day with *Plasmodium vivax* and *Plasmodium ovale*, and every 3rd day with *Plasmodium malariae*. At this stage, symptoms may be very similar to influenza. Rigors followed by profuse sweating occur, more so in *Plasmodium vivax* and *Plasmodium ovale* malaria. Malaria must be considered as a cause of any febrile illness in anyone who could have been exposed. Fevers can be less severe in those with some immunity or those on partially effective prophylaxis, which may confuse the unwary. A wide range of other symptoms can occur including diarrhoea, abdominal pain and a dry cough.

JAUNDICE AND CEREBRAL MALARIA

Jaundice, which may make the unwary think the patient has hepatitis, and rapidly progressive anaemia owing to massive haemolysis are usually the next major signs, followed by impaired conscious level, coma (cerebral malaria) and circulatory collapse. In malignant infections caused by *Plasmodium falciparum*, the illness can very rapidly progress. It is particularly fulminant in those who have had a previous splenectomy. The death rate at this stage even with the best intensive care can be up to 10%.

OTHER COMPLICATIONS

These include haemoglobinuria (blackwater fever) which may be followed by renal failure, and pulmonary oedema (presenting as adult respiratory distress syndrome), often after the initial recovery phase. Convulsions and hypoglycaemia occur and are sometimes related to

---

> **Box 13.1 Common clinical features of malaria**
>
> - Fever
> - Rigors
> - Jaundice and anaemia
> - Splenomegaly and thrombocytopaenia
>
>   The following occur in malignant *Plasmodium falciparum* but are unusual in benign malaria:
> - Confusion, coma and convulsions
> - Haemoglobinuria (blackwater fever)
> - Renal failure
> - Respiratory failure.

drug treatment. Secondary bacterial pneumonia or urinary tract infections can occur. In benign malaria, if the illness is not promptly treated, thrombocytopaenia and splenomegaly are common with a possible danger of splenic rupture. Anaemia may develop, but life-threatening complications are unusual.

The laboratory diagnosis

The diagnosis is confirmed by examining blood films, although treatment may have to be started before these can be examined. Both thin and thick films should be prepared. Thin films allow identification of species. Thick films, where the blood is clotted, allow more rapid examination of large volumes of blood for parasites but the cells are distorted. More recently PCR and simple stick tests have become available and their role is currently being evaluated (see p. 325 on recent advances).

Parasites can normally be visualised at any stage of the red cell cycle although the trophozoites may be larger and easy to make out just prior to a fever. Gametocytes do not cause illness and are usually not destroyed by first-line antimalarial treatment.

There is progressive normochromic anaemia, which is more rapid in malignant disease. Thrombocytopaenia is usually present. The blood white cell count is usually normal or depressed. As complications develop, serum bilirubin is elevated as a result of haemolysis and biochemical evidence of renal failure may be evident. Hypoglycaemia is common and may become worse during treatment.

Drug treatment

Antimalarial drugs can be more toxic than many other antimicrobials. Doses, contraindications and side effects must be carefully considered. If fever continues after adequate dosage, or if parasitaemia fails to decline by more than 75% after 48 hours, drug resistance should always be considered.

PLASMODIUM FALCIPARUM

Treatment of *Plasmodium falciparum* infection, especially in the non-immune, is a medical emergency and if complications are developing, intensive care should be considered. In more severe cases, exchange transfusion may need to be considered, for example when parasitaemia is greater than 10%. While expert medical advice should always be sought as soon as possible, emergency self-treatment (see Box 13.2) may be necessary as an immediate life-saving measure.

Drugs destroy the parasites but supportive care may be required for complications such as convulsions, hypoglycaemia, anaemia and renal or respiratory failure. It is essential to choose a drug or usually a combination of drugs, which will make drug resistance unlikely.

Quinine (10mg/kg orally, three times daily for 3–5 days) is the usual first-line drug for serious disease since resistance is rare. In adults it should be combined with tetracycline (250mg four times daily) or doxycycline (100mg twice daily) continued for 7 days, unless tetracyclines are contraindicated, for example in pregnancy. Fansidar is an alternative second drug in areas where resistance is not likely.

Oral treatment is preferable in order to minimise side effects, but parenteral treatment may be necessary if there is any doubt about rapid absorption, for example when there is evidence of cerebral involvement or uncontrolled vomiting. A very common side effect of quinine is tinnitus, which resolves when the drug is stopped or the dose reduced.

Alternatives are sulphadoxine with pyrithamine (Fansidar), mefloquine, halofantrine, artemisinin (Qinghaosu) and atovaquine with proguanil (Malarone). Artemisinin, not currently licensed in the UK, is becoming a drug of first choice in many countries but should always be combined with other drugs.

PLASMODIUM VIVAX AND PLASMODIUM OVALE

Chloroquine (10mg base/kg initially followed by 5 mg/kg, 12-hourly for a further two doses) is the

---

Box 13.2 Guidelines for travellers who may need to use emergency 'self-treatment'

- **Malaria is a disease that can be fatal within a few days.** Since it is spread by infected mosquito bites, you should cover up with suitable clothing, use insect repellents and a mosquito net when necessary. Preventive, anti-malarial tablets are important when you are at high risk. They are never 100% effective, so always seek prompt medical attention if you get a fever.
- **You may be advised to carry with you a course of emergency malaria treatment** if travelling to areas more than 24 hours from medical attention.
- **Your doctor will discuss suitable treatment for you.** Make certain that you fully understand the correct dosages, possible side effects, storage of tablets and when you should use it.
- **Malaria almost always starts with fever, often with marked shivering or chills.** The most serious form can begin a few days after an infected bite or up to 2 or 3 months later. Illness can occasionally start after you have finished taking your preventive tablets. A few days after the fevers begin, jaundice (a yellow colour first seen in the white of your eyes), dark urine and mental confusion can develop. Muscle pains, vomiting and occasionally diarrhoea can occur.
- **Emergency treatment often includes quinine and sometimes also tetracyclines or sulphadoxine with pyrimethamine (Fansidar).** You may be advised to take two drugs together. Quinine can cause tinnitus, a buzzing in the ears, which can be controlled by reducing the dosage. Tetracycline and Fansidar sometimes cause rashes. Remember always to make sure you are clear about how to use your emergency treatment before you leave and check any instructions given on the bottle or packet.
- **It is usually safer to take treatment unnecessarily than to risk becoming seriously ill** when no medical facilities are available.
- **If you have taken emergency treatment you must still seek medical advice as soon as possible** to ensure your treatment has been adequate and that no other illness is involved. The doctor will also check that no complications have occurred and you may need to discuss whether to change or start taking preventive, anti-malarial tablets.

---

first drug of choice, although resistance has occasionally been reported in Papua New Guinea and other parts of Oceania.

Primaquine may be used in addition, to attempt eradication of any remaining liver hypnozoites. Glucose-6-phosphate dehydrogenase levels should be checked before using primaquine since haemolysis may occur in those who are deficient in this enzyme.

Follow-up

Relapse can occur after apparently successful treatment if partial drug resistance is present or treatment has been inadequate. This usually occurs after about 3–6 weeks.

Recovery from the anaemia, owing to poor erythropoiesis, can take up to 2–3 months and does not usually respond to haematinics. Occasionally, after serious *Plasmodium falciparum* infection, some disturbance of renal, pulmonary or neurological function may persist.

Further episodes of *Plasmodium vivax* or *Plasmodium ovale* can occur as a result of reactivation of hypnozoites. The need for the traveller to comply carefully with chemo-prophylaxis may need to be reinforced and the choice of drugs may need to be reconsidered.

PRACTICE POINTS

- *Plasmodium falciparum* malaria can kill very rapidly, within days, and is a medical emergency, which may require intensive care.
- Symptoms and signs of *Plasmodium falciparum* infection in the non-immune, progress rapidly from fever, through to haemolytic jaundice, confusion and coma.
- Prompt treatment, at the onset of the first fever, usually prevents progression and allows rapid recovery.
- Treatment should always take into account the possibility of drug resistance.
- Consider supplying emergency stand-by treatment for those at risk who are also likely to be away from skilled medical facilities.

BIBLIOGRAPHY

World Health Organization. International travel and health. Vaccination requirements and health advice. (The 'yellow book'.) Geneva: World Health Organization. This is an annual publication available through HMSO. Useful for updates on malaria risk areas.

Cook GC. Manson's tropical diseases. 20th ed. London: WB Saunders; 1996. The malaria chapter in this book is an invaluable source of detailed information on all aspects of malaria. It is well referenced and frequently provides answers to 'those difficult questions'.

Guidelines for malaria prevention in travellers from Britain. These reports are summaries of findings of an expert committee convened by the Malaria Reference Laboratory and more recently the Public Health Laboratory Service. Treatment is discussed as well as prevention. The latest report, at the time of writing, was included as a supplement in the Communicable Disease Surveillance Centre Weekly Report 1997; 7 (19 Sept).

Prevention for travellers

Jane Chiodini

Introduction

Each year, in the developed world, returning travellers die from malaria. The numbers involved are a very small fraction of the terrible burden of malaria deaths reported from malarious countries, but such deaths are usually avoidable, given adequate resources, good care and advice. This section discusses malaria prevention advice for travellers while acknowledging that the international community must also focus control measures on the tropics to achieve any major reduction in the number of malaria cases worldwide.

While the approach and advice given here is based on UK guidelines, most of the principles involved will apply to travellers from other countries. Different countries do sometimes vary in 'official' recommendations on chemoprophylaxis depending upon availability of drugs and different assessment of risk, both from the disease itself, and from drug side effects.

History of the development of guidelines in the UK

A policy for malaria prophylaxis for travellers has to reflect changes in malaria epidemiology, travel habits and resistance of the parasites.[1] Healthcare professionals giving malaria prevention advice need to be aware of these issues.

WHO has laid down guidelines for malaria prevention, covering general considerations, protective measures against malaria, stand-by emergency treatment, special groups and special situations, including multi-drug-resistant malaria.[2] Individual countries often develop their own sets of guidelines, which may differ from those made by WHO.

In the UK, a committee of experts was convened by the Malaria Reference Laboratory (MRL) and met at intervals to set down guidelines for the choice of chemoprophylaxis, mosquito-bite prevention and advice regarding recognition, early diagnosis and treatment of malaria. Such meetings have been held since 1980 and regular reports have been published. The views expressed in the guidelines reflected experienced professional opinion and there was often a range of acceptable options.

The guidelines tried to give a recommended option and state alternatives, suggesting when and how different regimens can be used to good effect.[3]

Public awareness of the importance of malaria and prevention is not high, although media coverage in 1995 increased this awareness by focusing on potential drug side effects, particularly in relation to mefloquine.

In 1998, a more formal committee was established to be convened by the Public Health Laboratory Service in collaboration with the MRL.

The principles of prevention

The latest published guidelines identify four principles of malaria prevention that should receive attention from both travellers and their advisers.

- Awareness: know about the risk of malaria
- Bites by mosquitoes: prevent or avoid
- Compliance with appropriate chemoprophylaxis
- Diagnose breakthrough malaria swiftly and obtain treatment promptly.

AWARENESS: KNOW ABOUT THE RISK

It is essential that those visiting malarious areas are aware that there is a risk.

A detailed knowledge of the malaria distribution within a country is important. WHO annually publishes maps and details of regional variations.[2]

This knowledge can influence advice. In Kenya, for example, Nairobi itself is malaria free whereas there is significant transmission on the coast and in safari parks.

Thus it is essential that those giving advice are knowledgeable[4] and have access to up-to-date information. The advisers need skill in conveying this information clearly to the traveller.

The degree of risk is also dependent on a number of other factors:

- whether the area to be visited is urban or rural
- the length of the stay
- previous travel experience
- whether travel is during the wet or dry season
- the likelihood of staying in unprotected accommodation (e.g. basic guest house, camping)
- any previous problems with antimalarial drugs which might affect future compliance
- pre-existing medical conditions (e.g. previous splenectomy) may affect the severity of possible illness
- age: children may be at greater risk of severe illness
- possible or planned pregnancy.

BITES BY MOSQUITOES: PREVENT OR AVOID

It is clear from the malaria parasite life cycle that, apart from rare instances of transmission by blood transfusion, or shared needles, most malaria is transmitted by mosquito bite. Thus, preventing or minimising bites has a significant impact upon malaria transmission.

Unfortunately, it is not possible to rely upon the absence of obvious mosquito bites as an indication of no risk. Individuals may be bitten without being aware of it and without any 'sore' or rash developing at the site of the bite. This varies considerably from person to person and women appear to be more likely to be hypersensitive to mosquito saliva.

Mosquito-bite prevention is as important as compliance with chemoprophylaxis and a variety of strategies are available. Malaria-carrying mosquitoes bite mostly between dusk and dawn. Light-coloured, long-sleeved clothing, long trousers, and socks should be worn during this period. Insect-repellent sprays and solutions are manufactured specifically for clothing.

The use of insect repellents on the skin, for example diethyltoluamide (DEET) or eucalyptus-oil-based preparations, can significantly reduce the frequency of mosquito bites.[5, 6] The concentration of these repellents varies, but application of the lowest effective dose (e.g. 30% DEET), depending on formulation, is sensible[7] and the manufacturer's instructions should always be read carefully. Repellents must be applied regularly, particularly in a very hot and humid climate when the 'sweat off' time is shorter.

In sleeping areas, personal, mosquito-bite prevention methods vary according to the type of accommodation provided. 'Air conditioning' usually means the room is 'sealed' and cool which deters entry of mosquitoes, as long as the system is operating. If the windows and doors of the room are screened with wire or plastic mesh, screens must be closed well before dusk and ideally the room sprayed regularly with knockdown insecticide spray. Electrical vaporising pads releasing pyrethroid insecticides reduce the mosquito population in 'sealed rooms' provided they are used correctly and there is a constant power supply. Large-sized rooms may need more than one device operating. There is no scientific evidence that electronic buzzers, vitamin B and garlic are effective in deterring mosquitoes.

Bed nets were traditionally used before the advent of effective, antimalarial chemoprophylaxis[5] and remain important. A significant point in their favour is that they have no side effects! They also provide protection against biting insects other than mosquitoes.

Insecticide-impregnated nets have a significant advantage over untreated bed nets. Such nets allow larger mesh size in the netting for greater ventilation and comfort. Nets can be purchased already impregnated or with a kit to do so. The effects of impregnation last for 6 months unless the net is washed. Nets are available to purchase in cot, single and double bed size. They can be suspended above the bed with a variety of fixings and the hanging net is best tucked under the bed mattress. Any tears or holes that appear in the netting should be repaired. Those sleeping outdoors or camping in a malarious area should always sleep under an impregnated net and could use an outdoor vaporising coil.

COMPLIANCE WITH APPROPRIATE CHEMOPROPHYLAXIS

The four most commonly used drugs for malaria chemoprophylaxis in the UK are chloroquine, proguanil, mefloquine and doxycycline. Chloroquine, mefloquine and doxycycline act as suppressive prophylactics inhibiting replication in blood. Proguanil also acts as a causal prophylactic preventing liver phase development. Some other drugs are under development and include Malarone and long-acting 8-aminoquinolones.

The most effective regimens are usually defined by geographical area, and consider the prevalent species of malaria parasite and the likely extent of drug resistance.

Pre-existing medical conditions, other medications and factors affecting compliance, as discussed above, may also influence the choice of drugs.

When to use chemoprophylaxis, and the choice of drug, are difficult and sometimes controversial areas of malaria prevention. In the 1950s and 1960s chloroquine was almost universally effective and very well tolerated with a simple once weekly regimen. However, large-scale use for prophylaxis, therapy and empirical treatment eventually led to the appearance of chloroquine resistance. This has spread substantially so that now almost all *Plasmodium falciparum*-affected areas of the world have chloroquine-resistant strains.

The failure of chloroquine has led to the use of alternative drugs, sometimes more toxic and with potentially serious, and occasionally fatal, side effects.

Fansidar initially appeared an attractive, once a week, agent for antimalarial chemoprophylaxis

but, particularly when used with chloroquine, was followed by a number of cases of exfoliative dermatitis with fatalities. It was estimated that for American visitors to East Africa, the mortality rate from Fansidar chemoprophylaxis exceeded the mortality from malaria in that particular group.[9]

Twice weekly use of Maloprim has been thought to be associated with cases of agranulocytosis.[8]

Amodiaquine was used extensively for treatment in French-speaking West Africa. It was adopted in the UK for prophylaxis in the mid-1980s. However, agranulocytosis, which had been a previously recognised side effect of this drug, appeared even at this lower dosage.

The tendency for previously uncommon or unrecognised side effects to appear once an agent is used on a large scale for chemoprophylaxis continued when mefloquine was introduced and side effects were brought to public attention through the media.

In 1986, Peto & Gilks[10] published an article on risk–benefit analysis for antimalarial chemoprophylaxis. They argued that, when dealing with a healthy population, there is an obligation to use the least toxic regimen compatible with protection in a given area. For example, in those areas of the world where transmission is low, use of less toxic regimens is justifiable, provided there is not substantial drug resistance. However, in areas where there is a high-level transmission of chloroquine-resistant *Plasmodium falciparum*, the argument for more toxic antimalarial agents becomes stronger when less toxic alternatives are not available. The balance of risk is then in favour of giving the prophylaxis.

This balance of risks and benefits should be discussed openly with the traveller. It also has to be borne in mind that it is sometimes preferable for a traveller to take a less than ideally effective drug, rather than no prophylaxis at all. If the traveller decides to opt for a less effective, but possible safer, regimen, this should not be seen as a failure on the part of the adviser as it usually means better compliance.

While no antimalarial chemoprophylaxis ever gives 100% protection, the risk of contracting malaria can be substantially reduced by effective regimens and the likelihood of life-threatening illness, when prophylaxis is being used, is also reduced.

Health advisers must have access to an up-to-date reference source and know where to contact expert medical advice in the event of a complicated problem.

Notes on individual prophylactic drugs

These notes are brief guidelines only and manufacturer's literature should always be consulted for detailed and up-to-date information.

Chloroquine. Caution in hepatic and renal impairment; G6PD deficiency; may exacerbate psoriasis; avoid if history of epilepsy; may aggravate myasthenia gravis.

Side effects include gastrointestinal disturbances, headache, convulsions, visual disturbances such as temporary blurred vision, depigmentation or hair loss, skin reactions (rashes, pruritus), rarely bone marrow depression. Chloroquine is very toxic in overdose – warn parents with young children. It is generally accepted, as a result of long usage, to be safe in pregnancy.

Preparations available – Avloclor (Zeneca) and Nivaquine (Rhône-Poulenc Rorer). Nivaquine is available in syrup form.

Proguanil. Caution in renal impairment.

Drug interactions – anticoagulant effect of warfarin may be enhanced.

Safe in pregnancy, but folate supplement is advised.

Side effects include mild nausea and diarrhoea, apthous mouth ulcers and stomatitis.

Preparation available – Paludrine (Zeneca).

Mefloquine. Caution in severe hepatic and renal impairment, and cardiac conduction disorders.

No preparation is available for children and infants under 5 kg in weight.

In the UK, it is advised that mefloquine should not be used in the first trimester of pregnancy and that pregnancy should be avoided for 3 months after completing a course. Avoid when breast-feeding and when there is a history of neuropsychiatric disorders, including depression and epilepsy or epilepsy in a first degree relative.

Side effects, mostly rare, include nausea, vomiting, diarrhoea, abdominal pain, headache, loss of balance and dizziness – caution with

driving and using machinery, sleep disorders (insomnia, drowsiness, abnormal dreams), neuropsychiatric reactions (including sensory and motor neuropathies, tremor, ataxia, anxiety, depression, panic attacks, agitation, hallucinations, psychosis, convulsions).

Preparation available – Lariam (Roche).

Doxycycline. Side effects include nausea, vomiting, diarrhoea, photosensitivity (discontinue if unexpected erythema occurs, use effective sunscreens), vaginal candidiasis, oesophagitis (take with a full glass of water while sitting upright). Caution in hepatic impairment, avoid in porphyria.

Contraindications include pregnancy (including 1 week after completing the course), breast-feeding, children less than 12 years of age, systemic lupus erythematosus and history of allergy to other tetracyclines.

Preparations available – doxycycline (non-proprietary) and Vibramycin (Invicta). Doxycycline is currently not licensed in the UK for antimalarial chemoprophylaxis (1998).

How to take chemoprophylaxis

Chemoprophylaxis should be started 1 week before entering the malarious area, except for mefloquine which should be started ideally $2\frac{1}{2}$ weeks before departure to allow time to change the regimen if side effects develop. All regimens should be taken throughout exposure and for 4 weeks afterwards to cover the hepatic 'incubation' phase of *Plasmodium falciparum*.

Mild symptoms from tablets are not normally an indication to stop taking the medication. For example, those suffering from mild nausea and/or diarrhoea should persist, but seek medical advice if the symptoms continue. Stopping the tablets when the risk of disease is high is extremely unsafe.

The importance of compliance

Compliance is vitally important. Appropriate chemoprophylaxis substantially reduces the chance of contracting malaria, and if illness occurs, death is less likely in those taking chemoprophylaxis.

Travellers who return to their homelands to visit friends and relations are at particularly high risk of malaria.[3] Many immigrants from the Indian sub-continent settled in the UK at a time when the risk of malaria, for example, in Asia was low. Some think immunity to malaria is lifelong, but immunity is rapidly lost after exposure ceases.

DIAGNOSE BREAKTHROUGH MALARIA SWIFTLY AND OBTAIN TREATMENT PROMPTLY

The minimum incubation period of malaria is 8 days. Most *Plasmodium falciparum* malaria presents within 1 month of being in a malarious area, occasionally longer. *Plasmodium vivax* and *Plasmodium ovale* illness can be delayed up to 1 year or occasionally longer because of the presence of hypnozoites. The clinical features of malaria can be non-specific and are easily confused with other diseases, most dangerously influenza. The illness and its treatment are described on pages 309–315. It is vital that if travellers become unwell during or following exposure that they report their history of travel to their doctor.

Most tragedies occur because the traveller does not report symptoms to the doctor who may then, if not prompted, fail to take a travel history or consider malaria. Inquests provide graphic evidence of this.[11] It can be very difficult to distinguish early *Plasmodium falciparum* malaria from influenza on clinical grounds.[12, 13] Even microscopic diagnosis of malaria[14] may be difficult. This is achieved by examination of thick and thin blood films. New immunochromatographic strip tests are now available and are likely to be widely used.

Malaria prevention advice for special groups

EPILEPSY

Travellers with epilepsy need careful consideration. Mefloquine and chloroquine are unsuitable. Proguanil alone is advised for areas without resistance. For higher-risk areas, doxycycline is an alternative. Phenytoin, carbamazepine and barbiturates reduce the half-life of doxycycline.

Theoretically the dosage of doxycycline should therefore be increased but there is insufficient evidence on this as yet.[3]

PREGNANCY AND BREAST-FEEDING

Malaria in pregnancy increases the risk of maternal death, neonatal death, spontaneous abortion and stillbirth. Pregnant travellers should try to avoid malarious areas where there is substantial transmission of chloroquine-resistant *Plasmodium falciparum*. If travel is unavoidable, stringent mosquito-bite-prevention measures should be taken.

Chloroquine and proguanil chemoprophylaxis is considered safe for the fetus in pregnancy, and mefloquine in the second and third trimesters. In the USA, mefloquine is used in the first trimester if the risk is considered substantial. Doxycycline should not be used. However, in the case of an inadvertent pregnancy, malaria chemoprophylaxis is not considered an indication for a termination of pregnancy.[2]

Antimalarial drugs are secreted in the breast milk of lactating mothers, but the amounts involved are thought to be of no harm to the baby but at the same time they are inadequate for protection. Breast-fed infants in malarious areas, therefore, should be given chemo-prophylaxis.

CHILDREN

Children are at special risk because they can become seriously ill with malaria in a very short period of time. Travel to areas where there is substantial transmission of chloroquine-resistant *Plasmodium falciparum* should be avoided if at all possible with very young children and infants. Mosquito-bite prevention measures are very important. Choice of chemoprophylaxis and dosage must be carefully considered. Administration of the drugs can present problems. Chloroquine is the only antimalarial drug available in elixir form and the others must be crushed and the bitter taste disguised, for example, in jam. When both weight and age are available, weight is a better guide to dosage than age for children over 6 months old.[3]

SPLENECTOMY

Although the traveller who has undergone splenectomy is at no greater risk than others from being bitten by an infected mosquito, the illness is likely to be far more severe. Avoiding unnecessary trips to malarious areas should be strongly advised, especially those with chloroquine-resistant *Plasmodium falciparum*. Stringent mosquito-bite protection is necessary, full compliance with chemoprophylaxis carried out, and prompt medical attention sought in the event of any febrile illness occurring.

HEPATIC FAILURE

All antimalarials are contraindicated in those with severe liver failure. Chloroquine and proguanil can be used in mild hepatic failure, but specialist advice is best sought in this type of traveller.

RENAL FAILURE

Proguanil is excreted by the kidneys and the prophylactic dose may need to be less in renal failure. For high-risk, chloroquine-resistant areas, mefloquine or doxycycline may be used since they are excreted through the liver. However, in all cases, specialist advice should be sought.

Sources of advice on malaria prevention

ONLINE DATABASES

In the UK continually updated advice may be obtained by healthcare professionals from the online databases TRAVAX and MASTA (see Ch. 2).

TELEPHONE SUPPORT FOR HEALTHCARE PROFESSIONALS ONLY IS AVAILABLE FROM:

PHLS Malaria
Reference
Laboratory   0207 636 3924
     (weekdays 9 am–4.30 pm)
Birmingham   0121 766 6611
Glasgow   0141 300 1130
Liverpool   0151 708 9393

London
PHLS Communicable
Disease Surveillance
Centre   0208 200 6868 ext. 3412
     (9 am–12.30 pm weekdays)
Hospital for Tropical   0207 387 4411 (treatment)
Diseases   0207 388 9600 (travel prophylaxis)
Oxford   01865 225217

Recorded advice for travellers from the PHLS Malaria Reference Laboratory is available on 0891 600350 (calls are charged at 49p per minute, standard rate and at 39p per minute, cheap rate).

Advice on malaria chemoprophylaxis is given in Table 13.1. Further information can be obtained from the British National Formulary.

PRACTICE POINTS

Awareness – avoid bites – prompt treatment – chemoprophylaxis
- Check, not only, whether malaria is present in the country(s) concerned but also whether there are any regional variations, the species involved and is it common?
- Loose, light-coloured clothing, which covers as much skin as possible, should be worn especially between dusk and dawn to help prevent mosquito bites.
- In the evening, ankles under dining tables are very vulnerable to bites from mosquitoes. Cotton socks sprayed with insect repellent or insecticide are helpful.
- If accommodation is not going to be screened against mosquitoes, use an impregnated mosquito net and make sure you know in advance how to put it up correctly.
- Those going to be away from medical care should consider carrying emergency stand-by treatment. Be sure the traveller knows how it should be used and what to do if side effects occur.
- Choose prophylaxis carefully and make sure the traveller agrees with your choice. Discuss possible side effects. Remember chemoprophylaxis taken correctly gives excellent but never complete protection.

TABLE 13.1 Easy guide reference to malaria chemoprophylaxis

Generic name	Chloroquine	Proguanil	Mefloquine	Doxycycline
Proprietary name	Avloclor (Zeneca) and Nivaquine (Rhone-Poulenc Rorer)	Paludrine (Zeneca)	Lariam (Roche)	Doxycycline (non-proprietary) Vibramycin (Invicta)
Availability	Not on FP10, purchase over the counter at chemist	Not on FP10, purchase over the counter at chemist	Only on a private prescription	Only on a private prescription
Presentation	Tablets, but Nivaquine also available in syrup form	Tablet only	Tablet only	Capsules, Vibramycin also in dispersible form
Caution in use	• Hepatic and renal impairment • G6PD deficiency • May exacerbate psoriasis • May aggravate myasthenia gravis	• Renal impairment • Drug interaction – effect of warfarin possibly enhanced	• Pregnancy • Severe hepatic and renal failure • Cardiac conduction disorders • Children under 5 kg	• Hepatic impairment • Avoid in porphyria • Rarely causes photosensitivity
Contraindications	• For prophylaxis if history of epilepsy		• Pregnancy in first trimester and for 3 months after completing course • Breast-feeding • History of neuropsychiatric disorders including depression or convulsions • Epilepsy in patient or 1st degree relative • Hypersensitivity to quinine	• Pregnancy including 1 week after completing course • Breast-feeding • Children under 12 years of age • Systemic lupus erythematosis • History of tetracycline allergy
Most common side effects	Gastrointestinal disturbances and headache	Mild gastric intolerance and diarrhoea Occasional mouth ulcers and stomatitis	Gastrointestinal disturbances Headache Loss of balance, dizziness	Gastrointestinal disturbances Vaginal candidiasis Oesophagitis (unless taken correctly)
Less common side effect	Visual disturbances Convulsions Depigmentation or loss of hair Skin reactions (rashes, pruritus) Rarely, bone marrow depression	Skin reaction and hair loss reported	Sleep disorders (insomnia, drowsiness, abnormal dreams) Neuropsychiatric reactions including anxiety, panic attacks, hallucinations	Erythema (stop medication and contact medical help)
Dosage	300 mg (2 tablets) weekly	200 mg (2 tablets) daily	250 mg (1 tablet) weekly	100 mg (1 capsule) daily
Commencement of medication	1 week before entering malarious area	1 week before entering malarious area	2½ weeks before entering malarious area	1 week before entering malarious area
Duration of course	All time in malarious area and four weeks after leaving	All time in malarious area and four weeks after leaving	All time in malarious area and four weeks after leaving	All time in malarious area and four weeks after leaving
Special notes precautions	Safe for use in pregnancy Extremely toxic in overdosage Keep away from children Chloroquine and proguanil are now available to purchase in a combined bubble pack for easier compliance	Safe for use in pregnancy but folate supplement needed	Advise patient to contact medical adviser if side effects develop so that medication can be reviewed prior to departure	Not licensed in the UK for malaria chemoprophylaxis Take capsules after food in an upright position, do not lie down afterwards for at least 30 mintues Avoid excessive exposure to sunlight and use high factor sunscreen
Duration of prescribing	Several years – seek specialist advice	Several years – seek specialist advice	1 year	3 months

REFERENCES

1. Bradley DJ, Warhurst DC. Malaria prophylaxis: guidelines for travellers from Britain. British Medical Journal 1995; 310: 709–714.
2. World Health Organization. International travel and health – Vaccination requirements and health advice. Geneva: WHO: 1997.
3. Bradley DJ, Warhurst DC. Guidelines for the prevention of malaria in travellers from the United Kingdom. CDR Review 1997; 7(10): R137–R152. WebSite: http://www.phls.co.uk/advice/cdrr1097.pnf/ (requires Acrobat reader)
4. Reid AJC, Whitty CJM, Ayles HM, et al. Malaria at Christmas: risks of prophylaxis versus risks of malaria. British Medical Journal 1998; 317: 1506–1507.
5. Zucker JR, Carnevale PJ. Malaria: epidemiology and prevention of exposure In: DuPont HL, Steffen R, eds. Textbook of travel medicine and health. Hamilton, Ontario: Decker 1997: 101–108.
6. Collins DA, Brady JN, Curtis CF. Assessment of the efficacy of quwenling as a mosquito repellent. Phytotherapy Research 1993; 7: 17–20.
7. Goodyer L, Behrens RH. Short report: the safety and toxicity of insect repellents. American Journal of Tropical Medicine and Hygiene 1998; 59(2): 323–324.
8. Hutchinson DBA, Whiteman PD, Farquhar JA. Agranulocytosis associated with Maloprim: review of cases. Human Toxicology 1986; 5: 221–227.
9. Chiodini PL. Problems with antimalarial chemoprophylaxis In: Pounder RE, Chiodini PL, eds. Advanced medicine 23. Royal College of Physicians of London. London: Baillière Tindall; 1987: 362–371.
10. Peto TE, Gilks CF. Strategies for the prevention of malaria in travellers: comparison of drug regimens by means of risk–benefit analysis. Lancet 1986; 1: 1256–1261.
11. Anon. Malaria death ruling. The Times 1992; September 29.
12. Anon. Lack of medical care contributed to malaria death of MP's brother. The Guardian 1992; September 29.
13. Anon. Doctor negligent in not diagnosing malaria. The Times 1975; November 5.
14. Milne LM, Kyi M, Chiodini PL, Warhurst DC. Accuracy of routine laboratory diagnosis of malaria in the United Kingdom. Journal of Clinical Pathology 1994; 47: 740–742.

FURTHER READING

Bradley DJ, Warhurst DC. Malaria prophylaxis: Guidelines for prevention of malaria in travellers from the United Kingdom. CDR Review 1997; 7(10): R137–R152.

World Health Organization. International travel and health – Vaccination requirements and health advice. Geneva: WHO: 1998.

Future prospects

Peter Chiodini

Vaccination against malaria

Of the four species of malaria parasites infecting humans, *Plasmodium falciparum* is responsible for the overwhelming majority of deaths. Efforts to develop an effective malaria vaccine have therefore focused almost entirely upon this species, although work is also underway on a *Plasmodium vivax* vaccine.[1]

The malaria life cycle is complex, alternating as it does between a mosquito vector and a mammalian host, in which it invades liver parenchymal cells then erythrocytes. While this complexity increases the difficulty of producing a vaccine, it does offer a variety of targets, against one or more of which a vaccine can be aimed.

PRE-ERYTHROCYTIC VACCINES

During the 1970s, sub-lethally irradiated sporozoites, injected by the bite of irradiated mosquitoes, were shown to protect humans against challenge with viable sporozoites of *Plasmodium falciparum* or *Plasmodium vivax*. However, such immunity was short-lived and the mode of vaccination was clearly impracticable for wide-spread use. Subsequent cloning of the gene for the circumsporozoite protein (CSP) of *Plasmodium falciparum* was followed by trials in humans of recombinant and synthetic preparations of CSP with the aim of inducing neutralising antibodies. The results showed an inadequate degree of protection for clinical use. Once it had become apparent that antisporozoite immunity acted against the infected hepatocyte, greater attention was directed at the induction of cellular immunity. There is a clear need to induce CD8+ T cells and to identify all the CD8+ T cell epitopes expressed in *Plasmodium falciparum*-infected hepatocytes. Recombinant CSP, fused to hepatitis B surface antigen in an oil-in-water emulsion, plus the immunostimulant monophosphoryl lipid A and the saponin derivative QS21, produced encouraging antibody responses, T cell proliferation and interferon-gamma production in vitro in immunised volunteers.[2]

DNA vaccines against pre-erythrocytic stages are also being studied. Parasite DNA injected into a muscle is taken up into cells where the gene instructs the cell to produce antigen. This in turn is recognised by, and elicits a response from, the immune system. DNA vaccines have the potential to mimic natural infection and are relatively easily produced. Potential disadvantages are integration into the cell genome, induction of anti-DNA antibodies and autoimmunity. Hoffman's group[3] constructed DNA vaccine plasmids which encoded four *Plasmodium falciparum* pre-erythrocytic antigens: circumsporozoite protein (Pf CSP); sporozoite surface protein 2 (PfS SP2); carboxyl terminus of liver stage antigen 1 (Pf LSA-1 C-term); and exported protein 1 (Pf EXP-1). Injection of these plasmids into mice elicited antigen-specific antibody and cytotoxic, T-lymphocyte responses.

Pre-erythrocytic vaccines have the potential to prevent infection with sporozoites, or to eradicate infected liver cells. Thus, the infection could be aborted before the asexual erythrocytic stage (which results in clinical illness) is reached. Such a vaccine would be of value to both visitors to, and residents of, malaria-endemic areas. However, failure of the vaccine in an individual with no previous experience of malaria would leave that person fully susceptible to the clinical effects of malaria.

BLOOD-STAGE VACCINES

There are two possible types of blood-stage vaccines.

The first aims to reduce the number of parasitised cells. Since the likelihood of a severe, complicated or fatal attack of *Plasmodium falciparum* malaria increases with higher parasitaemia, such a vaccine might be expected to reduce mortality. This would be potentially very important for the residents of malaria-endemic areas, who experience repeated challenge with new malaria infections. The vaccine might still be of value in this context, even it if led only to reduction, rather than clearance, of the parasitaemia.[4] However, travellers from non-malarious to malaria-endemic areas would still be susceptible to malarial illness if only some of the parasites were removed.

The second type of vaccine can be classed as an 'antidisease' or 'antitoxic' vaccine which would reduce clinical symptoms but not parasitaemia. Whether deployed in semi-immune or non-immune individuals, this type of vaccine would need to be combined with other vaccine components as reduction in symptoms, but not parasitaemia, would potentially delay clinical diagnosis, allow substantial build-up of parasitaemia and permit malaria transmission in endemic areas.[4]

Candidate, blood-stage vaccine antigens are:

- merozoite surface protein-1 (MSP-1) which is protective in monkeys and under study in humans
- apical membrane antigen-1 (AMA-1) which is protective in both mice and monkeys.[4]

TRANSMISSION-BLOCKING VACCINES

These vaccines are directed at the gametocyte or ookinete stages of the malaria parasite or against mosquito proteins, and designed to prevent further development of the parasites in the mosquito vector, preventing its becoming infective. Such vaccines would produce no resistance to malaria infection nor malarial illness in the recipients, and benefit would accrue to individuals only via an overall reduction of malaria transmission in their community. It is likely that they will be incorporated into multi-antigen vaccines which include epitopes from other stages of the parasite life cycle.

Pfs 25, a recombinant protein from the zygote surface, is in the early stages of human clinical trials.[5]

COMBINATION VACCINES

SPf 66, a synthetic peptide vaccine, included sporozoite and merozoite stage antigens. Early promise in field trials against human malaria in South America and in Tanzania was not fulfilled in studies from The Gambia.[6, 7]

The vaccine NYVAC-Pf7, a highly attenuated vaccinia virus with seven *Plasmodium falciparum* genes encoding proteins from all stages of the life cycle inserted into its genome, has undergone a safety, immunogenicity and efficacy trial in human volunteers. More than 90% of the subjects produced detectable, cellular immune responses, though antibody responses were reportedly poor. There was significant delay in time to parasite patency compared with controls and one volunteer was completely protected against *Plasmodium falciparum*-infected mosquito challenge.[8]

New methods for the diagnosis of malaria

Romanowsky-stained blood films have been used to detect malaria parasites for more than a century.[9] In expert hands, they provide rapid, accurate, species-specific diagnosis of human malarial infection. But malaria diagnosis requires significant laboratory skills, including individual interpretation of parasite morphology, such that standards can vary significantly between laboratories.[10] Furthermore, expertise in malaria microscopy is unevenly spread, with many highly malarious areas having no provision for laboratory diagnosis. There was, therefore, a need for rapid, sensitive and specific, non-microscopic methods for detection of malaria parasites which could be used in the field, as well as in the laboratory. Much effort has gone into the development of rapid, dipstick tests for use on finger-prick as well as venepuncture blood samples. Three such products have now been developed.

1. The ParaSight F™ test (Becton–Dickinson) detects histidine-rich protein 2 (HRP-2) from *Plasmodium falciparum* using an immunochromatographic antigen capture technique. The test is specific for *Plasmodium falciparum* and does not claim to detect the other malaria parasites of humans. There have been many studies of its use, both in the tropics and in the temperate zone. For example, in a UK-based, multi-centre trial, co-ordinated

by the Hospital for Tropical Diseases, London, ParaSight F™ was 92% sensitive and 98% specific compared to microscopy for the initial diagnosis of *Plasmodium falciparum*.[11]

2. ICT malaria Pf™ (ICT Diagnostics) is a card-based, immunochromatographic test for the detection of HRP-2. It too has performed well in detecting *Plasmodium falciparum*; Singh et al.[12] reported sensitivity of 100% and specificity of 84.5% versus microscopy in a study based in India.

3. OptiMAL™ (Flow Inc, Portland, Oregon, USA) detects a different parasite antigen, lactate dehydrogenase (pLDH), using monoclonal antibodies which are specific for the parasite enzyme and can thus detect it even in the presence of human LDH. Unlike HRP-2 based assays, OptiMAL™ can detect *Plasmodium vivax* as well as *Plasmodium falciparum*. Having tested it at the Hospital for Tropical Diseases, London, Hunt Cooke et al[13] conducted a trial of its performance in The Gambia. OptiMAL™ was 91.3% sensitive and 92% specific for the initial diagnosis of *Plasmodium falciparum*, the predominant malaria species present in the locality. John et al[14] showed OptiMAL™ to be 98.2% sensitive for the detection of *Plasmodium vivax* in south India.

Palmer et al[15] compared the performance of the OptiMAL™ test with the ParaSight F™ test and the ICT malaria Pf™ test on blood samples from Honduras. OptiMAL™ showed sensitivities of 94% and 88% for detection of *Plasmodium vivax* and *Plasmodium falciparum* respectively, compared to 65% sensitivity for *Plasmodium falciparum* obtained with both ParaSight F™ and ICT malaria Pf™, a contrast to the results from other studies on HRP-2-based dipstick tests.

Jelinek et al[16] reported 88.5% sensitivity and 99.4% specificity using OptiMAL™ to detect *Plasmodium falciparum* compared to 92.5% sensitivity and 98.3% specificity using ICT malaria Pf™. In the same study, OptiMAL™ was only 61.5% sensitive, though 100% specific, for the diagnosis of *Plasmodium vivax*. Discrepancies between the results of studies, such as those cited, indicate a need for further, larger comparative trials in different geographical regions.

Each test has its own advantages and disadvantages. The HRP-2-based assays detect only *Plasmodium falciparum*, but that is the parasite which accounts for the vast majority of malaria deaths. After the thick blood film has become negative, there may be some persistence of HRP-2 antigenaemia for a few days in some instances and for up to 4 weeks in very occasional patients, which can give a false impression of persisting parasitaemia. However, this could be advantageous in the event of a patient attending for diagnosis soon after taking self-medication for possible malaria, when recent *Plasmodium falciparum* malaria can be diagnosed even if the blood film is negative. ParaSight F™ has given false-positive results in patients with rheumatoid-factor-positive rheumatoid arthritis, despite their never having been exposed to malaria.[17]

OptiMAL™ has the advantage of being able to detect *Plasmodium vivax* as well as *Plasmodium falciparum*, though its published sensitivity for detection of *Plasmodium falciparum* is lower than the stated sensitivity of the ParaSight F™ or ICT malaria Pf™. pLDH does not usually remain detectable for more than a day after successful treatment of malaria.

Should rapid diagnostic tests such as these be used by travellers? There are important issues to consider. Self-treatment for malaria based on a lay person's self-diagnosis (albeit with written instructions provided for use in aiding self-diagnosis) will inevitably be less accurate than a properly performed, dipstick test result. But how well will the traveller be able to undertake the test and how well will the kit itself perform after, say, 3 months in a rucksack in the tropics? What if the traveller uses the test very early in a malarial infection, when the parasitaemia is still very low and thus might be below the limit of detection of the test? Does the traveller take empirical treatment anyway, or repeat the test in 2 days' time, or set off to seek (possibly distant) medical attention without taking treatment, in which case why use the dipstick test at all? What if a local laboratory result disagrees with a stick test – which one is correct? Well-designed studies to answer such questions are required, so that a clear policy on the use or otherwise of these stick tests by travellers to malarious areas can be written.

There are, however, other scenarios where dipstick tests have an important part to play.[18, 19] A WHO, informal consultation group reported that a dipstick antigen-capture assay might be cost-effective for the management of *Plasmodium falciparum* malaria in epidemics and emergencies; where laboratory services are inadequate; in mobile clinics; where levels of malaria transmission are low and levels of antimalarial drug resistance are high; where first-line treatment is much more expensive than the dipstick assay; and, in severe cases where blood films may be negative, to provide evidence of antigenaemia.[18] In well-resourced countries, where malaria is relatively uncommon, lack of familiarity with malaria parasite morphology may lead to difficulties. In such areas, one of the immunochromatographic dipstick tests should be used as a back-up to microscopy, especially if there is a non-specialist microscopist on call.

Diagnosis of malaria by microscopy is subjective, relying as it does on individual interpretation of parasite and red cell morphology. Speciation, for example of *Plasmodium ovale* from *Plasmodium vivax*, or detection of mixed infections with two or more species present, can be difficult, and even in the best laboratories the limit of sensitivity for detection of parasites is 10 parasites/μL.[19] An alternative method objectively read, which can address these limitations would be very attractive.

Snounou et al[20] described a nested, polymerase-chain-reaction (PCR) method for the detection of all four human malaria parasites using oligo-nucleotides based on small, sub-unit ribosomal RNA genes. The first cycle of amplification uses genus-specific primers and rPLU5 and rPLU6. The product of this amplification is then placed in a second amplification cycle with separate species-specific primers. Agarose gel electrophoresis followed by ethidium bromide staining is used to demonstrate the presence of any amplification product, the size of which is different according to the species present. The nested, PCR assay examines approximately 200-fold more erythrocytes than does conventional microscopy and the authors report their nested PCR capable of detecting 10 parasites per sample. Using this method, Snounou et al[20] demonstrated the

presence of a greater number of mixed infections than were detected by light microscopy, a finding confirmed on a different set of patients at the Hospital for Tropical Diseases, London (Moody & Chiodini 1999, unpublished data).

Cheng et al[21] reported a nested, PCR method to amplify the sub-telomeric, variable, open, reading frame (STEVOR) of *Plasmodium falciparum*. Each *Plasmodium falciparum* genome contains approximately 100 STEVOR copies. They report the assay as 1000-fold more sensitive than microscopy for the detection of this parasite; it was able to detect a single ring-infected red blood cell and, tested against pure parasite DNA, was able to detect 0.002 pg of parasite DNA, equivalent to one-tenth of a parasite. The authors were able to detect asexual parasites in the peripheral blood of two infected volunteers, for 6 and 7 days respectively before they were detected by thick film microscopy and symptoms appeared.

PCR is in use in the UK National External Quality Assessment Scheme for Blood Parasitology to confirm the identity of the malaria parasites in blood films sent out for microscopic examination by scheme participants.

PCR is not yet in routine use for the diagnosis of malaria in hospital laboratories, but the trend towards automation of PCR diagnostics and the use of colorimetric systems to detect PCR product make this a real possibility in the foreseeable future. Earlier laboratory diagnosis will thus be achieved and it is possible that the results may show more mixed infections than have hitherto been recognised. Given the costs involved and the sophisticated laboratory facilities required for PCR, not least to minimise the chance of cross-contamination of samples, deployment for routine use in the tropics is most unlikely. Microscopy and, if affordable, dipstick tests will provide the basis for diagnosis in endemic areas.

REFERENCES

1. Arevalo-Herrera M, Roggero MA, Gonzalez JM, et al. Mapping and comparison of the B-cell epitopes recognized on the *Plasmodium vivax* circumsporozoite protein by immune Colombians and immunized Aotus monkeys. Annals of Tropical Medicine and Parasitology 1998; 92(5): 539–551.

2. Stoute JA, Kester KE, Krzych U, et al. Long-term efficacy and immune responses following immunization with the RTS,S malaria vaccine. Journal of Infectious Diseases 1998; 178(4): 1139–1144.

3. Hedstrom RC, Doolan DL, Wang R, et al. In vitro expression and in vivo immunogenicity of *Plasmodium falciparum* pre-erythrocytic stage DNA vaccines. International Journal of Molecular Medicine 1998; 2(1): 29–38.

4. Good MF, Kaslow DC, Miller LH. Pathways and strategies for developing a malaria blood-stage vaccine. Annual Reviews of Immunology 1998; 16: 57–87.

5. Barr PJ, Green KM, Gibson HL, et al. Recombinant Pfs25 protein of *Plasmodium falciparum* elicits malaria transmission-blocking activity in experimental animals. Journal of Experimental Medicine 1991; 174: 1203–1208.

6. D'Alessandro U, Leach A, Drakely CJ, et al. Efficacy trial of malaria vacccine Spf66 in Gambian infants. Lancet 1995; 346: 462–467.

7. Bojang KA, Obaro SK, D'Alessandro U, et al. An efficacy trial of the malaria vaccine SPf66 in Gambian infants – second year of follow-up. Vaccine 1998; 16(1): 62–67.

8. Ockenhouse CF, Sun PF, Lanar DE, et al. Phase I/IIa safety, immunogenicity, and efficacy trial of NYVAC-Pf7, a pox-vectored, multiantigen, multistage vaccine candidate for *Plasmodium falciparum* malaria. Journal of Infectious Diseases 1998; 177(6): 1664–1673.

9. Gilles HM. Milestones in the history of malaria and its control. In: Gilles HM, Warrell DA, eds. Bruce-Chwatt's essential malariology. 3rd ed. London: Edward Arnold, 1993: 1–11.

10. Milne LM, Kyi M, Chiodini PL, Warhurst DC. Accuracy of routine laboratory diagnosis of malaria in the United Kingdom. Journal of Clinical Pathology 1994; 47: 740–742.

11. Chiodini PL, Hunt Cooke A, Moody AH, et al. MDA evaluation of the Becton Dickinson Parasight F test for the diagnosis of *Plasmodium falciparum*. MDA/96/33. London: HMSO; 1996.

12. Singh N, Valecha N, Sharma VP. Malaria diagnosis by field workers using an immunochromatographic test. Transactions of the Royal Society of Tropical Medicine and Hygiene 1997; 91: 396–397.

13. Hunt Cooke A, Chiodini PL, Doherty T, et al. Comparison of a parasite lactate dehydrogenase-based immunochromatographic antigen detection assay (OptiMAL®) with microscopy for the detection of malaria parasites in human blood samples. American Journal of Tropical Medicine and Hygiene 1999; 60(2): 173–176.

14. John SM, Sudarsanam A, Sitaram U, Moody AH. Evaluation of OptiMAL®, a dipstick test for the diagnosis of malaria. Annals of Tropical Medicine and Parasitology 1998; 92(5): 621–622.

15. Palmer CJ, Lindo JF, Klaskala WI, et al. Evaluation of the OptiMAL test for rapid diagnosis of *Plasmodium vivax* and *Plasmodium falciparum* malaria. Journal of Clinical Microbiology 1998; 36: 203–206.

16. Jelinek T, Grobusch MP, Schwenke S, et al. Sensitivity and specificity of dipstick tests for rapid diagnosis of malaria in nonimmune travellers. Journal of Clinical Microbiology 1999; 37(3): 721–723.

17. Laferi H, Kandel K, Pichler H. False positive dipstick test for malaria. New England Journal of Medicine 1997; 337: 1635–1636.

18. WHO. A rapid dipstick antigen capture assay for the diagnosis of falciparum malaria. Bulletin of the World Health Organization 1996; 74: 47–54.

19. Chiodini PL. Non-microscopic methods for diagnosis of malaria. Lancet 1998; 351: 80–81.

20. Snounou G, Viriyakosol S, Zhu XP, et al. High sensitivity of detection of human malaria parasites by the use of nested polymerase chain reaction. Molecular and Biochemical Parasitology 1993; 61: 315–320.

21. Cheng Q, Lawrence G, Reed C, et al. Measurement of *Plasmodium falciparum* growth rates in vivo: a test of malaria vaccines. American Journal of Tropical Medicine and Hygiene 1997; 57(4): 495–500.

REGIONAL TRAVEL

A perspective from sub-Saharan Africa

Alan Pithie

Introduction

Sub-Saharan Africa (SSA) covers a vast land area, ranging from Senegal in the north-west, through southern Chad, Sudan and Ethiopia to Somalia in the west and southwards through Kenya, Zaire, Zambia and Zimbabwe to the Republic of South Africa (RSA). Several different geographical and climatic zones are encompassed, each harbouring specific health risks to the traveller. Within SSA, the pattern of endemic and epidemic disease varies greatly. Furthermore, the prevailing socio-economic and political situation contrasts greatly between different countries and significantly influences the pattern of disease and the local provision of healthcare. Consequently, there exists widely variable access to medical care of varying standards.

In many large cities throughout the region, excellent, private, healthcare provision is readily available, and can be accessed by visitors with adequate finances or medical insurance. Visitors may also use government hospitals, but in general, private care facilities are better equipped and are more readily accessible. Outside larger cities, particularly in the poorer countries, no private healthcare exists. Healthcare is generally provided by a combination of government and voluntary (mission) hospitals. Such facilities are often sparsely distributed, inaccessible and have persistent problems with drug supplies. For instance, in Zimbabwe, a stable country with relatively good infrastructure and economy, a single government hospital staffed by three doctors provides care for over 300 000 people living in a land area approaching the size of Belgium. In poorer and strife-ridden countries such as Rwanda and Zaire, medical care is likely to be much less accessible.

The risk to health of travellers is related to factors described above and to the duration and nature of stay in SSA. Generally speaking, the backpacker is at greater risk of acquiring a tropical infection than a package holidaymaker. A prior knowledge of locations to be visited, duration of stay and proposed activities is necessary to provide correct advice to travellers. The requirements for the backpacker, the business traveller, the package holidaymaker and the long-term visitor may vary greatly depending on the location they are visiting. These aspects will be discussed further below.

POTENTIAL HEALTH RISKS

Infections that can be acquired while abroad are foremost in the thoughts of travellers who are seeking pre-travel advice. However, other problems may present equally great risks to health while abroad. The traveller with chronic conditions, such as diabetes, asthma and congestive cardiac failure, may find climatic change difficult. Difficulty in obtaining regular supplies of certain medications is a common problem for long-term visitors. These issues are dealt with fully in specific chapters.

Road conditions are highly variable throughout Africa. In many countries, no test is required to obtain a driving licence. Vehicles are frequently in a poor state of repair, have inadequate brakes and lighting, and are overloaded with passengers. As a result, accidents are very common and serious injury all too frequent. Visitors travelling in local buses and taxis are especially at risk of injury. These are a cheap and entertaining means of transport, but whenever possible they should be avoided. Special care is also required when travelling by private car at night. Other vehicles may have no lights. Roads in rural areas have no fencing and wild animals frequently stray onto roads.

Muggings and other violent crimes are common in many African countries. Tourists are an obvious target. It is inadvisable to give lifts to strangers. Car doors should be locked when driving. Hotel room doors should be kept locked and windows closed in cities. These topics are also dealt with more fully in other chapters. The remainder of this chapter will concentrate on specific infectious risks to travellers.

The list of infectious diseases potentially acquired in SSA is large and daunting (see Table 14.1).

In practice, a small number of infections are recurrently found in travellers. For many of these conditions effective prophylaxis or vaccination is available. Box 14.1 summarises general pre-travel advice which might be offered. As in Table 14.1 these conditions will be discussed by routes of transmission.

> **Box 14.1 Checklist for pre-travel advice for visitors to sub-Saharan Africa**
>
> 1. Long-sleeved shirts and trousers for evening wear
> 2. Wide-brimmed hat
> 3. Good footwear for walking in bush and rough terrain
> 4. Correct immunisations
> 5. Correct antimalarials
> 6. Mosquito nets, insect-repellent spray
> 7. First-aid kit, including IV set , syringes, needles (see p. 168)
> 8. Adequate supply of regular medication.

Insect-borne infectious conditions

Infection transmitted by biting insect

MALARIA

Malaria is a major cause of morbidity in visitors to SSA. It is also the major infectious cause of mortality in visitors returning from Africa to the UK.[1] Malaria can affect all visitors, including package holiday-makers, backpackers and expatriates, to endemic areas. In 1992, 12 UK residents died of *Plasmodium falciparum* malaria after returning home. All had visited SSA, the majority to tourist destinations in Kenya.[1]

Transmission of malaria occurs throughout SSA (with the exception of most of RSA, Southern Botswana and Namibia, and in some other elevated locations). Transmission rates vary greatly, being highest in low, humid areas, but few areas are absolutely free of malaria. Visitors from the UK frequently visit areas of high transmission such as coastal resorts in Kenya, the Zambezi valley, The Gambia and Nigeria.

Plasmodium falciparum accounts for almost all cases of malaria contracted in SSA. Some infection with *Plasmodium vivax* occurs in the Kruger Park area of RSA, though even here infection with *Plasmodium falciparum* predominates. Chloroquine resistance in *Plasmodium falciparum* is prevalent throughout East, Central and, increasingly, West Africa. Resistance to chloroquine has also been documented in Transvaal and Natal provinces in RSA. The rising incidence of chloroquine resistant malaria has resulted in significant increases in malaria-related mortality in several African countries.[2] Clearly chloroquine can no longer be relied upon to provide adequate chemoprophylaxis in any part of SSA.

The prevalence and clinical severity of malaria mandates that all visitors to SSA, no matter the duration of stay, need to consider antimalarial chemoprophylaxis. Recommendations for chemo-prophylaxis have recently been revised by the UK expert group on malaria (see Table 14.2).[3] These recommendations take account of the changing epidemiological situation, particularly regarding chloroquine resistance, and increasing concern over the safety and efficacy of mefloquine.

Essentially mefloquine is advised for travel to areas of high transmission and widespread chloroquine resistance, while chloroquine plus proguanil may be preferred for visits to areas of less intense transmission and patchier chloroquine resistance. Examples of the former include Nigeria, Uganda and Malawi, while Botswana, Zimbabwe (excluding the Zambezi valley) and malarious areas of RSA are included in the lower-risk group.

Importantly visits of less than 2 weeks to tourist resorts in coastal Kenya and Tanzania, and similar trips to The Gambia through January to May, are thought to constitute a low enough risk

TABLE 14.1 Infectious conditions potentially acquired in sub-Saharan Africa

Condition	Geographical location
Insect–borne	
Malaria	Widespread
Trypanosomiasis	Patchy distribution, rural
Leishmaniasis	Localised, rural
Arboviral diseases	Widespread, rural
Yellow fever	Mainly West and Central Africa
Typhus	Mainly East and South Africa
Filariasis	Discrete localised areas
Faecal–oral transmission	
Hepatitis A	Widespread
Typhoid fever	Widespread
Non-typhi salmonella	Widespread
Shigellosis	Widespread, poor socio-economic conditions
Cholera	Widespread but limited to poor socio-economic conditions
Helminth infection	Widespread but limited to poor socio-economic conditions
Sexually transmitted diseases/direct contact	
HIV infection	Widespread, common
Chancroid	Widespread, common
Gonorrhoea	Widespread, common
Syphilis	Widespread, less common than previously
Airborne particle	
Tuberculosis	Common, close contact required
Diphtheria	Only commonly found in locations with failure of vaccination policy
Meningitis	Most common in 'meningitis belt', close contact necessary
Measles	Widespread
Others	
Schistosomiasis	Widespread

TABLE 14.2 Recommendations for malarial prophylaxis in visitors to malarious areas of sub-Saharan Africa (see also Ch. 13)

Type of visitor	Recommendation
Package holiday maker	Usually mefloquine (alt. chloroquine/proguanil)
Backpacker	Mefloquine (alt. chloroquine/proguanil)
Long-term/expatriate	Chloroquine/proguanil or Maloprim (consider taking supply of effective antimalarial)

to make chloroquine plus proguanil more preferable than mefloquine. Clearly, this is a rapidly changing situation, and recommendations will undoubtedly change again. For the long-term visitor, it is always worth while seeking local advice before travelling.

Many elevated urban locations, such as the major cities in Zimbabwe and Kenya, are relatively malaria-free or have only seasonal transmission. Long-term visitors who find chloroquine plus proguanil too demanding or unpleasant, and who are wary of long-term mefloquine, may consider prophylaxis with pyrimethamine and dapsone (Maloprim, Deltaprim). This regimen is very popular in Zimbabwe and Zambia, where it is of proven efficacy and minimal toxicity so long as the dose does not exceed one tablet every 5–7 days. Other long-term visitors may be advised to take prophylaxis only when travelling to malarious areas. Many expatriates elect to take no anti-malarial chemoprophylaxis even while residing in highly malarious areas. The reasons given for this action include a reluctance to take long-term medication, known or perceived drug toxicity and the limited efficacy of currently available anti-malarials. While these reasons are entirely under-standable, it is also clear that after residence for many years in endemic areas, expatriates remain susceptible to, and occasionally die from, *Plasmodium falciparum* malaria. Such individuals should be urged to seek medical attention for any severe or prolonged febrile illness. Alternatively, and particularly for expatriates working in remote rural areas, self-treatment of suspected malaria with an effective agent (quinine, mefloquine, halofantrine [not recommended by UK guidelines]) can be recommended.

It is always important to emphasise the effectiveness of bed netting and other measures to prevent mosquito bites (see p. 318). It is worth while stressing that such measures also protect against other infections that are transmitted by biting insects.

Other infections acquired from biting insects

YELLOW FEVER

Yellow fever is the most common cause of viral haemorrhagic fever (VHF) found in SSA. It is a serious disease, particularly in adults, with a case fatality rate of between 5 and 60%. The 17D strain vaccine, available for travellers from the UK, is very safe and provides effective immunity for at

Malaria – an overview	
Distribution	Widespread, sparing most of RSA and other areas of high altitude. Mainly *Plasmodium falciparum* malaria.
Symptoms	Initially fever, headache, rigors. Later drowsiness, confusion and focal neurological signs.
Prevention	Rigorous application of measures to avoid mosquito bites. Antimalarial prophylaxis.
Emergency measures	Seek medical help. Consider self medication.

least 10 years. Certain African countries require an International Certificate of Vaccination from all visitors before entry. Other countries require documented evidence of vaccination from visitors entering from another country within the yellow fever endemic zone. It is recommended, however, that all susceptible individuals travelling to yellow fever endemic areas should be adequately immunised before departure (Table 14.3).

Yellow fever transmission follows two distinct patterns. Endemic yellow fever occurs in rural, particularly jungle, areas throughout SSA, with the exception of countries in the southern part of the continent (RSA, Botswana, Namibia, Zimbabwe, Zambia, Malawi and Mozambique). Monkeys form the major reservoir and the forest-dwelling mosquito is responsible for transmission. Other vectors, principally *Aedes simpsoni* and other *Aedes* species transmit yellow fever from tree-top-dwelling monkeys to ground-dwelling humans. Sporadic cases of human disease are most frequently seen in forests and rural areas bordering jungle. In recent years, fatal, sporadic cases of yellow fever have occurred in unvaccinated travellers visiting rural areas within the endemic zone.

Urban yellow fever is an epidemic disease where vectors such as *Aedes aegypti* directly transmit the virus from infected to non-infected humans. Massive epidemics have occurred in SSA, particularly in Ethiopia and Senegal in the 1960s. Recently, smaller outbreaks of yellow fever have been recorded in the rift valley area of Kenya, and

TABLE 14.3 Yellow fever immunisation for visitors to sub-Saharan Africa (1999)

Certificate of vaccination necessary for entry
Burkino Faso, Cameroon, Central African Republic, Congo, Cote D'Ivoire, Gabon, Ghana, Liberia, Mali, Mauritania (unless staying less than 2 weeks), Niger, Rwanda, Sao Tome and Principe (unless staying less than 2 weeks), Senegal, Togo, Zaire

Certificate necessary if entering from infected country
Angola, Burundi, Equatorial Guinea, Ethiopia, The Gambia, Guinea, Guinea-Bissau, Kenya, Lesotho, Malawi, Mozambique, Namibia, Nigeria, Sierra Leone, Somalia, Republic of South Africa, Sudan, Swaziland, Tanzania, Zimbabwe

Vaccination recommended on clinical grounds
Angola, Burkina Faso, Burundi, Central African Republic, Chad, Congo, Cote D'Ivoire, Equatorial Guinea, Ethiopia, Gabon, Ghana, The Gambia, Guinea, Guinea-Bissau, Kenya, Liberia, Mali, Niger, Nigeria, Rwanda, Sao Tome and Principe, Senegal, Sierra Leone, Somalia, Sudan, Togo, Tanzania, Zaire

Yellow fever – an overview	
Distribution	Mainly rural and forest areas of West, Central and East Africa. Recent outbreaks have occurred. Epidemiology changing, risk increasing.
Symptoms	Fever, headache. Haemorrhagic shock and liver failure in severe cases.
Prevention	Effective and safe vaccine available. Precautions to avoid mosquito bites.

pose potential risk of transmission to visitors.[4] There has as yet not been a recent urban epidemic to match earlier outbreaks. However, comprehensive vector control measures are necessary to effectively eliminate the urban transmission of yellow fever. The potential for urban outbreaks exists when vector control measures are not maintained. The encroachment of unplanned urban areas on jungle is associated with population crowding, poor water supply and waste management. Discarded plastic containers and rubber tyres provide ideal breeding grounds for mosquitoes. These factors plus a lack of effective mosquito control measures have seen mosquito densities increase dramatically, significantly increasing the risk of further yellow fever outbreaks.[5]

Other viral infections including Lassa and Ebola

A bewildering number of other potentially serious viral infections are potentially transmissible to humans by arthropod vectors (arboviruses). With few exceptions (e.g. O'nyong-nyong), these are zoonoses, which mainly affect wild animals. Humans are an incidental host, most often becoming infected when they intrude into the habitat of the natural maintenance host. The arthropod vectors include mosquitoes, sandflies and ticks.

The arboviruses known to cause human disease in SSA include Chikungunya (widely distributed), O'nyong-nyong (East and Central Africa), yellow fever (see above), dengue fever (localised areas in coastal West and East Africa), Rift Valley Fever (broadly distributed through Central and Eastern areas, epidemics in Egypt), Crimean–Congo (widely distributed) and Hantaan (widely distributed).

Lassa fever virus, an arenavirus, is not transmitted to humans by insect vectors, but is included in this section as a potentially dangerous zoonosis. In the case of Lassa fever, humans acquire infection through direct or indirect contact with urine from infected rats. Furthermore, Lassa can be directly transmitted from person to person, and there have been a number of well-publicised, nosocomial outbreaks in West African hospitals.[6] Ebola shares Lassa's ability to be transmitted directly from person to person, and also lacks an insect vector. The natural reservoir for Ebola is unknown, although various monkey species are suspected and recently a zoologist acquired Ebola after dissecting a monkey captured in Cameroon. Like Lassa, Ebola is capable of causing large, but localised, human outbreaks, and there is a particular danger of transmission within hospitals.[6]

There is an ongoing, global epidemic of arboviral diseases.[5] There has been an explosion of dengue fever, particularly in the Far East and Central and South America. Dengue is also more prevalent in Africa, which has also seen increasing incidences of yellow fever, and Rift Valley fever.[5] An outbreak of Rift Valley Fever in 1997 is thought to have caused approximately 500 deaths in north-eastern Kenya–southern Somalia.[7] The case fatality rate for this infection is thought to be 5%, which indicates the likely massive scale of this outbreak. This normally drought-stricken area has been affected by uncommonly severe floods, which has resulted in population dislocation and increased mosquito densities. Few travellers reach such remote areas, and as a result Rift Valley fever does not currently pose much risk to them. However, with increasing mosquito densities, the risk of Rift Valley fever, and other arboviral infections is increasing.

Arboviral infections (including Lassa fever) are generally feared because of their reputation for causing severe illness, including haemorrhagic fever and meningoencephalitis, and the lack of effective therapy. In reality the majority of infections are mild and self-limiting. For example, as mentioned above, 95% of infections with Rift Valley fever virus result in a short febrile illness often associated with headache. In only 5% of cases do severe complications, such as haemorrhagic shock, acute hepatic failure or retinitis with blindness occur. Furthermore, serological surveys suggest that unrecognised arboviral infection is common in the indigenous human population. For instance, Lassa fever is thought to cause up to 100 000 new infections each year in the West African states of Nigeria, Sierra Leone and Liberia. The vast majority of infections are sub-clinical or cause a mild, transient disease. Ebola fever is the exception. Outbreaks of Ebola have been associated with mortality rates greater than 50%.[6]

At this time, few Western visitors to Africa appear to acquire arboviral infection. However, as enzootic infection in wild animals cannot be eradicated, the potential for human transmission, including to travellers, does exist and will continue. For reasons discussed above, populations of the key mosquito vectors are increasing, and epidemics of yellow fever, Rift Valley fever and dengue fever have recently occurred. An effective vaccine is widely available for yellow fever only. Measures to prevent infection with other arboviruses include the avoidance of endemic areas and, most particularly, general measures to avoid bites by mosquitoes and other insect vectors.

The risk from Lassa or Ebola fever is tiny, and essentially is restricted to individuals, such as doctors and nurses, working in rural healthcare situations.[6,8]

Returning travellers who develop a febrile illness within 21 days of leaving endemic areas must be considered for the possibility of Lassa, Ebola or Crimean–Congo fever.[6,8] The UK Advisory Committee on Dangerous Pathogens has recently revised their recommendations for management of such cases.[8] All cases should be discussed with an infectious diseases consultant, and high-risk cases should be transferred to a high-security infectious diseases unit (in the UK, sited at Coppetts Wood Hospital, London and Newcastle General Hospital).

Arboviral infection – an overview	
Distribution	Widespread, increasing prevalence, but currently exceedingly rare in travellers. Consider in special-risk situations.
Symptoms	Usually mild. Suspect with unexplained febrile illness associated with pharyngitis, conjunctivitis and myalgia. Haemorrhagic fever in severe cases.
Prevention	Avoid endemic areas. Measures to prevent insect bites.

Rickettsial infection

Tick-borne rickettsiosis is a common, seasonal disease throughout East (Kenyan tick typhus) and southern Africa (South African tick typhus). A Swiss report identified rickettsial diseases as the third most common cause of imported febrile illness.[9] Infection with *Rickettsia conori*, acquired in southern Africa, was the most frequently identified pathogen. In the UK, imported tick typhus also appears to be increasing and our unit has seen six cases of tick typhus, all from southern Africa, over the last 5 years.[10]

Tick typhus is usually a relatively mild disease, transmitted to humans by ixodid ticks. Typically, after an incubation period of approximately 1 week, an eschar develops at the site of infection and is followed by a febrile illness associated with a maculopapular rash. The clinical symptoms may suggest malaria or enteric fever, but the finding of an eschar (often small and unnoticed by the patient) and rash are highly characteristic of tick typhus. The illness is usually mild and self-limiting, but occasionally renal, hepatic or neurological complications arise.[10] Doxycycline is effective treatment.

Ixodid ticks infest domestic and wild animals. In humans, urban tick typhus is acquired from dog ticks, while rural tick typhus is acquired from bush ticks normally affecting game. Consequently all visitors to endemic areas of SSA might be considered at risk. Visitors walking through and camping out in the bush are at particular risk. Measures to avoid bush ticks include the wearing of long trousers tucked into socks, sleeping on cots above ground level and regular self-examination and deticking. Control of urban disease depends on avoiding contact with dogs and regular deticking of domestic pets.

Epidemic typhus is a considerably more severe disease, but now very rare. Infection with *Rickettsia prowazeki* is transmitted by the human louse, *Pediculus humanis corporis*, and is most likely to occur at times of severe socio-economic deprivation. The disease has most recently been recognised in rural, highland areas of Rwanda, Uganda and Ethiopia.

Holidaymakers are extremely unlikely to encounter any risk of acquiring infection. Backpackers also are unlikely to acquire infection, unless they spend extensive time in close proximity with the indigenous population in remote, rural areas. Any significant risk is likely to be limited to aid workers within disaster zones where epidemic typhus is present. A formalin-killed tissue culture vaccine and an attenuated live vaccine are produced but are unavailable in the UK.

Trypanosomiasis

Trypanosomiasis was once common in many parts of SSA, but the prevalence of the disease has fallen dramatically in recent decades. Even so, over 10 000 cases are reported annually, and the real number of affected individuals is likely to be considerably higher. The disease is now principally found in Sudan, Uganda and Zaire, but occurs in isolated foci in many other countries in East, Central and West Africa. There is evidence of a recent resurgence of infection in Uganda. Most of southern Africa, with the exception of northern areas of Botswana and Zimbabwe are free of trypanosomiasis.

The two forms of human trypanosomiasis, West African (Gambian) and East African (Rhodesian), caused, respectively, by *Trypanosoma brucei gambiense* and *Trypanosoma brucei rhodesiense*, are transmitted by the bite of infected tsetse flies. West African trypanosomiasis is largely a human disease. It affects people living in close proximity to tsetse-fly-infested woodland along river banks. East African trypanosomiasis principally affects wild animals in open savannah grassland. Humans entering such areas are at risk. Those affected include fishermen, hunters and, increasingly, tourists on safari.

There is no effective vaccine for trypanosomiasis. Control has depended on surveillance and early therapy, destruction of tsetse flies through trapping and spraying, and eradication of game. Personal prophylaxis relies on protective clothing and insect repellents. Short-stay visitors on safari holidays are at minimal risk of infection in the established tourist areas. Backpackers and longer-term visitors are more likely to enter and stay longer in endemic areas. If infected, early trypanosomiasis is likely to be indistinguishable from other febrile, tropical conditions. Therefore, a careful geographical history and a high index of suspicion are necessary to make the correct diagnosis. For individuals thought to be at high

Rickettsial infection – an overview	
Distribution	Tick typhus widely distributed through southern and East Africa. Murine and epidemic typhus restricted to poor, rural areas.
Symptoms	Fever and headache. Typical eschar and rash with tick typhus.
Prevention	Protective clothes when walking in bush. Deticking of domestic animals.
Treatment	Doxycycline or chloramphenicol.

Trypanosomiasis – an overview	
Distribution	Isolated patchy affected areas.
Symptoms	Painless chancre (boil) at site of infection. Fever and erythema. Later neurological manifestations.
Prevention	Wearing of protective clothing and insect-repellent cream.
Treatment	Requires specialist referral for investigation and therapy.

risk of trypanosomiasis, pentamidine prophylaxis, given intramuscularly every 3 months, may be considered.

Filariasis

Three filarial parasites, *Wuchereria bancrofti*, *Onchocerca volvulus* and *Loa loa*, cause human disease in SSA.

Wuchereria bancrofti, the cause of bancroftian filariasis, is widely distributed in rural areas of East, Central and West Africa. Infection is transmitted by several species of mosquito, including *Culex* and *Aedes* in urban areas and *Anopheles* in rural areas. The classical textbook picture of gross elephantiasis affecting limbs and genitalia occurs only after repeated infections, and the acquisition of a heavy worm burden, over many years. In the previously unexposed adult, such as a visitor entering an endemic area, symptoms may develop from 3 months after infection. Such individuals may present with an acute, febrile illness associated with lymphadenopathy and possibly cellulitis, lymphangitis, epididymo-orchitis or oedema. The febrile episode may be recurrent. Diagnosis rests on a high index of suspicion and the finding of peripheral eosinophilia, filiarial antibodies and microfilaria on blood film.

Tropical pulmonary eosinophilia, presenting with cough, wheeze and transient pulmonary infiltrates, is also thought to be a manifestation of infection with *Wuchereria bancrofti* (and other filarial parasites). This is occasionally seen in visitors to East Africa. An associated eosinophilia

and elevated IgE occur, and the finding of antifilarial antibodies confirms the diagnosis. Bancroftian filariasis presents a remote risk to package holidaymakers visiting established destinations. However, those spending longer time in endemic urban or rural areas are at some risk, and Bancroftian filariasis is well described in backpackers. No effective vaccine exists. However, measures to prevent mosquito bites are effective in preventing transmission of infection.

Infection with *Onchocerca volvulus* occurs in many sub-Saharan countries. Greatest transmission occurs in West Africa, where onchocerciasis is a leading cause of blindness. Onchocerciasis is extremely rare in East African countries, and is not found throughout southern Africa.

Infection of man occurs through the bite of *simulium* (black) flies. This vector breeds only in fast-flowing rivers and hence the greatest prevalence of human disease occurs in populations living beside rivers in endemic areas. For this reason, the disease is commonly called 'river blindness'.

Blindness and other severe consequences of this disease only occur with a heavy microfilarial burden as a consequence of repeated infections over many years. Expatriate workers and other travellers to endemic areas may acquire infection with *Onchocerca volvulus*, but clinically apparent disease rarely occurs. The most common symptom in expatriate workers is pruritus, although ocular symptoms (e.g. blurred vision) have been described. Examination may reveal minor skin changes, the presence of skin nodules (which need to be carefully searched for) and evidence of corneal inflammation. No effective vaccine exists. However, ivermectin is a safe and effective treatment which is gradually replacing diethylcarbamazine (DEC). Returning expatriate workers and other travellers who have resided in endemic areas for long periods may warrant screening for *Onchocerca volvulus* infection by specific serology, examination of blood for eosinophilia and microscopic examination of skin snips taken from the shoulders, buttocks and thighs.

Infection with the cutaneous helminth *Loa loa* is confined to the rain forest areas of West and Central Africa. Human infection occurs by day-biting *Chrysops* flies. Expatriate workers and others visiting these rural areas are at risk of infection. Infection is often asymptomatic, but understandable alarm may occur when the adult worm migrates under the conjunctiva. Other symptoms include tender swelling over pressure points (Calabar swellings) and joint effusions. Infection can be prevented by avoiding bites of *Chrysops* flies which live in the forest canopy and are attracted by dark colours.

Filarial infection – an overview	
Distribution	Onchocerciasis mainly in localised areas of West Africa. Bancroftian filariasis patchy distribution throughout the region. Loasis confined to jungle areas of West and Central Africa.
Symptoms	Infection with *Onchocerca volvulus* usually asymptomatic. Pruritus most common. *Wuchereria bancrofti* infection associated with fever, lymphadenopathy and cellulitis.
Prevention	Avoid bites of insect vectors.
Treatment	Specific antihelminth therapy available.

Leishmaniasis

Both cutaneous and visceral leishmaniasis are found in SSA. All forms of leishmaniasis are transmitted to man by the bite of female sandflies. Sandflies breed in moist, dark areas, are inactive in bright sunlight and generally bite at night. Measures to prevent sandfly bites, such as adequate evening clothing, bed netting and elevation of bedding, offer protection against *Leishmania* infection.

In SSA, cutaneous leishmaniasis is caused by *Leishmania major* and *Leishmania aethiopia*. The former is widely distributed throughout East and West Africa, and various wild rodents act as a natural reservoir of infection. Unlike infection with *Leishmania tropica*, which is mainly found in urban areas of the Middle East and Asia, *Leishmania major* is a rural disease. Infection of hunters, tourists and others entering endemic areas is common. The lesions of *Leishmania major* are large, wet and often multiple, but rarely disseminate.[11] In contrast, infection with *Leishmania aethiopia* is found in a limited distribution in highland areas of Ethiopia

and Kenya. The natural reservoir of this infection is the rock hyrax. Because opportunity for transmission is infrequent, infection of tourists is rare.

Visceral leishmaniasis (Kala azar) is caused by infection with *Leishmania donovani* and is a common infection in areas of Kenya and Sudan, but is much less frequently found in western African countries. In East Africa, humans are thought to be the only host and direct human-to-human transmission has resulted in large epidemics. However, transmission is generally restricted to isolated locations and consequently infection of tourists rarely occurs. Infection in non-indigenous visitors to endemic areas often presents as an acute illness after an incubation period of 4–6 months. Typical clinical features include a high, remitting fever, without associated rigors, and severe sweats. Progressive illness is associated with the development of significant splenomegaly, hepatomegaly, lymphadenopathy, and if untreated, eventual emaciation and anaemia. However, it is estimated that only 5% of those infected will go on to develop significant disease. It should be remembered that immunosuppressed individuals, (e.g. the HIV infected traveller) are at particular risk of developing serious disease following infection with *Leishmania donovani*.

Visceral leishmaniasis – an overview	
Distribution	Mainly in localised rural areas in Kenya and Sudan.
Symptoms	Prolonged febrile illness. Most common in immunosuppressed traveller.
Prevention	Avoidance of sandfly bites.
Treatment	No emergency measures. Expert advice needed for diagnosis and management.

Infection transmitted by the faecal–oral route

GASTROENTERITIS (see also Ch. 11)

Gastrointestinal infections with bacteria and protozoa are frequent causes of diarrhoeal illness in SSA. Intestinal helminth infestations are also common, but rarely present with diarrhoea. Cholera and *Shigella* dysentery are endemic, and major epidemics occur in situations of socio-economic disorder produced by drought, famine and war. The seventh pandemic of El Tor cholera, which began in Celebes, entered West Africa in the early 1970s and has since spread across the continent from Angola to Tanzania. Epidemics have recently occurred in Sudan, Ethiopia and Rwanda and Zimbabwe.[12] The recent outbreak in Zimbabwe almost certainly began in refugee camps on the Mozambique border, but once introduced spread rapidly throughout the country.[12] Similarly, epidemics of *Shigella dysenteriae* have occurred throughout Central and southern Africa over the last 20 years.[13]

Package holidaymakers visiting established holiday destinations are frequently affected by travellers' diarrhoea. In most instances, this is caused by *enterotoxogenic Escherichia coli* [ETEC] or non-typhoid *salmonellae*. Such episodes are generally self-limiting and of short duration, but can considerably affect the enjoyment of a holiday. Cholera, although a widespread problem in the continent, is a much less frequent problem in this group of travellers. Similarly acute dysentery, caused by *Shigella dysenteriae* and other *Shigella* spp., occurs rarely in package holidaymakers. Prolonged watery diarrhoea, often associated with abdominal pain and bloating, in the returning traveller is often caused by giardiasis.

More adventurous travellers, expatriate workers and, most particularly, aid workers are at considerably greater risk of acquiring infection with *Vibrio cholerae, Shigella* spp. or *Entamoeba histolytica*. Cholera typically presents with high volume fluid stools, while the other two infections cause dysentery. These groups of travellers must be scrupulous in their efforts to avoid unsafe food and water. Consideration may be given to the provision of antibiotics for self-administration in the situation of severe or persistent diarrhoea. This is a particularly useful strategy in immunosuppressed travellers with increased susceptibility to gastrointestinal pathogens. A quinolone is a good, 'first guess' choice as this group of antibiotics has good activity against *salmonellae, shigellae* and

pathogenic *Escherichia coli*. Metronidazole may be needed for suspected amoebiasis or giardiasis. In some circumstances, such as short-term visits to areas where the provision of safe water cannot be ensured, prophylactic antibiotics (trimethoprim or a quinolone) may be considered.

ENTERIC FEVER

Typhoid is a common infection in economically deprived areas of SSA. Large outbreaks occur when water supplies become contaminated with faecal material from a chronic carrier of *Salmonella typhi*.

As with other gastrointestinally-acquired infections, the risk of *Salmonella typhi* infection is greatest in the more adventurous travellers, expatriate workers and especially aid workers. Nevertheless, several effective vaccines are available and all travellers to SSA should probably be advised to be immunised. Standard precautions to avoid infection through contaminated food and water should be employed.

HEPATITIS A

All travellers are at some risk of infection, particularly if they are unable to take adequate precautions with food and drink, and in most cases should be immunised prior to travel using active vaccine. Currently available vaccines are safe and effective, giving 10 years protection after a primary course plus one booster. Passive immunisation with gammaglobulin may be used for individuals in whom active vaccine is inappropriate.

INTESTINAL HELMINTH INFECTION

Ascariasis is endemic in SSA, and in some areas affects up to 90% of the local population. Infection is often asymptomatic, but heavy infection is associated with significant morbidity in children. Transmission is dependent on the ingestion of soil that has been contaminated by human faeces containing ascaris eggs. It is therefore a disease of poverty and poor sanitation.

Short-term visitors to tourist areas are rarely exposed to situations where there is any risk of acquiring infection. Longer-term visitors, and particularly those visiting or residing in endemic rural or urban areas, are at greater risk of acquiring infection. However, infection is rarely, if ever, heavy in the non-indigenous population. Therefore significant symptoms, possibly other than eosinophilic pneumonitis which occurs early in infection, are unlikely to develop. More commonly the passage of an adult worm, often weeks after returning from overseas, alerts the individual to asymptomatic carriage.

Hookworm disease is similarly extremely common throughout SSA. Transmission is also dependent on contamination of soil by permissive defaecation. Consequently, mixed infection with ascariasis, and occasionally other intestinal helminths, is common in children in endemic areas. Heavy infestation results in chronic blood loss and severe iron deficiency anaemia. Bearing in mind the means of transmission, visitors to SSA are rarely at risk of acquiring hookworm infection. A notable exception might be young children of expatriate workers working in rural areas and who are allowed to play barefoot with local children.

As noted above helminth infection in travellers is likely to be asymptomatic, and those individuals thought to be at risk can be easily screened on return.

Sexually transmitted disease (see also Ch. 10)

Sexually transmitted diseases are extremely common throughout SSA. Ulcerative conditions, such as chancroid, genital herpes, donovanosis, lymphogranuloma venereum and syphilis account for up to 70% of attendances at sexually transmitted disease clinics in some African countries. HIV-1 also has a high prevalence in many SSA countries and HIV-2 is found in West Africa. WHO estimates suggest that 21 million African adults and children are infected and living with HIV.[14] In East Africa, with an HIV prevalence of 20%, it is estimated that 75% of all deaths are HIV-related.[14] To underscore these shocking statistics, a recent report from RSA estimates that more than 3 million people were

infected and living with HIV at the end of 1997, and that the figure was likely to rise to 4.5 million by 2005.[15] The human and economic costs are already immense.[15] In Africa, HIV is largely transmitted through heterosexual intercourse, although blood borne infection through contaminated transfusions is also important. Concurrent, genital ulcer disease has been shown to be an important co-factor in HIV transmission.[16] Up to 90% of prostitutes serving popular tourist areas, such as the coastal region of Kenya, may be HIV-infected. Any traveller engaging in casual sexual intercourse must consider themselves at risk of acquiring an STD and/or HIV infection. Indeed, a recent review suggests that the majority of heterosexually infected individuals in England and Wales acquired their infection from abroad (predominantly from Africa).[17]

The sexual behaviour of travellers abroad is reviewed in Chapter 10. Most information is available on the behaviour of young travellers, mainly taking short holidays to well-developed tourist resorts. There is less information on long-term visitors, particularly expatriate workers and those working for intergovernmental agencies who have greatest contact with local communities, and may be at greatest risk of acquiring infection. Visiting servicemen would also appear to be at greater risk.

Hepatitis B may also be acquired sexually, and should be discussed along with other sexually transmitted diseases. The other major risk factor for hepatitis B is through contaminated blood, syringes and other medical instruments, a means of transmission shared with HIV and hepatitis C. A considerable number of UK residents have acquired HIV or viral hepatitis from blood transfusions in African countries. Clearly, travellers need to be alert to the risks of blood-borne viral infection from medical intervention in Africa. Longer-term visitors should carry a medical kit containing sterile needles, syringes and infusion sets. They should avoid blood transfusion if at all possible and have adequate insurance cover which provides immediate repatriation in the event of serious illness.

It is important to emphasise the high prevalence of sexually transmitted diseases, including HIV and hepatitis B, in SSA and the risk of heterosexual transmission to potential travellers. When offering travel advice, it is crucial to stress the dangers of casual sex (particularly with prostitutes) and to urge the regular use of condoms.

Infection transmitted, person to person, through air-borne particles

MENINGOCOCCAL MENINGITIS AND SEPTICAEMIA

Meningococcal disease is endemic throughout most of SSA. Within the 'meningitis belt', that band of land south of the Sahara and north of the tropical rainforest, stretching from Ghana to Ethiopia, major epidemics, affecting up to 100 000 people, occur every 5–10 years. Most outbreaks are due to infection with group A meningococci, although group C meningococci have also been implicated. Respiratory droplets from healthy nasopharyngeal carriers spread meningococcal infection. Transmission requires close physical contact and is greatest in areas of socio-economic deprivation and overcrowding.

Meningococcal infection is of little concern to package holidaymakers visiting established destinations. More adventurous travellers, especially within the 'meningitis belt', are at greater risk and immunisation against group A and C strains is advisable. Expatriate workers, particularly teachers, nurses and others closely involved with the indigenous population, are at greatest risk and vaccination should be strongly encouraged in this group.

DIPHTHERIA

Diphtheria occurs throughout SSA. It is most prevalent in countries where immunisation cover is inadequate. Transmission is mainly by infectious droplet from healthy carriers or cases. Unimmunised travellers may be at risk of infection. Booster doses should be considered for overland traveller and long-term visitors.

TUBERCULOSIS

Tuberculosis is common throughout SSA. In several countries, the incidence of tuberculosis is increasing at alarming rates. Many studies have documented the close association of rising numbers of tuberculosis cases with high HIV prevalence.[18] Indeed, tuberculosis is probably the most common HIV-related opportunistic infection in SSA.

Tuberculosis is only transmitted by droplet nuclei excreted by individuals with active pulmonary tuberculosis. Prolonged (greater than 4 hours) and close contact is required for transmission. Therefore socio-economic deprivation and overcrowding markedly increase risk of transmission. For this reason, visitors to tourist resorts are at a tiny risk of acquiring tuberculous infection. However, long-term visitors, particularly those with close contact with local communities (teachers, nurses, doctors, aid workers), may be at increasing risk of infection. For this group, BCG vaccination is recommended. Attempts should be made to ascertain if BCG was given as part of the routine school immunisations. If so, Mantoux or Heaf testing is not indicated and no further immunisation is required. If there is no documented history of BCG immunisation and no scar on the left deltoid area, then a Mantoux or Heaf test should be performed. An absent cutaneous response suggests no prior exposure to tuberculosis, and BCG vaccination should be given. There is no place for repeating BCG vaccination in individuals with a documented scar from previous vaccination.

Other infectious conditions

SCHISTOSOMIASIS (BILHARZIA)

Schistosomiasis is found throughout SSA. Infections with *Schistosoma haematobium* and *Schistosoma mansoni* are widespread, while infection with *Schistosoma intercalatum* is confined to relatively small areas of West and Central Africa. In many rural areas, microscopic haematuria, indicating urinary tract infection with *Schistosoma haematobium*, can be demonstrated in the majority of children.

Minor infection is usually without symptoms, and only after repeated, heavy infection are significant symptoms and potential severe complications likely to arise.

The life cycle of all species of *Schistosoma* require freshwater snails. When contamination of freshwater with human urine and faeces containing schistosome eggs occurs, miracidia are released from hatched eggs and infect susceptible snails. Within these snails, large numbers of sporocysts develop. Eventually, cercariae, the second larval stage which are infectious to humans, are released from affected snails and swim freely until a suitable host is found. Cercariae die after 2–3 days if no host is found. Contact with contaminated freshwater, through bathing, washing, swimming and drinking, is essential for human infection.

Exposure to contaminated freshwater is essential for the acquisition of schistosomal infection. Consequently, the risk of infection in travellers is limited to certain activities. However, substantial numbers of visitors to SSA acquire this infection.[19,20] Package holidaymakers, who visit only the major towns and safari camps, generally have a low risk of schistosomal infection. Exceptions, however, include the growing numbers of tourists who swim in contaminated freshwater lakes or rivers, or who raft or canoe on the African rivers, such as the Zambezi. Overland travellers, voluntary workers and other longer-term visitors to rural SSA may be at significantly greater risk of infection. The risk of acquiring infection is related to the duration and intensity of exposure to infected water. All river systems and especially lakes and irrigation systems with sluggish flows should be assumed to be a risk for schistosomal infection. Until recently, it was believed that Lake Malawi was free from schistosomiasis, but two reports in 1996 demonstrated a substantial risk from recreational water contact at a resort on the lake.[19,20] A clue to infection is the development of cercarial dermatitis (swimmers itch) within 24 hours of exposure. After a few weeks, a febrile illness characterised by toxaemia, eosinophilia and hepatosplenomegaly may develop (Katayama fever) in a proportion of those infected. Such symptoms, and a history of exposure, should lead to a thorough search for schistosomal infection. Praziquantel is effective therapy for all forms of schistosomiasis.

Travellers who have had recreational water contact should be offered screening for schistosomal infection on return.

Schistosomiasis – an overview	
Distribution	Widespread in lakes and river systems.
Symptoms	Swimmers' itch. Febrile illness. Haematuria.
Prevention	Avoid bathing and other recreational activity in rivers and freshwater lakes.
Treatment	Praziquantil is effective.

Cutaneous conditions

AQUATIC LEECHES

Aquatic leeches are found in freshwater systems throughout SSA. Young leeches can enter the mouth, nostrils and other orifices and attach to mucous membranes. They cause harm through blood loss and obstruction. Avoidance of exposure to freshwater and filtration of drinking water prevents leech infestation.

SUBCUTANEOUS MYIASIS

The tumbu fly is the major cause of subcutaneous myiasis in SSA. The female fly deposits eggs on the ground and on clothing lying on the ground to dry. After hatching, larvae attach to susceptible hosts and penetrate the skin. The developing larva initially produces a papule which develops into a large, boil-like lesion.

Infection is most likely in travellers visiting and residing for a period of time in rural areas. Infection can be prevented by sleeping on a bed elevated from the ground, and thorough drying of clothes on a line in bright light and carefully ironing before wear.

JIGGERS

In flea-infested environments, the adult, female flea attaches and penetrates the skin of the human host.

The feet, and in particular the soles and the toenails, are usually affected. Jiggers occur in socio-economically deprived areas and travellers are unlikely to be affected. The wearing of shoes, rather than open sandals, provides good protection.

CUTANEOUS LARVA MIGRANS

Cutaneous larva migrans (creeping eruption) is common in coastal areas of SSA. Dog and cat hookworm larvae are deposited in moist soil and sand on beaches. Visitors frequenting beaches acquire infection when walking bare foot or sitting in moist sand. The classical itchy migrating lesion is usually found on the foot or the buttock.

RABIES

Rabies is endemic and a rising problem in SSA, although relatively few human cases are reported.[21] The natural reservoir is mainly jackals and other small carnivores. However, the domestic dog appears to play the key role in maintenance and transmission of rabies, and is the main source of human infection. Immunisation should be considered for overland travellers, particularly when remote and inaccessible areas are being visited. Expatriate veterinary workers, and others with occupational risk should be offered vaccination.

SNAKE BITE

Venomous snakes are common throughout SSA, and in some countries snake bite is a common occurrence amongst peasant farmers and other rural workers. Farmers are commonly bitten by carpet vipers or puff adders while working their fields. Spitting cobras may enter homes at night and may strike humans if disturbed.

Tourists are in little danger of snakes. Other visitors should be aware of the dangers of disturbing snakes. When staying overnight in rural areas, they should carry a torch, wear adequate footwear, avoid walking through undergrowth and sleep in a cot raised above ground level. If bitten, the affected limb should be immobilised with a splint or crepe bandage and the individual should be taken urgently to a local hospital. Tourniquets are probably ineffective in preventing systemic envenomation and, if applied too tightly for too long, they can result in irreversible limb ischaemia. For these reasons application of a tourniquet is not advisable. If possible, the responsible snake should be taken to hospital for identification so that specific antivenom may be given.

Summary

Sub-Saharan Africa is an exciting destination which attracts increasing numbers of visitors. The package holidaymaker usually visits established resorts for short periods and is relatively well cushioned from the realities of African life. The business traveller is similarly unlikely to be exposed to exotic conditions. However, all travellers must be alert to the risk of HIV infection. The overland traveller, however, has a far greater risk of exposure to tropical disease. Expatriate workers often live and work for several years under basic conditions in rural areas. The specific requirements needed to remain healthy differ for each group. Priority should be given to malaria prophylaxis. Yellow fever is the only vaccine for which a certificate of vaccination is required for entry to certain countries. Other vaccines, (e.g. polio and tetanus) are generally recommended for all travellers. Typhoid immunisation is generally recommended for all visitors, although the value of this policy has recently been questioned. Hepatitis A immunisation is usually necessary for visits to established tourist areas, and certainly, non-immune individuals visiting poor rural areas for short periods, and all longer-term visitors should be actively or passively immunised. Meningococcal immunisation is not required for package holidaymakers to any part of SSA, but is important in certain high-risk groups visiting countries in the meningitis belt. Hepatitis B immunisation is important for long-term visitors, especially those involved with medical or nursing care.

Discussion of immunisation requirements can sometimes blur the indisputable fact that *Plasmodium falciparum* malaria is, by far, the greatest infectious risk for **all** groups of visitors to SSA. All travellers should be aware of this danger.

They should be advised of the effective measures which are available to avoid mosquito bites as well as the importance of taking antimalarials. Avoidance of mosquito bites will offer additional protection against other infections for which no chemoprophylaxis is available.

Visitors planning to remain in SSA for longer periods should anticipate difficulties in obtaining certain medications. Therefore, those with chronic disorders requiring regular medication should ensure that they take adequate supplies from the UK. It is also advisable for the longer-term visitor to have a supply of antibiotics (a penicillin, a quinolone and metronidazole are most versatile) and, of course, effective antimalarials. They should be aware of the high prevalence of sexually transmitted diseases, and advised on ways to protect themselves from infection. In light of the high HIV prevalence in many African countries, it is also advisable for the longer-term visitors to keep a supply of sterile needles, syringes and giving sets. In the event of accident or serious illness, blood transfusions should be avoided if at all possible.

PRACTICE POINTS

- *Plasmodium falciparum* malaria is the predominant malarial species and is widespread in tropical and sub-tropical regions of Africa throughout the year. The most highly endemic area is West Africa. Volunteers in rural areas and expatriate workers are especially at risk.
- Lassa and other haemorrhagic fevers are very rare in travellers but must be considered as a cause of fever especially in those who have been in rural West and Central Africa.
- Yellow fever is unusual in East Africa and is most common in rural parts of West African countries.
- Lake Malawi is a very common source of schistosomiasis in travellers and is a popular tourist area.
- Tick typhus may occur in travellers to southern African countries who have been walking through scrub land.

- Onchocerciasis is a risk in West Africa and may not present with symptoms for more than a year
- HIV infection is widespread and usually spread heterosexually, although there is also a risk to healthcare workers undertaking surgical procedures.
- Security and personal safety is a problem in many areas and travelling alone at night and in isolated areas is not advised.

REFERENCES

1. Malaria imported into the UK during 1991. CDR Review. 1991; 3(2): 25–28
2. Marsh K. Malaria disaster in Africa. Lancet 1998; 352: 924–925.
3. Bradley DJ, Warhurst DC. Guidelines for the prevention of malaria in travellers from the United Kingdom. CDR Review 1997; 7(10): R137–151.
4. Yellow fever in Kenya. CDR Weekly 1993; 3: 33.
5. Gubler DJ. The global resurgence of arboviral diseases. Transactions 1996; 90: 449–451.
6. ONG ELC. Imported fever from abroad – when to consider VHFs? CME Bulletin of Infectious Diseases and Tropical Medicine 1998; 1: 6–8.
7. World Health Organization. An outbreak of Rift Valley fever, East Africa, 1997–1998. Weekly Epidemiological Record 1998; 73: 105–109.
8. UK Advisory Committee on Dangerous Pathogens. Management and control of viral haemorrhagic fevers. London: HMSO; 1996.
9. Raeber PA, Winteler S, Paget J. Fever in the returned traveller; remember rickettsial disease. Lancet 1994; 344: 331.
10. McCarron B, Clelland SJ, Kennedy D, Pithie A. Visual loss in a returning traveller with tick typhus. Scottish Medical Journal 1998; 43: 116–117.
11. Develoux et al. Diffuse cutaneous leishmaniasis due to *Leishmania major* in Senegal. Transactions 1996; 90: 396–397.
12. Bradley M, et al. Epidemiological features of epidemic cholera [El Tor] on Zimbabwe. Transactions 1996; 90: 378–382.
13. Iversen EF, et al. Epidemic *Shigella dysenteriae* in Mumias, Western Kenya. Transactions 1998; 92: 30–31.
14. UNAIDS. Report on the global HIV/AIDS epidemic. UNAIDS/WHO June 1998.
15. Baleta A. South Africa holds crisis summit on HIV. Lancet 1998; 352: 968.
16. Wasserheit JN. Epidemiological synergy. Interrelationship between human immunodeficiency virus infection and other sexually transmitted diseases. Sexually Transmitted Diseases 1992; 19(2): 61–77.

17. HIV Infection in travellers. CDR Review 1991; 1(4): 39–43.
18. Elliot AM, Hawkins MP. The changing pattern of clinical tuberculosis in the AIDS era: the role for preventive therapy. In: Malin A (ed): Mycobacterial diseases Part I: Clinical frontiers. Baillières Clinical Infectious Diseases 1997; 4(1): 63–76.
19. Day JH, et al. Schistosomiasis in travellers returning from sub-Saharan Africa. British Medical Journal 1996; 313: 267–268.
20. Cetron MS, et al. Schistosomiasis in Lake Malawi. Lancet 1996; 348: 1274–1278.
21. Cleaveland S. The growing problem of rabies in Africa. Transactions 1998; 92: 131–134.

A perspective from the Indian sub-continent

Eric Walker   Santanu Chatterjee

Introduction

The Indian sub-continent includes India, Pakistan, Bangladesh, Sri Lanka and Nepal. All the countries, but especially India and Nepal are popular tourist destinations, both for those on organised tours with a planned itinerary staying in high-class accommodation, and by those intending to be more adventurous. 'Adventure' trips usually involve cheaper accommodation and more opportunities to integrate with the local population. Specialised trips include activity holidays, such as trekking, white-water rafting or canoeing in the Himalayas and there is a developing tourist industry of 'sea and sun', economy package holidays, especially to Goa and Kerala.

Increasingly large numbers of younger visitors travel alone purchasing only their return air flights in advance and then spending months or longer exploring and making all their own accommodation and internal travel arrangements. Frequently they visit adjoining countries like Thailand and Myanmar.

The Indian sub-continent is one of the more industrialised, 'developing' regions of the world and hence there are substantial short-term and long-term business visits. Recent economic liberalisation and relaxation of government regulations have resulted in many international companies relocating expatriate staff and their families to India. Given the tremendous, dynamic, market potential of a 250 million middle class, this largest functioning democracy is attracting many potential investors. Moreover, substantial emigration from the Indian sub-continent to Western countries during the 1950s and 1960s, particularly from the Punjab areas of India and

Pakistan, means that many immigrants return to the region to visit family and friends. This is becoming less so as younger generations of immigrants have fewer direct family connections.

Geographical and sociocultural background

The region has a wide variety of terrain and climate. Lying entirely in the Northern Hemisphere, the mainland covers an area of 3 287 273 km² with a land frontier of 15 200 km. The Himalayas in the north comprise three, almost parallel, ranges interspersed with valleys and plateaux extending over 2400 km and include the highest mountain peaks in the world at permanent sub-zero temperatures. They form a natural border separating India from China. The rain-laden clouds of the south-west monsoon are confined to these ranges and forced to condense over the Gangetic plains. In the south, the land is mostly flat with outcrops of rocks and a few mountain ranges. This area known as the Deccan peninsula is separated from the Indo-Gangetic plains by rocky valleys and bounded by the Eastern and Western Ghats which are low-lying, rounded hills running parallel to the east and west coasts. Being near the equator, temperatures can vary from comfortably warm to unbearably hot. The Great Northern plains extend across the breadth of the country. They are formed by basins of three distinct river systems – the Indus, the Ganga and the Brahmaputra which is one of the most densely-populated areas in the world. The Great Indian desert in the north-west comprises huge stretches of desert in between rocky wasteland and limestone ridges. Rainfall is dominated by monsoons which come from the south-west between May and July and from the north-east between October and December. The south-west or summer monsoon blows from sea to land and brings most of the rainfall whereas the north-east monsoon blows from land to sea and brings rainfall mostly to the southern peninsula. Much of the local lifestyle revolves around water either because of shortage or, in some areas like the north-east, from flooding.

The climate can broadly be described as tropical monsoon. There are four seasons – winter (January to February), hot weather summer (March to May), rainy south-western monsoon (June to September) and post-monsoon (October to December), which is also known as north-east monsoon in the Deccan Peninsula. The whole region, except for the mountains and a few deserts, are heavily populated. For example, according to the last census in 1991, the population of India was 846.3 million. A more recent estimate in 1994–5 was 915.9 million with an increase of 17 million every year. India is the second most populous country and accounts for 16% of the world's population but has only 2.42% of the total world area. The majority are deeply religious which has direct influence on daily life and moral attitudes: Buddhism predominates in Nepal; in Bangladesh and Pakistan, most are Moslems; in India and Nepal, the majority are Hindu. In India, there is substantial Moslem influence in the north and a small Christian presence in the south. In Nepal, there are Buddhists, especially towards Tibet.

The diversity in culture, people and language is unique. One interesting feature is the coexistence of the traditional with the contemporary. Many centuries seem to exist side by side. There are very obvious extremes of affluence and poverty which many visitors find difficult to adjust to. Cities have a highly urbanised social structure with modern amenities and a hectic, stressful lifestyle. In comparison, life in rural India has a slow, easy pace which has not changed over years and is characterised by a traditional, agriculture-based economy and low levels of productivity. Poverty and unemployment in rural areas lead to increasing urban migration. This results in a burgeoning slum population and puts considerable pressure on the already overstretched, urban, civic infrastructure. Poor accessibility to healthcare in this marginalised group further contributes to the problem. Visitors because of transport, accommodation and language difficulties infrequently explore truly rural areas. In the villages, poverty is frequently less obvious because traditional social structures provide family and social support. However, in the city slums, thefts and begging are frequently encountered.

All travellers will experience some form of culture shock from the constant, human activity, noise, dust and frequently, very obvious human and animal excrement and open sewers.

In most parts, including cities, animals mix closely with the human population. Cattle wander the streets during the day scavenging for food and returning to their owners at night. Dogs frequently with only temporary owners wander around often in poor states of health. In rural areas, rodents, snakes and scorpions usually cause more anxiety than any associated health risks warrant.

Those staying in good or luxury hotel accommodation can expect clean surroundings and reliable food but they must be conscious of hygiene risks when venturing out. Water should always be considered unsafe to drink unless reliably bottled, boiled or filtered. Swimming pools should be treated with caution and the water not swallowed.

Public transport is cheaply available and often exciting. It ranges from reliable trains where seats are normally booked in advance, to busy buses that run frequently in all directions. Indian roads teem with cycles, handcarts, motorcycles, cars and buses. Moreover, cows and pedestrians compete for the same space causing driving to be a daunting experience for the unprepared. Accidents on the road are common and many visitors find the speed of transport in rural parts alarming. When planning a travel itinerary, it is wise to allow three or four times the time that you might allow at home because of delays, breakdowns and traffic jams.

Politically, India is a union of 26 states and 6 union territories with a central government in New Delhi and state governments in each of the states. The President is the constitutional head and exercises political functions only on the advice of the Council of Ministers which consists of elected representatives and is headed by the Prime Minister. India is a secular country with no official religion. The constitution grants certain fundamental rights to the people including freedom of expression, occupation, religion, culture and education.

Social adaptation problems

Many visitors are overwhelmed by constant 'new images' which include noise, 'hustle and bustle', climate, transport, food, smells, dust and dirt, lack of toilet facilities, animals and insects. Many find being approached by beggars distressing. Adjusting to the haunting spectre of poverty is difficult. It is not uncommon for new visitors, especially if they have no local personal contacts, to spend much time in their hotel, venturing out only for brief explorations, perhaps overindulging in alcohol and taking risks with food, water and hygiene which they might not do in more familiar surroundings. People are naturally curious and visitors may find themselves being stared at with uninhibited curiosity and crowded around especially in smaller cities and towns. For the uninitiated, such a close physical proximity may seem uncomfortable.

On the whole, visitors are treated by locals with great respect and often overwhelming hospitality. Given the extensive economic links with foreign traders over centuries, Indians have never suffered from xenophobia. Traditionally, the guest is always welcomed and honoured. It is a privilege within Hindu circles to entertain guests and it may cause distress if guests offer money in return. English, which is included under the Official Language Act 1963, is widely spoken by an estimated 28 million people in the country. Since English is accepted as the language of business and communication, visitors may find that they are included in animated discussions with total strangers. Politics and religion are hotly debated issues and conversation remains part-ritual and part-entertainment.

Except in the few supermarkets, bargaining is normal when making purchases. It is a way of establishing the best possible price and involves some amount of pre-negotiation planning, considerable patience and a sense of humour. Malicious bribery should be politely refused.

It may be wise to take care when giving to beggars, since there are professional begging groups, particularly in cities, which may use self-inflicted injuries as bait or young children as 'go betweens'. Many travellers therefore prefer to make donations to recognised charities or buy handicrafts from organisations involved in social welfare. Attacks on foreigners are very rare, although occasionally mugging is reported. Pickpocketing and petty thefts are problems in the crowded markets. It may be wise to avoid travelling alone at night in taxis, especially for single women in big cities. Depending on the outlook and attitude, the sub-continent can present a unique, once-in-a-lifetime opportunity to experience a fascinating culture. Thus, a positive attitude is essential to overcome the initial culture shock often experienced by newcomers.

Available medical care

The standard of medical care is of prime concern, particularly for the elderly and in those accompanied by young children. Children adapt much quicker than adults but are particularly prone to stomach and respiratory infections. Medical care can vary from excellent to very poor, but overall the standard of medical proficiency is high with a good choice of physicians available. Many of them are trained abroad and any criticism regarding the level of medical care is usually confined to the general hospital environment and aftercare, the standard of which may not conform to Western expectations. Frequently drugs, normally only available on prescription in the UK, can be obtained over the counter in chemists, including many antibiotics and antimalarials. Pharmacists are general practitioners, although the appropriateness of certain remedies may sometimes be questioned.

Many visitors needing medical attention go to private clinics which are found in most cities and small towns which often offer an excellent service. They usually have friendly and helpful staff. It is however important to differentiate those providing only outpatient care and diagnostics from the ones having indoor facilities. Some clinics are equipped to handle emergencies and often one needs to buy the prescribed medicines from local chemists since a dispensing service may be unavailable. It is worthwhile requesting a 'cash memo' when purchasing such medications. The costs of medical care may be small compared with private clinics at home but comprehensive health insurance should always be obtained prior to travel. Physicians and hospitals often expect cash payment for services rendered. Medical care can often be arranged through hotel receptions, travel agents, tourist offices or by explaining the problem to English-speaking staff in the bigger shops, post offices or government hospitals. Missionary hospitals usually provide a standardised level of care and personal recommendations from local expatriates are often helpful.

Care should be taken to ensure, if possible, that sterile needles are always used (disposables can often be bought) and that any blood transfusions have been adequately screened for HIV and hepatitis B which is not always done although legally it is required. There is a real concern about the quality of blood supplies and most embassies usually have a list of expatriate blood donors in case of need. Major dental treatment should be done on return home.

Modern amenities are generally available in most urban centres. People are warm and friendly and the lifestyle usually relaxed. English is spoken and understood by most educated Indians. The markets are a shoppers' paradise and display a wide range of affordable merchandise. Supermarkets are relatively uncommon and daily provisions are usually available at the local bazaar. For the spouse, managing children, domestic staff and the household needs patience and resilience. The cost of living is low compared with European standards. Though accommodation is available, finding something acceptable can be time-consuming and occasionally frustrating. Rental costs differ greatly between regions and can be prohibitive in certain cities like New Delhi and Mumbai. Premiums are expected for proximity to commercial centres, schools and shopping complexes. Hotels and clubs offer a wide range of leisure facilities and provide ample scope for fitness activities and general socialising. Temporary membership can easily be arranged. Golf, tennis and cricket are popular outdoor sports. Weekends are relaxing and balance the stressful work environment. The country abounds in numerous palaces, temples, forests, beaches and forts and offers exciting vacation options for those interested in history and heritage. Most importantly, working in the sub-continent, provides a unique opportunity to observe a fascinating and vibrant culture.

Working in India

For many, working in India can be a challenging and memorable experience. Technical expertise, cultural sensibility, adaptability and flexibility are essential personal attributes for those intending to work here. Previous relevant experience in a developing country is desirable. Family support is a great help and relocating expatriate staff accompanied by a spouse or partner is preferable to a single status assignment since this offers a greater degree of stability and lessens the sense of isolation. Given the choice, cultural awareness briefings and pre-assignment visits often help to provide a balanced picture of daily life.

Health problems the traveller may encounter and their management

1. Psychological and social adaptation can be helped by the traveller being prepared in advance for the almost inevitable 'culture shock'. A carefully planned itinerary will help reduce undue stress caused by too much travelling. It is advisable to allocate some time for relaxation around the end of the first week, if possible, especially for commercial delegations and cultural groups with fairly complex and extended itineraries. Excessive exposure to heat and unfamiliar, unhygienic accommodation may worsen adaptation. Local

customs should be respected and it is best to avoid becoming frustrated when things do not turn out as expected. The traveller on a tight budget should take sufficient emergency funds to cover good medical care if this is needed and also an occasional 'convalescent' night in good hotel accommodation can help those 'roughing it' when exhaustion sets in.

2. Those trekking at high altitudes in the Himalayas should ascend slowly to avoid developing altitude sickness and should understand emergency treatment should it occur. Heat exhaustion is common, especially during the first 2 or 3 weeks of a visit and can be reduced by drinking copious fluids and adding additional salt to meals. It is common for people to feel unexpectedly 'faint' owing to vasodilation after physical exertion. Air-conditioned rooms at night can be especially helpful for short-term visits when acclimatisation is impossible. Sunbathing, especially around noon, can be dangerous in the tropics. It is normal practice to stay indoors or in the shade during the hottest times of the day. Just 20 minutes' unprotected sunbathing in Goa at midday, for example, can incapacitate the traveller for days.

3. Diarrhoea and vomiting are by far the most common illnesses encountered. This is not always due to infection and can be brought on by unfamiliar oily or spicy foods. Dehydration on arrival (after inadequate fluid intake during a prolonged air flight) followed by the hot climate can cause constipation.

Enterotoxigenic *Escherichia coli* (ETEC) are the commonest infective cause of travellers' diarrhoea followed by *Shigella* and amoebic dysentery. Non-vegetarians may contract *Campylobacter* or salmonellosis from poorly cooked meats. Water-borne infections including cholera are most common during the monsoons when contamination of drinking supplies is more likely.

Cholera is rarely diagnosed amongst travellers, perhaps, because it is most frequently associated with poverty, heavily contaminated water and is due to an organism usually killed easily with all the traditional ways of sterilising such as heat and chlorine.

Of more insidious onset is giardiasis. This is extremely common among longer-stay travellers in the Indian sub-continent, probably because it is contracted through cysts in food and water, can be passed on through contaminated eating utensils and is resistant to many sterilising methods. Giardiasis causes nausea, anorexia and abdominal discomfort after food. It is associated with frothy, unpleasant-smelling motions, normally only passed a few times each day, often in the morning. These features distinguish a giardiasis infection from others previously mentioned, which usually cause acute watery diarrhoea.

FIRST-AID FOR DIARRHOEA

As diarrhoea is so common among travellers to this part of the world, carrying emergency treatment is a wise precaution. Antidiarrhoeals such as Immodium or Lomotil are especially helpful in relieving colic. Rehydration is essential, particularly with young children, and if vomiting makes this impossible for any prolonged period, medical attention should be sought. Rehydrating fluids should be sterile and contain approximately 1 flat teaspoon of salt per litre plus sugar and flavouring. Coconut milk is a local favourite – it is normally sterile and contains a balance of electrolytes. Banana, soups, salted crackers, tea and toast are reasonable diet alternatives when recovering from diarrhoea when fatty foods may prolong the symptoms.

Antibiotics such as the 8-aminoquinolones can shorten illnesses due to *Escherichia coli*, *Shigella* and possibly *Salmonella*. Most shigellosis in India is now resistant to co-trimoxazole. Persistent diarrhoea, especially if associated with fever and blood and mucous in the stools, may be due to amoebiasis and should respond quickly to metronidazole or imidazole (as does giardiasis, although repeated courses may be necessary). Some travellers carry small supplies of these drugs in their first-aid kit and should be advised carefully on indications for their use.

Other faecal–oral infections such as typhoid, poliomyelitis and hepatitis A are rare among travellers who are adequately immunised. Imported cases of these illnesses often occur in immigrant families visiting their country of origin when immunisations have not been considered.

4. Of insect-borne diseases, the most important life-threatening infection remains malaria (see Ch. 13) but an increasing problem in the sub-continent is dengue. This causes fever, muscle aches and pains and sometimes serious haemorrhagic complications. It is most common in the north-east. Since there is no available vaccination against dengue, its presence is another reason for giving special attention to avoiding mosquito bites. Treatment of the infection is symptomatic and directed towards preventing complications. Japanese B encephalitis is also spread through mosquitoes and the illness is endemic throughout India although less common in Pakistan and the north-west (Punjab regions) of India. Epidemics occur every year in the low-lying plains (Terrai) of Nepal. Mortality and morbidity from this disease are high, especially in children.

A lot of morbidity from mosquito bites is due to local skin hypersensitivity to their saliva and secondary infection of the bite area. Hypersensitivity is difficult to treat, but tends to resolve after a month or two of exposure. Antihistamines seem to have little effect, and prevention of bites is therefore of utmost importance for those known to have this problem. Secondary infection may need treatment with local, and sometimes systemic, antibiotics.

Longer-stay travellers and those living in poorer accommodation may contract skin and head lice or scabies. Spraying insecticides under the mattress and on 'the bathroom corners' is suggested. Itching is a common symptom and treatment is normally straightforward with skin insecticides. Conjunctivitis can be spread by eye flies and is most common during the dry seasons.

A localised, indurated, slow-growing skin lesion is characteristic of dermal leishmaniasis, most common in Pakistan and north-west India. Systemic leishmaniasis causing a serious febrile illness with anaemia and hepatosplenomegaly occasionally occurs in eastern India.

5. Respiratory tract problems such as asthma and bronchitis, aggravated by heat and dust, are common and there is no shortage of respiratory tract infections such as colds and influenza that occur mostly during the cooler months from November to February. Pollution is a major problem and many visitors develop a cough or itching in the throat upon arrival. Salt-water gargles and throat lozenges offer partial relief. Persons suffering atopic asthma should carry an adequate stock of inhalers since exacerbations are known to occur. Tuberculosis is extremely common as is reflected in the high incidence of this disease among immigrants to the UK. Surprisingly, it is seen infrequently in travellers to the sub-continent, perhaps because of the relative shortness of their stays, usually transient contact with the local community and previous BCG vaccination.

6. In long-term expatriates, substantial weight loss can be due to a variety of causes including diet, chronic intestinal infections and occasionally illnesses such as tropical sprue which normally warrants specialised medical care. Weight loss often improves rapidly after a traveller returns home and if this is not the case, it should be investigated.

7. There is a growing sex industry, mainly in bigger cities. It is not always as obvious as in some other parts of the Far East. Sex-workers are often illiterate and suffer from a variety of sexually transmitted diseases including HIV and some studies report that up to 60% of prostitutes are affected. In addition to 'red light' districts, advances may be made to tourists in hotels although this more particularly applies to the local travelling business communities.

Points for the traveller to consider prior to departure

CLOTHING

Apart from specialist equipment needed for adventure holidays, most items can be purchased easily and cheaply if required on arrival. Preparation should take into account the need to cover as much of the body as possible, especially after dark to prevent mosquito bites. The traveller wishing to respect local traditions should cover shoulders and legs with loosely fitting clothes which is also advised for female travellers who do not want to invite excessive attention, particularly if travelling alone. It should also be remembered that light cotton fabrics can become transparent in bright sunlight! Although open sandals are comfortable and airy, there are times when more solid footwear may help to avoid injuries, mosquito bites and excessive contact with dirt and excrement. Shoes are frequently removed when entering houses, for hygienic reasons. Although in the south, warm clothing is rarely required, nights can be unexpectedly cold in the north during the 'winter' months of December and January.

MONEY AND INSURANCE

Comprehensive travel insurance is essential and additional cover for medical evacuations, if the situation arises, is a definite necessity. It is important to choose insurance companies which not only assist in locating and evaluating medical care but also provide cover for trip interruption, baggage loss and make arrangements for direct payment of hospital bills. Travellers should remember that medical care can only be as good as the facilities available.

Local currency can only be obtained after arrival. Travellers' cheques can be encashed at most major cities with the branches of international banking groups usually providing more efficient services. Occasional cash dispensers are available in bigger cities. Credit cards are now widely used in larger shops and hotels. International telephone calls are expensive from hotels since taxes are levied. Reasonable rates for such calls are often found at STD/ISD telephone booths that are government-licensed but operated by private individuals.

FOOD AND WATER HYGIENE

The traveller should carry some means of sterilising water (unless only staying in 5-star hotels and not travelling far from base) and care should be taken to confirm food is freshly prepared and to avoid risky salads and unpeeled fruit. Bottled water is usually available in cities and tourist hotels. The purity of bottled water is doubtful in certain situations. Portable water filters are advisable especially for those travelling for extended periods under difficult circumstances.

MOSQUITO PRECAUTIONS

No antimalarial chemoprophylaxis is fully effective and there are other serious diseases spread by mosquitoes such as dengue for which there are no vaccines or effective chemoprophylaxis. Barrier prevention such as sensible clothing, repellents and mosquito nets are essential equipment for the self-organised traveller staying in basic accommodation. Mosquito repellents in cream, spray or roll-on formulations can be procured locally. Early morning golf or an evening out on the lawns of the hotel are ideal situations for mosquito bites.

FIRST-AID KIT

A good first-aid kit including sterile syringes and needles is important for the more adventurous traveller since there may be difficulty in obtaining these in an emergency. The first-aid kit should include emergency treatment for skin infections, antidiarrhoeals and possibly antibiotics to be used in clearly defined circumstances after discussion with your doctor. Sunscreens and blocks are essential for sunbathers as they are for mountaineers. Rehydrating fluids can be prepared locally or by using tablets or sachets.

VACCINATIONS (see also Ch. 12)

All travellers to the Indian sub-continent should be up to date with vaccinations for life in the UK. They should make sure that they have had boosters of polio, tetanus and diphtheria vaccines within 10 years and BCG is a wise precaution, especially for children. In particular, it prevents miliary and meningitic disease. Tuberculosis is extremely common in this part of the world and is likely to become more so with the spread of AIDS.

Typhoid vaccination is important although it must be remembered that this does not cover the rarer paratyphoid infections.

Hepatitis A is an extremely common endemic infection to which most of the local population is 'naturally' immune as a result of usually asymptomatic infection by the age of 10 years and vaccination of visitors is recommended.

Hepatitis B is rare in travellers who take care to avoid unhygienic injections and unsafe sexual practices; however, long-stay visitors may wish to be immunised because 2–5% of the local population carry HBsAg. Vaccination is important for at-risk occupational groups such as doctors, nurses and volunteers intending to join social welfare projects or providing healthcare in mission hospitals. Visitors contemplating acupuncture therapy should also be vaccinated.

Meningococcal A and C vaccine is probably overused as there is little evidence of outbreaks in the Indian sub-continent caused by type A and C strains. The disease is very unusual in the southern parts of the sub-continent. A few tourists in Nepal were infected during an outbreak in 1986 and although no outbreak has occurred since, it may be prudent to immunise travellers going on treks and away from immediate medical care. Yellow fever vaccination is only mandatory for travellers arriving or in transit from endemic countries in Africa and South America.

Japanese B encephalitis vaccine should be considered for those staying primarily in rural areas or for prolonged periods, or in accommodation that is not likely to offer effective mosquito protection. The vaccine is not freely available in the sub-continent. Japanese B encephalitis is endemic in India, low-lying parts of Nepal and in Bangladesh, although it is less common in Pakistan, the Punjab areas of India and is rare in the Highlands of Nepal. Outbreaks do occur, in low-lying eastern areas of Nepal and in the north-east and western parts of India following the monsoon in June to September. In other parts of the country, sporadic outbreaks occur but are less predictable. The virus is maintained in nature by the bird–mosquito–ovid cycle with pigs acting as the amplifier host. Herons and egrets are commonly implicated and the mosquito predominantly breeds in rice fields or large water surfaces.

Rabies is widespread among both wild and domestic animals. There is a large, roaming dog population, both in rural and urban areas. The disease affects all mammals although dogs are the main source of human cases because of their frequent contact with people in populated areas where they scavenge and are kept in houses as pets. Monkeys are another common source of rabies and they are usually found in aggressive groups, foraging for food, around temples. Bites

from cats, jackals, mongooses and sometimes rats are other sources of human infections. Although recorded cases of rabies in travellers are rare the majority of cases imported into the UK have been contracted in the Indian sub-continent.

Post-exposure vaccine should be started within 24 hours of a bite or lick on broken skin or mucous membrane and should ideally be given with rabies hyperimmune globulin. The only vaccine widely used in the region for post-exposure is the traditional, inactivated, neural tissue vaccine (Semple) manufactured in goats and sheep. Although this is cheap and affordable, the vaccine is not of the same proven efficacy as some more modern vaccines and involves a series of 2–5 mL injections. The purified chick embryo and the vero cell vaccine are available at cost in most cities. To avoid a usually fruitless search for rabies hyperimmune globulin and modern vaccines, it is now common to advise pre-exposure vaccination for those travelling outside main cities so long as this can be done without prohibitive cost. Pre-exposure vaccination can also avoid the anxiety and panic that may follow an 'at-risk' situation, even though the likelihood of the offending animal being infected is small. Booster(s) can then be sought calmly over the next few days and there is no need for hyperimmune globulin.

MALARIA PREVENTION (see also Ch. 13)

The risk from malaria in the Indian sub-continent is not as high as in Africa. The disease was almost eradicated 20 years ago but has since spread again into all areas and there is an increasing incidence of malignant *Plasmodium falciparum* cases, especially in the north and east of India.

Those flying straight into the Himalayas, above 2000 m (including Kathmandu) are not normally at risk unless they then travel into more low-lying areas. Overall, malaria is endemic in the sub-continent except for mountainous regions and the Ladshadweep islands. Some isolated coastal areas around the Western Ghats and the Andaman and Nicobar islands have low transmission.

The majority of infections contracted in this region are due to *Plasmodium vivax*, although in some parts up to 35% are now due to *Plasmodium falciparum*. It must be remembered that prophylaxis will not prevent *Plasmodium vivax* infections with a prolonged hypnozoite phase, which may result in symptoms, after prophylaxis has been discontinued.

Every year officially approximately 2 million new cases are reported. Actual estimates however are 10 to 15 times higher. The incidence increases following the monsoons when there are many pools of rain water which allow breeding sites for the anopheline mosquito. Urban malaria is the major problem with 15 major cities contributing 80% of the urban malaria cases. Migration of labour, emergence of insecticide resistance and rapid urbanisation contribute to this phenomenon. The north-western plains, the semi-arid climatic zone with annual rainfall up to 100 mm and the Indo-Gangetic plains in the north-east are the major epidemic areas. Transmission begins with the onset of monsoon rains in mid-June. Initially, *Plasmodium vivax* predominates, while *Plasmodium falciparum* cases are increasingly reported from August onwards, rising to a peak around September and then declining with the onset of winter in December. Desert areas of Rajasthan which were traditionally non-endemic are now reporting *Plasmodium falciparum* cases. This results from a marshy environment conducive to mosquito breeding created by unseasonal rainfall and increasing irrigation activities.

Since chloroquine-resistant *Plasmodium falciparum* has been observed in most areas, chloroquine plus proguanil is still the recommended regime together with careful precautions to avoid mosquito bites and being aware of the need for prompt treatment. The level of resistance is not yet high enough to warrant the use of mefloquine as first-line choice. If the traveller is intolerant of these drugs taken together, one of them taken alone will often give substantial protection. Compliance with the taking of antimalarials among budget travellers is poor. They usually discontinue the advised drugs either because of confusion arising from alternate regimens among co-travellers or because of perceived uselessness. There are few parts of the sub-continent where the traveller will be away from medical care, therefore emergency stand-by treatment is rarely essential. Those who are passing through malarious areas on their way to remote parts of the Himalayas, may be wise to carry a course of self-treatment as described in Chapter 13. Note that proguanil cannot be obtained in the Indian sub-continent.

PRACTICE POINTS

- The Indian sub-continent includes India, Pakistan, Bangladesh and Nepal.
- Roads are often crowded and accidents common.
- Diarrhoea in travellers is very common.
- Extreme economic and social contrasts, heat, changes in food, hygiene, mosquitoes and crowds make culture shock almost inevitable for the first-time traveller.
- HIV is becoming widespread especially among commercial sex-workers and other high-risk groups.
- Rabies is common in animals and modern vaccines may be difficult to obtain in an emergency.
- Trekking in Nepal is very popular and altitude acclimatisation problems can occur.
- Good healthcare is available but advice on where to go should be sought from reliable sources.
- India is one of the most popular destinations for travellers from the UK. It has been said that 50% cannot wait to return, the other 50% would not want to go back but the experience always 'changes you'!

FURTHER READING

Bell DR. Lecture notes on tropical diseases. 4th ed. Oxford: Blackwell Science; 1995. An excellent introduction to tropical diseases, their clinical aspects and prevention.

Center for Disease Control and Prevention. Health information for international travel. Atlanta: International Medical Publishing.

International Society of Travel Medicine 'News Shares' have included useful contributions from India on accidents and malaria in cities.

'Lonely Planet' guides to India, Pakistan and Nepal are very useful sources of general reading about the sub-continent.

Neuman K. Illness from water-related recreational activities. Travel Medicine International 1996; 14 (Mar/Apr): 69–73.

Walker E, Williams GR, Raeside F, Calvert L. The 'ABC' of healthy travel. 5th ed. London: British Medical Journal; 1997.

World Health Organization. International travel and health – vaccination requirements and health advice. Geneva: WHO.

UK Departments of Health. Immunisation against infectious diseases. (The 'green book'.) London: HMSO; 1996.

A perspective from South and Central America

G. B. Wyatt

Introduction

For many short-term travellers who live under good conditions in South American cities, the risks will chiefly be of mugging, road accidents, sexually-transmitted diseases and from previous medical conditions. Only basic updates of childhood immunisation, cover for hepatitis A and for some areas yellow fever immunisation are needed. Backpackers and other adventurous tourists, especially those travelling to Amazonia, will need careful evaluation, advice, malaria prophylaxis and a range of immunisations which are likely to include yellow fever, typhoid, rabies and meningococcal meningitis. Visitors to the Andes should be educated about the hazards of altitude sickness.

Introduction

Conditions in South America vary enormously from highly sophisticated city environments, especially in the south of the continent, to areas where health hazards are considerable as in parts of the Amazon basin. This is the region where there is most concern about infections such as yellow fever and malaria.

Even in cities, the rapid growth of population and the influx of people from rural areas has led to large 'septic fringes' or favellas where basic services are lacking and communicable disease is rife. For wealthy travellers to major cities, communicable diseases are not a great problem but risks from mugging or accidents are always present

and are a worldwide problem wherever poverty comes face to face with affluence.

For the backpacker in more remote rural areas, a wide range of communicable diseases warrants careful preventive measures and take care to avoid physical dangers such as water hazards and bites from venomous animals.

Many tourists and scientists visit the Andes mountain range along the west side of the continent where acute mountain sickness is a real possibility. Some flights land directly from overseas into cities at high altitude when the symptoms may not be recognised for what they are.

Gastrointestinal infections

Travellers' diarrhoea is common and such colourful names as Montezuma's revenge are used. Enterotoxogenic *Escherichia coli* (ETEC) are the most frequent cause, especially during the rainy season, but *Giardia* and *Shigella* species are also common. While careful hygiene is the chief preventive measure needed, treatment with antibiotics will quite often be required. There is evidence that trimethoprim plus sulphamethoxazole is effective in interior Mexico during the rainy summer months[1] whereas in other areas an 8-aminoquinolone is more likely to be successful.

Cholera was absent from South America this century until it was newly introduced into Peru in 1991. It has subsequently caused epidemics in most countries in South and Central America. Peru, Ecuador, Colombia and north-east Brazil have been particularly affected. The predominant organism is

El Tor, serotype Inaba. The disease is not a major hazard for the tourist who is prepared to take sensible hygienic precautions with food and drink.

Cholera immunisation certificates are now no longer officially required by any country. It is essential that the traveller is aware that the level of protection from immunisation is minimal. It is not now normally available in the UK.

Typhoid is a problem in some areas. In 1975–84, North American travellers to Peru with an incidence rate of 174 cases/million were at greater risk than elsewhere.[2] In the contrast, typhoid is said to be uncommon in Argentina but food-borne salmonellosis is frequent. The risk of antibiotic-resistant strains of *Salmonellae* should also be considered.

Amoebiasis is widespread and should be considered in travellers returning with bloody diarrhoea, prolonged fever or liver pain.

Soil-transmitted helminths including *Ascaris*, *Trichuris*, *Strongyloides* and hookworms are quite common.

Viral hepatitis

Hepatitis A transmission is relatively high throughout the region and most travellers will require protection with active vaccine or if this is contraindicated, pooled immunoglobulin.

Hepatitis B and delta hepatitis are commonest in the Amazon region. Risks of transmission are chiefly from sex and shared needles. Hepatitis B immunisation should be considered for people expecting to spend prolonged periods (e.g. more than 6 months) in South America as well as those who may otherwise be at high risk.

Arthropod-borne infections

Malaria is widespread in the northern half of South America and *Plasmodium falciparum*, *vivax* and *malariae* infections are all present. Chile and Uruguay are malaria-free and Argentina only has malaria in the northern provinces of Salta and Jujuy. Brazil is free of malaria along the south-eastern coastal areas, including the cities of Rio de Janeiro,

Sao Paulo and Belo Horizonte. Amazonia has a considerable malaria problem including chloroquine- and Fansidar-resistant *Plasmodium falciparum* infections. The risk is highest in gold mining and new, agricultural settlements. Mefloquine is the first choice for prophylaxis in the Amazon basin. Chloroquine plus proguanil are sufficient in some rural areas west of the Andes. Areas in the Andes above 1500 m are usually malaria-free (see also Ch. 13).

American trypanosomiasis (Chagas' disease) is spread by contamination of mucosae or bites with the faeces of cone-nosed bugs infected with the metacyclic forms of trypanosomes. The triatomine bugs live in cracks in mud walls or in vegetation and seek blood at night. Blood transfusion is another important method of transmission. Chagas' disease exists in all the countries of South America but there is considerable progress in its eradication. Tourists living rough are at risk but can be protected by the use of insecticide-impregnated bed nets.

Leishmaniasis exists in three main clinical forms. Travellers are most likely to be infected with cutaneous leishmaniasis and present with slowly evolving skin ulcers. There is always the concern that skin leishmaniasis may lead on to the destructive mucocutaneous variety associated with *Leishmania braziliensis* infections. For this reason, accurate diagnosis and full treatment of skin leishmanial lesions acquired in South America are important. Visceral leishmaniasis is chiefly endemic in north-east Brazil but there are foci in Venezuela and Colombia and rarely elsewhere. Prevention of all these varieties of leishmaniasis depends upon avoiding bites of Phlebotamine sandflies by the use of protective clothing, repellents and insecticide-impregnated bed nets.

Bartonellosis or Oroya fever is another sandfly-transmitted infection caused by the bacterium *Bartonella bacilliformis*. It is confined to certain valleys on the western slopes of the Andes and presents with fever, bone pains and anaemia or sometimes with a miliary or nodular skin eruption. It is rare in expatriate travellers.

Yellow fever exists chiefly as a zoonosis of rodents with fatal epizootics in monkeys in the tropical forests. Small outbreaks occur amongst people working in the forests and bitten by the vectors, *Haemagogus* mosquitoes. There have been recent fatal cases in tourists to the areas. Where *Aedes* mosquitoes breed in urban areas, there is always the risk of major human epidemics from introduced yellow fever. Travellers entering the endemic areas of Brazil and the other northern countries, up as far as Panama, should be fully immunised.

Dengue is found chiefly in the northern countries of South America, Central America and the Caribbean. It is spread by *Aedes* mosquitoes. Dengue haemorrhagic fever is unlikely to occur in the traveller experiencing dengue for the first time. Other causes of haemorrhagic fever, not strictly owing to arboviruses, should be borne in mind. They include Argentinean haemorrhagic fever caused by Junin virus which is transmitted from rodents either directly or by food contamination in the pampas area north-west of Buenos Aires, and Bolivian haemorrhagic fever caused by Machupo virus in rural, north-east Bolivia. This is also transmitted from rodents.

Equine encephalitis including Western Equine, Eastern Equine and Venezuelan Equine varieties are all transmitted by various varieties of culicine mosquitoes and occasionally affect travellers. This is yet one more good reason for protective measures against mosquito bite.

Bubonic plague occurs in small outbreaks in Peru, Brazil, Bolivia and Ecuador, but will rarely be a danger to tourists.

Rabies

Rabies is present both in the dog population throughout the region and in bats in South America. Vampire bats (*Desmodus rotundus*) are known to transmit rabies to cattle and humans. Bats with the virus remain healthy. Rabies has even been recorded in people visiting a bat-infested cave but who were not bitten; presumably infection was from inhalation of the virus. Rabies infection from bats often produces a paralytic rather than a furious presentation of disease. Pre-exposure rabies immunisation should be considered for long-term residents and for shorter-term travellers who will be remote from good health facilities.

Venomous bites

Although there are many highly venomous snakes in tropical South America, most tourists are at very low risk. The use of protective boots and a torch at night are important for adventurous hikers. Scorpions, leeches, aggressive bees and poisonous spiders could also be encountered.

Skin problems

The usual problems of sunburn, prickly heat, pyogenic infection, superficial fungal infection and scabies may all present in travellers. Larva migrans infections are common in people who have walked barefoot on beaches in Venezuela and elsewhere. Myiasis is most often due to *Dermatobia hominis* which exists throughout the area, but is particularly prevalent on the eastern slopes of the Andes in Colombia. Jigger flea (*Tunga penetrans*) lesions usually on the feet are also found. Onchocerciasis is present in scattered rural areas of Ecuador, Colombia, Venezuela and northern Brazil. Leprosy remains an important problem in Brazil and elsewhere but is very rarely contracted by the short-term traveller. Dermal leishmaniasis is relatively frequent in the traveller but has been mentioned above.

Subcutaneous and deep mycoses should be borne in mind. Paracoccidioidomycosis is commonest in Sao Paulo state, Brazil and may present with skin or mucocutaneous as well as pulmonary involvement. Mycetoma is relatively common in Venezuela but also occurs in much of the continent. Chromomycosis and sporotrichosis are also well recognised.

HIV infection

By late 1993, WHO estimated that there were 1–1.5 million HIV-infected adults living in South America and the Caribbean. Most of the infections have been contracted through sexual intercourse, predominantly heterosexual, and by intravenous drug users sharing equipment, particularly in cities. Commercial sex-workers including transvestite prostitutes are frequently infected. A worrying feature is the number of homeless street children in many cities who are forced to live by prostitution and who are often also involved in the drug scene. The risks of HIV infection need to be emphasised to travellers who may be anticipating sexual adventures.

Other diseases

Tuberculosis is highly prevalent in much of the sub-continent.

Poliomyelitis has been officially declared eradicated by WHO from all of South and Central America.

Meningococcal meningitis. Although there have been major epidemics during the last decade (e.g. in Brazil), most travellers are at low risk.[3]

Environmental toxins

There is concern about the widespread use of mercury in gold mining in the Amazon basin. River fish may contain excessive amounts of mercury.[4] Air pollution can be a problem in major cities such as Sao Paulo.

PRACTICE POINTS

- *Plasmodium falciparum* malaria and yellow fever are serious problems in Amazonian forested regions.
- The Americas have been declared free of poliomyelitis.
- Dengue has become more common in Central America, the Caribbean and northern parts of South America in recent years.
- Altitude problems can occur in those trekking in or visiting the Andes.
- Most major cities will have good medical facilities available.

REFERENCES

1. Bandres J, Mathewson J, Ericsson C, Dupont H. Trimethoprim plus sulfamethoxazole remains active against enterotoxigenic *E. coli* and *Shigella* spp. in Guadalajara, Mexico. American Journal of the Medical Sciences 1992; 303: 289–291.
2. Ryan CA, Hagrett-Bean NT, Blake PA. *Salmonella typhi* infections in the United States,1975–84: increasing role of foreign travel. Reviews of Infectious Diseases 1989; 11: 1–8.
3. Koch S, Steffen R. Meningococcal disease in travellers: vaccination recommendations. Journal of Travel Medicine 1994; 1: 4–7.
4. World Health Organization. Gold, mercury and health. Weekly Epidemiological Record 1994; 69: 275–278.

A perspective from South-East Asia

A. J. Hedley   A. S. M. Abdullah

Introduction

Travel and tourism are among the world's largest and fastest growing industries. People travel for leisure, recreation, study, business, medical treatment, work, conferences and religious pilgrimages. Travelling to and in regions such as South-East Asia now includes large numbers from populations in developed countries as well as people from the region itself. Although travelling is essentially a pleasurable activity, it is associated with many potential hazards and measurable risks for a wide spectrum of both communicable and non-communicable diseases, and health problems. Like other developing regions, many infectious and parasitic diseases are endemic in South-East Asia. However non-communicable diseases, principally trauma and other injuries, including those from natural disasters, are also very important and often present the greatest hazard.

South-East Asia is defined as the association of the following countries/territories: Bangladesh, Bhutan, Brunei, Darussalam, China, Cambodia, DPR Korea, Hong Kong, Indonesia, India, Lao People's Democratic Republic, Maldives, Malaysia, Myanmar (Burma), Macao, Mongolia, Nepal, the Philippines, Sri Lanka, South Korea, Singapore, Thailand, Taiwan and Vietnam.

Appropriate information and pre-travel health advice may reduce the risk of health problems during travel. This chapter aims to provide an overview of travel health risks in the South-East Asian region.

Background information on travel to South-East Asia

Heavenly Father, look down on us your humble, obedient tourist servants, who are doomed to travel this earth, taking photographs, mailing postcards, buying souvenirs and walking around in drip-dry underwear.

Art Buchwald

A Greek philosopher once advised: 'The world is a book. If you have not travelled, you have only read page one.'

The 'glamour girl' of the tourist business is international travel. The traveller budgets, plans and anticipates the prospect of changing scenery, people, food and customs. Travel is challenge: a new exciting experience of coping; the challenge of stepping into a new environment. Travel is usually fun but can also be very frustrating and it may be expensive in terms of its consequences. Worldwide the figure for expenditure on international travel is about $100 billion.[1]

People are travelling from region to region, country to country or within countries to explore variations of culture, people, lifestyle and environment, and to seek sun, sea, beaches and sometimes (or often) sex. Both international and domestic tourist arrivals worldwide are on the increase. Current projections suggest that world tourist arrivals will reach 666 million in the year 2000, with nearly one-third of these landing at

Asian destinations.[2] This estimate anticipates an annual growth of 4.5% for the whole world between 1988 and 2000, with the highest growth (12.1% per annum) expected to occur in Asia.

Overdevelopment and the 'predictability' of tourist destinations in developed countries have attracted travellers from many Western countries to Asia. Modernisation and changing economic and sociopolitical conditions in South-East Asia together with its historical and natural attractions have attracted travellers from all over the world into the region. Increased business possibilities and lower living costs induce people to stay either for short or long periods in these countries.

Tourism has become one of South-East Asia's foremost industries. Although the region receives less than 11% of the world's international tourist trade, the members of the Association of South-East Asian Nations (ASEAN) are experiencing a boom in both foreign and domestic tourism. The number of foreign visitors has doubled, receipts from tourism have tripled during the last decade, and tourism has become the leading source of foreign exchange in countries like Thailand. Tourism is the second largest industry in the Philippines and the third largest earner of foreign currency in Singapore.

Even the previously non-ASEAN nations such as Cambodia, Laos, Vietnam and Myanmar (Burma), where the income derived from tourism is low, are attempting to expand their own tourism industries. Vietnam has enjoyed an exponential growth in tourism over the last few years, rising from a meagre 20 000 visitors in 1986 to 187 000 in 1990, and projected to increase further to half a million by 1995. It is estimated that tourist arrivals in the Asia–Pacific region will increase 7% annually until the end of the century. This rate is much higher than the global average of around 4.5% per annum.[3]

Before the late 1960s, only relatively few travelled to South-East Asia, principally from the wealthy industrialised countries of Western Europe, the United States and Australasia. Then tourists came from those social groups who could afford the considerable cost of sea and later airborne travel to the Far East. The advent of cheap charter flights and package holidays changed international tourism, creating opportunities for

mass travel, respectively, to the periphery of Europe (e.g. Spain, Portugal, Greece), Central America and the Caribbean. Later opportunities included more distant destinations in Asia, the South Pacific and elsewhere.

The increase of tourism in South-East Asia relates to several factors including:

- the development of a tourism infrastructure adapted to current tourist interests
- historical, cultural and environmental attractions
- promotional activities
- advertising campaigns
- cheaper lifestyle
- easy and convenient access to hospitality services
- a proliferating sex industry, including escorts, massage parlours and child prostitution.

Every sexual preference is catered for at relatively low cost with virtual anonymity. In Thailand, these opportunities are considered to be a principal reason for visits by a large proportion of the annual total of 5 million visitors.

Intra-regional tourism is also on the increase in South-East Asia. This may be due to indigenous people's ability to travel, facilities to travel within the region and people's changing attitudes to explore even the same culture but in a different environment. In 1977, 6 million tourists visited the member countries of the ASEAN and one-third of these tourists were from ASEAN countries.

Health implications of travel to South-East Asia

General considerations

There are many potential, travel-related health issues for Asian travellers (as for those elsewhere) which may be viewed from several perspectives including environmental, sociocultural, political, physical, psychological, epidemiological and legal.

Many countries in the region are typical of warm-climate developing countries but many are now experiencing very rapid change through industrialisation, urbanisation, and commercialism.

The health problems in South-East Asian countries include communicable diseases such as diarrhoea, respiratory infections including tuberculosis and pneumonia, sexually transmitted diseases, vector-borne diseases such as malaria, and immunisable diseases, such as diphtheria, measles and polio. Some South-East Asian countries are also experiencing a rising trend of non-communicable diseases such as cancers, cardiovascular diseases, accidents, and drug dependence, as already experienced by the more developed and industrialised countries.

In this section, the focus is on those health risks that are more common in the South-East Asia region. However, it should be remembered that, as most of these countries are a long way from the West, the oriental traveller might be at risk from health problems that are related to long distance travel.

ROAD TRAFFIC ACCIDENTS

Road traffic accidents (RTAs) are one of the most important causes of death worldwide. Even in South-East Asian, warm-climate countries, they are the commonest cause of death under the age of 50 – although in Thailand that position has recently been replaced by HIV-related illnesses. A large number also sustain significant injuries from RTAs each year. In terms of years of potential life lost and thus of productivity, traffic injury exceeds in importance any other single cause of death, including cardiovascular disease, cerebrovascular disease and neoplasia. Age and gender, alcohol, drugs, medical conditions, roads, speed, vehicle and urban–rural differences are associated with RTAs in this region.

Many travellers (and perhaps their medical advisers) may consider exotic infections as the biggest danger to their health in Asia, but these represent only a small proportion of medical problems involving travellers. Half of all medical incidents notified to repatriation companies such as 'Europe Assistance' are accidental injuries, and 60% of those result from RTAs. Developing countries have increasing crash rates and increasing death rates whereas industrialised countries are experiencing marked declines in RTAs and deaths.[4] In 1998, there was an exhibition of smashed road vehicles, staged by the government in Beijing to raise public awareness about carnage on the roads. Most of the countries in South-East Asia will not have industrialised and developed environments for another 20–30 years.

In a study of deaths in Hong Kong travellers (based on causes of death in those repatriated), the causes were:

- pre-existing medical problems and heart disease and stroke
- road traffic accidents and injuries on work sites
- murders
- no deaths from communicable diseases.

There are multiple reasons for the high rate of RTAs in some South-East Asian countries.

The transportation system in many countries is not well developed. Many roads are being converted from predominantly dirt tracks, designed for pedestrians, oxcarts and cyclists, to thoroughfares for motor vehicles in a relatively sudden and uncontrolled fashion. All these forms of transport share roads where motor driving is often undisciplined and erratic. Dangerous obstacles, construction work, low levels of illumination and improper location of signs and lamp-post increase the risks. In rural areas (target destinations for many travellers), road junctions are often 'home made' and unmarked. Street lighting is in its infancy and night driving or driving during monsoons can be treacherous. Inadequate segregation of pedestrians is also very common, increasing the risk of accidents for cyclists, rickshaws, pedicabs and light public vehicles.

A 'macho' attitude among drivers is a well-established sub-culture in Asian countries. Drivers may have high social standing but adopt deplorable and inconsiderate attitudes to other road users. Competitions between drivers are commonplace.

In Chiang Rai in north Thailand at 01.00, three groups of European tourists boarded pedicabs (samlors = three wheels). The drivers were drunk as it turned out. A race through the dimly-lit streets developed. When negotiating a tight corner, one cab overturned dragging one occupant along the road on his elbow. He sustained a compound fracture contaminated by road dirt.

Unskilled and unlicensed drivers; careless and dangerous driving; outdated vehicles and vehicles with inadequate design, inadequate maintenance, in a poor state of repair; faulty construction of vehicles; inadequate traffic rules and negligent attitudes to traffic regulations are important factors in RTAs in some South-East Asian countries. Many drivers of long-distance transport such as trucks and coaches work long, uncontrolled shifts, at times round the clock with only catnaps at stopovers. The use of amphetamines and other stimulants is common. The time schedules to be met are unrealistic in terms of road and traffic conditions.

In Thailand, it is common to see bus drivers apparently sitting sideways to the steering wheel. This we are told is the driver's way of acknowledging that the Lord Buddha is really controlling the direction of the bus and the driver is simply holding the wheel for him. Divine intervention of this kind is obviously considered to be protective, but the outcome of this form of faith is frequently catastrophic. Presumably the followers of the faith consider that there would be far more and worse accidents if they did not involve the Lord Buddha's help.

The practice of fast driving (100–120+ km/hour) on narrow, congested roads in rural areas means that the joining speeds of colliding vehicles travelling in opposite directions may be of the order of 240 km/hr (160 mph). It has been commonplace to hear reports of coaches ripped open 'like sardine cans' and up to 80 people killed or maimed. Emergency services and the capacity of a local district hospital to handle such an emergency may be very limited. The need for a blood transfusion incurs other obvious risks.

In 1996 Thailand introduced legislation to require the wearing of hard hats for motor cyclists. This is now in operation in Bangkok but not yet in the provinces. In January 1996, scores of Western and other tourists on the island of Ko Samui were observed riding around on hired motorcycles without head protection.

In Thailand, a backpacker took the front seat on a long-distance bus used by the local population to travel the 800-km distance from a northern district to the capital Bangkok. The seat afforded panoramic views of rice paddy fields, water buffalo and villagers going about their tasks throughout the day. It was ideal for compiling a video album of the journey. 6 hours later she was dead. The driver fell asleep and the bus slammed into the back of a ten-wheeler rice truck.

A Dutch volunteer working in a church-sponsored community project in Thailand rode as a pillion passenger on a light motorcycle. The driver swerved to avoid a collision. The passenger fell backwards, her feet held in stirrups, and was dragged with her head impacting on the ground. She underwent three craniotomies for evacuation of subdural haematomata. A slow, but eventually satisfactory, recovery occurred over 2 years.

A middle-aged woman was walking across the road somewhere between Nanning and Beihai (Guangxi province, China); she was pushed in to a canal by a minibus that was overtaking another vehicle. The driver ignored the incident and the condition of the woman and accelerated the minibus, in which one of the authors was sitting on a front seat.

Road safety precautions

Preventive measures could decrease the risk of road traffic accidents and travellers should be made better aware of the following:

- Rail travel is safer than road, usually as affordable and just as interesting and exciting.
- Travellers should note carefully any traffic rules.
- Continuous sounding of horns can identify cities where people ignore the traffic rules.
- Travellers who wish to drive by themselves should understand the road signs of the country.
- Local insurance often does not exist or is worthless.
- If you are involved in an accident, whether it is your fault or someone else's, travellers are often attacked. Immediate payment of a very large sum of money may be a life-saving measure, especially in a remote rural area.
- In many countries in the region, road signs only appear in local languages.

Road safety precautions *cont'd*

- Alcohol increases the risk of road traffic accidents, travellers should not drink alcohol before or during driving or take journeys in vehicles with drivers who may be alcoholics or drug users.
- Travellers should be careful crossing roads because traffic rules are frequently not observed, and malfunction of brakes in outdated vehicles is common. Until recently, buses in Rangoon were vintage Second World War Canadian trucks. It is advisable, if possible, to cross streets while vehicles are stopped entirely.

Communicable diseases

This section outlines general risks from infectious diseases in South-East Asian countries. It aims to give a brief description of common conditions that may affect a traveller in the region. Arthropod-borne diseases are an important cause of morbidity throughout the area.

Malaria is endemic in many parts of the rural areas in countries such as Burma, Indonesia, Malaysia, the Philippines, Thailand, Cambodia, Laos and Vietnam. Malaria is not a public health problem in Hong Kong, Brunei Darussalam and Singapore, where normally only imported cases occur.

Travel advice on malaria for this region is of very variable quality and often misleading. Insufficient emphasis is placed on the need to avoid insect bites. If more travellers were assiduous about the use of protective clothing and insect repellent, rather than depending on uncertain ingestion of prophylactics, travel-related malaria would be less of a problem. The liberal use of an effective repellent such as neat (95%) diethyltoluamide (DEET) on skin and clothing by backpackers would offer protection against a range of insect bites, in addition to malaria-carrying, anopheline mosquitoes.

Travel advice on malaria, based on charts stating whether or not malaria is present, may encourage misleading assessments of risk. For example, advice on malaria prophylaxis in Thailand based on this approach may encourage the view that it is either essential or unnecessary. Malaria risks in Thailand are now largely confined to the border areas with Burma and Cambodia. Infection here may be dangerous because the prevalence of drug-resistant *Plasmodium falciparum* malaria is high. The implications for low-cost travellers are obvious. Travellers in the rest of low-risk, central, southern and northern regions need not be advised to take prophylactic medication. Exceptions occur and although malaria is very rare in Bangkok, recently a senior British diplomat's daughter arrived in Bangkok with the family. Within 2 weeks she had contracted malaria. Generally, the most important advice concerns avoiding mosquito bites and the need for prompt investigation of fever.

Filariasis in South-East Asian countries is caused by *Wuchereria bancrofti* (bancroftian filariasis) and *Brugia malayi* (Malayan filariasis), which are the tissue-inhabiting nematodes localised in the lymphatic system of humans (see Table 17.1). The nocturnally periodic and the nocturnally sub-periodic forms of microfilariae are the two types of Malayan filariasis. The former is generally distributed throughout the Asian region, while the latter is limited to some forested areas in Malaysia, Indonesia, and the Philippines. Filariasis caused by *Wuchereria bancrofti* is widely distributed in tropical and sub-tropical parts of Asia. A new kind of filariasis caused by *Brugia timori* has been found on the island of Timor situated in the eastern part of Indonesia. Short-term travellers are not at risk of developing chronic complications of filariasis such as lymphoedema but paroxysmal dyspnoea with cough and eosinophilia may occur – so-called pulmonary eosinophilia. Diethylcarbamazine is effective treatment. Prevention is through minimising mosquito bites.

Japanese B encephalitis is prevalent in many rural areas of the South-East Asian region. Mosquitoes, with farm animals and sometimes birds as intermediate hosts, transmit it. Culicine (*Culex tritaenorhyncus*) mosquitoes are the principal vectors for Japanese B encephalitis and they frequently breed in paddy fields. Japanese B encephalitis is the leading cause of viral encephalitis in Asia. About 50000 epidemic and sporadic cases occur each year in China, Korea, Japan, the South-East Asia and Pacific Rim and parts of Oceania.

TABLE 17.1 Filariasis in South-East Asia

Species	Strains	Geographical Distribution	Animal resereoirs	Mosquito vectors	Breeding grounds
Brugia malayi	Periodic	Throughout Asian region	Nil	Anopheles sp., Mansonia sp.	Open swamps, rice fields
	Sub-periodic	Malaysia, Indonesia, the Philippines	Domestic cats, leaf monkeys	Mansonia sp.	Swamp forests
Wuchereria bancrofti	Urban	Widely distributed in tropics and sub-tropics including Asia	Nil	Culex quinque-fasciatus	Urban areas
	Rural	Widely distributed in tropics and sub-tropics including Asia	Nil	Anopheles sp. (Malaysia, the Philippines)	Rural areas
				Aedes sp. (Thailand, the Philippines)	

The risk to travellers in the region, however, is extremely low but depends of course on locations visited, activities, season (mostly May to December), and time spent travelling in endemic or hyperendemic areas. It is reported that the attack rate ranged between 0.05 and 2.1 per 10 000 per week with a median of 0.9 among Western military personnel in Asia.[5] As with malaria and other insect-transmitted diseases, the first rule is not to be bitten.

Should travellers to these regions be vaccinated? The risk is small but the disease is serious. Symptomatic cases have a 30% mortality with others left with neurological disability. Leaving aside issues relating to vaccine efficacy and side effects, package holidaymakers to developed resorts usually do not require vaccination. Backpackers spending weeks in the rural regions of China, Thailand, Vietnam, Nepal, Philippines and Pacific territories such as Okinawa, usually should be vaccinated.

As new tourist destinations open up, including China and Vietnam, the pattern may change and the present reports probably understate the risk, particularly for children and elderly travellers who are more likely to have severe illnesses.

Since 1978, around 23 cases of Japanese B encephalitis have been recognised in Western travellers to the region; one case occurred in an Australian traveller who made only a few excursions into rural areas of Bali while on a 2-week vacation.

Dengue and dengue haemorrhagic fever have become important causes of childhood morbidity and mortality in South-East Asia. It is caused by arboviruses and transmitted by mosquitoes (Aedes species).

Epidemics can occur in both urban and rural areas in the South-East Asian region and dengue is an increasing threat to travellers in this region. The outbreaks usually start with the rainy season and last until it finishes. Most cases are mild in travellers, unless they have been infected previously, when haemorrhagic fever may occur. Vaccines are under development but at present the only available advice is to avoid mosquito bites. Neglected culverts, untidy villages littered with tyres, tin cans and other receptacles creating breeding sites are typical hazards for the unwary, low cost traveller.

Mite-borne typhus has been reported in deforested areas in most countries in the region.

A Hong Kong physician went on vacation to Thailand and travelled through rural areas. On return home, she became ill with malaise, fever, extreme tiredness and shortness of breath. Extensive investigation over many weeks was inconclusive. Eventually a colleague suspected a rickettsial infection. Tests proved positive and appropriate treatment eliminated the symptoms.

A further detailed history revealed that, during one tourist entertainment, the party sat in barbecue pits in which the diners legs dangled in a deep recess, while the table and cooking facility were above ground level. It is surmised that scraps of food were not properly cleaned out of the pits. Rats frequented the pits and were the source of rodent mites, with rickettsial infection, in the pits. The diners were at risk of being bitten by hungry larval mites waiting for a blood meal.

Those who hike in South-East Asia are at risk of scrub typhus, but so too are other conventional travellers if they indulge in adventurous walking in rural areas.

Plague has been reported in some countries in the area and endemic areas have been identified in India, China, Mongolia, Burma, Indonesia and Vietnam. Bubonic plague is more common in summer and autumn months because a cool climate and high relative humidity support the spread of the disease. Given that rats and the *Yersinia pestis*-carrying fleas are ubiquitous, the risk is ever present. There are probably more rats than people in some Asian urban environments.

Rats are a major problem in Vietnam. Rodent control has been the target of massive aid programmes over the past decade. Rats eat up to one-third of the rice crop. Rats in Hanoi hotels are common, even in the 4-star deluxe hotels charging US$ 100 per night. One of the authors on a WHO assignment in Hanoi, dined each evening with *Rattus norvegicus* scampering around the dining room. It remains to be seen whether the new 5-star hotels remain rodent-free.

Food- and water-borne diseases

Cholera and other watery diarrhoeas, amoebic and bacillary dysentery, typhoid fever and hepatitis A and E may occur in all countries in the area. Among non-immune travellers, infection by hepatitis A virus occurs 40 times more frequently than typhoid fever and 800 times more frequently

than cholera. No-one should be travelling in this region without hepatitis A vaccination or knowing they are immune. Among helminthic infections, fasciolopsiasis (giant intestinal fluke) may be acquired in most countries in the area; clonorchiasis (oriental liver fluke) and opisthorchiasis (fish liver fluke) in the Indo-China peninsula, the Philippines and Thailand; and paragonimiasis in most countries.

Eating is generally safe in South-East Asian countries in the Indo-China peninsula and if basic rules are followed ('cook it, boil it, peel it or forget it'), then most travellers have little to fear. There are, however, some exceptions.

The eating of certain types of raw food is often considered a delicacy. Most travellers would probably avoid such a risk, but backpackers staying in a village might easily eat raw fermented food inadvertently. *Opisthorchis* infestation in north-east Thailand is the commonest cause of malignancy and death from malignant disease in that community at present. It leads to the development of cholangiocarcinoma in early adult life. Thai villagers in some areas have 100% prevalence of *Opisthorchis* infestation.

A Thai University microbiologist had frequently eaten in village settings. In her late 30s, she developed mid-back pain and cholangiocarcinoma was diagnosed. Radical hepatic surgery did not prevent death in 6 months. Opisthorchiasis is contracted by eating raw freshwater fish and prevented by lightly poaching the fish. However, because the raw fish is considered a delicacy, there is resistance to this simple, preventive approach.

A Thai radiologist in his 40s developed epileptiform seizures. Brain scans revealed cystic space-occupying lesions and aspirates at surgery showed that the infestation was cysticercosis, contracted from eating raw pork.

Enteric infections will of course be avoided by ensuring that all cooked food has reached a temperature of at least 61°C. However, typical hazards for the unwary include seafood hot pot that is often placed on the table for cooking; the aroma tempts sampling before the stew is ready.

In many Asian communities, fish and other sea creatures are kept alive in the restaurant in tanks for selection by customers. The water in these tanks may, especially if the restaurant suppliers are unscrupulous, be drawn from heavily contaminated river or harbour water, polluted from sewage outfalls. Epidemics of hepatitis and cholera have occurred, even in well-regulated Hong Kong, because of this practice.

Forewarned is forearmed but tourist-dependent economies will not always report outbreaks of diarrhoeal and other health problems. There is no doubt that government information units in many countries have suppressed data (most recently in Thailand in early 1998) on cholera in recent years. Any indications that there have been outbreaks of diarrhoeal disease in 'rural' areas *alone* should be treated with suspicion. (The colloquial Thai name for severe diarrhoea sounds like *Aach-i-Wah* and probably often reflects cholera outbreaks.)

Travellers should maintain personal hygiene, avoid eating from unlicensed or street vendors and ensure that thoroughly cooked food and clean drinking water is taken at all times.

Sexually transmitted diseases (STDs) are a prominent feature of communicable disease patterns in Asia and considered as a major public health threat in some countries in the region. STDs and their complications are common in South-East Asia and this is an increasing threat to travellers' health. The relationship between tourism and STDs is now well established. Because travellers are out of their normal environment and often in circumstances that allow anonymous promiscuity, many become involved in high-risk sexual behaviour. Some groups of travellers travel from country to country solely to exploit the sex life of people from different races and nationalities. Such travellers are at special risk of STDs, as their sexual relations are often with persons who have a high prevalence of these diseases. Poor economic conditions, low costs and easy availability of sex-workers establish them as popular, sex-holiday destinations.

An advertisement in a Hong Kong newspaper (translated from Chinese) is seen in Figure 17.1:

Human immunodeficiency virus (HIV) infection and acquired immunodeficiency syndrome (AIDS)

Ticket for direct flight to Ho Chi Minh City ($3600) or to Hanoi ($3700)

Leisurely trip for men to Vietnam
    5 days for $4590
    7 days including Thailand $5990
- Direct flight
- Attractive female tour guide with warm hospitality
- Taste Vietnam-style cuisine and games
- Stay in the top new hotel

Fig. 17.1 'Sex-holiday' advertisement.

are becoming important STDs in the South-East Asian region as elsewhere in the world. AIDS is the commonest cause of death under the age of 50 in Thailand and HIV-positive individuals are conservatively estimated at 500 000–800 000 (probably over 1 million) in a population of 60 million. This is probably a gross underestimate. It may be at least as common as treated diabetes in the UK (1%) or even as high as 2%. After it was first recognised in 1984 in Thailand, HIV was reported from all other countries in the region except North Korea.

In 1993–94, there was an eight-fold increase in the number of AIDS cases in Asia and from 1990 to July 1995 the cumulative total of AIDS cases in Asia increased dramatically by over 20-fold, compared with 3.2-fold in Africa. By mid-1996, a cumulative total of 5 million adults and children were infected with HIV in South and South-East Asia and about 90% of the HIV-infected adults in South and South-East Asia live in India, Thailand, Myanmar and Cambodia.

By the end of the century, WHO predicts that the current total of 5 million infections in South and South-East Asia will increase two-fold to over 10 million infections.[6]

The epidemics of HIV in the countries of the Asia–Pacific region are diverse, localised and have different trends over time. In some countries, the prevalence of HIV infection is high and increasing while in some countries the prevalence is low and stable (Table 17.2).

The main modes of transmission of HIV in Asia were originally via needle-sharing amongst injecting drug users, and unprotected sexual

TABLE 17.2 HIV penetration into Asia and the Pacific countries*

Country	Current HIV epidemic trends		Main populations affected	Projected HIV epidemic trends (3–5 years)
	HIV incidence	HIV prevalence		
With epidemic spread				
Australia	Low and decreasing	Low and stable	MSM*	Decline
Cambodia	High and increasing rapidly	High and increasing	Individuals with high-and moderate-risk, heterosexual behaviour	Sustained upward trend
China	Low except in Yunnan	Low and increasing	IDU*	Increasing
India	Moderate and increasing (significant regional variation)	Still low but increasing (significant regional variation)	Individuals with high-risk, heterosexual behaviour and IDUs	Increasing
Malaysia	Moderate and increasing	Low and increasing	Principally IDUs but increasing among individuals with high-risk, sexual behaviour	Increasing
Myanmar	High and increasing	High and increasing	Individuals with high-risk, heterosexual behaviour, IDUs and their spouses	Increasing
New Zealand	Low and decreasing	Low and stable	MSM and IDU	Decline
Papua New Guinea	Moderate and increasing	Low but increasing	Individuals with high-risk, heterosexual behaviour	Slowly increasing
Thailand	Moderate and stabilising in specific groups	High but stabilising	IDUs and individuals with high- and moderate-risk, heterosexual behaviour	Tending to stabilise
Vietnam	Moderate and increasing	Still low but increasing	Principally IDUs but increasing among individuals with high-risk, sexual behaviour	Increasing
With low transmission				
Bangladesh	Low	Low	Individuals with high-risk, heterosexual behaviour	Slowly increasing
Indonesia	Low	Low	MSM, bisexual and high-risk, heterosexual behaviour	Slowly increasing
Japan	Low	Low	Previously blood-product-related, currently sexual	Slowly increasing
Hong Kong	Low	Low	IDU, MSM	Slowly increasing
Nepal	Low except in IDU	Low except in IDUs	Individuals with high-risk, heterosexual behaviour and IDUs	Slowly increasing
Philippines	Low	Low	Individuals with high-risk, heterosexual behaviour	Slowly increasing
Singapore	Low	Low	MSM, IDUs	Slowly increasing
Sri Lanka	Low	Low	Individuals with high-risk, heterosexual behaviour and MSM	Slowly increasing

The following countries in the region have minimal spread of HIV infection: Bhutan, Brunei, DPR Korea, Macao, Mongolia, Pacific Island countries and areas, Republic of Korea.
*MSM, men having sex with men; IDU, injecting drug users.

Source of extract: Provisional report of the official satellite symposium on 'Monitoring the AIDS Pandemic (MAP). The status and trends of the HIV/AIDS/STD epidemics in Asia and the Pacific.' Manila, Philippines; 25 October 1997: 10.

intercourse between men. However, heterosexual transmission is now the main mode of transmission, with relatively high levels of infection among female commercial sex-workers and their clients in several states in India, in various cities of Myanmar, and across Thailand, Cambodia and Vietnam.[7] (Table 17.3).

It is argued that travel and tourism combined with a proliferating sex industry have played an important role in maintaining the high level of

TABLE 17.3 HIV distribution among selected Asian and Pacific populations

Country	IDU	HET	MSM
Australia	+	+	++
Bangladesh	+	+	+
Cambodia	+	+++	+
China			
Yunnan Prov.	+++	+	+
Hong Kong	+	+	++
Rest of China	++	+	+
India			
West and South	+	+++	+
Central and East	+	+	+
Northeast	+++	+	+
Indonesia	+	+	++
Japan	+	+	+
Laos	+	+	+
Malaysia	+++	++	++
Myanmar	+++	++	++
Nepal	+++	++	++
Papau New Guinea	+	++	+
Philippines	+	+	+
South Korea	0	+	+
Sri Lanka	0	+	+
Thailand	+++	++	+
Vietnam	+++	+	+

+++, high or rapidly growing; ++, relatively low or plateauing; +, not a major component; 0, no evidence of spread.

IDU, injecting drug users; HET, heterosexual men and women; MSM, men having sex with men.

Source of extract: Provisional report of the official satellite symposium on 'Monitoring the AIDS Pandemic (MAP). The status and trends of the HIV/AIDS/STD epidemics in Asia and the Pacific.' Manila, Philippines; 25 October 1997: 11.

transmission of STDs in South-East Asia. The prevalence of HIV infection in massage parlour girls and other prostitutes is up to 80% in some countries in the region. In north-east Thailand, it has been estimated at 40–80%.

The irony for countries such as Thailand is that the massive economic growth experienced in the past two decades is attributable in large measure to the sex attractions of the hospitality industry.

Surveys of travellers' perceptions of risk and high-risk behaviour are difficult to carry out. The evidence available suggests that many are oblivious to (or choose to ignore) the risks. A recent study among international travellers at Kai Tak airport (Hong Kong SAR) established that 44% of the respondents (168/383), who had entered at least once within the previous year, had had sex with a stranger during their travel and 37% did not use condoms.[8]

Hepatitis B (HBV) is highly endemic in South-East Asia and is a major cause of chronic liver disease and liver cancer in this region. Hepatocellular cancer is the second commonest cause of death by malignant disease in Hong Kong. All newborn infants are now vaccinated at birth against hepatitis B. The proportion of the population who are carriers of hepatitis B virus is as high as 20% in some countries in the region.

HBV is spread through body fluids and thus by transfusion of contaminated blood and blood products and unprotected sexual contact, both homosexual and heterosexual. However, this may not explain all of the observed prevalence of HBV antibodies in Asia. An effective vaccine is available against HBV.

Precautions such as careful and safe sex, avoidance of transfusion with unscreened blood or blood products, use of disposable syringes and medical and dental equipment are important. There is a strong case for vaccinating long-term travellers and residents in this region.

Other communicable diseases

Schistosomiasis (bilharziasis) is endemic in the southern Philippines and in central Sulawesi of Indonesia and occurs in small foci in the Mekong delta. It is acquired from water containing larval forms or cercariae, which have developed in snails. Bathing in rivers while backpacking is a typical hazard.

Poliomyelitis is reported from Cambodia, Indonesia, the Lao People's Democratic Republic, Myanmar and Vietnam. The incidence of poliomyelitis is low in Malaysia, the Philippines and Thailand because of effective vaccination programmes but the environmental risks remain. In 1988, the WHO Western Pacific Region adopted a resolution to eradicate poliomyelitis from the region by the end of 1995. This goal is not yet achieved but circulation of wild poliovirus has been dramatically reduced in Vietnam and China. No-one should be travelling in this region without protection.

Trachoma is reported in Indonesia, Myanmar, Thailand and Vietnam. It is believed that the trachoma agent is spread from person to person by several means such as contaminated fingers and towels. Eye flies (*Musca sorbans*) also play an important role as vectors.

Rabies is common in some parts of the region. Rabies has a wide range of animal hosts, both domestic and wild. These include dogs, wolves and foxes. Wild dogs and monkeys can be observed in the streets and parks of many countries in the region. Many South-East Asian countries have cultural and social centres of activity, which attract dogs. These include market places and temples where there are scraps of food lying around. Exposure to saliva from animals, not necessarily a full bite, is common among travellers and a risk cannot be totally excluded in these circumstances when open cuts and scratches may be present.

In Bhuddist countries such as Thailand and Burma, temple (stray) dogs are commonplace.

In north-east Thailand, Khon Kaen province, a Scottish visitor was walking through the temple grounds. The grounds were home to Macaque monkeys who fed on surrounding fruit trees and food left as offerings. The monkeys became aggressive when visitors arrived because they were accustomed to competing for the food offered by tourists. The visitor was attacked by a large male monkey and bitten on the buttocks before others came to her aid.

Snake bites and leeches are also hazards in some areas.

A backpacker in Sakon Nakorn, north-east Thailand, stayed in a village on the banks of the Mae Kong river. In the early morning, he went out to the water jar to wash and stepped on a cobra. The snake struck and he was bitten on the thigh.

Despite emergency treatment and antivenom in the local district hospital, he developed neurotoxic symptoms, swelling and later gangrene of the leg and died 1 week later from septicaemia and disseminated intravascular coagulation.

OTHER TROPICAL AND PARASITIC INFECTIONS

Intestinal parasitic infections such as ascariasis, hookworm, trichuriasis, amoebiasis and giardiasis are still a problem in some areas where environmental hygiene and sanitation are inadequate. In such areas, high rates of infection may occur. Travellers to such areas should be careful with food, drinks and walking barefoot or in flip-flops through rural areas.

A UK visitor from Oxford University visiting Hong Kong went to Guangzhou for 2 days. She ate three meals in restaurants and drank water once from a pitcher in her hostel bedroom. 2 days later in Hong Kong she presented in the night with acute left lower abdominal pain and bloody diarrhoea. Stool smears revealed *Entamoeba histolytica*.

Environmental and social hazards

GENERAL CONSIDERATIONS

Travellers are exposed to many environmental hazards during their travel when they explore new cultures or gather new experiences in a new environment. The hazards that travellers are usually exposed to may arise from altitude, heat and humidity, sun, cold, water, insects, culture, political conditions, health and safety regulations, unhygienic and insanitary conditions, food and drink, routes of transportation, robbery or assault and other travellers' behaviour.

ALTITUDE

Illness related to altitude is becoming commoner among adventurous travellers. Thousands of visitors now journey to high-altitude areas in the

South-East Asian region, including the Himalayas in Nepal and most areas of Tibet. Staying at high altitudes poses a potential health risk to travellers, caused by lack of oxygen. It is potentially life-threatening to those with existing medical problems (e.g. cardiac or respiratory illness). Emergency medical assistance companies in Hong Kong SAR and Mainland China deal with several cases of altitude-related illness each year and some of these require evacuation. Among trekkers in Nepal the risk of dying while trekking is reported as 15 deaths per 100 000 trekkers.[9]

Trekkers and travellers intending to visit high altitude areas in the South-East Asian region as well as elsewhere in the world should be provided with proper medical advice for the prevention of severe incidents caused by reduced oxygen at altitudes. These include acute mountain sickness and high-altitude pulmonary oedema, and high-altitude cerebral oedema.

> A physician and his wife flew to Lhasa from Chengdu. They did not use acetazolamide as a prophylactic against altitude sickness. They spent most of the visit inhaling from oxygen bags in their hotel room.

> A team from a British military force in the Far East flew to Kenya to climb Kilimanjaro. The only member of the team who did not take acetazolamide had to be carried down the mountain on a stretcher.

WATER

There are examples of transmission of a number of diseases from contaminated water in South-East Asia. In many countries, there is a significant incidence of disease and other health disorders caused by or known to be associated with bathing in polluted seawater or with the consumption of contaminated seafood. In certain countries, El Tor cholera has been reported in villages along the lower course of rivers. Cholera and other diarrhoeal diseases were also reported after heavy rains that caused flooding and contamination of water wells. Outbreaks of 'red eye' disease were also reported after swimming in the pools or beaches. Shark attacks are also frequently reported from beaches in South-East Asia.

Three people were eaten alive swimming from Hong Kong beaches in 1995 and 1996. The sharks used to be policed by dolphins but destruction of the dolphins' habitat and food sources by urban development, pollution and over-fishing has depleted their numbers.

CULTURAL

Cultural differences between two societies sometimes increases risk for travellers. For example, showing a thumb (e.g. 'thumbs up') is interpreted as 'good' in most Western societies; while in some countries in the South-East Asian region, showing a 'thumb' is interpreted as 'penis' and is shown for insulting purposes only.

In some countries, women are sensitive to visitors and have a very sheltered status in society. Even a courteous attempt to shake hands with a woman may be seen as outrageous and offensive. It is wise for travellers to understand the culture of the country they want to travel in. This may minimise the risk of unwanted problems.

TERRORISM AND BANDITRY AND THE MILITARY

Politically unstable areas where there is violence, bombing, violent strikes and or attacks on vehicles or public property may pose important risks for travellers. Travellers should avoid such areas, if possible. Statements or informal discussions with local people about politics may cause problems for travellers in certain countries in the region, especially if it is brought to the attention of the authorities. There are often reports that travellers have paid penalties for ignoring local rules for accidentally entering prohibited areas or taking photographs of certain restricted items. Recently travellers have been threatened by the military and had film confiscated in Nepal and Tibet. Travellers should be very careful in dealing with such situations. Nervous, trigger-happy, young, inexperienced conscripts have killed many travellers.

Travellers are the target population for robbery or assault in certain countries in the South-East Asian region. Travellers are robbed for foreign currency or other valuable items, the resale of which can be lucrative. Women (especially Western women) tourists are in more danger of sexual assault. Western pornography and magazines have created the wrong impression about foreign women to locals in some areas. Backpackers are in more danger than the package tourists in regard to robbery or assault.

> A monk in Kanchanaburi province killed a British woman tourist in Thailand after an attempted rape in December 1995, 130 km from Bangkok. The woman's body was hidden in a cave near the temple and the monk unsuccessfully attempted to rape another Australian woman just a month after the previous incident. The monk was then arrested and sentenced to jail after the Australian woman filed a complaint of attempted rape with police.

> Travellers should take care of their valuable belongings as well as their own safety in the areas where robbery is frequent or where local laws and police corruption favour criminals. In some areas, local women are involved in deceiving travellers by offering sexual favours and then taking them to a place where there are other members of the group. They are not only robbed or blackmailed (a relatively benign outcome) but also often murdered.

> In early 1996, the mass public execution took place in Guangdong province of a gang of men and women who had decoyed and murdered business and commercial travellers.

Automatic weapons such as Kalashnikov and M16 rifles are freely available in many parts of Asia. Many were sold when defeated rebel groups (like the Khmer Rouge) sold their guns for money to buy food or safe transit.

> Several years ago, a Nottingham man was machine-gunned to death in a beach chalet in Phuket.

In the past 5 years:

> A bullet through the chest killed a German tourist travelling with her husband on a boat down the Fang river to Chiang Rai when bandits, known as Chinese Haws, shot up the boat and robbed the passengers.

> Recently, two British women visiting the Thai island of Koh Samui were shot dead by young men while out walking in a woodland area.

OTHER HEALTH HAZARDS

Natural disasters may also create dangers for travellers to South-East Asia. Cyclones, tropical storms or floods occur frequently in some countries and create hazards for travellers. Travellers in such situations should follow the local health and safety regulations. Passenger ferries in the Philippines are frequently overloaded and sink in heavy seas with huge loss of life.

Some other factors such as crowding, unlawful and undisciplined activities, long hours of waiting, disruption of eating habits, and changes in climate and time zones may result in various forms of stress for travellers.

> Visitors to a South-East Asian country at the time of the traditional New Year festival became involved in a crowd crush. Two of them were badly injured and sustained rib fractures.

The behaviour of travellers sometimes increases the risk of health hazards to themselves. It is known that some backpackers like to spend the night in a tent or outside on their backpack. Some move to a room with a stranger or accept an offer of free accommodation from local inhabitants. This increases the possibility of robbery or assault and also increases the risk of being bitten by mosquitoes, insects or animals.

Overall, it is essential for travellers to obtain as much information as they can about their targeted travel destinations prior to their travel, assess risks, follow pre-travel health advice from registered travel clinics and take necessary precautions all of which may minimise hazards to themselves.

Tobacco-related health problems

Advertisements in the media and smoking on public transport or in public places are officially restricted in some South-East Asian countries but few have effective enforcement. People smoke on the streets, in restaurants, institutes, entertainment places, waiting lounges, offices and even hospitals. Smoking on public transport including aircraft is also very common despite being prohibited. The authorities do not regard control as a high priority and are afraid of losing customers. In some countries, the drivers smoke in public transport vehicles despite notices that 'smoking is prohibited'. There are reports of travellers being assaulted or being put off the transport for complaining about smokers in non-smoking vehicles.

Travellers are potentially at risk of passive smoking in this region for these reasons. Travellers with medical conditions such as respiratory diseases or cardiovascular diseases may thus be at increased risk in certain circumstances and should be cautious while travelling in public transport or in a crowd.

Sex-travellers to South-East Asia

Sex-tourism is an ugly but important side of travel to South-East Asia, which involves sexual exploitation of women and children in the region. In recent years, sexual exploitation of men has also developed in some countries. Both men and women travel for sex in the South-East Asian region. In general, understanding the life and culture of the people of the tourist destination is a genuine desire of many tourists, but sometimes it is completely replaced by the desire for sexual exploitation or experimentation.

Whether travellers are actively seeking sex or not, most tourists will immediately come into contact with commercial sex-workers of all ages, gender and sexual proclivities in countries such as Thailand, Vietnam, Cambodia, Nepal, Burma and the Philippines. Many low-budget hotels and hostels function as both daytime and night-time brothels. Apart from the risks of STDs to the unguarded and unwary, other hazards such as deception and robbery are important.

South-East Asia is of interest to sex-travellers because of the easy availability of young adults and child sex-workers who are very cheap. The services and perceived attractiveness of South-East Asian women in Japanese and European brothels may also be a reason for travellers choosing this region as a sex-holiday destination.

Some countries have encouraged the sex industry to attract travellers. For example, a Thai government spokesperson, Mechai Viravaidya, was quoted in *The Nation*, one of Thailand's English-language newspapers, on June 17, 1988, as saying, 'Let's be frank; if there is no sex, there wouldn't be much tourism.' O'Grady[10] and Jurgensen[11] argue that sex tourism is an overt component of the tourist attractiveness of several countries of South-East Asia, with the tourism flow from tourist-generating regions being partially motivated by prostitution.

According to Gay[12] 'Between 70 and 80% of male tourists who travel from Japan, the United States, Australia, and Western Europe to Asia do so solely for the purpose of sexual entertainment.' It is estimated that a large number of these tourists are travelling to countries in South-East Asia. According to the Australian Bureau of Tourism Research and Department of Immigration and Ethnic Affairs: 2304000 Australians went overseas for short-term trips in 1993–4, with more than one-third choosing Asia as their destination. Among these, there were 200265 departures from Australia to Bangkok. It is thought that a large portion of these is related to sex-tourism. As Matsui[13] mentioned, in many countries of the region, sex-tourism is becoming one of the most pressing social issues and it has become a multinational sex industry for the promotion of its tourism business.

In a paper by Sister Soledad Perpinan of the Philippines, presented at the World Council of Churches meeting as long ago as July 1983, she said that 'across Asia, prostitution has been transnationalised and has reached unimaginable proportions mainly because of sex tours.'

In South-East Asia, the institutionalisation of sex-tourism commenced with the prostitution associated with Japanese colonialism and American military bases and has now become transformed through the internationalisation of the regional economies into a major item of systematised foreign trade.[14] Thousands of women in South-East Asian countries are involved in sex industries as prostitutes, social escorts, massage parlour or beauty parlour girls, accompanying girls in karaoke bars, show girls, house maids and as waitresses in night-clubs or discos. This is due to their socio-economic circumstances and in some cases by force. Earning lucrative profits from the sex business has attracted certain business people who employ, cheat or kidnap women and children from different areas to provide services to their customers. Trafficking in women is also increasing in countries in the region. Technically, prostitution is illegal in many of these countries, but the law is poorly enforced. In some countries in the region there is no 'red light' district but services are readily available through hotels, beauty parlours, massage parlours, sauna houses, discos, karaoke bars or via some other sources.

Not only women but also children are attractive to sex-travellers and the numbers of child prostitutes are increasing in several countries in South-East Asia. Issues related to child prostitution are discussed in Chapter 21.

A sexually active person who is willing to travel or is encouraged to travel for the purpose of sexual entertainment should know the dangers of unprotected, casual sex. However, it is apparent that many do not or choose to ignore the risk. Paedophiles should also be warned about the ethical and legal issues of child prostitution. Now the tide may be turning. Paedophiles from Europe, Scandinavia and Australia have been prosecuted for using child prostitutes in Asia. Several countries in the region issued tough decrees to tighten up the control of the sex industry. It is questionable, however, whether this will have a lasting effect.

PRACTICE POINTS

- Facilities can vary greatly from the highly developed to the very primitive.
- Serious risk of malaria is confined to only a few common tourist areas such as northern, border areas within Thailand, parts of China neighbouring Vietnam, Sabah (eastern Malaysia) and rural Indonesia.
- Japanese B encephalitis is endemic in most of the region and epidemics occur after the rains in low-lying parts of Nepal and Northern Thailand. It is most common in rural areas and not normally a risk for tourists staying in good quality hotels in resorts.
- Dengue is becoming more common in tourists to the region.
- The risk of HIV infection among commercial sex-workers is high in many areas and sex-tourism is common.
- Many larger cities have serious air-pollution problems.

REFERENCES

1. Travel Industry World Yearbook – 1983. Somerset Waters, Child and Waters, NYC 1983.
2. Hiemstra SJ. World tourism outlook for 1990s. World Travel and Tourism Review 1991; 1: 62.
3. Hitchcock M, King VT, Parnwell MJ. Tourism in Southeast Asia. London: Routledge; 1993.
4. Hedley AJ, Cheng KK, Lam TH. Causes of mortality in Hong Kong travellers dying abroad. Data presented at the World Congress on Travel Medicine, Singapore, January 1993 (unpublished).
5. Tsai TF, and Yu YX. Japanese encephalitis vaccines. In: Plotkin S, Mortimer E, eds. Vaccines. 2nd ed. Philadelphia: WB Saunders; 1993.
6. The Joint United Nations Programme on AIDS (UNAIDS). Fact Sheet 1 July 1996.
7. Soerono AR. The HIV/AIDS situation in the world and South-East Asia. Report of the Technical Consultation on Information regarding Population Movements and HIV/AIDS, 24–26 May 1995: 23–24.
8. Abdullah ASM, Fielding R, Hedley AJ. Travel, sexual behaviour and risk to HIV infection. Hong Kong Medical Journal (in press).
9. Shlim DR, Houston R. Helicopter rescue and deaths among trekkers in Nepal. Journal of the American Medical Association 1989; 261(7): 1017–1019.
10. O'Grady R. Third world stopover. In: Proceedings of the World Congress on Tourist Medicine and Health, Singapore, 1993. Geneva: World Council of Churches; 1981.
11. Jurgensen O. Tourism and prostitution in Southeast Asia. The Manitoba Social Science Teacher 1987; 14(1): 5–12.
12. Gay J. The patriotic prostitute. The Progressive 1985; 49(3): 34–36.
13. Matsui Y. The prostitution areas in Asia: an experience. Women in a Changing World 1987; 24 November: 27–32.

14. Hall CM. Sex tourism in Southeast Asia. In: Tourism and the less developed countries. London: Belhaven Press; 1992: 64–74.

15. Collier A. Principles of tourism. New Zealand: Pitman; 1989.

BIBLIOGRAPHY

Dawood R. Travellers' health. Oxford: Oxford University Press; 1986.

Harrison D. Tourism and the less developed countries. London: Belhaven Press; 1992.

Lundberg D. International travel and tourism. Chichester: Wiley; 1985.

Phoon WO, Chen PC. Textbook of community medicine in Southeast Asia. Chichester: Wiley; 1986.

Travel in cold climates

Jane Weaver

Introduction

Travellers to cold climates may include medical, nursing and other volunteers working in the north of Canada or Alaska, students of early Scandinavian history involved in field studies or archaeological expeditions, winter sports enthusiasts, and scientists taking up a term of residence with the Antarctic Survey.

Increasingly, however, with the fall of Soviet Communism and the opening up of China to Western expertise, there is a need for travel health advice for those expatriates, mainly educational, business and technical personnel, who will be living and working in those Central and Eastern Asian countries which have winter conditions of extreme cold. It is with these travellers that this chapter is chiefly concerned.

Climate, history and culture

GEOGRAPHY

The countries which are located in or around the Gobi and Taklamakan deserts are Mongolia and the new Central Asian republics, Siberia and Sakhalin Island, and north and north-eastern China. Climatic conditions are extreme:

- harsh Siberian winds sweep the desert and steppe during the winter months, the daytime temperature reaching -30°C
- settlements in the Gobi desert such as Saynsand can have temperatures of zero and below at midday even in June, and in Ulaan Baatar night frosts continue while the summer days get warmer
- near the Arctic Circle, winter daylight hours are short, and depending on climatic variations, this

season can mean a period of long, dark days without sunshine.

The region has a varied landscape: from Siberian scrub and softwood forest to Mongolian pastureland; from high steppe in the Gobi to sandy desert in the Chinese Taklamakan; from the Altai range of mountains to the Turfan depression, more than 200 m below sea-level. Mongolia, in particular, supports a rich flora and varied wildlife, from small rodents, marmots and susliks to deer, wolves, bears and the elusive snow leopard.

This is an area rich in mineral deposits, including uranium, and oil, coal, copper and precious metals. Groundwater and deepwater samples taken from the southern arc of the Gobi have shown high concentrations of selenium and fluoride and low iodine levels, which have implications for the health of the local people.[1]

PEOPLE AND HOUSES

Central Asia has a tradition of nomads, a way of life still visible today in and around cities like Ulaan Baatar and Almaty. The horse is the normal form of transport, and the commonly-worn traditional 'dale' or fur-lined riding coat, worn with heavy Russian boots, is the usual dress in winter. Nomadic homes in this part of the world are 'gers', circular skin or felt tents, stabilised on a wooden framework, heated by a central turf or dung stove, and capable of easy dismantling and carriage on horseback to new grazing pastures as the seasons change.

- Water is scarce during most of the year as it is either frozen or concealed under thick surface ice, and in winter, therefore, is used only for essential purposes such as cooking.
- Waste disposal is a problem when the digging of night soil pits becomes impossible after the land freezes.

In north-east China, the more settled farming way of life led to the development of the traditional Chinese 'courtyard house'. Built of brick or clay blocks with its back to the piercing northern winds, its focal point is a raised, central living area, the 'kang', heated by means of a wood or dung fire underneath the platform. The courtyard house design allows for inner enclosures to accommodate the household's pig and ducks, essentially bringing them into the house's living space for warmth.

Older Russian settlements have a lingering sense of the pioneer; the tightly-designed wooden cabins have homely little verandahs and are usually very brightly painted. But in colonising the remoter regions for the exploitation of oil, mineral deposits, or for strategic importance, both the Soviet Union and China rapidly established modern cities to accommodate all grades of workers and technical staff.

These new towns, often isolated, rise out of the landscape as clusters of identical housing blocks on a uniform, architectural plan. Built using standardised, prefabricated materials, these are perhaps the least suitable of all building styles for guaranteeing indoor warmth. Public buildings such as post offices and opera houses are often grandly designed with porticos, and are colour washed. Many cities embraced socialist realism with splendid, morally improving murals and tile paintings and forceful, patriotic sculptures in public open spaces. Some cities became important centres of learning and research.

Although the technology used may appear wasteful and ugly to the Western eye today, heat and hot water was nevertheless provided free of charge to apartment blocks and public buildings in the former Soviet Union through a centralised city supply. Municipal systems like these are increasingly an economic headache, though some are being maintained with the help of aid projects.

FOOD AND DRINK

In these, as in other cold parts of the world, winter food means fat meat: mutton or goat in Central Asia and pork in China. Neither the nomadic way of life nor the exceptionally short growing season allows for fresh vegetables in the diet. Both Siberian and northern Chinese cuisines have a tradition of using pickles to liven up the meal: hot spiced onion or cabbage in vinegar.

Fresh dairy produce is seasonally available and provides variety in the diet except in those areas of northern China which have been settled by Han Chinese from the central provinces. Lactase deficiency is common within this group and they must rely on a nutritionally poor, winter diet, which is based on beancurd and rice-flour dishes.

Tea is the most common, non-alcoholic drink in the nomadic world, served in a brew with sugar and butter.

This whole region has a tradition of using strong alcoholic drinks to keep out the cold: vodka and arkhi, kumis or fermented, mares' milk, and mao tai jiu – the ferocious distilled millet of northern China.

Recent history

In considering travel advice for today's visitor to this part of the world, it is important to remember that what China, Mongolia, and the former Soviet Union republics have in common is not only defined by geography and climate. There are significant modern historical aspects to consider in that they are all presently, or were previously, influenced by the centralist administrative methods of Communist government and the competitive demands of the Cold War. Consequently, they share the visible scars of certain developmental patterns: ecological disregard and environmental neglect – the near destruction of the Aral Sea through diversion of its two main feeder rivers to supply irrigation water for cotton production being perhaps the most notorious; wasteful industrial development and a different system of values in industrial safety (the Chernobyl story making salutary reading in this respect) and reliance on a centralised provision of goods and services, including those concerning healthcare – most of which have either faltered or are failing rapidly.

Both China and the Soviet Union used their cold wastelands to develop nuclear technology, to transport and test nuclear weapons and to dispose of nuclear waste. Both saw these remote and inhospitable regions as suitable for the siting of gulags and labour camps.[2]

Health risks for travellers and expatriates in cold climates

Introduction

This is not yet a region with a fully developed, modern tourism industry, and at the present time most visitors are likely to be long-term residents. Their health risks stem from the extent to which they find themselves immersed in the indigenous lifestyle and culture:

- working in local factories and schools or on the land
- making new friendships and a new social circle
- eating local food
- becoming involved in local sports and recreations.

Practical advice on these risks comes from relating not only the local epidemiological map but also the changing economic and political situation to the expectations and unawareness of the individual traveller, who may well take safety at work and living in warmth for granted.

Environmental pollution

Environmental pollution is a serious problem for some cities in this part of the world which is unlikely to be resolved in the short-term. The Soviet Union and China designed traditional power stations to accommodate the burning of low quality, fossil fuel, 'brown coal', which together with poor emission control from chimneys, have resulted in many years of acid rain contaminating the environment, woods and rivers. Incomplete combustion of coal results in a 'London smog' complex of suspended particulates, including hydrocarbons and sulphur compounds which are readily inhaled and which predispose to chest infections and bronchitis.

An environment of uncontrolled atmospheric pollution is not suitable for young children or for adults with existing respiratory disease, and smokers should be advised of an increased risk of ill-health.

Fortunately, at the present time, the number of petrol and diesel vehicles in this region generally is not sufficient to significantly contribute to air pollution, but the situation is changing rapidly in China, where a dramatic advance in urban wealth has demanded more access to private cars. Traffic congestion and poorly refined vehicle fuels are the recipe for photochemical smog, which will doubtless become commonplace here as elsewhere.

Accommodation

At the present time, the majority of visitors are mainly concerned with development or business ventures:

- teachers
- banking and finance experts
- veterinary advisers
- engineers involved in major construction projects or improvements to airports and power stations
- oil and gas exploration personnel.

For many of these visitors, available accommodation is likely to be in hotels, apartment blocks, or rooms on a university campus. With the exception of the most modern hotels, in any of these, and almost certainly in student accommodation, heating will probably be inefficient if not absent.

The fact that the internal environment can be almost as hostile as the cold outside can take some time to assimilate. Risks to health resulting from an inability to keep warm include a tendency to clumsiness and inertia, an increased susceptibility to infection, and an increasing risk of those health problems which result from difficulties in keeping oneself clean. There is also a temptation to resort to alcohol for warmth and stimulation.

- Long-term travellers need to take a good supply of warm, layered clothing, including woolly hats and fingerless mittens which can comfortably be worn indoors.

- Cashmere or camel-wool jumpers may be available locally, but this is not so in all areas.
- The risk of chilling down is greatest when inactive, for example while sitting reading, or while asleep.
- Small children and older people are at higher risk, the latter because sensitivity to cold perception and to changes in room temperature diminishes with age.[3,4]

Poor quality concrete was extensively used in the 1960s in the rapid development of tower-block sites. Another building material was asbestos, and both the West and the former-Soviet bloc will continue to have problems resolving the inherent health risks caused by living and working with this substance. Defects in prefabricated construction have become ever more apparent after years of neglect: a prime example is the stairwell with crumbling steps which invite accidental falls. Lighting in stairwells was never very adequate and is now likely to be worse, given frequent failures of electricity supply. Dark entrances may attract petty criminals to take refuge.

Expatriates are recommended to:

- carry a strong torch and pack spare batteries
- be aware of the possibility of mugging and street violence.

Cold living-quarters do not necessarily mean dirty living conditions but the strategies required to conserve a reasonable indoor temperature such as sealing windows and using curtains to prevent draughts facilitate, over the years, the accumulation of dust and dust-loving creatures such as dust mites and bedbugs. Asthma may become worse, or may reappear in adults who were childhood sufferers. Neglected living accommodation is also likely to harbour noticeable infestations of cockroaches, mice and rats.[5]

Packs of roaming dogs in urban areas are another sign of the breakdown of Soviet control and these days, as in many other parts of the world, semi-starved dogs in garbage areas are a health risk to residents. A rather more bizarre scavenger, reported from Vladivostok, is the 'urban' bear (Stoddart G., personal communication, 1995).

The workplace

Whatever the workplace, industry or university, it can be expected to have different standards of safety to protect its employees than is acceptable in the European Union or the USA. In addition, whatever the standards originally in place, the combination of neglect and lack of maintenance of site or machinery will have had a serious effect over the past decade as will the lack of enforcement of safety regulations during the transition from Communism to the present regime.

Employers are required by workplace law in more industrial developed countries to retain certain health and safety responsibilities for their expatriate and travelling staff, and not to place them at an increased risk through exposing them to unsafe work practices overseas. This obligation is almost impossible to meet in circumstances, for example, where the employees are going in to inspect, for the first time, a malfunctioning power station built to an unfamiliar, non-European design with outdated technology.

The best that can be achieved is for the travel adviser to heighten the traveller's awareness of the potential health risks which may at home have been reduced or eliminated through legislation, and may, as a result, have slipped from the employee's awareness. These risks will include:

- the increased risk of falls from inadequately secured structures such as scaffolding or gantries
- exposure to chemicals including isocyanates, or to radio-active materials
- exposure to asbestos
- exposure to crude oils.

For many, whether working indoors or outside, the workplace will be cold. The coldest outdoor jobs are traditionally those in the construction industry, agriculture, and oil and gas exploration, but for those travellers going to relatively sedentary jobs in Siberian university departments or hospitals, indoor temperatures may be as low as -4°C.[6] Expatriates may notice a general slowing down in their workplace efficiency caused by a combination of diminished mental agility, diminished fine digital manipulation, and diminished powers of concentration. The inevitable result is an increased risk of accidents; more so, if the workplace is inherently unsafe.

- A cold working environment demands a fair degree of physical fitness and plenty of breaks for hot drinks.
- Several layers of thin, warm clothing are the most effective insulators, including long underwear, thermal socks, and hats which cover the ears.
- Safety clothing, if taken on the overseas tour, may well be unsuitable, for example steel toe-cap, safety shoes will freeze the feet.[7]

Veterinary services in the Soviet Union maintained the health of nomadic herds using the feldsher system, and, given the nature of the terrain, kept surprisingly comprehensive epidemiological records. This work is now opening up to Western aid and expertise.

Risks to veterinarians include:

- brucellosis
- anthrax
- plague
- hydatid disease which has a well-researched focus in Xinjiang province.[8]

Laboratory staff working in the region may be helping to restructure either hospital or animal laboratory services and their vaccination protection needs to be specific. Risks to laboratory staff include:

- lack of appropriate protective clothing, particularly gloves
- inadequate information on the prevalence of blood-borne infections such as hepatitis B, generally high in Asia, and HIV
- being hampered by cold-induced digital clumsiness when handling specimens and sharps.

Leisure activities and tourism

Tours of acknowledged historical and cultural centres were available to Westerners under the former regimes through the state tourism boards such as Intourist, but less structured tourism is a new venture in this region and tends towards the more adventurous, outdoor pursuits such as trekking by horseback or winter sports. Travel can be difficult if not arranged through the new national tourism organisations, but resident expatriates can be more flexible in their leisure plans and 4-wheel drive journeys into the steppe or forest by Russian jeep are popular, as are hunting and fishing trips.

Health risks for tourists include:

- the lack of a tourism infrastructure, including transport, medical rescue and healthcare facilities
- being unaware of the need to avoid types of accidents not usual in a Western setting.

Rain is rare during the winter months and snowfall variable, northern China taking the heaviest cover. In bright clear sunshine, accidents caused by cold and windchill are a distinct possibility. Roaming off the beaten track by horse or car, or off-piste on the newly opened Chinese ski slopes, can be dangerous. Hire cars have probably not been adequately maintained, may have a bizarre tyre configuration, and break down frequently. Horses may fall or may cause their riders to fall; they are probably working horses, and unaccustomed to an unsure hand. Risks of accident resulting from inexperience in horsemanship or from driving across unmapped frozen tundra are compounded by liberal use of alcohol by either tourist or tour guide.[9,10] Expatriates should know how to deal with suspected hypothermia and trauma first-aid.

The newest pastime for travellers is the very new nightlife scene; drinking clubs, dancing, drugs and prostitution have all flourished in post-Communist Asia. Street drunkenness is now a sadly familiar sight. There is a serious risk of assault and robbery for the unwary tourist here, as there is on previously safe, travel routes such as the trans-Siberian railway. Drugs are now easy to obtain; a semi-legal street market will usually offer benzodiazepines, amphetamines and even antibiotics, as well as a selection of used syringes and needles. More serious drugs are probably available from a hessian sack after a few enquiries. These stands are periodically raided by police, only to reappear on a different site.

Nutrition

Expatriates in this region tend to lose weight through a combination of reduced food intake, a different nutritional balance, and increased energy expenditure in keeping warm.

Travellers of Caucasian origin are physiologically equipped to survive on a Central Asian, high-fat, meat-based diet, but most find it intensely dull quite apart from the health risks. Expatriates in northern China will probably find a high-carbohydrate, low-fat diet alone inadequate for warmth and energy needs. The situation is much improved in the summer when fish is usually freely available from markets or friends.

Food supplies are generally improving; the newly independent market gardeners of China are exporting fruit and vegetables through Beijing northwards using the railway routes into Russia. This is not a region for the vegetarian, and travel advisers need to ascertain the degree of flexibility in a potential expatriate's commitment to vegetarianism, and give appropriate advice.

Medical care

Soviet medical and nursing care provision was comprehensive, and after 1946 adopted a different system of priorities to the Western model, having more of a focus on military and industrial health and on provision for remote communities, using feldsher workers. Always underfunded, since 1990 it has struggled to keep going with few drugs, reagents, and vaccines, with aging equipment, and a diminishing skilled workforce.

Expatriates will need to take local or company advice concerning which doctor, clinic or hospital is able to take foreign patients, and the extent to which they have the means to help with, for example, trauma or cardiac care, or children's medicine. Joint venture polyclinics are also beginning to become established and these may have better equipped facilities or English-speaking staff.

China has particular problems in the provision of medical care: a legacy of the Cultural Revolution is an expertise gap as some medical schools were closed for up to 20 years. It also has certain experience gaps. One gap is in working with Rhesus-negative blood groups which have an extremely low incidence among the Chinese; one gap for the future is multiparous pregnancy as practical obstetrics and midwifery education are dominated by the one-child policy.

This region has a tradition of using herbal medicines, Chinese remedies have become both famous and fashionable, and Tibetan-style traditional medicine is now becoming available in Mongolia from replanted monastic herb gardens. Travellers may warm to these medicines as 'holistic' and they can certainly sometimes be helpful. They can also be dangerous.[11]

Summary of illness risks for travellers

Infectious diseases

Recently health services in the area have faltered while in the former Soviet Union they collapsed, but the complex public health authorities tried to keep under control those infectious diseases of close contact which thrive in the colder regions of the world: tuberculosis, diphtheria and meningitis. The resurgence of epidemic diphtheria in this region is well known. Mongolia and northern China experienced a large outbreak of group A meningococcal meningitis in the winter of 1993, and tuberculosis remains endemic. As in other countries with cold winters and overcrowded conditions among the poor – the Britain of the 1930s – the USSR built sanatoria for the isolation and treatment of tuberculosis sufferers. These are now long since deserted but community surveillance systems struggle to keep going, some with Western aid, while actual numbers of cases rise, reflecting the worldwide trend. In this region, the impact of AIDS on tuberculosis is probably yet to come.[12,13]

Expatriates will almost certainly spend long hours in the company of local people who may have colds or influenza or whose home conditions may present a health risk.

SPECIAL VACCINATIONS

- BCG vaccine should be considered.
- Adult diphtheria vaccine and meningococcal A and C vaccine are strongly recommended.
- Some USA and European company travel policies also specify influenza vaccine for those of their expatriate staff who are resident in Asia and China.
- Pneumococcal vaccine may be appropriate for certain travellers.

Gut infections

Common gastrointestinal infections are caused by *Rotavirus*, *Campylobacter*, and *Yersinia enterocolitica*. Water-borne diseases which are unaffected by low temperatures include giardiasis, cryptosporidiosis, and entamoebasis.[14]

Insect-borne infections

The Mongolian steppe has stunning botanical variety and is home to many Alpine species. No doubt in time this will become a focus of tourism as will trekking in the Siberian forests. Summer sees the invasion of Arctic midges, and the awakening activity of ixodid ticks.

- The endemic area for Asian-type, tick-borne encephalitis (TBE) extends eastward from the European TBE belt as far as Vladivostok, and has in the past been the subject of public health intervention measures in Siberia resulting in the closing of forests and taiga to visitors. Its seasonal incidence is May to September, hence its common name of Russian spring–summer encephalitis.
- Scrub typhus is reported from the area around Vladivostok; the rickettsial infection North Asian tick typhus (*Rickettsia sibirica*) has a wider distribution from Armenia eastward throughout this region.
- Expatriates to many parts of China will require information on and protection from Japanese B encephalitis, the endemic area for which has apparently spread northward since the 1960s following agrarian experimentation.

Animal-borne diseases

- Brucellosis is a health hazard to nomadic families through their practice, in the cold winter months, of bringing labouring and newly delivered sheep into their living tents. Expatriate vets may also be put at risk. Other expatriates and travellers may contract the infection from untreated milk and dairy produce, which is plentiful in season and usually of very good quality. Mature yoghurt and cheese are generally too acidic for the organism's survival.
- In a hunting culture, leather clothing and collections of horns and antlers are commonplace, and anthrax is mostly a risk to those who prepare these trophies or handle animal skins. Three groups of expatriates are at risk: vets, those visiting rural tanneries and factories for commercial reasons, and those resident expatriates and tourists who are attracted by the idea of hunting trips.
- Pre-exposure rabies vaccine is strongly recommended for all travellers to this region.

Diseases carried by rodents

- Plague is carried by marmots and other small rodents which are hunted for their fur. Soviet public health regulations governed the procedures used in the preparation of skin for clothing and bedding, and any province suspected of supplying infected skins, or reporting sightings of infected rodents was isolated by a 'cordon sanitaire'. This is no longer economically possible, and marmot trapping, previously controlled by licence, has become deregulated. Those involved in supplying skins are no longer necessarily experienced in the recognition of animals which are sick or behaving in an abnormal way. The risk of plague to expatriates is very low, but those who decide to purchase cheap furs from unlicensed warehouses, either individually or commercially, should certainly know about this disease.

- Buyers handling musk rat fur may be at risk from contracting Omsk haemorrhagic fever or leptospirosis.
- In northern China, the fieldmouse-transmitted Korean haemorrhagic fever is a health risk to those involved in agricultural development or whose accommodation is in traditional housing.[15]

Skin problems

Health risks to skin include sunburn. Much of the steppe is at a moderate altitude and once away from urban pollution the air is clear and sharp. Summer sunshine can be fierce, in an area of generally low humidity.

Simple cold injuries and skin conditions associated with cold include chilblains, cracked skin and lips, a tendency toward skin infections, minor circulatory symptoms, and haemorrhoids. Herpes simplex and fungal infections are common. Dusty or dirty living conditions harbour fleas, bedbugs, and house dust mites, and sharing accommodation may bring the risk of scabies and lice.

Frostbite and trench foot are serious skin conditions from which travellers are most at risk during outdoor work or when trekking in winter.

Sexually-transmitted diseases

Sexually transmitted infections are an increasing problem despite the survival of clinics providing free diagnosis and treatment. Poverty and the rapid growth of drug-related crime, assisted by greater freedom of movement within and beyond the region, have made the Russian commercial sex-worker a very marketable commodity. The numbers of street children now seen in cities like Ulaan Baatar doubtless reflect a trend towards the commercialisation of child sex.

Statistics on HIV are not freely available at the present time, but WHO has made an estimate of 150 000 persons infected in Eastern and Central Asia.[16]

Psychological difficulties

Certain groups of workers are known to be at an increased risk of psychological disturbance triggered by a combination of living in remote, harsh, cramped or isolated conditions; a lack of natural daylight; the long-term removal from family and friends and the impossibility, because of either geographical constraints or the demands of the job, to escape from a narrow social group.

'Cabin fever'. What is colloquially known as 'cabin fever' may present as a schizoid-type picture: problems with judgement or logic, thoughts of persecution, and suspicion of colleagues. Signs of impending illness may easily be missed. The slowing-down effects of cold, and possibly a more liberal use of strong spirits are to be expected during the adjustment period. Work may not suffer immediately; the need for skilled help may, equally, not be recognised for some time.

For some potentially affected groups, such as survey team members, individual selection and specific training are possible. Other long-term travellers may either be self-selected or may have to travel at short notice. All should receive pre-travel advice on recognition and coping techniques.

- 'Cold countries' include the Antarctic, northern Canada, the Scandinavian countries, Iceland and Greenland, Siberia and Sakhalin Island, Kazakhstan, Mongolia and north and north-east China.

- The climate may be cold all year round or may have extreme variables between winter and summer. Winter temperatures are significantly affected by windchill, particularly those areas swept by Arctic winds, which penetrate as far south as the Gobi desert.

- A high intake of carbohydrate in a cold climate demands a regular balanced diet. However, traditional diets may be high in fat as an alternative source of energy, or, as in rice-based diets, be deficient in both energy and basic nutrients.

- Suitable cold climate clothing includes wearing several thin layers, preventing heat loss through the extremities including the head, and wearing a warm, windproof coat which does not restrict movement.

- Small children and older people are at greatest risk of hypothermia in the home because of their reduced ability to detect or adapt to a drop in ambient temperature. Indoor residential or workplace temperatures may fall to zero or beyond.

- Health and safety legislation in Asian countries may appear inadequate and safety may be compromised by cold and its effects such as digital clumsiness.

- It may be appropriate to recommend a pre-travel course in basic vehicle maintenance and in off-road driving and navigation skills, as well as survival first-aid and the emergency treatment of cold injury.

- Coping with long periods of cold, dark and isolation requires a high degree of psychological strength, adjustment and coping skills, and self-reliance.

REFERENCES

1. Tan Jianan, ed. Atlas of endemic diseases and their environments in the People's Republic of China. Beijing: Science Press: 1989.
2. Kosserev I, Crawshaw R. Medicine and the Gulag. British Medical Journal 1994; 309: 1726–1730.
3. The Midwinter Group. Cold exposure and winter mortality from ischaemic heart disease, cerebrovascular disease, respiratory disease, and all causes in warm and cold regions of Europe. Lancet 1997; 349: 1341–1346.
4. Exton-Smith AN. Accidental hypothermia. In: Medicine in old age. London: British Medical Journal Publications 1991
5. Lowry S, ed. Housing and health. London: British Medical Journal Publications 1991.
6. Henni F. La longue souffrance des chercheurs de Russie. Recherche 1996; 228(June): 38–41.
7. Health and Safety Executive. Health and safety in retail and wholesale warehouses. Health and Safety Executive Publications, Cold Stores no. 58; 1995.
8. Craig P S, Liu D, Macpherson CN, et al. A large focus of alveolar echinococcosis in central China. Lancet 1992; 340: 826–831.
9. Harding J. Slip, sliding away in Yabouli. Financial Times 1998; January 25.
10. Troy T. On the up in Uzbekistan. Guardian Travel 1998; January 29.
11. Chan T Y K, Chan J C N, Tomlinson B, et al. Chinese herbal medicines revisited: a Hong Kong perspective. Lancet 1993; 342: 1532–1534.
12. Davies PDO, de Cock KM, Leese J, et al. Tuberculosis 2000. Journal of the Royal Society of Medicine 1996; 89(August): 431–435.
13. Frazer Wares D, Clowes C. Tuberculosis in Russia. Corresp to Lancet 1997; 304: 957.
14. Jones K. Waterborne diseases. New Scientist (Inside Science suppl) 1994; 73(July).
15. Clement J, Heyman P. Hantavirus infection, a world-wide emerging zoonosis. Travel Medicine International 1996; 14(2): 59–66.
16. Communicable Disease Report. AIDS and HIV infection worldwide. Communicable Disease Report 1997; 7(51): 461–462.

SECTION 8

SPECIAL SITUATIONS

Expedition medicine

Mike Townend

Introduction

An expedition has been defined as an organised journey or voyage for a specific purpose, especially for exploration or for a scientific or military purpose (Collins English Dictionary).

Expeditions often take place in conditions which are demanding in terms of climate, terrain and the nature of the activities undertaken. They may involve a wide variety of health risks and other objective dangers. Their physically demanding nature and the remote and unfamiliar surroundings experienced may also make great psychological demands on their participants. Medical care on expeditions demands a high degree of planning and organisation and a structured approach is necessary. Planning the medical care of an expedition will bring together many of the elements of travel medicine discussed in other chapters.

Introduction

> I kept six honest serving men, they taught me all I knew. Their names were What and Why and When and How and Where and Who.
>
> Rudyard Kipling

Kipling's six honest serving men provide the questions that must be answered in planning medical care for an expedition:

- **Who** is taking part in the expedition? The age and state of health and fitness, both physical and psychological, of the participants, their vaccination status, the presence or absence of any ongoing or recurrent medical problems and requirements for taking medication must all be investigated and catered for in planning.
- **Where** are they going?
  Health hazards may exist in the countries to be visited and the degree of risk relevant to the specific type of journey must be evaluated.
- **When** are they going?
  The time of year and resulting weather conditions together with the length of stay may alter the risks of some of the health hazards that exist at the destination.
- **How** are they going?
  The mode of travel to and within the country of destination may introduce particular hazards which need to be taken into account in the planning process.
- **Why** are they going?
  The activities that are involved in the expedition may involve increased risk of such hazards as those of climate, altitude, close personal contact or contact with animals.
- **What** precautions and what equipment do they need to take?
  Pre-travel precautions may include a health check or questionnaire, provision of any necessary continuing medication, vaccinations and malaria prophylaxis and a pre-travel briefing for the team.

  The contents of the expedition medical kit will depend on:
  — a careful evaluation of all the risk factors
  — the level of care which the expedition doctor feels able to provide
  — the overall philosophy of the expedition
  — what can reasonably be carried.

Pre-expedition planning

CHARACTERISTICS OF THE EXPEDITION MEMBERS

A medical enquiry in the form of a questionnaire (Fig. 19.1) should be circulated to all participants. The nature of the information to be gathered will depend to some extent on the nature of the expedition, but some necessary information will be common to all.

Vaccination status and adverse reactions to vaccines or antimalarial drugs in the past should be included as should proneness to chronic or recurrent medical conditions and current medication. If medication is being taken, the individual should be advised to obtain enough supplies to last through the expedition with some to spare in case of loss.

If there are any potential health hazards from the intended activities of the expedition, enquiry should be made about any previous problems associated with these hazards. For example, it is particularly important to know about previous frostbite and about previous complications of high altitude as there may be a recurrence of these problems on subsequent exposure to similar conditions. For expeditions that involve a great deal of physical exertion the presence of musculoskeletal problems of otherwise relatively minor importance may be of

Medical questionnaire

The following immunisations are advised for this expedition. Please check with your doctor which you have had and arrange to have any which are not up to date.

Tetanus	Typhoid
Polio	Rabies
Hepatitis A	Hepatitis B

Please tick any of the following which you have had and give brief details including present treatment if any:

Asthma	Pneumonia
Recurrent bronchitis	Sinus problems
Heart problems of any type	Piles
Raised blood pressure	Constipation
Circulatory problems	Dysentery or recurrent diarrhoea
(e.g. 'dead' fingers or toes)	Unusual sensitivity to sunlight
Recurrent indigestion	'Cold sores' (herpes)
Stomach/duodenal ulcer	Any other skin disease
Appendicitis	Dizzy spells
Eczema/dermatitis	Difficulty in sleeping
Athlete's foot or other skin infection	Frostbite
Migraine	Hypothermia
Fits, faints or blackouts	Any other cold or altitude problem
Surgical operations	Muscle or joint pains
(including appendix)	Contact allergies
Mountain sickness	Other allergies
High-altitude pulmonary oedema	
High-altitude cerebral oedema	
Major fractures or other injuries	
Drug allergies	
Food allergies	

Do you have any other regular or recurrent medical condition? Please give details below.

Are you taking any regular medication? Please give details below and ensure that you have enough supplies for the whole expedition.

What is your blood group?

Thank you for your co-operation. These details will remain confidential and will help in the planning of your medical care and the expedition medical supplies.

Fig. 19.1 Medical questionnaire for expedition participants.

great significance. Food or other allergies should be documented.

THE PRE-TRAVEL BRIEFING

A pre-travel medical briefing may be appropriate for many expedition members. The members of different types of expedition may vary widely, from schoolchildren on their first trip abroad to experienced and well-travelled explorers, mount-aineers, canoeists or cavers. Those with a great deal of experience may be very well informed about the hazards of their chosen itinerary and activities, but this cannot be assumed. The activities undertaken by other expedition members may not be commensurate with their level of experience; for example, it is possible for those with little experience of high altitude to hire professional guides and travel into the world's high mountain ranges, perhaps even to attempt the ascent of Everest.

The pre-travel briefing must therefore be carefully tailored to the level of knowledge and experience of the expedition members. It should include:

- information on the degree of risk from health hazards peculiar to the country being visited
- explanation of the risks inherent in the expedition's chosen activities
- how these risks may be avoided or minimised.

INSURANCE

It is important for expedition travellers, as for all travellers, to obtain adequate insurance. They must ensure that they are covered for pre-existing medical conditions and for medical expenses and/or repatriation in the case of serious illness or trauma. It may be difficult to obtain cover for an expedition from many travel insurers and it may be necessary to approach a specialist insurance broker or company. The insurance schemes operated by the British Mountaineering Council[1] and the Expedition Advisory Centre[2] are examples of specialised insurance for expeditions.

HAZARDS INHERENT IN THE COUNTRY BEING VISITED

The expedition doctor will need to be aware of precisely which parts of a country will be visited and of the health hazards that exist in them. The assessment of risk is addressed in Chapter 4, but it will be necessary to consult a comprehensive, up-to-date database to check on the hazards likely to be encountered, unless the expedition doctor is already reliably acquainted with the destination.

Countries in which there is a low risk of malaria[3] for tourists may have a much greater risk for those on expeditions travelling into rural areas. Countries that carry a high risk of malaria in lowland regions are likely to have little or no such risk in their highland or mountain regions.

Travel to remote areas of a country poses particular problems which will be addressed in more detail later (p. 399) and which may need a considerable amount of forward planning.

High-risk factors

- Although the risk of rabies for travellers is extremely small, it is invariably fatal and expeditions may be far distant from access to post-exposure rabies vaccination.
- The expedition members may be at greater risk than other travellers of trauma and need medical treatment in poor medical circumstances.
  The expedition doctor is therefore likely to advise rabies or hepatitis B vaccination.
- Planning for independence from medical facilities may be essential. Even if available, they may not be of an acceptable standard.
- A plan for medical evacuation will need to be considered.

TIMING OF THE EXPEDITION

The time of year during which an expedition is planned to take place may influence the degree of risk of some of the inherent health and safety hazards. In the rainy season, river crossings may be more difficult and hazardous and contamination of drinking water may be increased as faecal material is washed into the source of supply by heavy rainfall. If the expedition is to visit South-East Asia in the wet season, the members may be at greater risk of Japanese B encephalitis, particularly if their stay is to be prolonged.

In the dry season in Nepal or in sub-Saharan Africa, for example, there may be an increased risk of meningococcal infection, particularly if the expedition members are likely to be living in close contact with indigenous people during their stay.

The risk of most of the health hazards, especially infectious and insect-borne diseases, will be increased by the length of the expedition.

HAZARDS INHERENT IN THE MODE OF TRAVEL

Many expedition travellers will use air transport to reach their starting point. If travellers are usually fit and healthy, this will not normally be a risk but usual advice about limiting alcohol, avoiding dehydration and prolonged immobility during long flights may need to be emphasised.[4]

Overland expedition travellers face a different range of risks, including the risk of injury in a road traffic accident, and they will need to consider how they will plan for dealing with the effects of major or minor trauma and casualty evacuation. Other hazards of overland travel, depending often on whether public transport is used, may include close proximity with fellow travellers and their droplet infections, fleas, lice and animals, food and water hygiene, dust and other irritants and allergens and poor or non-existent sanitation.

HAZARDS INHERENT IN THE EXPEDITION'S ACTIVITIES

Many expeditions take place in order to expand personal frontiers by satisfying their participants' need for adventure by doing something which has not been done before. Others are undertaken in order to expand the frontiers of human knowledge by exploring a remote area or by carrying out research into the environment, anthropology, archaeology or other areas of knowledge. Their activities are therefore so diverse that it would be impossible to detail all of them.

Expeditions on or in water involve risk of drowning, hypothermia and water-borne diseases such as faecal–oral infection, schistosomiasis and leptospirosis. Planning medical care will need these potential problems to be taken into account.

Expeditions with other objectives may travel into a wide range of high-risk environments (see pp. 395–400).

Some may have cultural objectives and these, and indeed all expeditions, would be well advised to learn as much as possible about the culture they will encounter at their destination. In doing so they will profit more from their experience as well as avoiding offending the cultural senstivities of their hosts. This will also help to make them aware of some of the potential health hazards to which local cultural demands may expose them.

PLANNING THE EXPEDITION MEDICAL KIT[5–7]

Figure 19.2 shows a scheme for planning the contents of an expedition medical kit. Suggestions for the actual contents of such a kit, logistics and packing of kits are discussed on pages 403–406 but early planning is necessary.

The experience of the doctor or other person in charge of first-aid will determine the extent to which medical care can be provided. It will not be possible for most expeditions to offer the type of comprehensive medical care that would be available to travellers at home, even with the most experienced expedition doctor.

A team decision must be taken about the levels of care that the expedition is able to accept and what minimum and maximum standards of care should be provided. The doctor will then be able to decide according to his or her level of expertise the equipment that will be needed. The carrying capacity of the expedition, the availability or otherwise of casualty evacuation and the availability and quality of secondary medical care will also influence the contents of the medical kit. The management of illnesses which may occur just as readily at home should be considered and expedition members may decide to carry simple self-medication according to their own preferences.

MEDICAL OR SURGICAL EMERGENCIES AND SERIOUS TRAUMA

Resuscitation and life-support equipment is impracticable for many expeditions, as it would

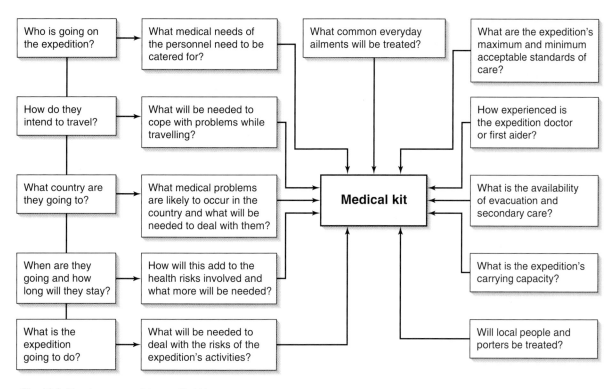

Fig. 19.2 Planning an expedition medical kit

use a great deal of the expedition's carrying capacity. There would often be little opportunity to provide intensive care after resuscitation or to transfer the patient on to a suitable secondary care facility. While intravenous fluids may be lifesaving they are heavy to carry and may be needed in large quantities. On such an expedition the doctor may be able to extemporise by, for example, rehydrating a patient using rectal fluids made up from more easily available water and salt.

CARE OF PORTERS AND GUIDES

Decisions may have to be taken about treating local people and porters or guides. When employing porters and guides, it is customary for the expedition doctor to treat them for any medical problems or trauma that arise during their employment. Some of them will be found to be suffering from chronic conditions that existed before the expedition arrived and will continue after it leaves. Local people will continue to be dependent on whatever medical services are normally available to them after the expedition

has left. It is advisable not to give them false expectations of what it is possible to achieve by attempting to treat them with expensive treatments which they do not understand how to use and will not be able to continue using.

Problems associated with specific environments

Hot climates

In temperate climates, heat loss from the body takes place by all available routes, that is radiation, convection and conduction, as well as by evaporation of sweat. In hot climates, the ambient temperature may approach or even exceed body temperature, and the only available method of cooling in extreme conditions is by evaporation of sweat. If the environment also has a high humidity, as for example in jungle regions, evaporation is greatly reduced, adding to the difficulty in maintaining body temperature. Exertion increases the loss of water from sweating.

PREVENTING DEHYDRATION[8]

A high intake of water, which may amount to several litres per day, is needed in hot climates and, at least until acclimatisation to the conditions is achieved, additional salt on food is advisable. Water should be taken in excess of what appears to be necessary from the sensation of thirst. The adequacy of hydration may be assessed by the output of pale-coloured urine. Acclimatisation takes place within about 2 or 3 weeks of arrival in a hot climate and involves an increased ability of the body to conserve salt and water while still retaining the ability to cool itself by sweating.

At least 10% of body water has probably been lost before clinical signs of dehydration such as loss of skin turgor appear, and death is likely when 20% has been lost. Earlier symptoms are a strong sensation of thirst (1% loss) and drying up of the saliva in the mouth (5% loss). Headaches, nausea, fatigue and confusion may follow.

Heat exhaustion[9] is the result of excessive loss of salt and water from sweating and/or inadequate salt and water intake. It is characterised by feelings of weakness and exhaustion and may lead to hypotension, faintness and collapse. There may be a sensation of extreme thirst and urine output is reduced. The body temperature is normal. If there is substantial loss of salt, there may also be muscle cramps. It may be avoided by an adequate intake of fluid and by adding additional salt to food. If this is done, salt tablets are seldom needed.

Treatment consists of rehydration with oral fluid made up as for the treatment of diarrhoea by giving copious drinks, each glass containing a small pinch of salt or by making up drinks with one teaspoonful of salt per litre.

Heat hyperpyrexia[9] occurs when the cooling mechanism of sweating breaks down and the body temperature rises unchecked. Headache, flushing and confusion may lead to drowsiness, delirium and coma, and convulsions may ensue. The subject's skin feels hot and dry. Rapid cooling by any means available is essential, as the condition is life-threatening. Removal from direct sources of heat such as strong sunlight, immersion

in cool water if available, covering with light-weight wet fabric or repeated sponging with cool water and exposure to a draught of air or a current from a fan are all useful in reducing the temperature.

Prickly heat is seen as a rash consisting of minute papules or vesicles with an intense prickling sensation. It appears to be caused by excessive sweating and obstruction of the outflow from the ducts of sweat glands. Good hygiene and frequent changes of sweat-soaked clothing may reduce the likelihood of its occurrence. There is no specific treatment, but careful washing of the skin, careful drying and wearing loose-fitting clothing made from cotton together with symptomatic treatment with an antipruritic such as calamine lotion will help to relieve symptoms.

Sunburn is frequently a problem in hot climates. It is discussed in detail in Chapter 9. Expedition members may need to be reminded about the dangers of exposure to ultraviolet light and to cover exposed skin and use an effective sunscreen cream. Apart from the short-term effects of sunburn and the long term effects of skin malignancy,[10] exposure to ultraviolet light may in susceptible individuals predispose to herpes simplex infection of exposed skin.

Exposure of the skin surface in hot climates also predisposes to insect bites and the resulting risk of insect-borne diseases. If insect repellents are being used, it is important that they are applied after the sunscreen cream, otherwise they will be ineffective.

Cold climates

Cold conditions are encountered at extremes of northern and southern latitudes and at high altitude. What may also be overlooked in planning an expedition is that in some circumstances such as in deserts and at moderately high altitudes, daytime temperatures may be high but night temperatures may be very low

Inadequate food intake and wet or inadequate clothing and sleeping bags predispose to cold-related illness. Those who are ill or injured are also more prone to both hypothermia and cold injury. It is important when travelling in conditions in which the air temperature may fluctuate suddenly from warm to cold that expedition members be reminded to carry layers of additional insulating clothing, hats and gloves and to put them on as soon as the temperature begins to fall. Travel in cold climates is considered in Chapter 18.

Hypothermia[11] is said to occur when the body core temperature falls below 35°C. At this temperature, some impairment of mental processes such as decision-making may already be impaired and excessive shivering may occur. Below this temperature, behaviour becomes inappropriate, clumsiness and confusion occur and as the body temperature falls lower, there is impairment or loss of consciousness and shivering stops. When the temperature has fallen to 30°C, it is difficult to detect vital signs such as pulse or respiration and below 28°C, death is a likely sequel unless warming is begun immediately.

The early signs of hypothermia may resemble those of altitude sickness or dehydration and it is important in cold conditions to operate a 'buddy system' in which expedition members look out for such signs in each other. Under expedition conditions, it is not likely that sophisticated methods of rewarming will be available. The victim should be insulated from further heat loss both above and below the body and sheltered from the cold environment as well as can be achieved. Sharing another person's body heat in a sleeping bag and breathing air in a tent which is heated by the presence of others and by, for example, a cooking stove or heat-emitting lantern are the most practicable methods of rewarming.

COLD INJURY

Frostbite[12] occurs when peripheral circulation is reduced in response to cold conditions and, ice crystals form within cells, causing tissue damage and in severe cases, gangrene of the extremities. Affected tissue has a pale appearance and a cold and dead feeling to the touch. It may be rewarmed by immersion in water at, or just above, body temperature but if a foot is affected and the victim needs to be evacuated on foot, it is better to allow walking on the frozen tissue before warming as less damage will be done to it. Re-freezing and thawing must be avoided as they also cause further

damage. There is no evidence to support the use of vasodilator drugs. As rewarming occurs, tissues become red, swollen and very painful and blisters may form. Apparently dead tissue should not be treated radically in the field, for example by debridement or amputation, as recovery may be greater than first appearances suggest. Decisions on radical treatment are best left to a surgeon experienced in the treatment of cold injury. Frostnip is a less severe form of cold injury in which tissues do not undergo necrosis.

Jungle environments

The jungle environment[13] is characterised by heat, which is usually not as extreme as in some other hot environments, usually up to about 35°C, and high humidity. The temperature does not fall to any great extent at night because of insulation by the tree canopy and cloud formation. Among the natural hazards present in the jungle an expedition may encounter are mosquitoes and other biting insects, leeches, snakes, animals and spiny or sharp-edged vegetation. Clothing should cover as much of the body surface as possible to avoid damage from these hazards and insect repellents are needed.

Leeches find their way with apparent ease into clothing and footwear. Pulling them off may leave portions of them embedded in the skin with resulting infection. If an alcoholic tincture of iodine is being carried for water purification, a drop or two placed on a leech makes it relax its grip and it may then be lifted off. Iodine may also then be used to clean the site of the bite, which may easily become infected, but other skin antiseptics should be used for those with a history of iodine sensitivity.

Insect bites produce unpleasant allergic reactions in susceptible individuals which may require the use of oral or topical antihistamines, though there is a small risk of skin sensitisation to topical antihistamine creams. Insect bites may become infected and topical or systemic antibiotic treatment may be needed.

In many jungle areas, there is a risk of malaria transmission from mosquito bites and dengue fever is a widespread and increasing hazard in many tropical and more temperate areas. In tropical areas of Africa and South America, mosquito bites are a potential means of transmission of yellow fever. Antimalarial drugs where appropriate and antimosquito precautions such as covering the skin, using insect repellents and sleeping under bed nets will reduce the risk of insect-borne diseases.

Snakes[14] are by no means all venomous and not all those which are venomous are life-threatening. They are best avoided and left undisturbed to go on their way. They will not usually strike at an immobile person or unless disturbed or attacked. If snakes are likely to be encountered, adequate footwear such as boots, and protection of the legs by tucking trousers into socks are advisable. In a majority of snake bites there is little risk to life, even from snakes known to be potentially harmful, as significant amounts of venom are not always injected. Calm reassurance and analgesics to relieve the pain of the bite may be the only treatment needed. The use of tourniquets to limit the spread of venom from the bite can result in ischaemia and gangrene and it is usually better to apply firm bandaging and to immobilise a bitten limb by makeshift splinting.

If venom has been injected, there may be an entirely local reaction with pain and swelling. Depending on the species of the snake, other reactions may include hypotension and shock, haemorrhagic manifestations or neurotoxic effects such as paresis of muscles. The administration of antivenom should be restricted to those with the more severe reactions as its use may be associated with allergic or anaphylactic reactions.

Local knowledge of snakes, the effects of their bites and the need for antivenom should always be sought, ideally in advance, and envenomed patients taken to hospital if possible. It is often recommended that the snake should be killed and captured for identification but this is often neither safe nor practical.

Animals are more likely to avoid humans than to attack them but it would be dangerous to assume that this is always the case. Apart from the dangers of attack by a large animal, there is the possibility of transmission of rabies from a variety of mammals to humans by bites or scratches and possibly by licking. If contact with animals is considered likely or if the objectives of an expedition involve contact with animals, pre-exposure rabies vaccination should be advised, particularly if the expedition will be more than 24 hours away from a reliable source of post-exposure vaccination.

SKIN PROBLEMS

In hot environments, particularly if they are also wet, fungal infections of the feet are common and foot hygiene is very important. Wounds and insect bites are also easily infected and healing may be prolonged.

Desert environments

In desert areas,[15] daytime temperatures may rise to very high levels but at night, in the absence of tree or cloud cover, night temperatures may fall very low and warm clothing and sleeping bags are needed.

ULTRAVIOLET RADIATION

During the day ultraviolet radiation is at a high level by direct radiation from the sun and by reflection from sandy or stony surfaces. Protection of the head by a wide-brimmed hat, light-coloured and loose-fitting clothing that covers as much as possible of the skin surface and application of a sunscreen will reduce the effects of exposure to the sun. Metallic 'space blankets' may be used as a shelter from the sun with the metallic layer outermost to reflect heat away.

Water supplies are scarce with long distances between them. A high fluid intake is needed in view of the high daytime temperature and careful planning of water supplies is necessary when water resources are scarce. A desert still constructed from a sheet of transparent polythene weighted in the middle and stretched over a hole dug in the sand enables condensate to be collected in a vessel placed in the centre of the hole to supplement water supplies.

Climbing at altitude

The problems specific to high altitude are discussed in more detail in Chapter 8.

ALTITUDE SICKNESS

Altitude sickness[16] may affect up to two-thirds of those ascending to altitudes of over 3–4000 m on some popular, Himalayan, trekking routes. It is caused by hypoxia and is precipitated or exacerbated by inadequate acclimatisation. Other factors leading to its development are dehydration and over-exertion. Symptoms include headache, dizziness, nausea, vomiting, lethargy, sleep disturbance, peripheral oedema and periodic (Cheyne–Stokes) breathing.

In aiding acclimatisation and avoiding altitude sickness the 'rules of three' should be followed:

• over 3000 m, ascend no more than 300 m per day, rest every 3rd day.

The use of acetazolamide[17] 500 mg daily may aid acclimatisation, particularly in those who have acclimatised badly in the past or whose itinerary or lie or the land does not allow the above rules to be followed.

PULMONARY AND CEREBRAL OEDEMA

These potentially fatal complications of high-altitude travel fortunately occur in only about 1–2% of those travelling to high altitude.

The earliest symptom of pulmonary oedema[18] is dyspnoea which does not subside on resting, with or without a persistent cough. Descent as far as possible as quickly as possible is essential, though nifedipine[19] is an adjunct to treatment with which it is useful to start treatment while evacuation is being organised. Oxygen and the pressurised Gamow bag are also of use prior to or during descent if they are available.

The earliest symptom of cerebral oedema[20] is often a headache which does not subside on lying down and taking analgesics, and which may in fact become worse when lying down. Other early symptoms and signs may include irrational behaviour, unforced errors of judgement, unsteadiness on the feet and apathy. Once again, rapid descent is essential, with the use of dexamathasone orally or intramuscularly as a useful adjunct. The Gamow bag may be used if available.

Climbing expeditions face the possibility not only of high-altitude problems but also of problems associated with cold, exertion, dehydration, ultraviolet radiation and trauma. Dehydration is often seen at altitude as it may be difficult to keep pace with increased water loss owing to exertion and a low partial pressure of water vapour when the only source of drinking water is melted snow. It may produce symptoms such as headache, fatigue and lethargy that may easily be confused with the effects of altitude.

Travel to remote areas

Remoteness is not measured solely in geographical terms. The traveller in such circumstances is separated, whatever the distance involved, from:

• home and family
• friends
• accustomed facilities
• communications
• medical help.

For the expedition doctor remote travel brings together all the strands of planning for the medical care of an expedition, including:

• What can the doctor, deal with in the field?
• What equipment will be needed?
• Can the expedition carry all that might be needed?
• Will medical evacuation be possible?
• How will evacuation be organised?
• Will secondary care be available? If so, of what quality and how long will it take to reach it?

PSYCHOLOGICAL EFFECTS OF REMOTE TRAVEL

In addition to whatever physical hazards the expedition may encounter, remote travel may carry psychological hazards for the expedition members:

Previous personality and psychological 'baggage' are of great importance in the success of an individual's participation in an expedition. Those who join an expedition in order to escape from problems will almost inevitably bring those problems with them. Personality traits previously kept in check may well come to the surface under the stress of remote expedition travel. It is advisable for expedition leaders or organisers to look carefully at what has prompted members to wish to join the expedition and at their personality and likely compatibility with other members.

Friction with companions. When expedition members are forced by circumstances to live in close contact for long periods, what may initially be charming eccentricities can change into intolerable irritation. Personal space and possessions become jealously guarded and apparent inequalities of any kind deeply resented.

Fear of the environment may interfere with the individual's ability to play a full part in activities, particularly when the surroundings carry objective dangers.

Fear of illness may lead to an almost paranoid suspicion of people, food and water.

Fear of the unknown. Unfamiliar surroundings, food, customs and climate may produce an anxiety reaction.

Anxiety about poverty, begging or theft may lead to extreme suspicion of the motives of local people encountered en route

Separation anxiety. Separation from friends and family may produce a reaction akin to the grief of bereavement.

General health risks

Food and water

Whatever the destination and activities of the expedition, the health risk most likely to be encountered is that of travellers' diarrhoea.[21] Expedition food is often cooked in less than ideal circumstances and if cooks are employed locally, little is usually known about their personal hygiene or carriage of pathogenic organisms. Water supplies

for expeditions must be obtained from whatever sources are available locally, with all the attendant risks of contamination with pathogens. Under expedition conditions, latrine arrangements are often less than ideal and personal hygiene such as hand-washing may be allowed to slip below customary standards. All these circumstances conspire to produce faecal–oral infection, which may be a greater threat to the success of an expedition than tropical diseases or objective hazards. Some ground rules may be laid down which would limit the likelihood of gastrointestinal infection;

- Local cooks should be hired, when possible, from a reputable or previously known trekking agency.
- Latrines should be dug away from camp sites and sources of drinking water, and be downwind from the camp.
- Cooks and expedition members should be encouraged to wash their hands after using the latrine and before preparing or eating food. A bowl of water reserved for hand-washing and containing a dilute solution of potassium permanganate should be kept near the latrine and outside the mess tent.
- Fresh produce should be washed in a dilute solution of potassium permanganate and fruit should be peeled before being eaten.
- Food should be thoroughly cooked and eaten when still hot.
- Food storage should take into account the possibility of access by flying and other insects and by rodents.
- Water for drinking should be boiled or purified chemically or by filtration.

WATER PURIFICATION

Water may be boiled, filtered or chemically treated.

- **Boiling** is a good method of destroying pathogens in water but may be very demanding on scarce fuel supplies. There is evidence that simply bringing water to boiling point is adequate to destroy most pathogens and that prolonged boiling may not be necessary. Longer boiling may be needed at higher altitudes, where water boils at a lower temperature, for example 80°C at 6000 m.

- **Filtration** may be used simply to remove debris from water or to remove pathogens. Removal of debris by a fabric filter such as the Millbank bag produces water which needs further purification; the removal of solid matter makes chemical purification easier to achieve. Ceramic filters remove most bacteria, *Amoeba*, *Giardia* and some but not all viruses. Other devices incorporate both filtration and exposure to an iodine-resin compound and remove most pathogens including viruses. The disadvantages of filtration devices include the slow speed with which they are able to produce a reasonable volume of drinking water and the limited life of the filtration unit that needs to be cleaned or replaced. Chemical contamination is not removed by filtration unless a carbon filter is also used.
- **Chemical purification** involves the use of tablets that release chlorine, iodine in liquid or tablet form and silver salts that are present in some filtration devices. Iodine has a wider spectrum of action against viruses and encysted forms of *Amoeba* than does chlorine.

Four drops of 2% tincture of iodine should be added per litre of water and the solution should be left for 20 minutes at room temperature and longer in cold surroundings before it is drunk. A plastic dropper bottle such as is used for eye drops makes an ideal container for the iodine. The addition of sodium thiosulphate, ascorbic acid or lemon juice after the purification period eliminates the taste of iodine.

Alternatively, a saturated solution of iodine may be prepared by putting iodine crystals into a bottle or jar, adding water and shaking. 10 mL of this solution added to a litre of water and left for 20 minutes will produce drinkable water and the iodine bottle is kept 'topped up' from whatever source of water is available. Iodine is of course not suitable for those who are allergic to it, are pregnant or have thyroid disease.

Sanitation

At base camps, latrines[22] should ideally be 'long drop' if there is enough depth of earth to allow a pit

to be dug to a depth of 2 or 3 m. Otherwise the site should be changed regularly, avoiding previously used sites, before it is full. Latrines should be downstream from sources of drinking and washing water and downwind from the camp. After each use, earth should be kicked or shovelled into the pit. From time to time, a flammable liquid such as kerosene may be poured into the pit and carefully ignited. Ideally, toilet paper should be burned, particularly after casual, wayside halts for defaecation. The use of toilet paper is controversial and is offensive in some cultures where the left hand is used for cleansing and is subsequently washed. There is no evidence that using paper is more hygienic or is associated with a lower risk of faecal–oral infection. Latrines may also be dug in snow when camping above the snow line. Here snow may be kicked into the pit after each use but when temperatures fall below freezing this will not be possible. They should be situated downstream from daytime meltwater sources used for drinking or washing and away from sources of snow used for melting to provide water supplies.

Emergency treatment

Medical emergencies

It has already been pointed out that expedition members cannot expect to have every conceivable medical and surgical emergency dealt with in the same way as it would be in the UK. The expedition doctor must also realise that it is not possible to allow for every eventuality. Given unlimited porterage for equipment there would be many emergencies which could be given excellent primary care only to perish through lack of facilities for safe evacuation or effective secondary care.

Asthma attacks[23] should be dealt with by giving oral corticosteroids (e.g. prednisolone 40 mg stat and daily) until the status quo is regained plus multiple doses (10–12 initially and up to 25 or more) of a beta-agonist inhaler through a large volume spacer which may be improvised using a plastic bottle or a rolled-up sheet of paper. The expedition doctor should have been alerted to the possibility of such an attack by prior knowledge of the condition.

Other respiratory problems. Pneumonia with pleurisy and pulmonary embolus may both occur at high altitude and may be difficult to distinguish at first sight. Clinical signs, pyrexia and systemic disturbance will usually help to distinguish pneumonia which is treatable with antibiotics from embolism for which little can be done under expedition conditions. Pneumothorax may also be a cause of chest pain and dyspnoea; the trachea will probably be displaced and the typical resonance to percussion with diminished breath sounds will assist diagnosis. Under trek conditions, increasing dyspnoea suggesting tension pneumothorax can be relieved by makeshift release using an intravenous cannula.

Epileptic attacks will usually stop in a few minutes; otherwise they will probably respond to intravenous or rectal diazepam. Once again the expedition doctor should have prior knowledge of the condition. Rectal tubes of diazepam should be made available to the immediate companions of an epileptic expedition member with detailed instructions on their use.

Myocardial infarction. Soluble aspirin 300 mg (preferably chewed) has a thrombolytic effect and should be given. Effective pain relief may be a problem as not all trek doctors are prepared to carry controlled drugs. Nalbuphine (Nubain)[24] is not a controlled drug and may be given by intravenous, intramuscular or subcutaneous injection; it is not as effective as diamorphine but avoids the necessity of obtaining a Home Office licence to export controlled drugs and the possible consequences of being found 'in possession' by inadvertently contravening import regulations elsewhere. Atropine may be used for bradycardia and lignocaine for tachycardia but no other drugs are appropriate under trek conditions. Prolonged cardiopulmonary resuscitation is unlikely to achieve positive results as it will not be possible on trek to correct the associated metabolic abnormalities and provide suitable aftercare.

Diabetic emergencies. Diabetic ketoacidosis or coma are fortunately not as likely to occur on an expedition as is hypoglycaemia caused by over-exertion and/or inadequate carbohydrate intake. Knowing that an expedition member is diabetic should warn the doctor that the early symptoms of what appears to be altitude mountain sickness, hypothermia or dehydration could instead be hypoglycaemia. Ketosis could however occur, especially if some other illness or infection occurs.

For the treatment of hypoglycaemia, ampoules of 50% dextrose are required but they have a tendency to break and convert the medical kit into a disgusting sticky mess; Glucagon injection, Hypostop oral gel and/or easily absorbable carbohydrate should be carried by diabetic expedition members and their immediate companions instructed on their use.

Surgical emergencies

There are few surgical problems that can be dealt with on trek, hence the scanty surgical kit advised.

Abdominal emergencies. There is little that can be done about problems such as appendicitis apart from giving a broad-spectrum antibiotic plus metronidazole in the hope of minimising the consequences of gangrene or perforation of a viscus. Ureteric or biliary colic will probably respond to diclofenac injections. Acute cholecystitis and urinary tract infections will need a broad-spectrum antibiotic, the former possibly with metronidazole added.

Serious trauma

The principles of dealing with serious trauma on an expedition are those of all good first-aid, namely to preserve life and to minimise further damage pending evacuation for secondary care. Immobilising fractures using Cas-Straps and when necessary improvised splints, preservation of the airway in the unconscious and pain relief for the conscious are the main achievable objectives. Ski sticks, tent poles, ice axes or other rigid pieces of equipment are useful as makeshift splints. Inflatable splints have the disadvantage of being easily punctured and being easy to over-inflate, to the detriment of the circulation in a limb. Broad-spectrum antibiotics should be given for open fractures.

Fluid replacement following serious trauma is a great problem as it may not be possible, especially on a small expedition, to carry large quantities of intravenous fluids. The logistics of an expedition will not always allow such fluids as are carried to be available when needed. If logistics allow, both electrolyte and plasma volume expanding fluids should be available in a mobile, emergency, medical kit with further supplies available at the most forward point possible for continuing treatment. In an emergency where no intravenous fluids are available, rectal fluids, which should be as far as possible pathogen-free but need not be completely sterile and pyrogen-free, may be given via a urinary catheter inserted into the rectum.

Medical and first-aid kits[5,25,26]

WHAT TO TAKE?

On many expeditions the most frequently used medications are likely to be oral rehydration solution, antidiarrhoeal drugs, simple analgesics and antibacterial drugs. The most frequently used first-aid items are also likely to be commonplace items such as adhesive strip bandages, antiseptic and simple dressings. For all these high-use items, it is best to assume that each member of the party will need them on at least one occasion or for one full course. For all other items, it is probably safe to assume that the quantities needed will be for about 10% of this 'worst case scenario'.

Allowances must be made for treating porters whose numbers will not be known before starting the expedition but will probably at least double the size of the party. Other passing travellers may also need emergency treatment which it would be difficult to refuse.

Policy about treating local inhabitants depends on the philosophy of the expedition and the individual doctor. Again, it would be difficult to withhold emergency treatment but any other treatment is probably best left to whatever local resources exist, however primitive they appear,

which will have to continue treatment after the expedition has moved on. The expedition doctor will make little impact on most problems without good communication with local people in their own language and knowledge of their culture and circumstances. Nor will the doctor be able to give continuity of care.

PACKING MEDICAL EQUIPMENT

In order to save space and weight, tablets and capsules may be removed from their original packs and put in small, self-sealing, polythene bags. Glass ampoules may be packed in cotton wool or bubble plastic in similar bags or left in their original packs. Damage is unusual if tablets and ampoules are packed tightly. Plastic food boxes with well-fitting lids make suitable containers and the lids may be held in place more securely by using stout rubber bands or Velcro-fastening, elastic tourniquets.

Each box should be labelled indelibly with its contents as should each bag, which should also carry details of dosage. The individual boxes are then packed into a crate or kitbag clearly labelled as medical equipment. A group check-in, if allowed, at the departure airport will usually ensure that there are no difficulties caused by this apparent excess baggage carried by the doctor, but if necessary the kit could be split between party members.

Large expeditions often favour stout plastic drums for packing supplies to be carried by porters and these drums are particularly useful if the kit is likely to be exposed to water or heavy rainfall. Smaller expeditions in relatively dry surroundings may find that a relatively small number of plastic boxes of equipment will suffice and can be packed in a single kitbag.

LOGISTICS EN ROUTE

Unless the expedition doctor intends to carry a substantial load, one or more porters will carry most of the doctor's equipment. It will therefore be necessary for the doctor to carry a smaller kit for use on the trail. The bulk of the kit should be made the responsibility of a single porter selected for reliability. The doctor should always know the porter's whereabouts and ideally the porter should never be far from the doctor, especially if the porter is carrying, for example, the only cylinder of oxygen for a trekking party on a high pass. If expedition members are likely to disperse widely, as on some climbing or fieldwork expeditions, it may be necessary to issue each member with an individual first-aid and medical kit to deal with the problems most likely to occur, at least until they are able to contact the doctor.

The contents of such a kit would depend on the nature of the expedition and contents would need to be clearly labelled with such details as indications and dosage. For an expedition with a fixed base camp, the bulk of the medical supplies should be kept at this fixed point, but if, again as in some climbing expeditions, the whole party moves onward in stages from its base camp, an advance base kit would be needed.

The doctor will usually need to compile a personal mobile kit to be carried at all times in order to be able to react rapidly to emergencies. The following are examples of medical kits that the author has used on many occasions for climbing and trekking parties. Their contents may be added to according to the preferences of the individual doctor, the specific needs of the expedition and its carrying capacity:

Doctor's kit. The contents of the medical kit shown in Box 19.1 can be fitted into two or three small to medium, sandwich boxes.

Main medical kit. The suggested contents are shown in Box 19.2.

Surgical kit. The suggested contents are shown in Box 19.3.

Other items that may be added to the medical kit are shown in Box 19.4.

Box 19.1 Doctor's expedition kit

Diagnostic
Stethoscope
Anaeroid sphygmomanometer
Lightweight auriscope/ophthalmoscope (optional)
Pen-torch
Urine dipsticks
Blood glucose strips
Tongue depressors
Fluorescein strips

Emergency drugs
Strong analgesic (e.g. diclofenac and nalbuphine injections)
Adrenaline injection 1/1000
Hydrocortisone injection
Dexamethasone tablets and injection (for high-altitude cerebral oedema)
Nifedipine capsules (for high-altitude pulmonary oedema)
Diazepam injection

Other drugs
Paracetamol tablets
Loperamide capsules
Rehydration sachets
Ciprofloxacin tablets
Metronidazole tablets
Acetazolamide tablets (for acute mountain sickness)

First-aid
Antiseptic sachets/swabs
Non-stick dressings
Sterile gauze swabs
Micropore tape
Elastocrepe bandage
Conforming bandage
Triangular bandage
Assorted adhesive strip plasters
Safety pins
Scissors
Airway
Set of Cas-Straps (carried in its own wallet)

Medicolegal considerations in expedition medicine

By undertaking to provide medical care for an expedition, a medical practitioner acquires a duty of care towards the expedition members.[27] Under UK law, the doctor can only be found to be negligent if a court establishes that the duty of care has been breached and that the breach caused or materially contributed to injury. In other words, a doctor who fails to provide proper care and attention during an expedition may be found to have been negligent if that lack of care or attention has resulted in damage to the health of an expedition member.

Defining proper care and attention under expedition conditions is not an easy task. The usual legal definition of what constitutes appropriate standards of care is that it should

Box 19.2 Main expedition medical kit

Eye preparations
Fluorescein drops
Amethocaine drops
Chloramphenicol drops or ointment
Aciclovir eye ointment

Ear preparations
NeoCortef drops

Nasal preparations
Otrivine drops

Analgesics
Paracetamol tablets
Ibuprofen (tablets and gel)

Anti-infective
Ciprofloxacin tablets
Metronidazole tablets

Antidiarrhoeal
Loperamide capsules
Rehidrat or Dioralyte sachets
Codeine phosphate tablets (also useful as a strong analgesic and cough suppressant)

Anti-emetic
Prochlorperazine tablets (Buccastem buccal preparation is very useful or metoclopramide tablets and/or injection)

Throat lozenges
Any variety (little therapeutic effect but a useful placebo)

Hypnotic
Zopiclone tablets (useful for short-term readjustment after crossing time zones)

Antihistamine
Chlorpheniramine (tablet and injection)

Skin preparations
Antibacterial (e.g. Flamazine or Bactroban creams)
Antifungal (e.g. clotrimazole cream)
Topical steroid cream (medium potency)
(e.g. betamethasone 0.1%)

Reserve supplies of all drugs and dressings in doctor's kit

Box 19.3 Expedition surgical kit

Disposable scalpel
Dissecting forceps
Small artery clip
Stitch holder
Scissors
IV cannula
Sutures
Local anaesthetic (e.g. lignocaine)
Stitch cutter
Steristrips
Lignocaine injection
Ketamine (if experienced in its use)
Skin-cleaning solution
Gloves
Foley catheter
Nasogastric tube

Box 19.4 Other equipment which may be added to the medical kit

IV fluid replacement
Normal saline
Plasma volume expander
IV cannula
IV giving set

Injections
Midazolam
Benzylpenicillin
Glucagon

Anti-infective
Penicillin V
Amoxycillin
Flucloxacillin
Erythromycin

Respiratory
Salbutamol inhaler
Large volume spacer

STD prevention
Condoms

conform to standards that would be accepted by a reasonable consensus of the doctor's peers. This need not be a majority consensus so long as there is an adequate body of opinion to support the doctor's actions.

It has been accepted in a UK court (Wilsher v. Essex Health Authority 1986) that 'an emergency may overburden the available resources, and if an individual is forced by circumstances to do too many things at once, the fact that he does one of them incorrectly should not lightly be taken as negligence.' This means that, the circumstances in which care is provided may influence the decision as to what constitutes a reasonable standard of care.

Expedition members in the field cannot reasonably expect to receive the same standards of care which they would receive in, for example, the accident and emergency department of a district general hospital at home. But they can and should expect that their doctor will act as would any reasonably competent doctor in the same circumstances. If a doctor professes or advertises to have special experience or expertise in a particular field, it is likely that higher standards of care will be expected of that doctor.

It is advisable that any doctor agreeing to provide medical care for an expedition should discuss in advance with the other members of the team the reasonable standards of care which can be provided and the limitations which the expedition conditions will place upon that care. Such considerations will determine the amount and type of medical equipment that the expedition wishes to carry. This in turn will involve discussion about the carrying or porterage capacity of the expedition and how such expedition logistics will influence the standards of care that the doctor will be able to provide.

In the event of litigation against an expedition doctor, it is of course possible that the case may be heard in another country in which case the provisions of UK law would not apply.

Liability on commercially organised expeditions

If a doctor is employed by the organisers of an expedition or trek, the organisers will be liable for any acts or omissions of the doctor in addition to the doctor's own professional liability. If, however, the organisers engage the doctor as a contractor, the organisers may not be liable unless it can be shown that they did not exercise reasonable care in selecting a contractor with adequate qualifications or expertise.

Provision of drugs for expeditions

On some occasions, a doctor may provide medical advice and/or drugs without personally accompanying an expedition. On other occasions, a doctor accompanying an expedition may provide drugs to be administered by others in his absence, for example when logistics demand that the team is widely scattered over a large area or on a large mountain. On all these occasions, the doctor retains a duty of care towards any individual to whom those medicines that the doctor has prescribed or advised are given and is responsible for the effects of all such drugs.

It is therefore essential that all drugs intended for administration by anyone other than the doctor are clearly labelled with their name, dosage, indications for use, contraindications and possible side effects and that all relevant members of the team are instructed in their use. While such precautions may reduce the possibility of damage to the recipients, they do not remove or alter the doctor's ultimate responsibility.

Medical defence issues

Doctors accompanying expeditions abroad will in most circumstances be covered by their defence organisations for any litigation arising out of their duty of care towards expedition members, but they should inform their defence organisation of their intention to act in such a capacity and ensure beforehand that they are covered.

It is unlikely that cover will be extended to include acting on the territory of the USA, on US aircraft, in US airspace or on any aircraft intending to land in the USA, or treatment of US citizens. In other words cover would not extend to any case which would be heard in a US court. In addition, the Medical Defence Union (personal communication) does not extend cover to cases which would be heard in courts in Canada, dependent territories of the USA and Canada, Hong Kong, Israel or Zimbabwe.

Treatment of local people en route to and from the expedition's destination is unlikely in most countries to result in litigation but would probably be covered by the doctor's defence organisation.

REFERENCES

1. British Mountaineering Council, 177–179 Burton Road, Manchester M20 2BB; Tel: 0161 445 4747.
2. Expedition Advisory Centre Insurance, AON Risk Services Ltd, Richmond House, College Street, Southampton, SO14 4ZB; Tel: 01703 225616.
3. Bradley DJ, Warhurst DC. Guidelines for the prevention of malaria in travellers from the United Kingdom. Communicable Disease Review 1997: 7(10): R137–R152.
4. Sahiar F, Mohler SR. Economy class syndrome. Aviation Space and Environmental Medicine 994: 65(10 Pt 1): 957–960.
5. A'Court CHD, Stables RH, Travis S. Doctor on a mountaineering expedition. British Medical Journal 1995; 310: 1248–1252.
6. Steele P. Medical handbook for mountaineers. London: Constable; 1988: 21–46.
7. Backer HD, Bowman WD, Paton BC, Steele P, Thygerson A. Wilderness first aid. London: Jones and Bartlett; 1998: 301–311.
8. Terrados N, Maughan RJ. Exercise in the heat: strategies to minimise the adverse effects on performance. Journal Sports Sciences 1995; 13 (Spec No): S55–S62.
9. Lee-Chiong TL Jr, Stitt JT. Heatstroke and other heat-related illnesses. The maladies of summer. Postgraduate Medicine 1995; 98(1): 26–28, 31–33, 36.
10. Naylor ME. Erythema, skin cancer risk and sunscreens. Archives of Dermatology 1997; 133(3): 373–375.
11. Segantini P, Horn R. Cold induced pathology at high altitude. Schweizerische Rundschau für Medizin Praxis 1991; 80(46): 1283–1286.
12. Foray J. Mountain frostbite. Current trends in prognosis and treatment. Journal of Sports Medicine 1992; 13 (Suppl.): S193–S196.
13. Chapman R, Jermy C. Tropical forest expeditions. London: Expedition Advisory Centre of the Royal Geographical Society; 1993.
14. Worrell DA. Venomous and poisonous animals. In: Worrell DA, Anderson S, eds. Expedition medicine. London: Profile Books; 1998.
15. Sheppard T. Desert expeditions. London: Expedition Advisory Centre of the Royal Geographical Society; 1988.
16. Milledge JS. Acute mountain sickness. Intensive Care Medicine 1985; 11(3): 110–114.
17. Bradwell AR, Wright AD, Winterburn M, Imray C. Acetazolamide and high altitude disease. International Journal of Sports Medicine 1992; 13(Suppl.): S63–S64.
18. Hultgren HN. High altitude pulmonary oedema: current concepts Annual Review of Medicine 1992; 47: 267–284.
19. Oelz O, Maggiorini M, Ritter M, et al. Nifedipine for high altitude pulmonary oedema. Lancet 1989; ii: 1241–1244.
20. Clarke C. High altitude cerebral oedema. Internat J Sports Med 1988; 9(2): 170–174.
21. Farthing MJG. Travellers'diarrhoea. Gut 1994; 35: 1–4.
22. Bennett-Jones H. Base camp hygiene and health, In: Worrell DA, Anderson S, eds. Expedition Medicine. London: Profile Books; 1998.
23. British guidelines on asthma management. 1995 review and position statement. Thorax 1997; 52(Suppl): S1–S21.
24. British National Formulary
25. Illingworth R. Expedition medical kits. In: Worrell DA, Anderson S, eds. Expedition medicine. London: Profile Books; 1998.
26. Hillebrandt D. Planning an expedition medical kit. Mountain 1989; 125: 38–39.
27. Duff A. Liability on commercial expeditions. Newsletter of the International Society for Mountain Medicine 1998; 8(2): 13.

Refugees, disaster relief and migration

John Howarth

Introduction

Every year between 1990 and 1995 at least 30 wars were in progress.[1] The majority were civil wars,[2] leading to a large increase in the number of refugees and internally displaced persons (IDPs) (see Fig. 19.3). The end of the Cold War did not lead to world peace. Conflicts instead became more regionalised, often ethnic in nature. Emergencies such as sudden population movements, wars, famine and epidemics are becoming more and more common. They frequently occur in the areas least able to cope as a result of poverty and longstanding under-development.

DEFINITIONS

Refugees are defined as those who have fled their countries because of a well-founded fear of persecution for reasons of their race, religion, nationality, political opinion or membership of a particular social group, who cannot or do not want to return.

This definition excludes the large number of economic migrants who have sought refuge in Western Europe and North America.

An **internally displaced person** is a person fleeing but remaining within his or her own country.

Since 1986, IDPs have outnumbered refugees. They represent possibly an even more vulnerable group as there is no international instrument or treaty that defines IDPs nor provides for their protection. IDPs often constitute a hidden and neglected population. Many move into remote bush areas or congregate on the outskirts of cities with little assistance. The return of Eritrean, Mozambican and Rwandan refugees has resulted in a fall in numbers since the mid-1990s but as

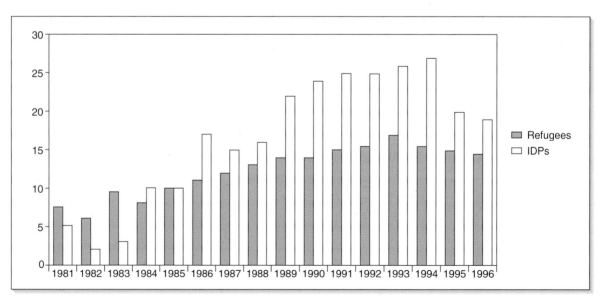

Fig. 19.3 Refugees and internally displaced persons (IDPs), 1981–96. (millions). (Source US Committee for Refugees)

Figure 19.3 shows, current totals still represent a significant increase from the early 1980s.

The relief environment

The 20th century has seen an institutionalisation of the care for refugees under the framework of the United Nations (UN). The UN High Commissioner for Refugees (UNHCR) was created by the UN General Assembly and began work in 1951. In recent years UNHCR's involvement with persons who have not crossed an international border such as IDPs, refugees who have returned home (returnees) and persons threatened with displacement has increased substantially. However, there remains huge gaps in provision for displaced populations with consequent high levels of excess mortality and morbidity.

A large number of non-governmental organisations (NGOs) responding to humanitarian crises were formed in the 1990s with varying degrees of professionalism and effectiveness. Many have their own agendas and there is a lack of accountability to the recipients of the aid. Worry over the quality and effectiveness of humanitarian aid led in 1994 to the development of a code of conduct in disaster relief by the International Red Cross, Red Crescent and major NGOs (Box 19.5).

PROBLEMS WITH HUMANITARIAN AID

There are many criticisms of humanitarian aid in emergencies. Humanitarian aid may be used as a substitute for political action, or as part of a policy where containment is the objective rather than resolution. It is often seen as rivalling rather than complementing development aid, and competes for the same funding. Poorly designed disaster interventions that flood the area with material resources can undermine existing development initiatives such as cost recovery in the health sector. Large quantities of food aid can put local farmers out of business and decrease overall food security. Emergency relief should build capacity not undermine local economic survival and coping mechanisms.

> **Box 19.5 Code of conduct in disaster relief (International Red Cross, Red Crescent and NGOs)**
>
> 1. The humanitarian imperative comes first.
> 2. Aid is given regardless of the race, creed or nationality of the recipients and without adverse distinction of any kind. Aid priorities are calculated on the basis of need alone.
> 3. Aid will not be used to further a particular political or religious standpoint.
> 4. We shall endeavour not to act as instruments of government foreign policy.
> 5. We shall respect culture and custom.
> 6. We shall attempt to build disaster response on local capacities.
> 7. Ways shall be found to involve programme beneficiaries in the management of relief aid.
> 8. Relief aid must strive to reduce future vulnerabilities to disaster as well as meeting basic needs.
> 9. We hold ourselves accountable to both those we seek to assist and those from whom we accept resources.
> 10. In our information, publicity and advertising activities, we shall recognise disaster victims as dignified human beings not hopeless objects.

The aid sector is largely unregulated. There is increasing competition and institutional survival of the agency may appear to be more important than the disaster affected population. Quality standards are also extremely variable[3] with too little investment in training. There has been considerable and justified criticism over the failure to involve the displaced populatons themselves in the planning and delivery of aid.

In every disaster, there are people who gain both politically and economically. Failure to recognise this has led to aid fuelling and prolonging conflict. Diverted aid may feed combatants and help finance the war – many of the military vehicles used in Somalia and Liberia originally belonged to humanitarian agencies.

Cultural differences between the displaced population and the relief workers inhibit understanding. Western aid-workers often find it difficult to know where power and influence lie in complex, clan-based societies and by negotiating with warlords may give them added legitimacy making resolution of the conflict less likely.

Finding a way through these pitfalls is not easy. Stakeholder analysis and political mapping[4,5] are tools that can help to describe the balance of power and influence in an area and help avoid unforeseen, adverse effects of the aid.

MORTALITY AND MORBIDITY IN DISPLACED POPULATIONS

Displacement is often the final act in a series of stresses on a population, that may already be malnourished, sick and has exhausted all its coping mechanisms. Displacement makes a population much more vulnerable. Refugees and IDPs frequently lose access to safe water, sanitation, food, shelter and healthcare.

In the emergency phases of refugee movements, mortality rates in all age groups appear to be higher than baseline rates but the excess mortality appears to be greatest in those aged 1–4 years and 5–14 years.[6] In the chaos and panic of flight, many children become separated from their parents. Unaccompanied children represent a particularly high-risk group.

In most wars, far more deaths are caused from disease than combat-related trauma. War-related material deprivation, displacement, overcrowding and disruption of water, food and sanitation systems have effects that last long after the combat has finished. In chronic, low-grade conflicts such as Angola and Mozambique, an estimated 14 people died from disease for every one killed in combat. [7]

The following illnesses acounted for 60–95% of deaths among refugee populations in the emergency phase.[8]

- acute respiratory infection
- diarrhoeal disease
- malnutrition
- measles
- malaria.

In long-term refugee camps, the major causes of death are acute respiratory infection and diarrhoea. While more exotic diseases (such as epidemic typhus in the former Yugoslavia) do occur during population displacement, the majority of deaths are from an increased incidence of common endemic diseases associated with an increased case fatality rate.[9] The stresses on the population caused

by lack of water for drinking and hygiene, crowding, and the movement of non-immune populations into high-risk areas all contribute to this excess mortality.

Nutritional status also significantly affects the case fatality rate with greatly increased death rates in the malnourished. Vitamin A deficiency is common in refugees and causes impaired T cell, humoral and mucosal immunity.[10] Vitamin A distribution and measles vaccination are probably the most effective, public health intervention in refugee camps in developing countries.

Conditions for respiratory infections are ideal in many displaced populations with overcrowding, increased poverty and poor living conditions. Bronchopneumonia is common and access to treatment is often limited.

Measles was a common cause of mortality in refugee camps during the 1980s. During a measles epidemic in Wad Kowli, Sudan in 1985 as many as 2000 children may have died with a case fatality rate of 32%.[11] Measles, however, seems to be less prominent a cause of death in refugees in the 1990s. Reasons for this are not clear but may include increased awareness amongst the aid community with early vaccination of refugees. It may also reflect the increased number of refugees and IDPs in the 1990s from more affluent countries such as the former Yugoslavia, Kuwait and Iraq.

Diarrhoeal disease from all causes is extremely common in displaced populations. They are particularly vulnerable to explosive epidemics of cholera with very high death rates. Amongst Rwandan refugees in Goma, Zaire during 1994 the first cases of cholera were reported on day 6 of the displacement and the epidemic had peaked by day 11. Epidemic dysentery was slower to start but persisted for months and was multi-drug resistant. Tens of thousands died. Other causes of diarrhoea in refugee populations include *Rotavirus*, enterotoxigenic *Escherichia coli* (ETEC), *Campylobacter* and *Salmonella*.

Plasmodium falciparum malaria is increasingly recognised as a major cause of death amongst war-affected populations in sub-Saharan Africa.[12] Refugee camps can often become ideal breeding sites for mosquitoes, especially in the rainy season. Non-immune populations may move from highland areas where there is little or no malaria to mosquito-infested, lowland areas and suffer catastrophic epidemics.[12] Drug resistance is causing increasing problems. In epidemics, it is particularly important to have an effective, first-line drug, especially for the under 5s and pregnant women in whom the case fatality rate can be particularly high.

It is important not to stereotype disasters. Massive population movements can have dramatically different mortality rates and the proportion of deaths from trauma can vary greatly. In the exodus of refugees from Rwanda in 1994, crude mortality rates peaked at over 40/10000 per day mainly because of cholera and dysentery.[3] In the return of 553000 refugees from Goma 2 years later, death rates within Rwanda were in the order of 0.5/10000 per day although 3586 bodies were counted in the abandoned refugee camps most of whom had died from trauma.[13] The returning population had benefited from a billion dollars worth of aid over the previous 2 years. They were well nourished with high vaccination rates. They had access to water and food stores right up until displacement and received a great deal of help from UNHCR and NGOs during thier return. In addition, they had a high level of immunity to cholera and dysentery because of the almost universal exposure 2 years earlier.

Wars and population movements in more affluent countries

Most of the current research and knowledge on refugee health comes from developing countries. While wars and disasters in more affluent countries share many characteristics such as the importance of adequate water, food, shelter, sanitation and security, there are crucial differences. First, the demographics of the population are entirely different with many more elderly. This presents problems related to the management of chronic disease and cancer which are less often an issue in developing countries. Health systems such as those in the former Soviet Union may be more doctor-based and centralised and it is far less clear which

interventions in an emergency will be effective. Early measles vaccination and vitamin A distribution are clearly best practice in African refugee scenarios but may be inappropriate in Chechnya where an elderly population is dying from lack of drugs for chronic diseases such as diabetes and ischaemic heart disease.[14]

Affluent countries frequently suffer a higher intensity conflict with more deaths and injuries from high explosives and fewer from knives and bullets. The capital of Chechnya, Grozny, suffered massive aerial and ground bombardment when it was seized by the Russians in early 1995 causing an estimated 30000 trauma-related deaths.

The onslaught caused most of the 400000 population to flee leaving an estimated 60000, mainly elderly, in the city during the 3 months of intense fighting. Many died from cold in temperatures reaching -20°C. In such a situation, a thorough needs and capacity assessment is essential as is the early establishment of a simple surveillance system to give early warning of epidemics.

Data collection in disaster relief

The importance of rapid and reliable data collection in emergencies cannot be overstressed. Massive aid efforts are often based on assumption of need. Aid is sent in on an ad hoc basis with individual agencies working with their own agendas and with little attempt at coordinating with the local health authorities. Huge amounts of resources can be wasted and lives can be lost. A rapid needs and capacity assessment combined with the early establishment of effective ongoing surveillance are critical to the success of the response.

In general, there are five major categories of data that are important in emergencies:[15]

1. mortality
2. morbidity
3. nutritional indicators
4. activities (e.g. number of outpatients, vaccination coverage)
5. vital sectors (food, water, shelter, sanitation).

1. MORTALITY

Crude mortality rates

Crude mortality rates (CMR) are often used to measure the severity of the situation (Table 19.1).

During the first month of the Rwandan refugee displacement into Goma, 50000 people died with the average CMR being between 20 and 35/10000/day.[16]

Calculating crude mortality rate

1. Total the deaths for a given number of days (e.g. 1 week).
2. Divide this total by the number of days data were gathered. This gives the average numbers of deaths per day.
3. Divide this figure by the size of the population.
4. Multiply by 10000 for the daily crude mortality rate.

If a system for mortality surveillance does not exist already, then it should be created. Methods include mandatory registration of deaths, 24-hour graveyard watches to count the number of burials, checking with clinic and hospital records, and interviewing local community leaders. The date of death, address, name, age and sex should all be noted. Community health workers can have a useful role in the collection of mortality data.

Population numbers are essential for checking CMRs. This is often difficult in the chaos of mass population movement and in the early stages, speed is more important than absolute accuracy.

TABLE 19.1 Crude mortality rates – benchmarks

	Crude mortality rate	<5 mortality rate
Normal rate for developing country	0.5/10000/day	1.0/10000/day
Relief programme under control	<1.0/10000/day	<2.0/10000/day
Relief programme: very serious situation	>1/10000/day	>2.0/10000/day
Emergency: out of control	>2.0/10000/day	>4.0/10000/day
Major catastrophe	>5.0/10000/day	>10.0/10000/day

Population can be estimated by projection of previous census data, registration figures in camps (but note that food registration figures are often overestimates), or in refugee situations counting of shelters and a simple survey of say 30 shelters to calculate the average household size. Other methods of population estimates using cluster survey techniques have been used.[17,18]

It does not always require a great increase in mortality to warrant a humanitarian response. The human rights' abuses in Kosovo are a good example where overall CMRs may not be high but a clear crisis exists nonetheless.

Case fatality rates

Major outbreaks of communicable diseases are common in emergencies and the case fatality rates (CFR) can be very high. This is especially true when there are also significant rates of malnutrition in children.

The measurement of CFR is particularly useful when looking at epidemics such as measles, cholera and meningitis.

Calculating case fatality rate:

1. Total the number of deaths from the specific disease over the last 7 days.
2. Divide this total by the total number of cases and multiply by 100.
3. This gives the case fatality rate.

---

2. MORBIDITY

Disease-specific incidence rate

Morbidity can be monitored by the disease-specific incidence rate:

Calculating disease specific incidence rate

1. Add up the number of cases of the disease during 7 days.
2. Divide by the total population.
3. Multiply by 100000 to get the disease specific incidence rate as cases per 100000.

In the absence of population figures the actual number of cases of each disease in the clinics can be plotted weekly on a graph to give early warning of epidemics. Consideration should be given to background rates of the disease in the area and seasonal variations. Many other factors can influence these numbers such as a change of staff, a change of population numbers, and the arrival of drugs when there were previously none. Of particular importance in disasters is the monitoring of diarrhoeal cases and fever cases with the rapid investigation of any apparent outbreak. Early laboratory confirmation of diseases such as cholera, dysentery and meningitis is essential to mobilise resources and determine antibiotic sensitivities. Data collection between clinics must be standardised with clear case definitions.

3. NUTRITIONAL INDICATORS

Malnutrition rates in the under-5s

The under-5s in the population are a vulnerable group sensitive to reduction in food availability. Changes in the nutritional indicators of this group are usually a sensitive indicator of the overall nutritional status of the population.

To calculate acute malnutrition, weight for height (W/H) is much better than weight for age. Weight for age as carried out in many clinics is more suited to longer-term growth monitoring and often indicates stunting rather than acute malnutrition.

Global acute malnutrition = <80% W/H or <-2 SD (Z-score)

Severe acute malnutrition = <70% W/H and/or oedema or <-3 SD (Z-score)

Nutritional surveys need to be carefully organised and usually it is best to seek the help of an experienced nutritionist. The measurement of mid-upper arm circumference (MUAC) however, is a useful rapid technique for assessing malnutrition rates in the under-5s. It can be used for screening new arrivals and gives a rough estimate of the nutritional status. Much rigour needs to be used, however, in carrying out the measurement properly and the teams undertaking the survey need to be carefully trained. This method is based on the observation that MUAC changes little between the ages of 6 months and 5 years so 'normal' ranges can be described. Different agencies have used different cut-offs[19,20] of MUACs to indicate malnutrition but a metanalysis[20] of how MUAC results relate to W/H suggests the following cut-offs are most accurate:

Global acute malnutrition = MUAC < 125 mm

(roughly equating to W/H of less than 80% W/H or - 2 SD)

Severe acute malnutrition = MUAC < 110 mm +/- oedema

(roughly equating to W/H of less than 70% or - 3 SD)

Measuring adult malnutrition

Body mass index (BMI) is frequently used for assessing adult nutritional status.

> **Calculating body mass index BMI = weight in kg / height in m^2**
> Adequate nutrition = BMI > 18
> Malnourished[20] = BMI < 16

Food

There is considerable debate as to what constitutes an adequate daily ration. It also changes depending on the demographic breakdown of the population (e.g. few children vs high numbers of children), temperature (more needed in cold conditions), overall malnuntrition rate (increased calories needed if a large percentage of the population is malnourished to allow for recovery).

TABLE 19.2 Malnutition – benchmarks

	Global acute malnutrition	Severe acute malnutrition
Normal rate in developing country	<5%	<1%
Under control	<10%	<2%
Very serious situation	>10%	<2%
Major catastrophe	<20%	>5%

Médecins Sans Frontières define rations as:

Adequate ration quantity => 2000 kcal per person per day

Marginal ration quantity = 1750–2000 kcal per person per day

Inadequate ration quantity = 1500–1750 kcal per person per day

Grossly inadequate quantity = <1500 kcal per person per day

Breast-feeding is particularly important in refugee situations with the risks asociated with bottle-feeding being dramatically increased as a result of poor hygiene, crowding and limited clean water.

4. ACTIVITIES

Consultation numbers at the health facilities

Often this is the only data available but these numbers are the least useful. So many factors influence the numbers of people seen (drugs available, cultural aspects, free prescribing or cost recovery, quality of service) that they are not a reliable indicator of the health of the population.

Vaccination coverage in mass campaigns

Measles vaccination is the number one, public health priority in a refugee camp. Other outbreaks such as meningococcal meningitis may need mass campaigns. Report weekly and monthly on the percentage coverage for measles and other diseases covered in the mass campaigns.

Coverage surveys using the Expanded Programme of Immunisation (EPI) cluster survey technique are relatively easy to organise.

5. VITAL SECTORS

Water quantity

An immediate assessment of water availability and projected need is essential in emergencies such as refugee displacement. Calculate the number of litres of water per person per day.

Minimum water needs[21]
Individuals   15–20 L per day
Health centres   40–50 L per patient/day
Feeding centres 20–30 L per patient/day

Water quality

The water should be palatable and safe to drink. 'A large quantity of reasonably safe water is preferable to a smaller amount of very pure water'.[21] New water sources should ideally be tested. This can involve the local water authorities or the use of various kits from agencies such as Oxfam.

As a rough guide.[21]

Reasonable quality
         =   0–10 faecal coliforms/100 mL
Polluted   =   10–100 faecal coliforms/100 mL
Very polluted
         =   100–1000 faecal coliforms/100 mL
Grossly polluted
         = over 1000 faecal coliforms/100 mL

If the water is significantly polluted, it can be chlorinated with or without filtering.

Water access and sources

Available water sources and distribution points should be described and plotted on a map if possible and compared with the concentrations of population. Consideration should be given to seasonal factors, position of latrines, geography, and if possible an expert in water supply in emergencies should be called in. If the minimum quantities cannot be rapidly supplied, the possibility of moving the affected displaced population to a more suitable site should be considered.

Sanitation

To build a sanitation infrastructure takes time. Short-term solutions include screened-off defaecation areas or simple, pit latrines. Ventilated, improved, pit (VIP) latrines usually offer the best solution in the medium-term. Careful siting of latrines and water sources can avoid contamination of the water supply and help reduce the risk of sexual violence to women by reducing the distance needed to walk. It is possible to calculate a latrine-user ratio on a weekly basis. Divide the total population by the number of latrines in use. This gives the average number of persons per latrine.[22]

Aim for at least 1 latrine for 20 persons.

Shelter

The World Health Organization recommends a minimum usable floor space of 3.5 m² per person in an emergency.

Shelter should, where possible, be made of local materials with perhaps the addition of materials such as plastic sheeting.

Use of cluster sampling for household surveys

It is possible to gain useful baseline data on household characteristics such as fuel used for cooking, water source used, food source, demography, household size, percentage of female-headed households, and latrine use rapidly by use of a cluster sampling technique.[22,23] Results are possible within just a few days and can be invaluable in guiding the emergency response. This can then be repeated at intervals to evaluate the effectiveness of the aid effort.

The proper collection of data can guide the response to an emergency and use scarce resources efficiently. It is rarely done well. Presentation of the data should be clear, preferably by a bar chart or line graph and the data should be used and not just filed away. Well-presented data are a powerful tool to use when lobbying for more assistance.

Preparedness and logistics

In areas prone to emergencies, prior planning and organisation are advisable (see Box 19.6). To react

quickly to large refugee movements requires extremely good logistics, often with use of pre-packed kits of medicines and equipment which can be mobilised within hours (e.g. WHO/Médecins Sans Frontières Medical Kit for 10000 people for 3 months). While there is a need for rapid mobilisation of materials from abroad in large crises, the local resources and capacities are often underutilised. The best resource in any refugee crisis is the refugees themselves. Helping the refugees to help themselves will often be more effective than massive material responses.

The relative importance of interventions varies with the situation. Common mistakes, however, are to underestimate the need for shelter, blankets, ground insulation and fuel and overestimate the

---

Box 19.6 Response to sudden population movements – main principles

1. Security is paramount. Have a clear security policy. The death of an aid-worker can halt the whole aid effort.
2. Priorities are: blankets/shelter, water, food (including fuel and cooking utensils), sanitation, measles vaccination and vitamin A distribution.
3. Start with a rapid needs and capacity assessment. Include a careful assessment of the likely adverse impacts of aid (e.g. fuelling conflict, putting local farmers out of business).
4. Work with and through local structures where possible (capacity building). Build up a local team.
5. Understand existing development initiatives in the area and national health strategies and work with rather than against these. Aim for sustainability when feasible. Have a thinking approach to the situation.
6. Target women and children as they are likely to die first.
7. Primary health care is usually more effective than interventions at secondary level.
8. Establish surveillance early on.
9. Use only drugs on the WHO essential drugs list.
10. Work on the political and diplomacy aspects.
11. You may need to lobby and use advocacy to mobilise a much bigger aid effort.
12. Preparedness for a worsening of the situation is essential.
13. Rigorous audit, evaluation and monitoring are essential.
14. Good inter-agency coordination is critical.
15. Good leadership is needed to keep teams functional during extreme stress.

need for immediate food aid.[24] The largest component of energy expenditure is basal metabolic rate (BMR). This is equivalent to about 1600 kcal for a 65 kg person. A lightly clothed refugee exposed to ambient temperatures well below the thermoneutral range may need to increase energy expenditure to three or more times the BMR, that is, requiring up to 4800 kcal per day. It therefore follows that the first priority for refugees suddenly exposed to low temperatures (e.g. on a mountainside) is shelter and blankets. Next comes water with survival times without water being only a few days. Normally nourished adults with adequate fluid intake can survive over a month without food. Refugee populations, however, may already have significant levels of malnutrition even before displacement. Early attention to the general food ration is therefore the third priority. It is extremely important to address the vital sectors (shelter, water, food) together with measles vaccination and vitamin A distribution before focusing efforts on curative care.

Reproductive health in refugees

Since the 1994 International Conference on Population and Development, held in Cairo, and the mass rapes of Bosnian women, reproductive health for refugees has rightly had a higher profile.

Reproductive health consists of the following issues:

- safe motherhood
- sexual violence
- prevention and management of sexually transmitted diseases and HIV
- family planning
- other isssues such as female genital mutilation.[28]

Displacement can adversely affect all aspects of reproductive health. Women and girls are particularly vulnerable during flight. They may become targets of sexual violence from the military or border guards. They may be forced to exchange sex for food, water or protection. Amongst Mozambican refugees fleeing to Malawi, 8%

reported sexual abuse during displacement and 3% reported exchanging sex for money.[25] War and population displacement create ideal conditions for the spread of sexually transmitted diseases and HIV. There is frequently a mixing of low and high HIV-prevalence populations as happened in the Rwanda crisis in 1994. Urban rates of HIV were up to 30% and rural and semi-rural rates probably less than 1%. Following the massing of refugees in huge refugee camps outside Rwanda, the HIV risk increased in the rural and semi-rural groups to 8.2%.[26] According to the Rwandan Ministry of Health study released in May 1998, 11% of Rwandan adults are now infected with HIV compared to less than 2% in 1986.

Fertility rates tend to drop in the acute phase of refugee movements but despite this there is a continued need for contraception, especially post-coital contraception for rape victims. Basic reproductive healthcare cannot wait for the situation to stabilise. With this in mind, the Minimal Initial Services Package (MISP) was conceived (Box 19.7).

Box 19.7 The Minimum Initial Services Package – for use in the early stages of population displacement	
Prevention and management of sexual violence	• Careful planning of refugee camps to minimise risk of sexual violence
	• Physical, psychological and economic support to victims of sexual violence
Prevention of HIV transmission	• 'Universal Precautions'– gloves, protection of health workers
	• Minimise injection use and blood transfusions.
	• Syndromic* management of sexually transmitted diseases
	• Condom promotion
Reduction of excess maternal and neonatal mortality	• Early organisation of safe delivery service
	• Creation of referral system for high-risk pregnancies
Planning for the provision of more comprehensive services	• Training
	• Logistics
	• Coordination

* A syndrome-based approach to sexually transmitted disease management has been shown to be effective and to reduce HIV transmission.[27,28]

Evaluation and monitoring of aid programmes

Evaluation was defined in 1986 by the Organisation for Economic Co-operation and Development as 'an examination as systematic and objective as possible of an ongoing or completed relief project or programme, its design, implementation and results, with the aim of determining its efficiency, effectiveness, impact, sustainability and the relevance of its objectives'. Many agencies involved in relief programmes still do not evaluate the effectiveness or impact of their programmes.[5] The fact that the aid is well intentioned and delivered in difficult circumstances should not exclude it from rigorous evaluation. When mortality rates are high the difference between getting it right and getting it wrong may be counted in hundreds if not thousands of lives. Evaluation is critical for institutional learning and also facilitates accountability. In extreme emergencies, it is very difficult to apply cost–benefit analysis and controlled trials pose many ethical dilemmas. Appropriate data are often hard to come by and lack standardisation between agencies. In the chaos of large population movements where need always exceeds capacity, it is hard to convince aid-workers of the need to spend time on evaluation and audit. There is also little time to undertake baseline assessments of need and capacity. Evaluation and monitoring can sometimes get lost in the dynamic of the response. It is thereore important at the earliest design phase to build in appropriate and valid indicators of success. Various tools have been used to facilitate this. Logical framework analysis sets out clearly, and in a hierarchical fashion, the objectives, results and activities of the programme together with objectively verifiable indicators of success and is widely used in development and relief programmes.[5] There remains a considerable gap between what is desirable and what happens in practice.

REFERENCES

1. International Federation of Red Cross and Red Crescent. World Disasters Report 1996.
2. International Federation of Red Cross and Red Crescent. World Disasters Report 1995.
3. The international response to conflict and genocide: Lessons from the Rwanda Experience. Joint evaluation of Emergency Assistance to Rwanda.
4. Political mapping
5. Borton J assessing the impact and effectiveness of relief assistance. Paper prepared for the 1995 World Disasters Report.
6. Toole M, Waldman R. Prevention of excess mortality in refugee and displaced populations in developing countries. Journal of the American Medical Association 263: 3296–3302.
7. Garfield RG, Epidemiological analysis of warfare, Journal of the American Medical Association 1991; 266: 688–692.

8. Center for disease control and prevention. Famine affected refugee and displaced populations: recommendations for public health issues. MMWR. Morbidity and Mortality Weekly Report 1992; 41(RR-13): 1–76.

9. Lollibridge S, Noji E, Burkle F. Disaster assessment: the emergency health evaluation of a population affected by disaster. Annals of Emergency Medicine 1993; 11: 1715–1720.

10. Semba R. Vitamin A, immunity and infection. Clinical Infectious Diseases 1994; 19: 489–499.

11. Shears P, Berry AM, Murphy R, Nabil MA. Epidemiological assessment of the health and nutrition of Ethiopian refugees in emergency camps in Sudan, 1985. British Medical Journal 1987; 295: 314–318.

12. Allen R. Malaria control in complex emergencies, Dialogue Child Health in Emergencies, Special Supplement in Emergencies. (in press)

13. Banatvala N, Roger A, Denny A, Howarth J. Mortality and Morbidity among Rwandan refugees repatriated from Zaire, November, 1996. (in press).

14. Howarth J. Field visit report – Chechnya 1996. Merlin internal report.

15. Hakewill PA, Moren A. Monitoring and evaluation of relief programmes. Tropical doctor 1991; 21(Suppl 1): 24–28.

16. Goma Epidemiology Group. Public health impact of Rwandan refugee crisis: what hapenned in Goma in July, 1994? Lancet 1995; 345: 339–344.

17. Moren A. Rapid assessment of the state of health of displaced populations or refugees. MSF Medical News 1992; 1(5):

18. A survey of the Western area. Sierra Leone: Sierra Leone Ministry of Health.

19. Metaanalysis of MUAC. MSF Medical News, Holland.

20. Young H. Food scarcity and famine. 1992 Oxfam Practical Health Guide

21. Handbook of emergencies UNHCR

22. Hausman B, Ritmeijer K. Surveillence in emergency situations. Médecins Sans Frontières, Holland July 1993

22. Drysdale S, Howarth J, Powell V, Healing T. The use of cluster analysis to determine aid needs in Grozny Chechnya in 1995. (in press)

23. Hilady WG, Quenemoen LE, Armenia-Cope RR, et al. Use of a modified cluster sampling method to perform rapid needs assessment after Hurricaine Andrew. Annals of Emergency Medicine 1994; 23: 719–725.

24. LaMont-Gregory E, Henry C, Ryan TJ. Letter to Lancet 1995; 356: July 29.

25. Cossa HA, Gloyd S, et al. Syphilis and HIV infection among displaced pregnant women in rural Mozmbique. International Journal of STD and AIDS 1994; 5(2): 117–123.

26. Rwanda National AIDS Control Programme 1996.

27. Grosskurth, Hiner, et al. Impact of improved treatment of sexually transmitted diseases on HIV infection in rural Tanzania: randomised controlled trial. Lancet, 1995; 346: 530–536.

28. Reproductive health in a refugee setting – an inter-agency field manual. UNHCR.

Ethnic minority and immigrant travellers

Pradhib Venkatesan   Martin Dedicoat

Introduction

In 1948, the *Emperor Windrush* sailed to the UK from the Caribbean, bringing a group of migrants seeking work. Labour was in short supply in the UK at that time and further immigration followed from the Caribbean and other Commonwealth countries. In the ensuing decades, migration occurred for other reasons, such as the expulsion in 1972 from Uganda of peoples with an Indian–Asian background.

Over the years, economic and political migration has led to the emergence of ethnic minority groups of African–Caribbean, African, South Asian and Chinese backgrounds. In addition to peoples who have settled in the UK, there are also a significant number of students and workers who come here from all over the world for limited duration.

From first-generation immigrants, we now have second and third generations born in this country. With each succeeding generation, intermarriage and social mixing are breaking down cultural barriers. Yet ethnic identities remain, characterised by ancestry, geographical origins, culture and language. Rigid categorising of ethnic groups is debatable but in the 1991 census the England and Wales population was categorised as in Table 20.1.[1] The main ethnic minority groups are African–Caribbean, South Asian and those from Commonwealth countries and these are the groups discussed in this chapter.

This chapter deals with health issues for ethnic minority groups as they travel abroad from the UK. As a result they may suffer illness, which may be infectious or non-infectious. The latter relates more to the individual, particular, medical history (e.g.

TABLE 20.1 Ethnic minority breakdown in the 1991 England and Wales census

	Number	%
Total population	49 890 273	
White	46 936 500	94.1
Black–Caribbean	499 000	1.0
Black–African	205 400	0.4
Black other	176 400	0.4
Indian	830 600	1.7
Pakistani	454 500	0.9
Bangladeshi	159 500	0.3
Chinese	147 300	0.3
Other		
Asian	193 100	0.4
Other	280 900	0.6

asthma or angina) that could be exacerbated by travel. It is infectious diseases peculiar to the travel destination that are usually highlighted in travel medicine.

Certain illnesses may have been present prior to first entry into the UK. Here some definitions are required. One definition of travel medicine is that it deals with the traveller departing from the country of domicile, requiring advice and prophylaxis and any illness on the traveller's return, requiring diagnosis and treatment. An 'imported' infection could have been acquired during a trip out of a new country of residence or prior to the original migration from another country. Strictly, the former should be included in travel medicine but not the latter. However, in real life this distinction is not distinct.

Case 1 illustrates that some infections are very chronic and may only present years after first infection. This usually involves helminthic infections such as strongyloidiasis, schistosomiasis and filariasis, all having prolonged adult life stages.

Case I

A 39-year-old headmaster from Sierra Leone presented with a hard lump near his right anterior superior iliac crest. This had been present for several years and was gradually increasing in size. It was now rubbing on his waistband and causing him discomfort. He had no other symptoms.

He was born in a small village in rural Sierra Leone, near a river, and had lived there until he came to the UK 9 years previously.

He mentioned that there were numerous, biting, black flies around the river near his village and that river blindness was a common condition amongst people in the region.

On examination, there were two, 2 × 1 cm, firm, non-tender lumps above the right iliac crest. These were fixed to deep structures but the skin over them was mobile.

The lumps were removed and histology revealed adult, nematode worms consistent with a diagnosis of onchocerciasis. The adults can live for over 10 years and produce microfilaria throughout this time.

Therefore, expatriates from sub-Saharan Africa remain at risk of eye and skin damage for many years after they have left an endemic area.

Pre-travel behaviour

ATTITUDE TO PROPHYLAXIS

Whatever their ethnic background not all travellers seek advice or prophylaxis prior to travel. Less than one-third of travellers receive vaccines,[2] if the number of travellers compared with the number leaving the UK with vaccine prescriptions dispensed is a true reflection of those who are unprepared.

There are few studies specifically looking at prophylaxis uptake by ethnic minority groups. Data from the Malaria Reference Laboratory show that only 19% of ethnic minority travellers used chemoprophylaxis when visiting friends and relatives in their countries of origin, compared with 73% of other tourists.[3] It is suggested that this lack of usage is paralleled by poor vaccine uptake and may relate to limited travel health consultation prior to travel.

In patients with *Plasmodium falciparum* malaria admitted to the Hospital for Tropical Diseases in London, Lewis et al[4] found that 10% of Africans living in Africa took chemoprophylaxis, compared with 50% of Africans living in the UK and 70% of whites. However, there are also studies which show that the uptake of travel health advice is comparable between ethnic groups and UK whites.[5]

Our experience is that returned ethnic travellers with typhoid, hepatitis A and malaria have invariably not received previous prophylaxis or advice. However, travellers with other presenting illnesses, such as gastroenteritis or self-limiting viral illnesses, do report having had vaccinations and malaria chemoprophylaxis. Thus, ethnic minority travellers do seek advice but not all, just like all other groups in the UK. However, the reasons for not taking up advice may differ. In general, lack of uptake may arise from inconvenience, concern over costs, lack of concern or lack of awareness of health risks.

ESTABLISHED BELIEFS

The ethnic traveller may be more aware of local health risks in their country of origin than the advising health practitioner and health beliefs dictate whether it is thought possible or worthwhile preventing illness. Thus, an attack of malaria may be an illness to be tolerated and treated once contracted rather than to be prevented. Our observation is that when families travel, the health beliefs of the head of the family determine prophylaxis uptake.

Thus, if the father, who was born abroad and has visited his country of origin several times, does not use chemoprophylaxis or have vaccinations then neither will his children, born in the UK and visiting their ancestral homeland for the first time. On return, it is often the children who present with, for example, hepatitis and typhoid fever.

However, health beliefs do change with generations and successive UK born ethnic minority travellers are converging in their behaviour with UK whites.

Patterns of travel

ACCOMMODATION

The traveller of Western origin frequently falls into distinct groupings: for example, a 2-week package tourist, a backpacker travelling for several months, a businessman travelling for a few days and the expatriate worker abroad for months or years. In their travels, they will stay in hotels of varying standard or expatriate accommodation which may be of a better standard than for local people.

In contrast, ethnic minority travellers may return to their country of origin to stay with family or relatives in rural or urban areas. These may not be in 'tourist spots' and the prevalence of disease may not be the same as in relatively sanitised tourist destinations. The accommodation, food and water will be the same standard as the local residents and may vary from excellent to poor. The duration of travel may be for a few months rather than a few weeks. These travellers are likely to return to the same destination at each visit. Thus many factors affect the risks of various illnesses.

PILGRIMAGES

Muslims going on pilgrimage demonstrate an example of difference between the travel patterns within ethnic minority groups.

Each year during the month-long period of the Haj, Muslims from around the world converge on Saudi Arabia. They visit the holy cities of Makkah and Medina. The population of Saudi Arabia swells, hotels are filled to capacity and temporary villages in the form of tent encampments are established. The heat and unusual activities can lead to exhaustion. Millions of people live in close confinement and also come together during the religious observations.

Conditions are very favourable to the spread of infections, particularly respiratory tract infections such as influenza and tuberculosis. Diarrhoeal illnesses result from poor hygiene as a result of the crowded conditions.

In 1987, an outbreak of Group A meningococcal infection among pilgrims, with several fatalities, resulted in the Saudi authorities introducing a requirement that all future pilgrims should produce a certificate confirming they have received meningococcal vaccination before arrival. Outbreaks of dengue during the Haj have also been reported.

Factors affecting illness while abroad

MEDICATIONS

Behaviour, exposure and pre-existing immunity to infections affect the spectrum of illness. One aspect of behaviour is compliance with regular medication. Practitioners will be familiar with diabetic patients forgetting to take insulin or oral hypoglycaemic agents with them and falling ill with a loss of diabetic control (Case 2).

Case 2

A 66-year-old Pakistani man was admitted shortly after returning from a trip to Pakistan. He had been an insulin dependent diabetic for many years but while away he had felt particularly well and had decided to stop his insulin.

At presentation, he had not taken insulin for 2 weeks and his family reported he had been deteriorating over this time with blurred vision, increasing confusion, polyuria and polydipsia.

On admission, his blood pressure was 250/125 mmHg and it was assumed he had also stopped his antihypertensive medication. He was not ketotic but his blood glucose was 46 mmol/L.

This case illustrates that some ethnic travellers may not appreciate the importance of their medication and may not consider it necessary to continue with it when returning home, especially if they feel well.

Other medication such as steroids may be stopped abruptly with serious consequences. If prescriptions are sought locally, there may be confusion over dosage and the identity of drugs. Problems with medications are more likely to affect the long-term traveller and those who do not have much credence for their efficacy. Again, health beliefs play a part and there may be ethnic differences in this area.

SEXUAL PRACTICES

It is well known that some travellers engage in unprotected sex and acquire sexually transmitted diseases (STDs) abroad, including HIV infection. Specific information on sexual behaviour has mainly looked at those of Caucasian origin, for example British, Swiss and German travellers.[6][7] To date, there is little detailed information on sexual behaviour in the various ethnic minority groups. Higher rates of STDs and HIV reported in sub-Saharan Africans may reflect the prevalence of these diseases in the countries of origin.[8]

It is difficult to extrapolate from such findings to say that some ethnic minority groups have more sexual contacts and take fewer precautions.

CLIMATE AND CULTURE

Extremes of climate and levels of physical activity while travelling can affect respiratory and cardiovascular disease. The transition from a cold, temperate climate to a hot, tropical climate, with the necessary exertion of travel, can precipitate cardiac ischaemia. However, travellers returning to warm, dry and stress-free villages in India or Africa may report an amelioration of their asthma or angina. In fact, some report discontinuing regular medication without detriment.

CULTURE

While difficult to quantify, the experience of travel overall may be less stressful to the ethnic minority traveller returning to a familiar environment, than a Caucasian traveller visiting a strange country and encountering a strange culture and incomprehensible language. However, this is not always the case with second and third generation immigrants who may have a very difficult time while abroad when their established lifestyle at home is now very different from that which may be expected of them in the country of their parents' or grandparents' origin.

'FAMILIARITY'

The traveller staying with family and relatives is more likely to behave 'as the locals do'. Walking barefoot runs the risk of acquiring soil-borne helminths or of leptospirosis. Insecticides and bed nets may not be routinely used. Water may come from household or portable sources. In rural areas, gastrointestinal pathogens are more likely to be acquired and more than one infection could arise (Case 3).

Case 3

A 56-year-old Pakistani woman was admitted to hospital with a 3-day history of fever, rigors, nausea, headache and bloody diarrhoea. She had returned 4 days previously from a 4-month trip to Pakistan.

Stool cultures revealed *Shigella boydii* and *Campylobacter jejuni* .

Her husband and children accompanied the patient to Pakistan. Subsequent inquiry revealed that they were also suffering from diarrhoea. The patient's husband was admitted to hospital for treatment of his diarrhoea. His stool cultures revealed he also had *Campylobacter jejuni.*

The index patient was later readmitted with further bloody diarrhoea and on this occasion *Campylobacter coli* was cultured from stool.

If family and relatives become ill, infections may pass onto the visitors. This pattern of intra-household transmission is unusual with non-ethnic travellers. In patients with hepatitis A or E, it is not unusual to hear of a history of household illness, although this may merely also reflects a common outside source of infection (Case 4).

Case 4

A 29-year-old Pakistani man presented with fever and jaundice 2 weeks after returning from a trip to Pakistan.

While in Pakistan, he had been visiting his mother and brother. His mother had been unwell with fever shortly before his return and his brother had developed jaundice. During his stay, he had mainly eaten at his mother's house.

Serology showed positive hepatitis E IgM, and blood cultures also revealed *Salmonella paratyphi* A.

ANIMAL BITES

Another exposure risk which increases with long-term visits and staying in rural settings is animal bites. Dogs are frequently seen in tropical countries and serve a protective function for households. However, many dogs become stray and live off rubbish heaps and roadside scraps. Rabies virus is transmitted amongst these stray and unvaccinated domestic dogs.

The risk of rabies has not been quantified in ethnic travellers, but may more closely approximate the risk of the local population than of the visiting Caucasian tourist staying in a city hotel. In India each year 25 000 people die from rabies and 0.5 million receive post-exposure prophylaxis.[9]

Over the past three decades, rabies has been reported with increasing frequency in Africa.[10] Partly this relates to surveillance but a true rise in incidence is thought to be present. Each year 200–300 confirmed cases occur in Kenya.

PREVIOUS EXPOSURE TO INFECTION

Pre-existing immunity dating from previous infection will protect the ethnic traveller. If the infection occurred in childhood, it may have been mild or asymptomatic. Thus, since childhood hepatitis A can be asymptomatic, many ethnic adults who have been raised in endemic areas may be immune without knowledge of illness. Children living in endemic areas almost invariably become seropositive by the age of 10 years and have lifelong immunity.

Hepatitis E is the commonest cause of faecal–orally-spread hepatitis in adults living in endemic areas. This is usually because infection is first encountered during epidemics in adult life.[11] Thus, enteric hepatitis in ethnic travellers is more likely to be hepatitis E if they had grown up abroad. In a seroprevalence study in inner city London, the antibodies to hepatitis A were present in 45% of UK-born subjects and 70% of non-UK born subjects, while antibodies were present in 4% and 9% respectively to hepatitis E.[12]

Immunity generated by a natural *Salmonella typhi* infection is more protective than immunity following vaccination. Second serious episodes of typhoid fever are rare. In endemic areas, infection does not always occur in childhood and therefore there are susceptible adults.

Another gastrointestinal pathogen that follows the same pattern of immunity is *Vibrio cholerae*. Second illnesses with classical cholera are very rare, while other strains do not confer significant protection against a second episode.[13] *Vibrio cholerae* 01 strains do not protect against the 0139 strain.

Recurrent attacks of malaria are evidence of the lack of complete protective immunity to infection. Infections can become chronic and be low grade.

However, immunity does develop against *Plasmodium falciparum*, following repeated attacks over many years, with subsequent attacks being of diminishing severity. In experimental situations this immunity is most pronounced against an homologous strain of parasite rather than an heterologous strain.[14] The immunity is T lymphocyte independent and thus lacks memory.

Once out of an endemic area, immunity diminishes and may be lost after around 2 years without the antigen stimulus from repeated infection. The ethnic traveller returning to an endemic area after a long spell therefore may be at the same risk of serious malaria as a Caucasian counterpart staying in the same conditions.

Illnesses seen in returning ethnic minority groups

While abroad, the pattern of illnesses seen will depend on disease prevalence in the countries visited.[15]

On return from abroad the pattern of illness reflects the ethnic mix, and country of origin of the infections, in a particular city or region. Throughout the UK, there are regional variations in the distribution of ethnic groups.[1] In some cities, ethnic residents are predominantly Pakistanis, in others Indians and in others African–Caribbeans. This ethnic diversity and distribution must be appreciated when looking at reviews of returned ethnic travellers at single study centres.

Information on certain infections is available through notification data. But this information is selective, incomplete, and does not provide an overview of all the illnesses seen in unwell, returned travellers.

To date only two prospective studies of infections in returned travellers to the UK have been published.

The first study looked at 195 febrile adult patients admitted to the Hospital for Tropical Diseases in London.[16] Of these, 108 were European, North American or Australian. Of the remaining 87 patients, 65 originated from sub-Saharan Africa, 9 from the Indian sub-continent and 6 from the

Caribbean. The main travel destination was sub-Saharan Africa, visited by 117, with 41 visiting Asia. The infections diagnosed were not distinguished between ethnic groups. This study predominantly reflects African travel. The principal diagnoses were *Plasmodium falciparum* malaria (71), non-specific viral infections (48), dengue fever (12) and dysentery (10).

The second study reported on 31 children admitted to Northwick Park Hospital, London, with fever on return from the tropics.[17] There were UK white children, with 19 being of South Asian and 8 African or African–Caribbean background. The principal diagnoses were non-specific fever (14) and malaria (4).

In Birmingham, we have reviewed 227 consecutive, returned, adult travellers (unpublished). There were more patients from ethnic minority groups (168) than UK-whites (59). The majority of ethnic minority patients were Asian (Pakistani 90, Indian 40, Bangladeshi 8, Thai 1), with only 15 from sub-Saharan Africa and 4 from the Caribbean. Therefore, this series predominantly reflects travel to the Indian sub-continent. The majority of diagnoses (85%) fell into one of five categories: malaria (77), gastroenteritis (50), unexplained, self-limiting fever (31), enteric fever (23) and hepatitis (12).

All three studies are concerned with hospitalised patients. However, many travellers with illness do not get admitted to hospital. Information on ethnic minorities attending outpatient departments and general practitioners is lacking. Nonetheless some general observations can be made.

Following Asian travel, *Plasmodium vivax* malaria appears to be more common in ethnic travellers than in UK whites. This may be because of longer durations of travel with an increased cumulative risk and less use of prophylaxis.

Following sub-Saharan African travel, pre-existing immunity in those of African origin may modify the presentation of *Plasmodium falciparum* malaria. Symptoms can be delayed by about 1 week and fever is less common than in non-immune travellers.[3]

In our experience, enteric fever and hepatitis A are common in ethnic groups and this may be due to poorer levels of hygiene where they stay. It may also be due to poorer vaccine uptake.

Many infections in ethnic groups are not rare parasitic or viral diseases, but bacterial infections of the respiratory tract, urinary tract and soft tissues, all of worldwide distribution.

It is important to be aware of the possibility of antibiotic resistance amongst bacterial pathogens abroad as illustrated by Case 5.

Case 5

A 62-year-old Pakistani man presented with a 1-week history of malaise, cough, fever and rigors.

He had previously been in good health and had just returned the previous day from a month's trip to Mecca for the Haj. While there, he had been moving in large crowds and at one point was crushed in a stampede sustaining minor injuries.

A chest radiograph revealed right lower lobe consolidation and sputum cultures grew *Haemophilus influenzae*, *Haemophilus parainfluenzae* and *Streptococcus pneumoniae*.

These organisms were probably acquired from close contact with other pilgrims in Mecca and were resistant to a number of antibiotics as shown below.

Antibiotic	Pathogen		
	H. influenzae	*H. para-influenzae*	*S. pneumoniae*
Penicillin			Resistant
Ampicillin		Resistant	
Tetracycline		Resistant	
Erythromycin	Resistant		
Trimethoprim	Resistant	Resistant	Resistant
Ciprofloxacin			Resistant

TUBERCULOSIS

The ability of *Mycobacterium tuberculosis* to cause rapid clinical illness or to remain dormant and reactivate after several years makes it difficult to clearly associate tuberculosis with a particular trip abroad or indeed with the travel itself.

Tuberculosis is well known to be an imported infection in immigrants, often from the Indian sub-continent, who acquired an inapparent infection in childhood, only developing the disease following emigration. In the majority, clinical disease, however, develops within 5 years of arrival.[18] In the new country, tuberculosis can then be transmitted within households and to social contacts.

A person visiting family and relatives abroad where tuberculosis is present could acquire infection and develop the disease after return. Quantifying the likelihood of local and foreign infection is difficult. However, in one study, about one-fifth of ethnic travellers notified to have tuberculosis had travelled within 5 years and probably acquired their infection abroad.[18]

Behaviour of ethnic minorities when ill

On being taken ill, individuals behave differently. Some present to their general practitioner promptly, while others wait to see if they recover spontaneously. This could be serious when febrile patients with *Plasmodium falciparum* malaria do not seek advice early. However, in a study of 301 patients with *Plasmodium falciparum* malaria, there were no differences in the times to presentation between whites and Africans.[4]

If taken ill while abroad, there are often easily available medicines for purchase over the counter and this has been blamed for inappropriate self-medication. However, in a recent community survey in Karachi, Pakistan of 2348 households, it was found that the purchase of antibiotics from pharmacies was 'on prescription' in 91.4%, following advice by pharmacists in 2.3% and only 6.3% represented self-medication.[19] Whether ethnic minority travellers, with perhaps no local trusted physician, are more likely to self-medicate is unclear.

INJECTIONS AND TRADITIONAL REMEDIES

Ethnic minorities often belief in the 'power' of injections and the use of herbal and traditional remedies.

The risks associated with re-used needles are well known. A variety of hepatitis viruses can be transmitted[20] and Case 6 illustrates the hazards associated with hepatitis B.

While the use of injected drugs may be necessary, there are occasions when individuals

Case 6

A 29-year-old Pakistani woman presented 2 months after a 5-month trip to Pakistan. While in Pakistan she had suffered with a febrile illness attributed to typhoid. This was treated with intramuscular injections and an intravenous infusion.

She presented with malaise, nausea and jaundice for a week and was found to have tender hepatomegaly. She had acute hepatitis B.

As there were no other risk factors it was assumed she had acquired hepatitis B from the injections received in Pakistan.

She made a full recovery but unfortunately during her convalescence, her husband became jaundiced and also proved to have acute hepatitis B. His only risk factor was unprotected sex with his wife. He had refrained from sex since his wife's diagnosis and probably acquired the virus before she became jaundiced.

This case highlights the importance of using sterile needles while overseas. There is also a cultural dimension, as medicines given by injection are often perceived as being stronger or superior to tablets.

seek injections for illnesses such as malaise and other minor symptoms. This illness behaviour is seen much more commonly in ethnic groups and less in Western whites who generally avoid injections abroad if at all possible.[21] They are also more likely to use local herbal and traditional remedies. Many of these do alleviate symptoms, but as there is little regulation some available preparations may not be properly formulated, may be out of date and may be mislabelled. There is potential for side effects and doctors need to be aware of this possibility when assessing an unwell returned ethnic traveller.

Conclusions

Some determinants of travel illness in minority groups do not primarily correlate with ethnicity. Socio-economic factors may determine whether the ethnic traveller returns to stay with relatives in a poor village or in a city with adequate sanitation and washing facilities. These socio-economic factors dictate the likelihood of illness. Therefore, there should be more focus on travel destinations, local conditions and health risks irrespective of the ethnicity of the traveller.

However, with prophylaxis and post-illness behaviour there is a need to distinguish between Western whites and immigrant groups as health beliefs and cultural and language differences do differ. As in other areas of medicine, understanding the diversity of health beliefs enables the formulation of solutions.[22] Encouragement to have vaccinations, to take malaria chemoprophylaxis and to avoid unnecessary injections while abroad needs to be conveyed in suitable languages, in a culturally acceptable form and by understanding advisers.

PRACTICE POINTS

- Visits are often to family and friends, unlikely to be taking the same precautions against illness that you are advising to the travellers – compliance may therefore be difficult to achieve.
- Decisions regarding advice and prophylaxis may have to be agreed to by the head of the family, who may be the father or grandmother.
- While 'first-generation' immigrants may be familiar with likely facilities and culture at their destination, younger members of their families may not and 'culture shock' can be very real.
- Close contact with local people may increase exposure to illnesses such as tuberculosis and typhoid.
- Special immigration requirements for pilgrimages may include meningococcal vaccination.

REFERENCES

1. Balarajan R, Raleigh VS. The ethnic populations of England and Wales: the 1991 census. Health Trends 1992; 24: 113–116.
2. Behrens RH, Roberts JA. Is travel prophylaxis worthwhile? Economic appraisal of prophylactic measures against malaria, hepatitis A, and typhoid in travellers. British Medical Journal 1994; 309: 918–922.
3. Behrens RH. Travel morbidity in ethnic minority travellers. In: Cook GC, ed. Travel associated disease. London: Royal College of Physicians; 1995.
4. Lewis SJ, Davidson RN, Ross EJ, Hall AP. Severity of imported falciparum malaria: effect of taking antimalarial prophylaxis. British Medical Journal 1992; 305: 741–743.
5. Packham CJ. A survey of notified travel-associated infections: implications for travel health advice. Journal of Public Health Medicine 1995; 17: 217–222.
6. Kleiber D, Wilke M. Sexual behaviour of sex-tourists: conclusions from a study of the social and psychological characterisitics of German sex-tourists. In: Cook GC, ed. Travel associated disease. London: Royal College of Physician; 1995.
7. Hawkes S, Hart GJ, Bletsoe E, Shergold C, Johnson AM. Risk behaviour and STD acquisition in genitourinary clinic attenders who have travelled. Genitourinary Medicine 1995; 71: 351–354.
8. Hawkes S, Hart GJ, Johnson AM, et al. Risk behaviour and HIV prevalence in international travellers. AIDS 1994; 8: 247–252.
9. Dutta JK, Dutta TK. Rabies in endemic countries. British Medical Journal 1994; 308: 488–489.
10. Cleaveland S. Epidemiology and control of rabies. The growing problem of rabies in Africa. Transactions of the Royal Society of Tropical Medicine and Hygiene 1998; 92: 131–134.
11. Skidmore SJ. Hepatitis E. British Medical Journal 1995; 310: 414–415.
12. Bernal W, Smith HM, Williams R. A community prevalence study of hepatitis A and E in inner-city London. Journal of Medical Virology 1996; 49: 230–234.
13. Clemens JD, Van Loon F, Sack DA, et al. Biotype as determinant of natural immunising effect of cholera. Lancet 1991; 337: 883–884.
14. Miller LH, Good MF, Millon G. Malaria pathogenesis. Science 1994; 264: 1878–1883.
15. Wilson ME. A world guide to infections. Diseases, distribution, diagnosis. New York: Oxford University Press; 1991.
16. Doherty JF, Grant AD, Bryceson ADM. Fever as the presenting complaint of travellers returning from the tropics. Quarterly Journal of Medicine 1995; 88: 277–281.
17. Klein JL, Millman GC. Prospective hospital based study of fever in children in the United Kingdom who had recently spent time in the tropics. British Medical Journal 1998; 316: 1425–1426.
18. McCarthy OR. Asian immigrant tuberculosis – the effect of visiting Asia. British Journal of Disorders of the Chest 1984; 78: 248–253.
19. Sturm AW, Van der Pol R, Smits AJ, et al. Over the counter availability of antimicrobial agents, self-medication and patterns of resistance in Karachi, Pakistan. Journal of Antimicrobial Chemotherapy 1997: 39: 543–547.
20. Moatter T, Tariq SA, Fisher-Hoch S, et al. Hepatitis G virus in Karachi, Pakistan. Lancet 1996; 348: 1318–1319.

21. Dedicoat M, Ellis C, Abid M, Boxall E. Iatrogenic hepatitis B in travellers. Transactions of the Royal Society of Tropical Medicine and Hygiene 1997; 91: 508 (abstract).

22. Greenhalgh T, Helman C, Chowdhury AM. Health beliefs and folk models of diabetes in British Bangladeshis: a qualitative study. British Medical Journal 1998; 316: 978–983.

Impact of tourism on host countries

A. J. Hedley   A. S. M. Abdullah

Introduction

The word 'tourism' is not very easy to define. The Concise Oxford Dictionary defines it as 'organised touring', that obviously begs more questions than it provides explanations. Professor Hunziker of Berne University defined tourism as:

> the sum of the phenomena and relationships arising from the travel and stay of non-residents, in so far as they do not lead to permanent residence and are not connected with any earning activity.[1]

Alternatively, tourism may be a form of pilgrimage, a 'sacred journey',[2] a move from structured societies to unstructured communities, perhaps echoing rites of transition practised in some pre-industrial tribal societies.[3] Or tourism is the temporary movement of people to destinations outside their normal places of work and residence, the activities undertaken during their stay in those destinations, and the facilities created to cater to their needs.[4]

It does not matter what definition is used for tourism, as it is already recognised as one of the world's largest and fastest-growing industries and an economic and sociocultural phenomenon of major importance. Travelling is one of the characteristics of human nature. Human nature has as one of its inborn characteristics the need to change, to experience and to explore. Tourism allows people to do so by going from one place to another, one environment to another environment, one culture to another culture and so on. By the year 2000, the international travelling business will become the world's biggest industry In 1993, the World Tourism Organisation estimated the number of international tourists at 661 million by the year 2000 and 937 million by the year 2010.

Tourism is one of the most important export industries and foreign currency earners in many countries in the world. In countries such as Jamaica, Spain and Mexico, tourism is the largest earner of foreign exchange and the leading industry in terms of income and employment.[4] Tourism has become the leading source of foreign exchange in countries like Thailand; it is the second largest industry in the Philippines and the third largest earner of foreign currency in Singapore. In Indonesia during the 1980s, when revenues from the country's main export commodity, petroleum, had fallen, tourism helped to boost foreign exchange earnings. Similarly in Malaysia, when foreign exchange earnings from the country's primary industries such as tin and rubber were decreased, tourism was expanded as another source of foreign exchange.

Most of the countries in the world have given a high priority to the growth of tourism business, as an important factor in the growth of economic development. This can be seen in governments' expansion of tourism departments, encouragement and sponsorship of tourist developments, promotional activities and expanding facilities for tourists. It is less fashionable, however, to highlight the negative impact of tourism in host countries. Most countries are attracted to the possibility of increasing the number of travellers or attracting an increasing amount of dollar earnings from the tourism business. It is often only later when travellers are arriving with their own culture, their own behavioural traits, and a large proportion are arriving with their own health problems, that the interaction of these factors with those of the host countries is fully recognised. It has an impact on a wide range of economic, social, cultural, environmental and health areas. The aim of this section is to highlight some of these issues and describe their effects on host countries.

Economic impact of tourism on host countries

While describing the economic development of tourism, Fox[5] stated:

> Tourism is like fire. It can cook your food or burn your house down.

There are different arguments about the economic impact of tourism on host countries. Some have considered it as a stimulus for economic development, as was the case in Spain; while others considered that tourism does not confer economic benefits and is socially very damaging, as was the finding in the Caribbean. Thus we can say that the potential impacts of tourism on the economy of the host country include both 'positive' as well as 'negative' effects which are illustrated below:

POSITIVE EFFECTS

Governments often encourage tourism as an alternative means of economic development. It represents an important source of foreign currency income for host countries. With the increases in tourist arrivals, a wide range of new demands on a country's systems and infrastructure arise. Both existing activities and different demands create new opportunities. The creation of new job opportunities plays an important role in the countries' developing economies. Both skilled and first-time employees benefit from the creation of new posts directly within the sector and indirectly in other sectors. Construction companies benefit from hotel and other infrastructure projects; hotels, food and catering companies benefit from the increasing demands of their services and some other sectors also benefit, either directly or indirectly, such as taxis and other forms of public transport, restaurants, bars and retail outlets, theatres, cinemas and other places of entertainment, arts and crafts

industries, agriculture and manufacturing industries. Establishment of new services such as hospitality services provides income sources, particularly to unskilled women, that also play an important role in domestic economies.

The tourism industry in Thailand was a source of direct employment for 460 000 people, and of indirect employment for an additional 1 million.[6] Carver[7] noted that each nine tourists in the country were estimated to create one job.

In developing countries, tourism has been encouraged by governments to provide financial resources so that they can pull the country towards industrialisation. Brownrigg & Greig[8] argued that tourism has been viewed as a means of introducing new growth into declining rural economies in developed countries. Peters[9] summarised the views of the proponents of tourism as an agent of economic development as follows:

> The economic gap between rich and poor countries has widened over the past ten years. But to create new industries and to transform rural life in Asian, African and Latin American countries is a gigantic task. The relevance of tourism to this situation is that income from international travel can bring the foreign exchange essential for major investment. There is a widespread awareness of the potential benefits, but little has been done in practice to provide the means of expansion of tourism plans in most of the developing areas of the world.

Given that there is nothing so inhibiting to an improvement in public health as poverty, the development of education and creation of work opportunities, improvements in per capita GDP must all be seen as powerful, beneficial, socio-economic influences. They are likely to be reflected in improvements in infant mortality, age-specific mortality rates and life expectancy.

NEGATIVE EFFECTS

Although tourism can create many economic benefits for the host country, it may also have its disadvantages. There are a lot of arguments or criticisms about the benefits from tourism. Bryden,[10] Economist Intelligence Unit,[11] Perez,[12] Rivers,[13] Marsh[14,15] and Turner[16] are among those who have expressed reservations concerning the benefits of tourism. Tourism has contributed a little to economic development in Turkey[17] and in the West Indies.[12]

Tourism often has only medium- to long-term effects on the host country as most of the currency earned from tourist sources goes to foreign corporations and relatively little is left to the host country. To attract tourists, the country has to invest a large amount of money in the development of infrastructure. That includes airport expansions, major roads, police and emergency services, medical services, water supply and drainage facilities, recreation areas and parks, educational materials, and training for skilled and multilingual workers. This in turn may disrupt people's lives, the environment, culture and society.

Employment vacancies created by tourism industries are sometimes filled by immigrants as the local population is insufficiently educated and without adequate technical or managerial skills. Thailand had only one hotel school in 1988 and in the 1970s and 1980s relied on foreign labour to meet its skill shortages, particularly at management level.[6] Indonesia has experienced a considerable shortage of skilled labour. Singapore, Malaysia and Hong Kong also hire a reasonable number of foreign workers each year to meet its labour demand.

Sometimes commissions have to be paid to overseas tour operators and a wide variety of items have to be imported to meet the demands from tourists. All of these lead to a large outflow of currency from the country. Another downside of tourism is that it influences people from other sectors to change their jobs because of the attractiveness of its wages and opportunities that often creates new problems in other sectors of the host country, particularly agriculture. The following example was cited by Professor Jaime De Los Santos at the Symposium on Tourism Management, Kathmandu, Nepal in 1982 about the Banaue rice terraces in the Philippines:

> The main attraction in the area is the centuries-old rice terraces carved in the mountainside by the Igorots, an ethnic minority tribe. With the influx of visitors following the construction of roads and hotels in Banaue, the young men started to shun agricultural manual labour. Those who could not find employment in tourism-oriented establishments chose to migrate to other areas rather than return to farming. As a result, the terraces are crumbling due to the lack of manpower needed to reinforce the mountainsides.

Mings[18] argued that as the labour requirements of the tourist industry are often especially suited to conditions prevailing in developing countries, developed countries are less likely to benefit from the tourist industry.

Job-seekers entering a country as tourists may be a factor in the creation of a local unemployment situation that has an adverse effect on a country's economy. Epidemics, or new health problems, that may be introduced to the country by tourists, are a potential cause of economic and other problems for the host country.

The increase of tourism business creates requirements for new services that may affect a country's economy. In Thailand, the government created a new division of the police force, the tourist police, to deal with tourist-related problems of crime (by or against them) and other issues.

Social impact of tourism on host countries

Tourism has a profound impact on the society of the host country. It brings both advantages and disadvantages for the host society.

SOCIAL ADVANTAGES

Tourism is not without redeeming social and cultural values. The World Tourism Organisation asserts that tourism contributes 'to international understanding, peace, prosperity and universal respect for, and observance of, human rights and fundamental freedom for all, without distinction as to race, sex, language or religion'. To describe social advantages, if we focus on poverty and its elimination, then it is probably fair to state that the society of the host country benefits from the business of tourism in at least some aspects. It often increases employment, increases revenue to the government and stimulates the country's economy. The increasing revenue can be used to the benefit of the host society.

The development of tourist attractions and facilities is accompanied by the development of the country's transportation, communication and recreation facilities. The whole society is benefited, as it may (but not always) also enjoy the same facilities. Employment and business opportunities and development of the area can have a positive impact on the society and lead to improved lifestyles. Developing countries in particular benefit by improving their living and sanitary conditions which can be expected to have an impact on public health. Local people come in contact with tourists and it may allow them to better understand other societies and lifestyles. A tourist who can afford a vacation usually dresses well, lives an attractive lifestyle and dines well while in the host country, which may increase the desire of local people in less developed areas to aspire to a higher standard of living. After all, although vows of poverty may be virtuous for individuals, there is no merit in poverty (from a public health viewpoint) in populations.

SOCIAL DISADVANTAGES

Parkinson[19] considered tourism as a social evil. Both economic and social benefits are, it is argued, associated with disadvantages.

While it is true that employment opportunities increase with the increase of tourism business, it often provides only low-paid employment with poor working conditions and leads to the development of a more unskilled, service oriented or tourist-dependent population.

It is inevitable that the tourism industry depends to a great extent on the economic, social and political conditions of the society and any changes may affect the tourism business. As a result, local society will in turn be influenced. China's tourism industry was affected in this regard after student demonstrations and the resulting deaths at Tiananmen Square in June 1989. Similarly, the outbreaks of 'bird-flu' in Hong Kong in early 1998 affected the tourist arrivals in the territory during that period.

Another problem of the tourism business in relation to the host community is that of inadequate facilities and services. There is often inequity in developments to improve them. It is recognised that local communities are often given a much lower priority in the provision of new services. With the increase of the tourism business, the importation of products (industrial, agricultural and recreational) also increases. In most cases, the products imported are targeted at travellers but later, products which are attractive (and affordable) to local people are imported in large quantities which may sometimes cause the death of local industries and affect the local job market.

Real estate value is very sensitive to tourism development. It is argued that property prices increase with the increase of tourism business and that this has an adverse effect on the living standards of the community. For example, in Bali, Indonesia which has the reputation of being the paradise of the East, there has been an increase in malnutrition in the poorer uplands of the island because of the rising cost of living caused by mass tourism. Inadequacies of commodities like food often result in higher prices for the local population. Nepal with its too rapid tourism growth is experiencing problems of supply and rising prices.

Another downside of tourism concerns some aspects of the hospitality services (e.g. massage parlours, night clubs, karaoke bars or escort services) which increase. This may be associated with crime, illegal activities, divorce and disease. Local people are encouraged, influenced or sometimes forced into these services. In certain developing countries, people are interested to become associated with tourists in order to earn foreign currency or to have an opportunity to emigrate. This may lead them to be involved in sexual activities or crime. Dr Francis Cottington (*New York Times*, 9 August 1970) considered tourism as a cause of the increasing rate of divorce among the residents of the island of Hawaii.

Social norms may be affected by tourists who are considered as stimulants of unwanted trends such as prostitution and alcoholism.

A survey study in Sri Lanka showed that 92 per cent did not openly resent the arrival of tourists, but about 71 per cent felt that the indiscriminate entry of tourists caused or enhanced existing social problems such as:

Prostitution, homosexuality (or possibly its externalisation), nudism and other sexual deviations; erosion of traditional values, attitudes and norms among the indigenous people; increase in drug addiction, alcoholism and school absenteeism and emphasis on commercial art that leads to the gradual disappearance of traditional arts and.[22]

This statement obviously reflects the perceptions of local people as well as any real trends in social behaviour.

Cultural impact of tourism on host countries

Culture is a powerful attraction for tourism. The following extract from its advertising campaign for 'Visit Malaysia Year 1990', that was made by the Malaysian Tourist Development Corporation highlights its importance to and for culture:

> Malaysia has a wonderful pot-pourri of different races comprising three main groups – Malays, Chinese and Indians – in Peninsular Malaysia, and numerous indigenous groups ... in Sabah and Sarawak ... Visitors from all over the world can ... expect to always feel at home and welcome in this vital, colourful and kaleidoscopic nation of ours.

Urry[20] argued that tourism is socially grounded, 'imaginative pleasure-seeking' but others have argued that a tourist is 'a person at leisure, who also travels' or that tourism is not a unitary phenomenon, and therefore its effects will be various. It may have an effect, both positive or negative, on the culture of the host community.

POSITIVE IMPACT

In addition to economic benefit, tourism may also bring some cultural benefits for the host country. It can enrich, add to or strengthen local customs and tradition, much as it has been doing on a different scale for centuries. Host countries may pay more attention to their cultural development and regeneration of cultural practices; restoration and preservation of historical places, national parks, museums, buildings, fauna and flora, traditional foods and dress, with the development of tourism businesses, which were previously neglected. So tourism may save local customs, arts and crafts and traditions from dying out. In general, tourists have a curiosity and interest about culture, arts and crafts and traditions of the country they visit. With the increasing demands and interest in cultural events and traditions, people experienced in the area such as artists, crafts people and traditional dancers get opportunities to work which would not otherwise have existed. This development of 'culture' may play an important role in adjusting a country's unemployment or underemployment situation.

On the other hand, it provides the host community with the opportunity to come in contact with people from different cultures that may help them to enrich their knowledge and insights into the wider world. The culture and tradition of minority tribes and ethnic groups who very often are neglected also benefit from tourism as they also come into focus as tourist attractions. A few observations about the positive impact of tourism on the culture of the host country are illustrated below:

> Tourism can foster the individuality of culture as well as provide an avenue for cultural exchange.

> Tourist interest in local culture, arts and crafts, historical places etc. may lead to a generation of awareness, interest and pride in their culture among the local people.

> Lundberg noted the following views while explaining how the culture of Bali, Indonesia was strengthened by tourism:

> > In exchange for his money the tourist was allowed to enter the mythic realm of the Balinese cosmos. He was welcomed as a spectator at well staged aesthetic events. Rather than diluting the island's culture and fostering the development of 'pseudo cultural events' which would have destroyed the indigenous tradition or 'homogenised' the cultures, the Balinese culture suffered not at all. The people welcomed outside participants in their ritual performances which in the

Balinese tradition enhanced their ceremonial value. The income from tourist tickets to watch a temple performance was welcomed and used to improve both performances and equipment needed for them.

NEGATIVE IMPACT

Beside positive impacts, tourism may also have a profound negative impact on host society and culture. In his book, Adler[21] uncompromisingly termed tourists as 'cannibals' of culture. Tourism can affect an individual, a group of people or the whole society. People in the host country may become attracted to a culture or tradition that may divert them from their own tradition or culture. To cope with the interest of tourists from different cultures, the modernisation and artificialisation of a culture (which happens often) may destroy the native culture of a country. Alan Moorhead titled his book on the history of Western arrival in the South Pacific islands as *The Fatal Impact*.

It is postulated that when two cultures come into contact for any duration, both parties become part of a process of borrowing. Since tourists are a medium of the more dominant cultures, they are less likely to borrow from their hosts than their hosts are from them. The chain of change, therefore, is precipitated more in the host country.[22] So tourism may act as a medium for social and cultural change. The regeneration of cultural monuments may lead to cultural involution and may peg people to the old ways of life because tourists demand the old ways.

The increases in beggars, thieves, touts, pimps and prostitutes may also destroy the traditional pride of the host country. Promotion of sexual services, child prostitution and drug-trafficking that increases with the tourism business may also destroy the culture of a country or create bad impressions about a country. For example, Bangkok is no longer known to visitors as a city of monks or temples or angels (or canals) but a city of prostitution and pollution – both, however, indicators of its successful economy.

Aggressive behaviour that tourists would not resort to in their own country, but often do so in a host country, may influence the local culture. Some other factors that very often arise in developing countries to fulfil the increasing demands of tourists, such as selling a daughter or other children to a brothel, or allowing a wife to earn money as a sex-worker, may hamper the cultural norms of a community and destroy the lives of families and individuals.

In a well-known, slum area of Manila, a couple and their children lived in a packing case on stilts over water. Both parents worked as prostitutes in the evening in bars and brothels while the grandmother minded the children.

The religion of a country may also be affected by tourism in various ways. For example, the religion of Islam prohibits alcohol drinking, free mixing between men and women (except in a marital relationship), and prostitution. However, to encourage travellers with different interests, some of these countries allow such activities among foreign travellers which eventually become patterns for local inhabitants.

Finally, the cultural impacts of tourism can be summarised as De Kadt[23] states:

> The frequent charge that tourism contributes to a degeneration in this field appears to be an exaggeration. Even though curio production, 'airport art', and performances of fake folklore are of course stimulated by tourist demand . . . frequently arts, crafts, and local culture have been revitalised as a direct result of tourism. A transformation of traditional forms often accompanies this development but does not necessary lead to degeneration. To be authentic, arts and crafts must be rooted both in historical tradition and in present-day life; true authenticity cannot be achieved by conservation alone, since that leads to stultification.

Environmental impact of tourism on host countries

> Tourism is potentially the least damaging of the profit-making initiatives, because it is in its own interests to preserve the environment.[24]

The environment of the host country plays an important role in tourist attraction. It offers attractions that the tourist is looking for and needs.[25] Environment now includes not only land, air, water, flora and fauna, but may also encompass 'people, their creations and the social, economic and cultural conditions that affect their lives'.[26]

NEGATIVE IMPACT

The geographical distribution of people often changes with an increase in the tourism business and this has an effect on the environment; in particular, pollution increases from different aspects of development. Some authors argue that it brings disruption of animal life cycles, the extinction of fragile plants, and the pouring of human waste into rivers and upon beaches.[27–30]

All countries in the Asia–Pacific region, Latin America and elsewhere are now experiencing serious pollution of air, water and open terrain. Much of this is directly related to tourism as well as other industrial developments. While describing the negative impacts of tourism, the English Tourist Board's 'Tourism and Environment' Working Group on Historic Towns in 1991 highlighted traffic congestion and parking; the congestion, noise, pollution and resident hostility created by coach tours; and crowds and queues of pedestrians.

The host countries in which coastal tourism is the principal attraction are experiencing water pollution. The over-use of sea beaches, recreational boating on waterways and litter nuisance that increases with the increase of tourism contribute to water pollution and may contribute to the destruction of the marine environment.

The environmental impacts from tourist activities on water are:

- pathogens from raw or inadequately treated sewage
- the release of sewage onto beaches and into lakes and rivers
- fluctuation in dissolved oxygen has implications for aquatic plant and animal life
- oil from recreational boats causing detrimental effects to local plants and wildlife.

Tourism involves travelling. There are various modes of travelling such as by car, ship, train, bus or aeroplane. All of these modes are associated with air pollution and the level of pollution may be increased with the increase in the number of these forms of transport.

Noise pollution also increases with the increase of tourism business. It may arise from over-population, increased vehicular traffic, recreational facilities and aircraft. Residents have battled in several countries against noise from aircraft and also against night-time recreational facilities.

Construction work for hotels, restaurants, shops and roads which increases with tourism business may increase both air and noise pollution and sometimes destroy natural scenery and spoil the natural state of the surroundings.

Host countries, which attract tourists because of their wildlife, may be affected by increased numbers of tourists leading to the inevitable destruction of habitat. The loss of wet lands, forests, grasslands, mangroves, the pollution of rivers and estuaries are often the result of tourist-oriented developments. Equally, these effects may result from developments which are made possible by a successful economy dependent or partially dependent on tourism. How much can tourism be blamed for that?

The host countries, however, often argue that the West has been through similar periods in which long-standing natural environments have been completely transformed and that now it is the turn of the developing countries to profit and otherwise benefit from their natural resources.

POSITIVE IMPACT

Although there are significant, negative, environmental effects of tourism, the positive impact of it cannot be ignored. Tourism encourages conservation and preservation of natural areas, archaeological sites and historical monuments. Preservation of animals and forests are also another positive side that increases environmental stability.

It has also been argued that the need to preserve a commercially viable environment leads to research on air pollution, water pollution and this may initiate conservation measures sooner than would otherwise have occurred.

Overall, it is probably the case that host countries experience more negative than positive impacts from tourism in terms of its effects on the environment. Proper planning for a tourism infrastructure may decrease the negative impacts of tourism on host countries.

Impact of health issues on host countries

The mobility of people plays an important role in determining the health of travellers, their hosts and the health services of both native and host countries. Travellers travel to a country for leisure, for fun, for business or for other reasons but they cannot leave their health problems at home. Both communicable and non-communicable health problems may develop in travellers. Non-communicable health problems cause logistic problems to the host country.

Communicable diseases, food- and water-borne diseases, arthropod-borne diseases and sexually transmitted diseases (STDs) can be introduced to the host country by travellers. Epidemics of certain diseases have been both imported and exported by travellers. Within the incubation period of some diseases, a traveller can travel through several countries or areas and may spread the disease within the host community. Malaria, yellow fever, Ross River and dengue virus are recognised as imported problems in many countries. For example, in 1979, an epidemic outbreak of Ross River virus infection occurred in Fiji with 30 000 clinical cases, caused, it was later suggested, by an infected tourist who arrived by air from another country. In the 19th century, Westerners imported measles into the South Pacific and completely decimated some populations. It killed about 250 000 Fijians. Travellers exported plague from South China in the 1880s and caused 2 million cases worldwide.

Tourist destinations with a growing sex-industry and hospitality services are likely to have increased rates of STDs, including AIDS. The rapid increase of STDs and AIDS in certain areas following the rapid growth of tourism is a threat to the public health of the host country.

The outflow of travellers causes overcrowding, congestion and environmental pollution all of which may cause public health problems.

All communicable diseases that may be transmitted to or infect the host community may become a major public health problem for the host country. If any outbreaks occur, they may affect a whole community, the whole country, the public health policy of the host country and may bring unwanted pressure on that country's economy. The current AIDS crisis in Thailand which is the major public health problem in the country apart from road accidents is believed to be related in part to its booming tourism business in the early 1980s and its popularity as a sex-holiday destination.

Tourism not only has a negative impact on public health, it can also contribute to the maintenance and improvement of public health facilities in host areas because it provides additional sources of revenue. This extra source of income may be used for the establishment of new hospitals and medical centres, for upgrading the existing medical facilities, the improvement of community sanitary conditions and may be used for providing better maternity and child health-care facilities in developing countries. The establishment of travel health clinics monitored by international experts has become a common feature for most developing countries in recent years. Local people could benefit from the services of these clinics that provide an international standard of medical services.

Impact of sex-tourism on host countries

Sex-tourism is a contemporary feature of tourism that has a profound impact on host countries. It is related to other legal, ethical, economical and health issues.

Sex-travel may be defined as travel where the main purpose is to have sex with local people or with other tourists, either by paying money or in kind. It may also be a prominent part of business travel or attending conferences.

Most sex-travellers travel on their own or in small groups of between 2 and 5 or sometimes on a larger scale, involving special charter flights. Travel agencies have organised group tours and charter flights for sex-travellers where the package includes the price of the sex-worker. There is one report in the Hong Kong press that sex-travel was offered and people were sent for sex-holidays by their employers as a form of company bonus.

It is reported that 1.5 million Japanese men go on holidays to South-East Asia every year on 'sex-tours' organised by tour operators and large corporations.[31] These often masquerade as golfing holidays although the clubs usually stay in their bags. However, golf is a major growth industry in Asia and other parts of the world and provides a potential convenient platform for other tourist diversions. We do not have any statistics concerning sex-travellers from other countries, but it is already recognised that a large number of tourists travel to a country only for sex purposes or to provide an opportunity to have new sexual experiences. For example, the Hong Kong annual rugby sevens competition is a noted, annual, sporting festival attracting visitors from over 30 countries. A group of Australians flying to attend the 1995 tournament, travelled via Manila to visit bars and massage parlours before continuing to Hong Kong.

While most of the impact that sex-tourism has on host countries is negative, there may be a positive impact from economic benefit. With the increase or promotion of sex-tourism, the unskilled women and men who are willing to serve as commercial sex-workers obtain a source of income that may be helpful both for them and for their families. The establishment of night clubs, bars, karaokes and sauna houses that increase with the promotion of sex-tourism provide more job opportunities for locals. Several authors have studied the positive economic effects of sex-tourism in different countries. For instance, in the case of Fiji in the early 1970s, Naibavu & Schutz[32] argued:

> Prostitution is a fully localised industry which gives employment to unskilled female workers for most of whom no other jobs are available. It requires no investment of foreign capital, yet it brings in large amounts of foreign exchange with a minimum of leakage back overseas.

Many Thai sex-workers, for example women from north-east villages, would probably defend their right to earn money in this way. Those who manage their business safely, protect their health, invest earnings and 'retire' early may be found in new lifestyles and houses with successful businesses. Others of course may squander their new income, become involved with drugs and face a miserable future with serious health problems and an early death.

There are many descriptions of the negative impact of sex-tourism on host countries. It relates to disease, race relations issues, crime (both national and international), and cultural and religious issues. Developing countries are more affected than developed countries. O'Grady[33] pointed out that the relationship between tourism and prostitution in the Third World is very strong.

Sex-tourism increases the demands for prostitutes and other hospitality services. Lucrative income related to sex-tourism attracts people from various sectors of the community to these services. Housewives may become involved as part-time sex-workers which may lead them to divorce, with effects on the social stability of families and communities. Under-aged young people become involved with an industry that diverts them from schooling and higher education. The service providers or the owners of the hospitality industries involve criminal elements for finding women, children and sometimes men to serve in the industry, for example the Mafia and triads. It may be associated with kidnapping and enslavement.

The demand for sex and the lucrative income from it leads people in the host community to shed religious affiliations. Despite Islamic laws that prohibit prostitution, there are major, 'red light' districts in Bangladesh and Pakistan. Tourism prostitution also exists in other Islamic countries such as Malaysia, Indonesia and some countries in the Middle East.

Child prostitution and child abuse have become established as a negative impact of tourism on host countries. The AIDS epidemic in some popular, sex-holiday destinations has now diverted sex-tourists towards the countries where child prostitutes are available or easy to obtain (Fig. 21.1). The increasing number of child prostitutes in certain countries is a cause for alarm. There are an estimated 60 000–100 000 child prostitutes in the Philippines (*Asia Week*, August 25, 1995),

Paedophiles' new stopover in child prostitution market

INDIA

From **RAHUL BEDI**
in New Delhi

THE country is fast replacing Southeast Asian nations as a stopover for paedophiles.

The introduction of stricter laws against child abuse and the growing incidence of AIDS in the traditional sex bazaars of Thailand, Cambodia and the Philippines has led to an increasing number of Westerners seeking child prostitutes in India.

Social workers attempting to increase public awareness about child abuse, say foreigners have realised that Indian child prostitutes are cheaper and AIDS is not so widespread as it is in Southeast Asian flesh pots.

The fact that there are fewer laws against child abuse is one of the principal reasons for the increasing numbers of paedophiles visiting India and other South Asian countries.

Abject poverty and illiteracy are the other factors responsible for perpetuating the practice.

And, though no definite statistics exist on the number of child prostitutes across India, surveys by social organisations estimate there to be about 300,000.

Many are lured away from their villages by prostitute syndicates, often with the approval of their parents who are either too poor to care or have more children than they are able to look after.

And, though there are no organised "sex tours" for paedophiles in India yet, social workers fear they may start if this practice is not curbed soon.

The beaches of Sri Lanka are a favourite stopover for child abusers, mostly from Western Europe.

But in India, the languid beaches of Goa in the west and Kovalam in Kerala state to the south are the main destinations for tourists seeking child prostitutes.

The easy availability of drugs like hashish and heroin are an added attraction.

Matters came to a head in Goa with the arrest of an Anglo-Indian who ran an ashram or charity home for "destitute" boys for allegedly "supplying" them to German, French, British, Scandinavian and Swiss tourists.

But such incidents are infrequent as offenders are rarely arrested by the corrupt police force.

According to recent news from Kovalam, a German man was caught having sex with a boy, but managed to bribe his way out.

Reports about the prevalence of child prostitution from the eastern beach town of Puri recently led to protests from priests who forced police to charge the culprits.

The South China Morning Post, 18 November 1995 (Reproduced with the permission from the editor).

Fig. 21.1 Report of child prostitution in India (reproduced with permission from *The South China Morning Post*, 18 November 1995).

30 000–800 000 in Thailand, 300 000 in India (*The South China Morning Post*, 1995) and 4000 children are involved in prostitution in Sri Lanka (*The Star*, March 14, 1984). This situation also exists in some other countries in the world and is increasing, for example in Kathmandu, Nepal. Ladawan Wongsriwong, the best-known woman politician in Thailand, warned the 1998 'Amazing Thailand' tourist campaign by saying that it may increase the child prostitution in the country (*The South China Morning Post*, 1997).

Prostitution related to sex-tourism is playing an important adverse role in the host countries' sociocultural environment and public health. Sex-tourism increases sexual assault, changes in behavioural patterns and attitudes among host communities, increases the rate of STDs, kidnapping of children and young women and can cause incalculable stress among the sufferers and their families.

There are signs of a move by many governments to arrest and reverse these developments. Malaysia is tightening Islamic rules on extramarital relationships, with draconian punishments; Thailand's former prime minister Banharn (a reputed puritan) tried to legislate against night-life. However, given the economics of the sex-industry, it is unlikely that there will be lasting impact.

It is important to create awareness among the population by providing proper education and information about the rights of children as emphasised at the first World Congress Against the Commercial Sexual Exploitation of Children which was held in Stockholm, Sweden in 1996. Children should also be informed about the risk of STD infection from unprotected sexual intercourse and should be involved in the planning of prevention programmes.

Summary

The impact of tourism on host countries is well recognised. It brings both advantages and disadvantages from economic, social, cultural, environmental and health standpoints. It brings foreign exchange or other benefits for the country and plays an important role in economic development of the country as well as in the development of regional economies. But, it also causes harm to the host country by degradation of the landscape, cultural uniqueness, traditions, environment and sometimes women and children. Much negative impact of tourism on host countries derives from the behaviour and attitudes of both travellers and the faulty infrastructure of tourism development by local policy makers. Proper tourism development planning with special attention to local priorities and needs, public health issues and educational materials targeting tourists may play an important role in minimising the negative impact of tourism on host countries.

PRACTICE POINTS

- There are social, cultural, environmental and health impacts from tourism on the host countries.
- Travellers and locals may end up competing for scarce resources and capital.
- Income generation and employment potential are great for the local population but there can be considerable strain on local traditions, lifestyle norms and standards. This potential must be grasped in an environmentally and culturally sensitive way to be sustainable.
- Newly emerging and re-emerging infections are global concerns and the health of the traveller is closely linked to that of the host population.
- Improving access to quality medical care for travellers within the host countries is an important issue.

REFERENCES

1. Hunziker W. Social tourism: its nature and problems. Geneva: Alliance Internationale de Tourisme; 1951.
2. Graburn NHH. Tourism: the sacred journey. In: Smith V, ed. Hosts and guests: The Anthropology of tourism. 2nd ed. Philadelphia: University of Pennsylvania Press; 1989: 21–36.
3. Turner V, Turner E. Image and pilgrimage in Christian culture. Oxford: Blackwell; 1978; 34–39.
4. Mathieson A, Wall G. Tourism: Economic, physical and social impacts. New York: Longman; 1984.
5. Fox M. The social impact of tourism: a challenge to researchers and planners. In: Finney B, Watson KA, eds. A new kind of sugar: Tourism in the Pacific. Honolulu: East–West Center Press; 1976.
6. Barang M. Tourism in Thailand. South 1988; 71 (December): 73.
7. Carver E. Tourism: offers of natural delights. Far Eastern Economic Review 1987; February: 56.
8. Brownrigg M, Greig MA. Tourism and regional development. Speculative Papers No. 5. Glasgow: Fraser of Allander Institute; 1976.
9. Peters M. International tourism. London: Hutchinson; 1969: 10.
10. Bryden J. Tourism and development: A case study of the Commonwealth Caribbean. Cambridge: Cambridge University Press; 1973.
11. Economist Intelligence Unit. The role of tourism in economic development: is it a benefit or burden? International Tourism Quarterly 1973; 2: 53–68.
12. Perez LA. Aspects of underdevelopment: tourism in the West Indies. Science and Society 1974; 37: 473–480.
13. Rivers P. Unwrapping the African tourist package. Africa Report 1974; 19(2): 12–16.
14. Marsh JS. Hawaiian tourism: costs, benefits, alternatives. Alternatives 1975; 4(3): 34–39.
15. Marsh JS. Tourism and development: the East African case. Alternatives 1975; 5(1): 15–22.
16. Turner L. The international division of leisure: tourism and the third world. World Development 1976; 4: 253–260.
17. Diamond J. Tourism's role in economic development: a case re-examined. Economic and Cultural Change 1977; 25: 539–553.
18. Mings RC. Tourism's potential for contributing to economic development in the Caribbean. Journal of Geography 1969; 68: 173–177.
19. Parkinson K. Ireland: a model of planned tourism development. Department of Recreology, University of
20. To hell with paradise. New Internationalist 1974; February 12.
20. Urry J. The tourist gaze – Leisure and travel in contemporary societies. London: Sage; 1990.
21. Adler C. Tourists, cannibals of culture. West Germany: Ethno Verlag; 1981.
22. De Los Santos J. The economic and social impact of tourism development: Report of the symposium on tourism management, Kathmandu, Nepal, 1982.
23. De Kadt E, ed. Tourism: Passport to development? New York: Oxford University Press; 1979.
24. Hamilton A. Environmental Guardian 1990 10 August: 21.

25. Burmeister H. Mass tourism and the environment: a closer look. Travel Research Journal 1977; 21–30.

26. Lerner SC. Social impact assessment: some hard questions and basic techniques. Unpublished workshop paper. Ontario: University of Waterloo; 1977.

27. Goldsmith E. Pollution by tourism. The Ecologist 1974; 48(1): 47–48.

28. Crittendon A. Tourism's terrible toll. International Wildlife 1975; 5(3): 4–12.

29. Mountfort G. Tourism and conservation. Wildlife 1975; 17: 30–33.

30. Tangi M. Tourism and the environment. Ambio 1977; 6: 336–341.

31. Utusan Konsumer. The ugly side of tourism. In: See the Third World while it lasts – the social and environmental impact of tourism with special references to Malaysia. Penang: Consumers' Association of Penang; 1985.

32. Naibavu T, Schutz B. Prostitution: problem or profitable industry. Pacific Perspective 1974; 3(1): 59–68.

33. O'Grady R. Third World stopover. Geneva: World Council of Churches; 1981.

AFTER RETURN

Health screening and psychological considerations in the returned traveller

Ted Lankester

Introduction

In a traditional, medical model, post-travel screening implies question, examination and tests to exclude significant physical illness. This definition is useful as far as it goes, but we need a paradigm more in tune with the complex, post-modern understanding of health, so often exemplified in a range of health-related issues experienced by the returned traveller.

Those returning from overseas will often have experienced a range of illness, personal difficulty, psychological trauma or anxiety, each of which can affect their state of physical or mental well-being. For many, especially aid-workers, the military, missionaries, journalists or long-term expatriates, this can result in a cumulative loss of well-being which may present via physical or psychological symptoms weeks or months after returning home. Screening the apparently well within a few weeks of returning from overseas can help pick these problems up at an earlier stage when they are easier to treat.

Adequate post-travel screening needs to engage with these issues. We require a working model that includes traditional, post-tropical screening with selective blood and stool tests, as exemplified by the work of Carroll et al[1] but which moves beyond this into a more holistic approach to the traveller's well-being.

Doctors and other healthcare workers must prioritise time to work in partnership with returning travellers, so as to help identify and solve these wider health issues and concerns, until the returned traveller or expatriate feels mentally and physically, and where relevant spiritually, restored to health.

Of course, not all returning travellers will need or want this. Most asymptomatic, short-term tourists to exotic locations will need no screening at all, others will have a simple problem they wish to discuss in a short interview, or the reassurance of a normal test.

Who needs screening on return from overseas?

There continues to be debate about the value of screening the apparently well, returned traveller. Peppiatt & Byass[2] in a survey of the health of 212 returning missionaries found 6.5% of adults had an eosinophilia count and concluded that full blood count and absolute eosinophilia counts were useful tests. More importantly, they emphasised that in this sub-group of travellers the history and psychiatric examination were important and that psychiatric illness could easily be underestimated by doctors unfamiliar with people returning from overseas.

Carroll et al[1] examined the results of screening 1029 asymptomatic individuals returned from the tropics, who comprised diplomats, aid-workers, volunteers, British government employees and trekkers. In this comprehensive paper, eosinophilia was found in 67 out of 852 samples and positive schistosomal serology in 72 out of 676 tests. Cysts of *Giardia duodenalis* (*lamblia*) and *Entamoeba histolytica*/*dispar* were the commonest potential pathogens found on stool test. They concluded that screening for tropical disease can be efficiently carried out by an informed health professional using a structured history-taking and relevant laboratory tests, and that physical examination added little to the practical management of these patients. It has to be pointed out, however, that this survey was looking at health screening according to a traditional medical model with the aim of documenting abnormal physical signs and abnormal tests.

Churchill et al[3] concluded from their results that the value of screening depends to a large extent on the risk of exposure to infectious diseases of the individual traveller. However they acknowledged that two groups of asymptomatic travellers will commonly ask for screening – those concerned they may have latent infections which might give rise to problems later in life, and those wishing to have a retrospective diagnosis of an illness suffered abroad. Often concerns about infectivity to others or fitness to return to the tropics in the future underlie their concerns. This particular study illustrates the importance of considering the mind-set of the 'worried well' in deciding who to recommend for screening on return from overseas.

TRAVELLERS RECOMMENDED FOR SCREENING

In the light of published evidence and our own experience, we suggest the following might benefit from health screening on return from abroad:

1. **Those who are ill or who have significant symptoms** (see pp. 454–458)

2. **The 'worried well', or perhaps better described as the 'worried, probably well'**

Many travellers returning from a period overseas have some uncertainty whether they do feel as well and energetic as they might expect. Usually the 'worried well' will be reluctant to 'waste the doctor's time'. Alternatively, they may present with a variety of random symptoms at antisocial times.

These worries can cover a vast range of concerns and questions that reflect the complex health-related issues arising from international travel. Here are some examples:

- 6 months with a difficult colleague in a remote location that has undermined self-confidence and created cumulative stress
- the condom that slipped after 3 (or was it 4?) bottles of beer in Nairobi
- the threatened rape by a drunk soldier, still causing flashbacks
- the sights, sounds and smells of death and disease in the aftermath of civil war
- increasing addiction to the gin bottle after 12 months as the bored partner of an expatriate workaholic
- a failing marriage or increasingly dysfunctional family relationships after a difficult overseas placement
- the feeling of exhaustion after being home for a full 4 weeks
- the inability to face life in the UK: 'No-one is interested in what I've done and where I've been, and I haven't a clue what I should do next'
- being unable to sleep at night because of the doubling of debt during 6 months of backpacking
- an unsympathetic family sure that their son must have picked up a tropical bug travelling around Africa and worried they will become infected themselves
- concern about feeling so cross and irritable on getting back home
- wondering whether that single swim in Lake Malawi could have caused bilharziasis
- all these terrible dreams and feelings of doom: could it be the mefloquine?

These concerns and a hundred like them present to the health professional who has the time and willingness to move beyond stethoscope, stool tests and solar keratoses. Sensitive handling and creative referral of the real, and often subtly hidden, needs of the returned long-term traveller can help to identify and to treat a complex range of problems at an early stage, and before they become more established and harder to deal with.

3. **Those with a real or perceived risk of exposure to infectious or parasitic diseases, or to occupational hazards**

These risks are hard to define from an evidence-based viewpoint given the huge range of countries, occupations, and lifestyles travellers experience. Health professionals and travellers together need to assess the likely risks and decide on appropriate screening. Here are some common examples:

- *schistosomiasis*: a risk for travellers who have swum in freshwater lakes and rivers in Africa, and to a lesser extent in South-East Asia
- *infection with HIV*: travellers with at-risk lifestyles and health workers with occupational health risks will need counselling and where mutually agreed, HIV testing
- *tuberculosis*: health workers, anthropologists, aid-workers and others with prolonged contact with tuberculosis patients should consider Purified Protein Derivative (PPD) testing and possibly a chest radiography.

4. Those seemingly fit on return, who subsequently develop symptoms

The classic example is malaria and all travellers to malarious areas need to be advised verbally and in writing that any fever occurring within 3 months of leaving a malarious area requires a blood smear and medical consultation without delay. Schistosomiasis is another common illness which may present in a variety of ways after weeks or months (see Ch. 11).

A small but important group of travellers assume that any post-travel symptoms are obviously travel-related. Very often they are not. A change of bowel habit as the presenting symptom of malignant bowel disease is not infrequently assumed by the older traveller to be the result of a world tour, or a meal out in Bangkok.

5. Those who have been on high-risk assignments

This group is hard to categorise scientifically. It includes many aid-workers, missionaries, journalists, military personnel and volunteers working in conditions where stress, danger or tropical illness is prevalent. Employers should have guidelines on post-travel medicals for their staff and a management structure which encourages employees to be checked at the expense of the company or agency.

6. Those who have been living in a developing country for 12 months or more

This is an arbitrary, cut-off point, as many travellers will experience greater risk in a few weeks than others will over several years. For example, diplomats and their partners will generally be less prone to tropical illness, thought not necessarily to stress or boredom, than aid-workers or missionaries.

However, over a period of 1 year, unless a high standard of medical care is available locally without excessive cross-cultural differences, many expatriates and long-term travellers will have collected a symptom or worry list they would like to discuss with a health professional on return home.

7. Those who want to know the nature of the undiagnosed illness they suffered abroad

Even though it may be unnecessary or impossible to discover this, part of our duty as health workers is to reassure worried patients and discuss legitimate concerns.

What type of screening should be offered?

A post-travel consultation with a health professional is the traditional norm and is probably the best starting point for those in the categories above.

The time needed, and available, will vary greatly. Both traveller and health professional will need to adapt to a timeframe and style which is mutually acceptable. In our experience, 20 minutes is the minimum needed, and a full hour, including time for tests, is the ideal for many returning from long or difficult assignments. A family of five may need half a day. A short-term traveller with a specific concern may need only 10 minutes.

THE HISTORY

Taking an informed history as in all branches of medicine is the key to correct diagnosis and good management.

- Where has the traveller been? Obtain as full an account as time allows, including locations, elevations (malaria risk), predominant vegetation (strongyloides in tropical forest: tick bites, tsetse flies in the Savannah) and other geographically relevant data to help assess medical risk.
- What paid or voluntary work has the traveller been doing? Have there been any occupational health risks (HIV infection, hepatitis B or C, leptospirosis)?
- What types of leisure and recreational interests have been followed? Has the traveller been swimming in African lakes and rivers (schistosomiasis) or sleeping in 'adobe' (straw and thatched) huts in South America (Chagas' disease)?
- Are there any medical concerns the traveller would like to discuss, including sexual health risks?
- Has the traveller suffered any experience, acute or longer-term which has been painful, hard to reconcile and which still causes distress, anxiety or avoidance (post-traumatic or cumulative stress disorder)?
- Is there any sleep disturbance?
- Is the traveller feeling unusually tired?
- What was the average weekly consumption of alcohol? How many units have been consumed in the past 3 days?

As with all medical consultations, verbal answers, body language and the health professional's sixth sense are all vital in coming to an assessment of the real underlying problems.

THE EXAMINATION

This needs to be done but in practice little information is usually gained, with occasional vital exceptions. Some important areas to concentrate on are:

- signs of anaemia
- presence of enlarged spleen, liver or lymph glands
- signs of active naevi, solar keratoses or malignant skin conditions, especially in the older or well-seasoned traveller

- careful examination of any organ or body area which the traveller has mentioned in the history.

INVESTIGATIONS

These should be kept to the minimum necessary to satisfy the clinical judgement of the health professional and the wishes and concerns of the traveller.

Useful screening tests include the following:

- urine test by dipstick with referral to a laboratory to confirm any abnormalities; the presence of haematuria is useful as it can indicate possible *Schistosoma haematobium* infection
- full blood count, especially to detect anaemia, eosinophilia (for parasitic disease including schistosomiasis, filariasis and strongyloides), macrocytosis (to detect high alcohol consumption)
- schistosomiasis serology, dependent on risk, to detect present (or past) infection; alternatively, or in addition, ova can be sought in centrifuged, terminal, urine specimens and in stool examinations (see Ch. 11)
- stool tests for ova, cysts and parasites – is the commonest findings usually being cysts of *Giardia lamblia, Entamoeba histolytica/dispar*[3] and ova of *Trichuris* and *Ascaris*.

Other tests can be included depending on both the wish of the client and the clinical judgement of the doctor. They might include the following:

- Heaf or Mantoux test if significant contact with tuberculosis patients
- liver function tests, especially if there is a history, or suspicion of heavy drinking; this can easily be run through as part of an automated biochemistry or haematology screen
- serology for filaria and strongyloides if the traveller has been living in a known endemic area; alternatively, these can be performed on a saved serum sample if eosinophilia is detected.

In addition to post-tropical screening, it is worth considering other investigations in the case of older travellers, long-term expatriates or those who have not had regular medical care over a number of years. They will be chosen according to the situation, the doctor's judgement and patient's wish, but might include the following:

- cholesterol or (fasting) lipid profile; urea, electrolytes and blood sugar (these also can be run as part of a biochemical profile)
- prostate specific antigen in men with prostatic symptoms, or over the age of 45 or 50 (there is no consensus on this in the UK at present)
- cervical smear and mammography in women appropriate for age.

PSYCHOLOGICAL HEALTH ASSESSMENT

- During the course of the consultation, have you noticed signs of significant cumulative, post-traumatic stress, or re-entry stress?
- Are there other psychological problems that will need referring on for further debriefing, counselling or psychiatric assessment and care?
- Is there a felt or perceived need for marriage or relationship counselling?
- To help demystify the way forwards, would spiritual or career counselling be helpful? (See below for further details.)

CONSULTATION WRAP-UP

Before the traveller leaves, ask yourself if you have adequately answered the following:

- Have you addressed the real and perceived concerns of the traveller?
- Have you drawn up any necessary action plan?
- Have you explained when and how results will be sent through or reported back (including HIV where carried out)?
- Have you assessed and arranged for any necessary referrals?
- Have you assessed whether any personal debriefing, counselling or psychological support is necessary and made appropriate plans?
- For those returning from a malarious area, have you underlined the importance of seeking immediate medical advice if a fever develops?

Who should carry out the screening?

McIntosh et al[4] in a retrospective study of 1568 individuals aged 16 or over registered in one general practice found that in 1 in 5 of those who travelled outside the UK sought a general practitioner consultation on return home. They concluded that a large and significant population of travellers becomes ill while abroad (42%) and that travel-acquired illness has a large impact on general practice.

Recent years have seen a sustained increase in the number of travellers going to exotic destinations. There is a greater perceived risk, part-real, part-media-generated, of travel-associated illnesses such as malaria, dengue fever, schistosomiasis and other infectious diseases. We can therefore expect an increase in the number of those requesting 'post-travel/tropical check-ups'.

REQUIREMENTS FOR POST-TRAVEL SCREENING

In order for this to be done adequately, the following needs to be in place:

- a health professional with experience and expertise in travel or tropical medicine and the time and motivation to listen and engage with the real concerns of the returning traveller
- a laboratory with confirmed expertise in the recognition of tropical parasites on blood, stool and urine samples, and an adequate turn-around time for tests
- a counsellor able to offer personal debriefing, counselling or other appropriate forms of follow-up therapy
- a receptionist whose demeanour does not add to the traveller's reverse 'culture shock'.

LOCATIONS FOR POST-TRAVEL SCREENING

In practice there are three places where post-travel health screening takes place:

General practitioners' surgeries

Providing they have sufficient time, general practitioners and practice nurses are well placed to carry out post-travel check-ups. However, if health practitioners are unfamiliar with the health problems and concerns of returning travellers important features may be missed.[2]

Regional infectious or tropical disease units which may have a travel medicine clinic

Such centres will be able to carry out accurate medical examinations and parasitological screening but often have constraints in offering a more holistic healthcare approach.

Medical charities or private healthcare organisations

These may specialise in the needs of returning travellers and be well placed to carry out unhurried post-travel medical examinations according to the more holistic paradigm described above.

Psychological aspects of returning from abroad

Two trends in international travel point up the need for psychological issues to be addressed with greater care in the screening of the returned traveller. The first is the number of travellers exposed to a significant traumatic event when overseas. The second is the increasing number of adventure travellers, aid-workers and longer-term expatriates, a number of whom are returning with symptoms of cumulative stress from many apparently trivial but unresolved conflicts, often in the area of interpersonal relationships.

Looking at travellers' holiday photos or hearing them recount endless stories of their adventures abroad demonstrates the need we all have to make sense of the unusual, and to share these experiences with others. The wealth of books and diaries written by returned travellers echoes this. It

helps to demonstrate the particular importance of those returning with psychological trauma to have a chance to be heard, and to talk issues through with a trained and sympathetic listener, debriefer or counsellor.

For most, sharing their stories with family and friends will be all the 'debriefing' they will need. For those returning from overseas employment, writing a report or having an operational debrief by the company or agency can also aid understanding and integration of experiences (though for a minority this can make matters worse or bring unresolved conflicts to light).

An important minority of returned travellers do however suffer more profound reactions from their overseas experience or find that past conflicts and mental health problems, including depressive illness, can resurface. For this group, greater exploration and reflection with skilled help will be needed.

In writing about 'short-termers' returning from overseas mission, Adams[5] states that disillusionment can set in quickly if there is not a perceived way forwards in incorporating this experience into the totality of their life-meaning. He recommends personalised attention for these people in working through the implications of their experiences.

The reasons for returning from overseas are surprisingly varied:

- end of a holiday or job contract
- the need to enter a new stage of life, for example further education, marriage, the birth of children, retirement
- personal or family needs
- home leave
- enforced return, for example visa problems, financial insolvency, evacuation, ill-health.

Reactions on return are strongly influenced not only by location and experience but by the reason for return and whether this was planned or unexpected. There may be a sense of loss, akin to bereavement of what has been left behind and uncertainty, even anxiety, about the future, likely to be made worse if departure was sudden or unexpected. Many returned travellers feel an intense sense of alienation within their home culture, especially if returning after a prolonged or particularly significant time of travel overseas. What used to be familiar seems strange and sometimes threatening. A common example is the sense of being overwhelmed by the choice in supermarkets in those returning from poorer parts of the world.

In Lovell's study[6] of returned aid-workers, many reported their time overseas as a positive, fulfilling experience and 60% reported feeling predominantly negative emotions on returning home; only 15% felt glad or relieved to be back. The most common experiences were feeling disorientated and confused, and feeling a sense of bereavement or even devastation on leaving behind friends overseas.

Foyle[7] in looking at missionaries returning home after a period of overseas service found that the commonest reactions are insecurity, over-emotionalism, loneliness and a general sense of feeling lost. Macnair[8] found that 75% of a group of aid-workers said they had difficulty readjusting on their return. The commonest difficulties were feelings of disorientation, problems getting a job, lack of understanding from family and friends, and financial difficulties.

Experiences gained overseas may bring about quite profound changes in a person's outlook. Janoff-Bulman[9] has proposed the view that traumatic experiences alter the basic assumptions held by many people viz. that the world is benevolent and meaningful, and that they themselves have self-worth. Cumulative or chronic stress may also change these assumptions leading to an avoidance of associations with the unpleasant experience. Sometimes, if unresolved, this leads to an unwillingness to return overseas.

Although a successful overseas holiday can give us renewed strength to face the challenges of life at home, living abroad does not give immunity from normal life stresses nor from anxieties about life at home which are there to be faced on return. In a recent review of expatriate mental health, home country anxieties were one of four sources of stress positively associated with adjustment disorders. The others were occupational anxiety, acculturation and physical illness.[10]

Those who have had problems abroad or encountered difficulties readjusting are often very reluctant to seek advice. McConnan[11] found that 73% of aid-workers reported feeling inadequately debriefed and supported on their return. People may be reluctant to seek help because they feel they should be able to cope or fear that their present or future job could be at risk if they acknowledged problems, and had this noted on their medical records.

ROLE OF DEBRIEFING

Although it has not definitely been shown that debriefing prevents the later development of psychological problems, there is a perception on behalf of clients that it is helpful. A recent survey by a major aid agency suggested that 90% of those offered an hour-long confidential debriefing outside of their organisation felt positively about this.

One agency (InterHealth) specialising in the care of aid-workers, missionaries and long-term expatriates offers debriefing as an optional and separate part of the healthcare screening. This debriefing has two main functions: first, it is an opportunity to help the client readjust to life in the UK and to integrate experiences gained abroad. Second, it is a screening tool which identifies those with more serious psychological problems which may require further diagnosis and treatment.

Box 22.1 shows the explanatory leaflet sent in advance to all those who will be attending for personal debriefing, so as to explain its purpose and allay anxieties.

In a reflection on such debriefings, Hargrave (personal communication 1998) reports that those attending for such debriefings tend to fall into two broad categories:

People newly returned to the UK

Although many feel fine with no apparent problems, a significant number have burning issues, difficulties, questions, or worries to address. What all have in common are minds still largely engaged, with the situations they have left behind. She goes on to point out that the debriefers' limited knowledge and identification with the exact situation despite their best attempts to identify, can act as a prototype for the early disappointment many go through as they return to family and friends 'who don't understand or aren't interested'.

What is it?

- Up to 50 minutes for a confidential exploration of the experiences you have had during your recent assignment.
- A chance for you to raise any issues of importance to you.
- A time not so much concerned with what work you have done but how the experiences involved in carrying out that work have affected you.
- There is no report back to your agency or company.

Who is it for?

- Anyone returning from a situation of unusual or prolonged stress.

What is its purpose?

- To help you reflect on and understand your reactions and responses to your assignment.
- To consider any personal matters you may wish to talk over.
- To give you an opportunity to think about your next step.
- If appropriate, to consider your transition back to UK life.
- It is not an indication that you have failed or that anything is wrong with you.
- It is not a counselling session nor therapy, but a chance to look at how your experiences have affected you.
- It can be thought of as a time for exploring normal reactions to abnormal situations.

What happens?

- You can raise anything you wish.
- The debriefer may ask questions to help you recall more of your experience and reactions.

What happens next?

- This is up to you.
- Generally one session is sufficient but some find that issues are raised which they would like to explore further.
- When this happens, there are a number of options which the debriefer can explain to you.

People seen later after initial readjustment to life at home

By the time of their debriefing, most will have seen families and friends, may have had a holiday and begun the healthy leaving-and-grieving process of detaching themselves from the country they have returned from. These people are often more reflective. They are able to begin to assess their experiences and are beginning to put them into the overall context of their life: what they have learnt, what they have gained and lost, their disillusionment, joys and sorrows.

In a debriefing, Hargrave aims to:

- establish a personal empathy based on trust and rapport
- explore and share in the issues and feelings brought by the client
- hold and manage distress and pain
- move on to a discussion about meanings or the reaffirmation of meanings
- discuss appropriate ways forward.

Sometimes a further session is required and for a minority further counselling is indicated, especially for those who are suffering from symptoms of post-traumatic stress disorder, or from more severe psychological symptoms. A small minority needs referral on for psychiatric help, especially if serious anxiety or depression is uncovered or if there are suggestions of psychotic illness.

Finally, it is helpful to look briefly at children and couples returning from overseas as they may need special attention.

CHILDREN

When families have been abroad, it is easy to forget the readjustment children face on return home. In fact home to them may be where they have come from, or they may be unsure where it is or what it is. Often the culture in the UK will be more alien than it is for their parents. Their behaviour and accent may draw unwanted attention, and criticism from peers and teachers can add to their sense of alienation. They may react by trying to suppress all they have experienced abroad, for example by refusing to speak the language they were fluent in, or refusing to eat favourite foods they grew up with. They may be angry with their parents for causing them to feel so different. In the long-term, many children view having lived abroad as a positive experience but adjustment to returning home in the short-term and medium-term may be intensely painful at times.

For teenagers, where peer-group identification is so important, returning to the schools, pubs and clubs of their UK contemporaries may be especially daunting. This is even more the case if they are out of step with fashion, sport and the current film and music scene. Some may go on to identify with the fringe members of their peer group, other outsiders with whom they can identify, or withdraw into depression or antisocial behaviour. For most, there will be times of disorientation and loneliness. Meeting up with others of their own age group who have had similar experiences of living abroad may be the most useful help we can offer. This can enable them to see that their reactions are normal and shared by others in similar situations. The company or agency with whom their families were working may have details of helpful networks.

COUPLES

When one partner travels and the other remains at home, strains can quickly appear in even the most stable relationships. This is especially true when frequent absence by one or both partners leaves no time together for recreation, discussion or 'regrouping'. The returning partner may feel unwanted, the partner remaining at home bored or resentful, especially if the constant needs of young children or lively teenagers have to be borne alone. Health workers need to be aware of these dynamics and recognise early warning signs through a sensitive exploration during the post-travel health screening or debriefing.

Romantic attachments frequently occur abroad – from the casual holiday encounter neither partner expects to last, to the cross-cultural marriage. Differences may not become fully apparent until the couple returns to one of their home countries, when conflicts easily arise. These again will need early recognition and counselling, ideally with the help of an experienced couple who have been through similar experiences themselves.

Summary

This section has looked at common experiences of returning travellers. For many, the simple realisation that their reaction and feelings are normal may be all that is required to enable them to deal with the stresses of reverse 'culture shock'. Some will need only to share their experiences with an empathic listener, but a small majority require more skilled help as individuals and as families. It is essential that the health workers screening those returning from abroad learn to recognise this group.

PRACTICE POINTS

- Counselling and screening may be necessary for asymptomatic illnesses such as schistosomiasis and HIV infection.
- Debriefing with a trained counsellor can be helpful for those who have been under considerable stress while abroad or who have been away for long periods.
- Very close friendships often develop between expatriates and their colleagues overseas – this can cause 'bereavement' reactions and confused emotions after return.
- Culture shock on return can be real: there is often a natural wish to let friends and relatives know all about experiences abroad, and surprise that those with no similar background may not be so keen to listen!
- Jobs may be difficult to find. Older children may find it hard to adjust to new schools.

REFERENCES AND FURTHER READING

1. Carroll B, Dow C, Snashall D, et al. Post-tropical screening: how useful is it? British Medical Journal 1993; 307: 541.
2. Peppiatt R, Byass P. A survey of the health of British missionaries. British Journal of General Practice 1991; 41: 59–162.
3. Churchill DR, Chiodini PL, McAdam KP. Screening the returned traveller. British Medical Bulletin 1993; 49(2): 465–474.
4. McIntosh IB, Reed JM, Power KG. The impact of travel acquired illness on the world traveller and family doctor: the need for pre-travel health education. Scottish Medical Journal 1994; 39(2): 40–44.

5. Adams A. Pastoral care issues for short-termers in mission. In: Jones ME, Jones ES, eds. Caring for the missionary in the 21st century. Vol 2. Duns, Scotland: Care for Mission; 1996: 11–16. This is a collection of papers looking at pastoral and psychological problems facing missionaries and longer-term expatriates. Available from Care for Mission, Ellem Lodge, Duns, Scotland TD11 3SG.

6. Lovell D. Psychological adjustment amongst overseas aid workers. Unpublished thesis. Bangor: University of Wales; 1997.

7. Foyle M. Honourably wounded: Stress among Christian workers. Bromley, Kent: MARC Europe; 1997. A series of helpful pastoral and psychological insights from a Christian perspective into the health of long-term expatriates and missionaries.

8. Macnair R. Room for improvement: the management and support of relief and development workers. London: Overseas Development Institute, 1995. The report of a wide-ranging survey of the attitudes and perceptions of relief and development workers and how they were cared for and managed.

9. Janoff-Bulman R. Shattered assumptions: towards a new psychology of trauma. New York: The Free Press; 1992.

10. Foyle M, Beer MD, Watson JP. Expatriate mental health. Acta Psychiatrica Scandinavica. 1998; 97: 278–283.

11. McConnan I. Recruiting health workers for emergencies and disaster relief in developing countries. London: International Health Exchange; 1992.

Infection in the returned traveller

Christopher Ellis

Introduction

Awareness of the pattern of illness seen in returned travellers not only facilitates prompt diagnosis and treatment of disease that can rapidly be life-threatening, but must also inform the process of preventing disease in intending travellers.

Prioritising advice on healthy behaviour in those about to travel should be based on an appreciation of relative risk as should the calculation of risks and benefits of chemoprophylaxis and vaccines.

Practitioners should recognise that an illness is more likely to be associated with travel when the illness in question is not normally acquired in the patient's home country (e.g. malaria) or when the incubation period is relatively brief (e.g. dengue fever and typhoid). Conversely when the incubation period is long and variable (e.g. HIV infection) or the disease is ubiquitous (e.g. Legionellosis), that an illness was acquired during previous travel may not occur to the patient or doctor. Not only may this delay diagnosis for the individual patient but doctors may fail to consider some of the more obscure, travel-acquired infections when advising intending travellers of the risks they may be about to run.

This section is concerned with returned travellers displaying symptoms and will not, therefore, refer further to HIV infection (except for the so-called 'seroconversion' illness[1]) but those advising travellers should remember that HIV acquired during foreign travel probably eventually kills as many travellers as all other travel-acquired infections put together.

Introduction

Of the infections seen in returning travellers, malaria and Legionellosis are the main causes of death and neatly illustrate the biggest difficulty standing in the way of prompt diagnosis and treatment. This is because the diagnosis may not be made promptly, or at all, and appropriate treatment is unlikely to be given unless the diagnosis is considered.

This is not as obvious as it may seem. Common infections of the chest and urinary tract will usually respond to the most widely-used, broad-spectrum

Typical incubation period of some travel-related infections	
Cholera	1–3 days
Shigella dysentery	1–4 days
Amoebic dysentery	3–14 days
Salmonellosis	1–2 days
Campylobacterosis	2–10 days
Diphtheria	2–5 days
Dengue	2–5 days
Legionnaires' disease	2–10 days
Enteric fever	7–14 days
Tick-borne typhus	4–10 days
Lassa and Ebola fevers	3–21 days
Plasmodium falciparum malaria	8–28 days
Plasmodium vivax malaria	10–300 days
Hepatitis A	2–6 weeks
Hepatitis E	2–8 weeks
Hepatitis B	6–20 weeks
Schistosomiasis (acute)	4–6 weeks
Rabies	4–30 weeks
Onchocerciasis	1–3 years

antibiotics even if the precise pathogen is not known and the site of the infection unclear, not so Legionnaires' disease and malaria.

The most urgent infections in returned travellers virtually always present as febrile illnesses, the most common with diarrhoea. Jaundice and skin lesions are also commonly seen in returned travellers. Children present with a very similar range of conditions but are more likely to be pyrexial when suffering from travellers' diarrhoea or diarrhoeal illness caused by viruses.[1]

Infections presenting with fever

MALARIA

Exclusion or treatment of *Plasmodium falciparum* malaria remains the first priority in any patient who has returned from the tropics in the 3 months preceding the onset of symptoms.

During the 1970s, *Plasmodium falciparum* accounted for only around 15% of all imported cases of malaria into the UK. This proportion is now around 60% as a result of more travel to and from Africa (particularly West Africa) and fewer cases originating in the Punjab of India and Pakistan. Other than feverishness, headache and 'fluey' aches and pains are the most consistent other symptoms.

Paroxysmal fevers preceded by chills and rigors are suggestive of malaria but are not seen in the majority of returned travellers in whom the presenting illness suggests 'flu' although often with an unusually severe headache. The '3-month rule' is valuable since it reliably defines when *Plasmodium falciparum* malaria is a possibility since it virtually never presents later than 3 months after exposure except occasionally in pregnant women.

Diagnosis is made by identification of parasites within red cells in a blood film. Parasites are not recognised by mechanical cell counters so that this diagnosis will never be made incidentally in the laboratory as part of a routine blood 'count'. A standard sequestrine or heparinised sample is all the haematology laboratory requires to make the films but the practitioner must request malarial parasites specifically and should provide a contact number for receiving the report immediately.

Details of treatment are given in Chapter 13 but essentially all *Plasmodium falciparum* patients should receive at least two drugs. Otherwise, there is a higher rate of recrudescence since most infections consist of a mixed population of parasites with differing sensitivities.

In the UK, patients with *Plasmodium falciparum* malaria should ordinarily be admitted initially to hospital. All malaria from Africa, where benign forms of malaria are unusual, should be assumed to be *Plasmodium falciparum* unless the laboratory is absolutely confident that it is not. Patients with suspected malaria who have returned from other continents need not be admitted routinely unless they are unwell or are shown to have *Plasmodium falciparum* infection, provided a blood film can be reliably reported on within 24 hours.

LEGIONNAIRES' DISEASE

This disease[2] causes the death of between 4 and 10 returned UK travellers each year and is therefore in the same league as malaria. Like malaria, it often presents non-specifically and is readily misdiagnosed as flu or as an 'ordinary' chest infection, likely to be treated with a β-lactam antibiotic such as amoxycillin to which *Legionella pneumophila* is resistant. A clue to the diagnosis is an ill patient with flu and chest symptoms, who has stayed in hotel accommodation in Southern Europe during the 2 weeks before the onset of fever.

The most common sources are common destinations for UK holidaymakers with Spain responsible for most cases but Turkey currently having the highest attack rate. The most useful early investigation is a chest X-ray. If this shows an area of consolidation, then the returned traveller should be admitted, blood cultures performed for *pneumococci*, and treated with a macrolide (e.g. erythromycin). Sick patients, confused or hypoxic, often benefit from receiving rifampicin in addition.

THE PYREXIAL TRAVELLER RETURNED FROM THE TROPICS WHO DOES NOT HAVE MALARIA OR HAS NOT RESPONDED TO ANTIMALARIALS

Such patients should always be managed by, or in conjunction with, specialists. Priority as always must be given to potentially rapidly progressive, treatable conditions. Fortunately these are rare in travellers who have visited the common tourist destinations. Enteric fever and tuberculosis are more common in immigrants, especially those from the Indian sub-continent.

Enteric fever

This can be due to *Salmonella typhi* or *paratyphi* A, B or C. Fever is usually the first symptom with increasing malaise, headache and a 'toxic' appearance. After a week, the patient is obviously ill and the spleen tip may be palpable. 'Rose spots' are occasionally seen, usually on the trunk, in non-pigmented skins and more often in paratyphoid. As in malaria, the total white blood count is usually normal or low. Blood cultures are usually positive (90%) if no antibiotics have been administered.

Treatment is ideally with an aminoquinolone such as ciprofloxacin to which resistance is still rare. This also appears to reduce the chance of persistent gallbladder or faecal carriage. Fever normally takes around 5 days to respond by which time the patient is usually beginning to improve symptomatically.

If treatment is delayed, or the organism is resistant to the antibiotic prescribed, complications such as bowel perforation or haemorrhage are more likely (see also Ch. 11).

Tuberculosis

Tuberculosis can present acutely with primary infections, usually of the lungs, or more often insidiously with reactivation. Normal chest X-rays do not exclude the diagnosis as intra-abdominal tuberculosis is notoriously difficult to diagnose and may involve, for example, lymph nodes or the renal tract. In uncomplicated disease, the white cell count is often normal. It is important to try to obtain material for culture (e.g. sputum or lymph node biopsy) so as to be able to detect resistance. Treatment is initially with quadruple antituberculous drugs.

Viral haemorrhagic fevers

Although very unlikely to present in the returned traveller, these infections cause a lot of concern because of the potential to spread to close contacts and their high mortality.

There are three major African viral haemorrhagic fevers: Marburg disease, Ebola fever and Lassa fever. The last is acquired through exposure to the urine of multimammate bush rats whereas the animal reservoir and mode of transmission of the first two are unknown. Lassa fever caused a large epidemic in Nigeria in 1969 and a repatriated nurse and her 'specimen contacts' in the USA were involved. The disease has a high mortality in adults although many cases of Lassa fever in children are mild or asymptomatic.

Distribution of haemorrhagic fevers

Exact distribution is unclear but areas where human cases have occurred are described below. Those marked * have occasionally resulted in human-to-human spread, usually in conditions of very poor hygiene or to laboratory workers.

- Yellow fever (sub-Saharan Africa, Central and South America)
- Dengue (widespread in India, Asia, Central America and northern parts of South America, patchy in Africa)
- Rift Valley fever (Central, East and southern Africa) is spread by mosquitoes; Crimean–Congo* fever (Africa, Asia, Middle East, Iran, Pakistan, former USSR, Eastern Europe), Omsk* fever (Siberia) and Kyasanur fever (south-west India) are spread by ticks
- Korean and Hantaan fever (Asia, Europe, Scandinavia, Kenya), Argentinian fever (rural area north-west of Buenos Aires), Bolivian* fever (rural north-east), Venezuelan, Brazilian* fever (Amazonian region), Lassa* fever (West Africa, especially Sierra Leone, Liberia, Nigeria, and related strains in the Central African republics, Zimbabwe and Mozambique) are transmitted through excreta from rodents and through blood and human excreta from infected patients in conditions of poor hygiene
- Marburg* (Uganda) and Ebola* fevers (Zaire and southern Sudan) are of unknown origin, but can be spread through blood and human excreta from infected patients in conditions of poor hygiene

They are caused by a variety of viruses with the common feature that a severe illness can occur with haemorrhagic features. This possibility must always be considered when there is fever in a returning traveller.

The incubation period is usually 7–10 days with the maximum recorded being 17 days, but for management purposes limits of 3 days to 3 weeks are recommended. Lassa virus is pantropic and symptoms develop slowly with fever and a sore throat with increasing prostration with facial oedema, pleural effusions and ascites. Terminal haemorrhage is common.

While most fevers from Africa will be due to malaria or other causes, immediate consultation with an infectious or tropical disease consultant must take place so that the case can be categorised into low, medium or high risk of haemorrhagic fever. Such consultation and decision-making should be done urgently as delay in diagnosis of malaria may be fatal. In the UK, official guidelines are available[3] and possible cases must also be reported immediately to the local consultant in public health medicine.

Leptospirosis, tick typhus and amoebic abscess are the most urgent, other possible diagnoses in patients with fever without an obvious focus and their diagnosis and management are summarised in Table 23.1.

Other 'imported' infections not normally presenting with fever

ACUTE VIRAL HEPATITIS (see also Ch. 11)

Hepatitis A has become less common as a result of widespread immunisation of travellers while travellers who spent the early years of their lives in the Indian sub-continent or Africa are almost always naturally immune.

The most common, faecal–orally transmitted hepatitis is now **hepatitis E** which causes large epidemics in northern parts of the Indian sub-continent and principally infects backpackers and UK Asians visiting relatives. **Acute hepatitis B** is less common in returned travellers but may be contracted by unimmunised homosexuals, 'sex-tourists', and UK Asians who receive injections with contaminated needles from practitioners in the Indian sub-continent.

Other causes of jaundice and recognising when antimicrobials may be necessary

There is no specific treatment available for patients with any form of acute viral hepatitis so the priority in assessing returned travellers with jaundice is not only to recognise those requiring supportive therapy for dehydration and hypoglycaemia but also to identify those whose illness requires specific antimicrobial treatment. Most of such patients will also be febrile and the differential diagnoses include *Plasmodium falciparum* malaria, pneumonia and leptospirosis.

EOSINOPHILIA

This suggests an 'invasive' parasitic infection and causes include **schistosomiasis, Bancrofti filariasis, strongyloides** and **onchocerciasis**. Marked eosinophilia is unusual in non-invasive helminthic infections of the gut such as *Ascaris* (roundworm), *Ancylostoma* (hookworm) and *Enterobius* (threadworm) infections.

SKIN LESIONS

Generalised rashes

The erythematous rash of primary **HIV infection** is mentioned in Table 23.1.

About one-third of patients with **dengue fever** have a generalised erythematous rash which usually appears 4 or 5 days after the onset of fever. Diagnosis is serological and treatment supportive. Dengue is becoming more common in South-East Asia, the Caribbean and South and Central America which are increasingly popular tourist areas.

An itchy, erythematous rash, particularly around the upper leg and arm, may be due to the release of microfilaria from adult female worms in **onchocerciasis**. Eosinophilia is common; microfilaria may be visualised in skin snips. Serology may be helpful.

TABLE 23.1 Diagnosis of illness in returned travellers presenting with fever

Clues to the diagnosis	Effective incubation period (median)	Investigations indicated	Action required
Leptospirosis (see Ch. 11) Exposure to potentially rat-infested water; multi-organ involvement e.g. liver, renal tract, meninges.	Up to 3 weeks (1 week)	Leptospira serology	Empirical treatment (see text)
Tick typhus (see Ch. 11) Wandering in scrub in South-East Asia or southern Africa; eschar may be present	Up to 2 weeks (1 week)	Typhus serology, blood cultures	Empirical treatment (see text)
Amoebic abscess (see Fig. 23.1) Tender liver; leucocytosis; rapid response to treatment	2–4 weeks but up to 4 years	Liver ultrasound; amoebic serology	Metronidazole
Diagnoses that are usually less urgent			
Schistosomiasis (see Ch. 11) Swimming in lakes in southern Africa, such as Lake Malawi; Eosinophilia; haematuria or blood stools	4–6 weeks for fever, longer for renal tract or gut involvment	Schistosomal serology; ova in urine, stool or rectal 'snips' (see Fig. 23.2)	Praziquantel
Pulmonary eosinophilia Caused by filarial infection; cough and wheeze; eosinophilia	6–12 weeks or longer	Filarial serology	Di-ethylcarbamazine or ivermectin
Dengue Fine erythematous rash, low platelet count or white cell count.	5–8 days	Dengue serology	Symptomatic and supportive
HIV infection[4] Erythematous rash, lymphadenopathy, pharyngitis, headache; unprotected sex	4–6 weeks	HIV serology (but may be negative so repeat 1 month)	Consult specialist

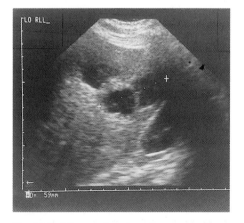

Fig. 23.1 CT scans of the liver showing amoebic abscesses. These cause fever, pain and if untreated, they can perforate externally or into the perineum.

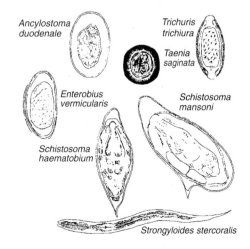

Fig. 23.2 An artist's impression of some of the more common ova and parasites which may be found in the stool or urine.

Generalised itchy papules may be caused by hypersensitivity to the **scabies** mite and specific lesions (burrows) should be sought between the fingers and on the wrists.

Localised and discrete lesions

Serpiginous, itchy, red lesions on areas where bare skin (usually feet but often buttocks) has been in contact with tropical soil are pathognomonic of **cutaneous larva migrans** caused by the arrested migration of the larvae of dog hookworm (see Fig. 11.8, p. 270). Mebendazole orally or thiabendazole locally is usually curative.

Infected insect bites are usually found on the limbs and are identified as such by the patient. The pathogen is usually *Staphylococcus aureus* but cellulitis owing to *Streptococci* can result.

An eschar is usually a single lesion with a necrotic centre and a rim of erythema. The surrounding skin may be oedematous and regional lymph nodes enlarged and tender. They should be sought in pyrexial patients who had been wandering in scrub in southern Africa or South-East Asia up to 3 weeks previously. If found, doxycycline should be prescribed and serology for **typhus** requested.

Diarrhoea

Diarrhoea in travellers is covered in detail in Chapter 11 but all practitioners should be aware that diarrhoea may be a presenting symptom of infection outside the gastrointestinal tract and that dual infections are common in travellers.

In practice, the presence of fever in a patient with diarrhoea should alert the practitioner to several possibilities:

- *Plasmodium falciparum* malaria
- prodrome of viral hepatitis
- bacteraemic diarrhoeal illness (e.g. salmonellosis)
- Legionellosis.

Therefore, whenever the travel history makes it appropriate, blood films for malaria parasites, blood cultures and chest X-rays may be indicated, in addition to stool culture and microscopy.

Screening and counselling (see also Ch. 22)

Those who have knowingly been exposed to certain infections but are asymptomatic often seek advice about screening. Examples include schistosomiasis in those who have been swimming in infected lakes (e.g. Lake Malawi), intestinal helminths in those who have been living abroad for prolonged periods, and those who have been bitten by a dog or other animal in a country where rabies is present. Sometimes, the possibilities of infection may have to be raised at a post-travel check-up (e.g. HIV infection).

A full history, examination and selected investigations such as a blood count for eosinophils, stool and urine examinations and sometimes serology may be required. Post-exposure rabies vaccination is covered in Chapter 11. Appropriate reassurance is essential and may be all that is necessary.

PRACTICE POINTS

- Always consider malaria first as a serious cause of fever in the returned traveller. Enteric fever and amoebic liver abscess are other possibilities.
- Fever persisting for more than a few days in a traveller with a normal or reduced blood white cell count, and with no obvious cause on clinical examination, should suggest malaria, enteric fever or tuberculosis.
- Dengue is becoming more common in travellers to Asia and Central and South America. The incubation period is short, so the illness often begins abroad.
- Remember Legionnaires' disease as a cause of fever and pulmonary signs in travellers who have been staying in hotels, especially around the Mediterranean.
- Important causes of jaundice in travellers are malaria, hepatitis A, B and E and less frequently leptospirosis.
- It is important to consider the possibility of infections such as schistosomiasis and HIV in the traveller who has been exposed even if asymptomatic.

REFERENCES

1. Riordan FA. Cases of fever in children who travelled to the tropics in the last 12 months. British Medical Journal 1998; 313: 1390.
2. Watson JM, MacFarlane JT. Legionellosis. In: Ellis M, ed. Infectious diseases of the respiratory tract. Cambridge: Cambridge University Press; 1998.
3. Advisory Committee on Dangerous Pathogens for DOH. Management and control of viral haemmorhagic fevers. London: The Stationery Office; 1996.
4. Kahu JO, Walker BD. Acute human immunodeficiency virus type 1 infection. New England Journal of Medicine 1998; 339: 33–39.

BIBLIOGRAPHY

Bell D. Lecture notes on tropical diseases. 4th ed. Oxford: Blackwell Science; 1995.
Benenson AS, ed. Control of communicable disease in man. Washington: American Public Health Association.
Cook GC, ed. Manson's tropical diseases. 20th ed. London: Baillière Tindall; 1997.
Walker E, Williams GR, Raeside F, Calvert L. The 'ABC' of healthy travel. 5th ed. London: British Medical Journal Publications; 1997.

EDUCATION

Education in travel medicine

Cameron Lockie   Jeannett Martin

Introduction

As discussed in the preface of this book, travel medicine is both an interdisciplinary and multidisciplinary specialty (Box 24.1). This can provide an opportunity for health professionals to share skills and expertise as well as the development of collaborative working between different areas that provide care to travellers such as general practice, occupational health departments and travel clinics. While many disciplines contribute to the whole of travel medicine, they are not necessarily involved in any process of education. The direction and content of any education are at the behest of those most actively involved in travel health.

> **Box 24.1 Interdisciplinary and multidisciplinary health professionals involved in travel medicine**
>
> **Nurses**
> - Practice nurses in general practice
> - Occupational health
> - Schools
> - Travel clinics
> - Health visitors
>
> **Doctors**
> - General practitioners
> - General physicians
> - Infectious disease physicians
> - Tropical medicine specialists
> - Clinical microbiologists
> - Genitourinary physicians
> - Public health physicians
> - Physiologists
>
> **Pharmacists**
> - Community
> - Drug information
> - Hospitals with travel clinics

The groups of health professionals in Box 24.1 perhaps contribute more to co-education in travel medicine; other groups may have a more peripheral involvement.

What is the best form of education in travel medicine?

Clearly different disciplines have different needs and it is hoped that individual education initiatives result in the gradual process of dissemination and cross-fertilisation of knowledge to the benefit of the traveller by developing the discipline of travel medicine, which Carroll et al concluded 'is becoming increasingly more specialised.'[1]

ACQUISITION OF KNOWLEDGE

There are several routes to approved knowledge:

- peer pressure
- in-house training
- mini-seminars, for example 1- or $\frac{1}{2}$-day settings usually organised at postgraduate centres and academic institutions
- joining a society or association, for example the International Society of Travel Medicine, British Travel Health Association, Royal Society of Tropical Medicine (see also Ch. 2)
- formal qualifications in the subject which may be targeted at specific groups or be multidisciplinary in nature

Many nursing students will have a clinical placement arranged in general practice and work alongside practice nurses and community nurses as part of their pre-registration course and can therefore develop an awareness of issues relating to travel health education and vaccination. However, a global search for references on the subject of medical undergraduate education in travel medicine proved negative.[2]

Nursing

It could be argued that nurses should be supported by a doctor with a special interest in the subject. Effective collaborative working and a team approach to education are then more likely to develop. In reality, this is often not the case. In the UK, it has been identified that nurses are the main patient contact for travel advice and that practice nurses are likely to be the main providers of travel health advice.

Many nurses attend 1-day seminars such as those organised by health authorities, the Royal College of Nursing or by pharmaceutical companies, but in addition longer courses in travel health are now much more available for nurses to access.

Recently, the United Kingdom Central Council for Nursing and Midwifery (UKCC) undertook a review of post-registration nurses' education and as a result established a new specialist practitioner, degree-level qualification for the eight branches of community nursing such as general practice nurses and occupational health nurses. Travel health and vaccination are included as topics to be studied within this degree programme, because it is such an important part of their role.

Not all nurses will want to become travel health experts, but they are all accountable for their actions. If they are involved in providing pre-travel advice to travellers, nurses should ensure that they access appropriate education to provide a safe and effective service.

1-day study courses are useful in the first instance to begin to develop knowledge, or as an update, but more extensive education will be required in order to meet the requirements of accountability and the high level of responsibility that is involved in a nurse-run travel clinic.

Undergraduate education in travel medicine

Medical and nursing schools have yet to determine where to introduce this subject into the undergraduate curriculum. It is often neglected. As it is interdisciplinary, there is no consensus as to whether training should be within public health, communicable disease, tropical medicine or general practice courses.

A simple study of 4th year medical students' knowledge in Glasgow showed there was good knowledge of illnesses that have a 'high profile' in the media such as malaria and HIV infection. There was much less appreciation of the risks from the common causes of diarrhoeal illness such as enterotoxigenic *Escherichia coli*, giardiasis and diseases such as poliomyelitis and tetanus. Many students, however, have personal experience of health problems that may be encountered overseas during or following their own 'elective' studies!

A multidisciplinary specialty

In this textbook of travel medicine, it is perhaps appropriate to mention that the UK achieved a world first with the development of a postgraduate diploma/MSc in travel medicine.[3] This course was constructed as a multidisciplinary, distance-learning course over 12–24 months at the University of Glasgow.

A great strength of the course is the multidisciplinary nature of the participants who are from a wide variety of disciplines and include nurses, general practitioners, armed forces doctors, occupational health professionals and public health physicians. The core tutors are made up of experienced nurses and doctors. A touch of realism to travel medicine is apparent when one becomes aware that a physician or general practitioner may have as a tutor a nurse who is a travel health specialist.

Multidisciplinary qualifications are challenging both in curriculum development and in the attention necessary for formative and summative assessment.

Doctors and nurses vary considerably in their skills between different areas of competence. There is more than one way to become a good travel medicine specialist.

Assessment

Recognition of this is vital for the assessment process in a multidisciplinary group and when constructing a multidisciplinary course, the process of assessment requires special consideration. In any assessment process, it is of prime importance to address:

- validity
- reliability
- feasibility
- generalizability.

VALIDITY

A test is valid if it tests what it is meant to test, but validity comes in many guises. Therefore the test has:

- *content validity* if it truly reflects the work of, in this case, the health professional in the field of travel medicine
- *face validity* if it is perceived to test this area but only careful analysis of the candidates' score will see if they actually reflect real world performance
- *construct validity* if what is to be assessed is not clearly visible in the natural world. Attributes such as empathy and communication skills cannot be measured with weights or yardsticks
- *predictive validity* if the course's success is to be capable of assessment. It is the essential attribute of any summative assessment and only accurate analysis of the data will give an indication if the course has been successful. Do candidates who pass the exam go on to perform better than those who fail to complete the course?

RELIABILITY

The test should produce the same results if used with different markers on different occasions. If the test is not reliable, it cannot be valid.

FEASIBILITY

It is important to consider whether the practical requirements of the examination can be met in terms of accommodation, students, examiners and simulated patients. In addition, time constraints may dictate certain actions.

Multiple choice questions (MCQs) can be marked with speedy reliability and indeed with an optical scanner if necessary but an objective structured clinical examination (OSCE) is more demanding both in time and resources.

GENERALISABILITY

Generalizability theory is based on the concept of finding out how many samples need to be taken from the universe of all travel medicine activities, before a clear and reliable picture of candidates' performance can be obtained.

Types of assessment that can be used to ensure validity and reliability

It is essential that in a multidisciplinary course assessment should give equal opportunities for all. This may require assessment that may appear, in the first instance, to be somewhat complex and may involve:

- MCQs to test knowledge
- modified essay questions (MEQs) to test application of knowledge
- OSCE is an approach to the assessment of competence in which the components of competence are assessed in a planned or structured way. By definition, the OSCE attempts to eliminate the subjectivity which besets most types of assessment and to focus on pre-determined areas for testing. It concentrates primarily on the doing and leaves the knowing to more traditional forms of assessment (see Fig. 24.1).

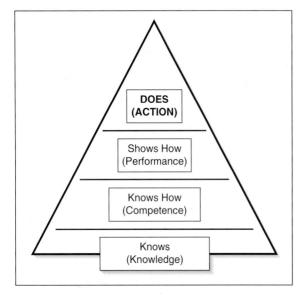

Fig. 24.1 Miller's triangle. This is in essence a framework for assessment. While recognising the importance of tests of knowledge such tests are incomplete tools in the holistic assessment of knowledge; that is if one believes that there is more to the practice of travel medicine (and indeed medicine in general) than merely 'knowing'. The travel medicine health professional should not only be someone who is well informed but who is also competent in a range of skills.

Level 1. Knows (Knowledge): Involves the assessment of factual knowledge e.g. by Multiple Choice (MCQ) or Extended Matching Questions.

Level 2. Knows How (Competence): The second level of Millers' triangle involves the assessment of the cognitive skills used in the application of knowledge or the technical abilities with which clinical procedures are carried out. The Modified Essay Question (MEQ) aims at assessing whether the student 'knows how'.

Level 3. Shows How (Performance): The assignment-based assessment (as in the Glasgow MSc/Diploma course) may be regarded as testing an aspect of level 3 of Millers' triangle in that the student 'shows how' he or she can critically evaluate and apply information from written material, i.e. course material provided, plus personally researched information.

Level 4. Does (Action): Ideally, to assess what the student actually 'does' in practice would involve direct observation in the travel medicine clinic. Both from the standpoints of generalisability and sheer logistics such an assessment would prove almost impossible. The Objective Structured Clinical Examination (OSCE) attempts to assess what the student actually 'does' in practice.

An alternative would be a video recording of the student at work. The OSCE has the advantage of allowing the assessors to construct a series of current and appropriate stations for objective assessment. The challenge at each station should as far as possible with the use of simulated patients, mimic situations experienced by the health professional in the real world of travel medicine.

Travel health courses available in Britain

University of Glasgow MSc/Diploma in Travel Medicine

The course is run from the Department of Public Health, University of Glasgow and in conjunction with the Scottish Centre for Infection and Environmental Health (SCIEH).

Students who complete the diploma to a high standard can proceed for a further year and obtain an MSc (Med Sci) in Travel Medicine. Nurses without a primary university degree can proceed to the MSc depending on research ability shown during the diploma year. In recent years, overseas students have been accepted on the course.

The course consists of:

— introductory week with attendance at the University of Glasgow with lectures and workshops
— two distance-learning, assignment-based modules on core subjects of travel medicine with study options
— a follow-up week at the university consisting of lectures and workshops
— a research project over 3 months with presentation of a mini-thesis.

Performance is assessed on quality of work throughout the course in written assignments and a mini-thesis and not just on the results of examinations. However, to allow unbiased assessments, the examinations comprise:

- MCQs (no negative marking)
- MEQs
- OSCE.

Further information. Mrs Maria Williamson, Department of Public Health, University of Glasgow, Glasgow, G12 8R2. *Tel:* 0141 330 5617, *Fax:* 0141 330 6303.

Royal Free Diploma in Travel Health and Medicine

This diploma from the University of London was developed by Jane Zuckerman and began in October 1997. It is based at the Royal Free Hospital within the Academic Unit of Travel Medicine and Vaccines and is supported by the Department of Microbiology and of Primary Care and Population Science.

The course runs for 1 academic year and requires attendance 1 day a week to study modules in:

— infectious diseases
— prevention of travel-related disease
— environmental hazards and travel
— practical issues for travellers
— evidence-based travel medicine.

The assessment for the diploma includes MCQs (30%), a written paper (40%) and a written research project (30%).

Further information. Dr Jane Zuckerman, Academic Unit of Travel Medicine and Vaccines, Royal Free Hospital School of Medicine, Rowland Hill Street, London, NW3 2PF. *Tel:* 0207 830 2999.

London School of Hygiene and Tropical Medicine Travel Medicine Course

A 1-week course in travel medicine developed by Bernadette Carroll and Ron Behrens from the Hospital for Tropical Diseases in conjunction with the London School of Hygiene and Tropical Medicine (LSHTM). The course requires attendance for 5 days at the LSHTM in London for lectures and workshops. The main objectives are to ensure practitioners are aware of:

— their role in protecting travellers' health
— major risks associated with travel
— methods for reducing and managing travel-associated hazards
— methods used in prioritising risk in travellers
— the role of information technology in travel medicine.

Further information. The administrative officer for short courses, Registry, London School of Hygiene and Tropical Medicine, Keppell Street, London, WC1E 7HT. *Tel:* 0207 927 2074.

Magister Travel Health Distance Learning Unit

Not all practice nurses will wish to become experts in travel health, but because most UK travellers will seek advice from their general practice, it is likely that most practice nurses will need to develop a level of competency in this subject in order to provide a safe service. This distance-learning course was developed by Jeannett Martin, Ursula Shine and Joan Sawyer to meet the needs of nurses in general practice.

Course content involves:

— accidents, food and water, sun exposure, sexual activity, sea and freshwater bathing, bites and stings, insurance
— immunisation and prophylaxis, malaria, communicable disease, vaccinations
— the environment and special groups of travellers
— providing a travel health service, professional issues, risk assessment, sources of advice, patient information.

The cost of the course does not include assessment. This is so students can choose and only have to pay for, the level of assessment they wish to undertake:

• no assessment
• RCN continuing education points (CEPs) (payment for this is to the RCN)
• an academic assessment by South Bank University (Level 2 CATS) (payment for this is to the university).

Further information. Louise French, Magister, Doral House, 2b Manor Road, Beckenham, Kent, BR3 5LE. *Tel:* 0208 650 0005.

Staffordshire University ENB Travel Health Promotion

This course was developed by Karen Howell, a UK representative on the Council of the International Society of Travel Medicine, and is open to all professionals who provide a travel health service. The day consists of 12 days' attendance at the university, for lectures and workshops on:

— epidemiology
— health promotion and health education
— risk assessment
— immunisation

— health and safety
— policies and protocols
— audit.

Further information. Karen Howell, Staffordshire University, School of Health, Beaconside, Stafford, ST18 0AD. *Tel:* 01785 353696.

Lancaster University Travel Medicine Course

This course runs over 6 months and aims to offer educational opportunity for all healthcare professionals who wish to further their knowledge and skills in travel health and medicine. The course is a combination of distance learning, workshops and tutor-led sessions to cover the following aspects:

— immunisation theory and practice
— sources of infection for the traveller
— problems of the individual traveller
— problems specific to the destination
— problems specific to activities undertaken
— problems of the returned traveller
— sexually transmitted diseases
— malaria
— running a travel service in general practice.

Students may choose the level of assessment:

• certificate of attendance/PGEA – MCQs
• level 2 CATS 30 points – 3000-word essay and 2-hour examination

Further information. Linda Sharpe, Registry (post-professional), Bowerham Road, Lancaster, LA1 3JD. *Tel:* 01524 384604.

Short course in travel medicine for nurses

This course is a continuation of courses previously held at the Scottish Centre for Infection and Environmental Health, which is now run by Queen Margaret College, Edinburgh, in continuing collaboration with SCIEH.

It is designed for nurses who have maintained their UKCC registration and are currently working in a related field. Participants attend the course on 2 separate, full days, 1 week apart.

Learning outcomes

By the end of the course, nurses should be able to:

— access and use up-to-date and accurate sources of travel health information
— carry out a comprehensive, pre-travel risk assessment
— deliver health advice specific to the needs of the traveller
— provide appropriate immunisations and chemoprophylaxis
— understand the basic principles of providing a travel medicine service.

Further information. Ms Shona Rattray, Department of Health and Nursing, Queen Margaret University College, Clerwood Terrace, Edinburgh EH12 8TS. *Tel:* 0131 317 3294. *Fax:* 0131 317 3573. *e-mail:* k.munro@mail.qmeced.uk

PRACTICE POINTS

• Increasingly, opportunities are becoming available for education in travel health at varying academic levels from basic courses in risk assessment and immunisation practices to advanced qualifications and research.
• General practitioners, practice nurses, occupational health staff and those involved in expeditions, voluntary work and repatriation may all require ongoing professional training.
• Education needs vary between countries. For example, the approach may be very different in countries where travel medicine is practised within a national health service and where it is practised only within private practice.
• Undergraduates often qualify with very little training in clinical, preventive medicine and vaccinology. Many, however, have practical experience of overseas health problems following elective periods overseas.

REFERENCE

1. Carroll B, Behrens RH, Crichton D. Primary health care needs for travel medicine training in Britain. Journal of Travel Medicine 1988; 5: 3–6.
2. Lockie C. Travel medicine – an integral part of the undergraduate curriculum. Scottish Medical Journal 1996; 41: 139–140.
3. Lockie C. A higher qualification in travel medicine – new established (abstract). First Asia Pacific Travel Health Congress, Hong Kong, March 1996.

APPENDIX OF MAPS
Bilharzia
Cutaneous leishmania
Dengue
Epidemic meningococcal infection
Japanese B encephalitis
Onchocerciasis
Tick-borne encephalitis

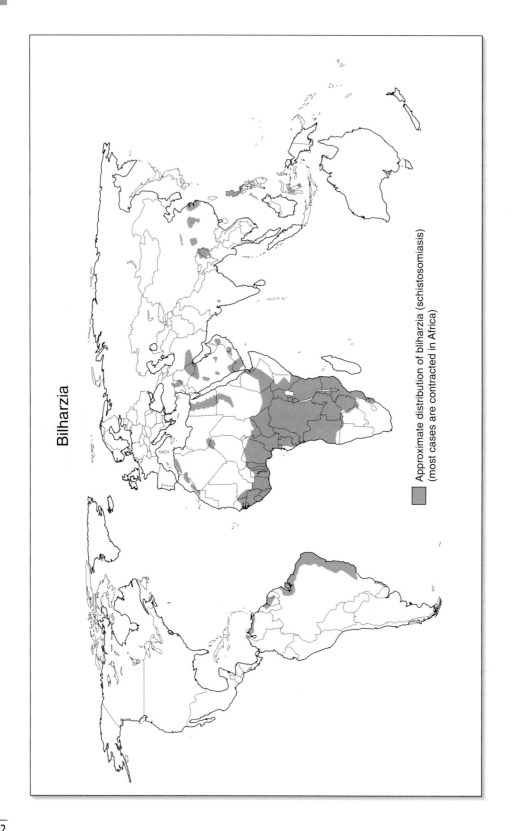

Bilharzia

Approximate distribution of bilharzia (schistosomiasis) (most cases are contracted in Africa)

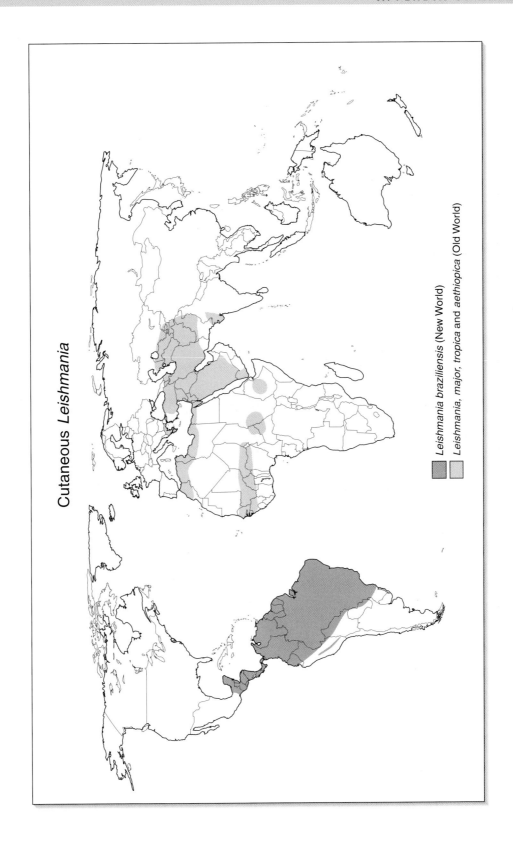

Cutaneous *Leishmania*

Leishmania braziliensis (New World)

Leishmania, major, tropica and aethiopica (Old World)

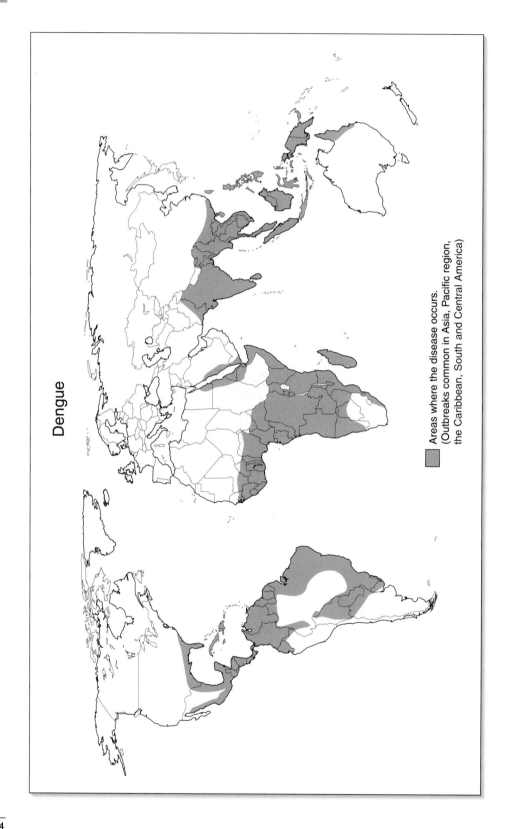

Dengue

Areas where the disease occurs.
(Outbreaks common in Asia, Pacific region,
the Caribbean, South and Central America)

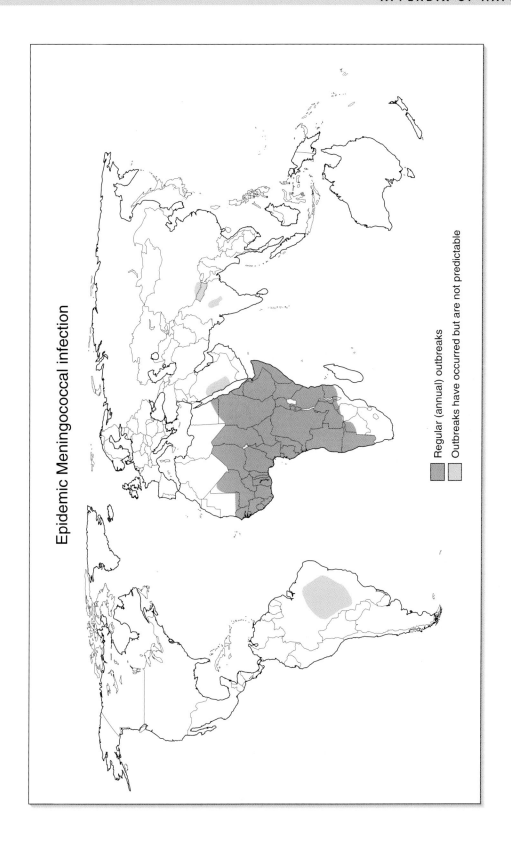

Epidemic Meningococcal infection

Regular (annual) outbreaks

Outbreaks have occurred but are not predictable

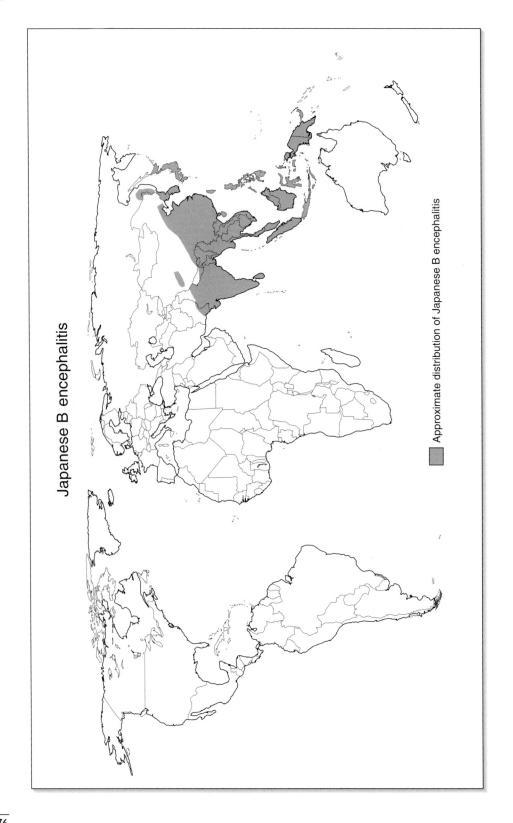

Japanese B encephalitis

Approximate distribution of Japanese B encephalitis

Onchocerciasis

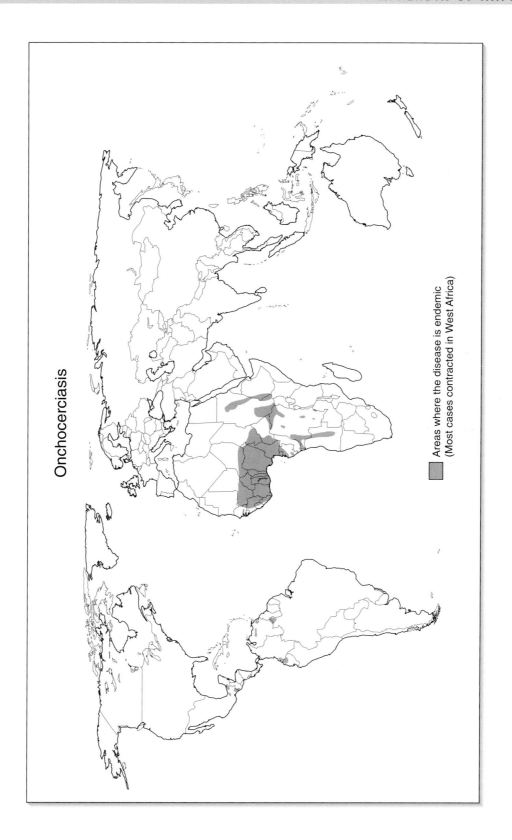

Areas where the disease is endemic
(Most cases contracted in West Africa)

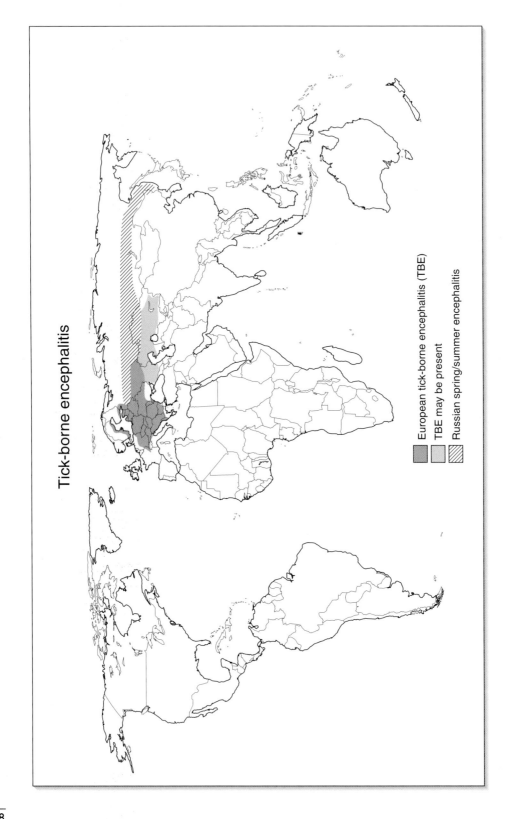

Tick-borne encephalitis

European tick-borne encephalitis (TBE)

TBE may be present

Russian spring/summer encephalitis

Index